AF831158

Smart Innovation, Systems and Technologies

Volume 259

Series Editors

Robert J. Howlett, Bournemouth University and KES International, Shoreham-by-Sea, UK

Lakhmi C. Jain, KES International, Shoreham-by-Sea, UK

The Smart Innovation, Systems and Technologies book series encompasses the topics of knowledge, intelligence, innovation and sustainability. The aim of the series is to make available a platform for the publication of books on all aspects of single and multi-disciplinary research on these themes in order to make the latest results available in a readily-accessible form. Volumes on interdisciplinary research combining two or more of these areas is particularly sought.

The series covers systems and paradigms that employ knowledge and intelligence in a broad sense. Its scope is systems having embedded knowledge and intelligence, which may be applied to the solution of world problems in industry, the environment and the community. It also focusses on the knowledge-transfer methodologies and innovation strategies employed to make this happen effectively. The combination of intelligent systems tools and a broad range of applications introduces a need for a synergy of disciplines from science, technology, business and the humanities. The series will include conference proceedings, edited collections, monographs, handbooks, reference books, and other relevant types of book in areas of science and technology where smart systems and technologies can offer innovative solutions.

High quality content is an essential feature for all book proposals accepted for the series. It is expected that editors of all accepted volumes will ensure that contributions are subjected to an appropriate level of reviewing process and adhere to KES quality principles.

Indexed by SCOPUS, EI Compendex, INSPEC, WTI Frankfurt eG, zbMATH, Japanese Science and Technology Agency (JST), SCImago, DBLP.

All books published in the series are submitted for consideration in Web of Science.

More information about this series at http://www.springer.com/series/8767

Álvaro Rocha · Daniel Barredo ·
Paulo Carlos López-López ·
Iván Puentes-Rivera
Editors

Communication and Smart Technologies

Proceedings of ICOMTA 2021

Springer

Editors
Álvaro Rocha
ISEG, Universidade de Lisboa
Lisboa, Portugal

Daniel Barredo
Universidad del Rosario
Bogotá D.C., Colombia

Paulo Carlos López-López
University of Santiago de Compostela
Santiago de Compostela, Spain

Iván Puentes-Rivera
Universidade da Coruña
A Coruña, Spain

ISSN 2190-3018 ISSN 2190-3026 (electronic)
Smart Innovation, Systems and Technologies
ISBN 978-981-16-5791-7 ISBN 978-981-16-5792-4 (eBook)
https://doi.org/10.1007/978-981-16-5792-4

© The Editor(s) (if applicable) and The Author(s), under exclusive license to Springer Nature Singapore Pte Ltd. 2022
This work is subject to copyright. All rights are solely and exclusively licensed by the Publisher, whether the whole or part of the material is concerned, specifically the rights of translation, reprinting, reuse of illustrations, recitation, broadcasting, reproduction on microfilms or in any other physical way, and transmission or information storage and retrieval, electronic adaptation, computer software, or by similar or dissimilar methodology now known or hereafter developed.
The use of general descriptive names, registered names, trademarks, service marks, etc. in this publication does not imply, even in the absence of a specific statement, that such names are exempt from the relevant protective laws and regulations and therefore free for general use.
The publisher, the authors and the editors are safe to assume that the advice and information in this book are believed to be true and accurate at the date of publication. Neither the publisher nor the authors or the editors give a warranty, expressed or implied, with respect to the material contained herein or for any errors or omissions that may have been made. The publisher remains neutral with regard to jurisdictional claims in published maps and institutional affiliations.

This Springer imprint is published by the registered company Springer Nature Singapore Pte Ltd.
The registered company address is: 152 Beach Road, #21-01/04 Gateway East, Singapore 189721, Singapore

Preface

This book is composed of the papers written in English and accepted for presentation and discussion at the International Conference on Communication and Applied Technologies 2021 (ICOMTA'21). This conference had the support of the Universidad del Rosario (Colombia, Bogotá), Universidad de Vigo (Galicia, Spain), Universidad de Santiago de Compostela-Equipo de Investigaciones Políticas (Galicia, Spain), Universidad de A Coruña (Galicia, Spain) and International Media Management Academic Association (IMMAA). It will take place at Bogotá, Colombia, during September 1–3, 2019.

The International Conference on Communication and Applied Technologies 2021 (ICOMTA'21), in its first edition called "Computation, Communication and fact-checking in the post-truth era", invites all those within the scientific, academic, and professional communities to present and discuss the latest innovations, results, experiences, and concerns in various fields of communication and technologies related to it.

The Program Committee of ICOMTA'21 was composed of a multidisciplinary group of 107 experts and those who are intimately concerned with communication and technologies. They have had the responsibility for evaluating, in a "double-blind review" process, the papers received for each of the main themes proposed for the conference: A) digital communication and processes; B) communication, health, politics, and technology; the other pandemic: disinformation in the age of coronavirus; and automation, bots, and algorithms; C) fact-checking experiences in Europe and Latin America at the service of journalism: a comparative perspective; D) persuasion and emotion: language and content analysis, and artificial intelligence; E) freedom of speech, ethics, and transparency in digital society; F) digital social media; G) software, big data, data mining, and intelligent systems; and H) miscellaneous (journalism, communication, advertising and public relations, political science, and other aspects of social and human sciences derived from the information and communication technologies).

ICOMTA'21 received 138 contributions from 15 countries around the world. The papers accepted for presentation and discussion at the conference will be published by Springer (this book) and will be submitted for indexing by ISI, Ei Compendex, Scopus, DBLP, and/or Google Scholar, among others.

Álvaro Rocha
Daniel Barredo
Paulo Carlos López-López
Iván Puentes Rivera

Organization

Honorary Committee

Daniel Barredo Ibáñez	Universidad del Rosario, Colombia; Fudan University, China
José Rúas Araújo	University of Vigo, Spain
Iván Puentes Rivera	University of Vigo, Spain

International Scientific Committee President

Nieves Lagares Díez	University of Santiago de Compostela, Spain

International Organizing Committee President

Paulo Carlos López-López	University of Santiago de Compostela, Spain

Local Organizing Committee President

Carlos Gustavo Patarroyo Gutiérrez	Universidad del Rosario, Colombia

Organizing Committee

Carlos Gustavo Patarroyo Gutiérrez	Universidad del Rosario, Colombia
Paulo Carlos López-López	University of Santiago de Compostela, Spain
Julia Fontenla Pedreira	University of Vigo, Spain
Juan Arturo Mila Maldonado	University of Santiago de Compostela, Spain
Talía Rodríguez Martelo	University of Vigo, Spain
Ángel Torres-Toukoumidis	Salesian Polytechnic University, Ecuador

Marco López Paredes	Pontifical Catholic University of Ecuador, Ecuador
José Ángel Fernández Holgado	University of A Coruña, Spain
Xiana Casas	University of Vigo, Spain

International Scientific Committee

Nieves Lagares Díez	University of Santiago de Compostela, Spain
Andreu Casero Ripollés	University Jaume I, Castellón, Spain
Paulo Faustino	University of Porto, Portugal
Laura Alonso Muñoz	University Jaume I, Castellón, Spain
José Manuel Rivera Otero	University of Santiago de Compostela, Spain
Erika Jaráiz Gulías	University of Santiago de Compostela, Spain
María Pereira López	University of Santiago de Compostela, Spain
Paulo Carlos López-López	University of Santiago de Compostela, Spain
Alfonso López Rodríguez	University of Santiago de Compostela, Spain
Ángel Cazorla	University of Granada, Spain
Iván Puentes Rivera	University of A Coruña, Spain
José Rúas Araújo	University of Vigo, Spain
Palmira Chavero Ramírez	FLACSO Ecuador
Pablo Escandón	Andina Simón Bolívar University, Ecuador
Verónica Crespo Pereira	Pontifical Catholic University of Ecuador, Ibarra Headquarters, Ecuador
Marco López Paredes	Pontifical Catholic University of Ecuador, Ecuador
Verónica Yépez Reyes	Pontifical Catholic University of Ecuador, Ecuador
Verónica Altamirano	Private Technical University of Loja, Ecuador
Abel Suing	Private Technical University of Loja, Ecuador
Mónica López Golán	University of A Coruña, Ecuador
Luis Cárcamo Ulloa	Austral University of Chile, Chile
Camila Cárdenas Neira	Catholic University of Temuco, Chile
Karen Tatiana Pinto Garzón	Universidad del Rosario, Colombia
Víctor Manuel García Perdomo	University of La Sabana, Colombia
Jorge Francisco Galán Montesdeoca	Salesian Polytechnic University, Ecuador
Daniel de la Garza	Autonomous University of Nuevo León, Mexico
María Isabel Villa	EAFIT University, Colombia
Elba Díaz-Cerveró	Panamerican University, Mexico
Belén Puebla Martínez	Rey Juan Carlos University, Spain
Silvia Maria Vega Saldaña	University of Cádiz, Spain
Narcisa Jessenia Medranda	Salesian Polytechnic University, Ecuador

Nicolás Sumba	Salesian Polytechnic University, Ecuador
Roberto López	Salesian Polytechnic University, Ecuador
Angel Torres-Toukoumidis	Salesian Polytechnic University, Ecuador
Andrés Bayolo	Salesian Polytechnic University, Ecuador
Ana Luisa Correa Cabrera	Salesian Polytechnic University, Ecuador
Andrea De-Santis	Salesian Polytechnic University, Ecuador
Fabián Villacrés	Salesian Polytechnic University, Ecuador
Jorge Cueva	Salesian Polytechnic University, Ecuador
Francisco Campos Freire	University of Santiago de Compostela, Spain
Xosé López García	University of Santiago de Compostela, Spain
Andrea del Carmen Mila Maldonado	University of Santiago de Compostela, Spain
Valentín Alejandro Martínez	University of A Coruña, Spain
Oscar Juanatey Boga	University of A Coruña, Spain
Laura Milagros Castro Souto	Universidade da Coruña, Spain
Ana Belén Fernández Souto	University of Vigo, Spain
Juan Manuel Corbacho	University of Vigo, Spain
Montserrat Vázquez Gestal	University of Vigo, Spain
Beatriz Legerén Lago	University of Vigo, Spain
Manuel Pérez Cota	University of Vigo, Spain
Mónica Valderrama Santomé	University of Vigo, Spain
Alejandro Romero Reche	University of Granada, Spain
Andrés Mazaira Castro	University of Vigo, Spain
Natalia Quintas Froufe	Universidade da Coruña, Spain
José Ángel Fernández Holgado	University of A Coruña, Spain
Carmen Costa Sánchez	University of A Coruña, Spain
Ana María González Neira	University of A Coruña, Spain
Eva Sánchez Amboage	University of A Coruña, Spain
María Magdalena Rodríguez Fernández	University of A Coruña, Spain
Clide Rodríguez Vázquez	University of A Coruña, Spain
Matías Membiela Pollán	University of A Coruña, Spain
Félix Bláquez Lozano	University of A Coruña, Spain
Clide Rodríguez Vázquez	University of A Coruña, Spain
Carlos Toural Bran	University of Santiago de Compostela, Spain
José Miguel Túñez López	University of Santiago de Compostela, Spain
Alba Silva Rodríguez	University of Santiago de Compostela, Spain
Jorge Vázquez Herrero	University of Santiago de Compostela, Spain
Julio Torrado Quintela	University of Santiago de Compostela, Spain
Nancy Graciela Ulloa Erazo	Pontifical Catholic University of Ecuador, Ecuador
Jenny Yaguache Quichimbo	Private Technical University of Loja, Ecuador
Teresa Augusta Ruão Correia Pinto	Universidade do Minho, Portugal

María Gabriela Cabral Bernardo Funk	Universidade dos Açores, Portugal
Fernando Vasco Moreira Ribeiro	Universidade do Porto, Portugal
Antonio Castillo Esparcia	Malaga University, Spain
Joan Cuenca Fontbona	Ramon Llull University, Spain
María del Carmen Carretón Ballester	University of Alicante, Spain
Salvador Alejandro Hernández Martínez	San Antonio de Murcia Catholic University, Spain
Kathy Matilla	Ramon Llull University, Spain
Concha Pérez Curiel	University of Seville, Spain
Julia Fontenla Pedreira	University of Vigo, Spain
Francisco Paniagua	Universidad of Málaga, Spain
David Cabrera Souto	University of A Coruña, Spain
John Wihbey	Northeastern University of Boston, USA
Daniela Rincón Reyes	Northeastern University of Boston, USA
Talia Rodríguez Martelo	University of Vigo, Spain
Berta García Orosa	University of Santiago de Compostela, Spain
Juan Cárdenas Tapia	Salesian Polytechnic University, Ecuador
Blas Garzón	Salesian Polytechnic University, Ecuador
Luz Marina Castillo	Salesian Polytechnic University, Ecuador
Pedro Colangelo-Kraan	Salesian Polytechnic University, Ecuador
Luis Bayardo Tobar Pesántez	Salesian Polytechnic University, Ecuador
Juan Pablo Salgado	Salesian Polytechnic University, Ecuador
Fernando Pesántez Avilés	Salesian Polytechnic University, Ecuador
Angel Torres-Toukoumidis	Salesian Polytechnic University, Ecuador
Luis Álvarez Rodas	Salesian Polytechnic University, Ecuador
Raquel Rodríguez Díaz	Rey Juan Carlos University, Spain
Anna Amorós Pons	University of Vigo, Spain
Alberto Pena Rodríguez	University of Vigo, Spain

Contents

Political Communication, Technology and Applications

About the Editors

Álvaro Rocha holds the title of Honorary Professor and holds a D.Sc. in information science, Ph.D. in information systems and technologies, M.Sc. in information management, and B.Sc. in computer science. He is Professor of information systems at the University of Lisbon—ISEG and Researcher at the ADVANCE (the ISEG Centre for Advanced Research in Management). He is also President of AISTI (the Iberian Association for Information Systems and Technologies), Chair of the IEEE Portugal Section Systems, Man, and Cybernetics Society Chapter, and Editor in Chief of both JISEM (Journal of Information Systems Engineering & Management) and RISTI (Iberian Journal of Information Systems and Technologies). Moreover, he has served as Vice-Chair of Experts for the European Commission's Horizon 2020 Program and as an expert at the COST—intergovernmental framework for European Cooperation in Science and Technology, at the Government of Italy's Ministry of Universities and Research, at the Government of Latvia's Ministry of Finance, at the Government of Mexico's National Council of Science and Technology, and at the Government of Polish's National Science Centre.

Daniel Barredo Ibáñez is Associate Professor in the Journalism and Public Opinion Program of the Universidad del Rosario, Colombia, and Director of the Journalism Laboratory of the same institution. He is currently Coordinator of the Working Group on Digital Communication, Networks, and Processes of the Latin American Association of Communication Researchers. In addition, he is Visiting Researcher at the Fudan Development Institute at Fudan University, China. He has written more than 100 works on topics related to social media, political participation, organizational discourse, or communication in Spain, Colombia, Mexico, or Ecuador. He has a Ph.D. in journalism from the University of Malaga, a master's degree and expert in communication, and a degree in Hispanic philology and audiovisual communication from the University of Granada, has an H index of 14, and is accredited as Senior Researcher, the highest qualification granted by the Science Ministry of Colombia.

Paulo Carlos López-López is Professor and Researcher in the Department of Political Science and Sociology at the University of Santiago de Compostela (USC), Ph.D. in communication, Journalist, and Political Scientist. He is Member of the International Research Network on Communication Management, the Political Research Team of the USC, and the Iberian Association of Information Systems and Technologies. He has published more than sixty scientific papers on topics such as communication, social media, and political science. He was Director of the group "Media, Applied Technologies, and Communication" and Director of a postgraduate degree in political communication in Ecuador. He was awarded the Drago 2019 research award for his study on transparency and has work experience in electoral campaigns, organizational communication, press office, and parliament management. He has an H index of 7 and is an accredited professor in the category Contracted Doctor by the Quality Department of the Galician University System (ACSUG).

Iván Puentes Rivera is Ph.D. in communication, a master in research in communication, and a graduate in advertising and public relations from the University of Vigo; he is Professor in the area of audiovisual communication and advertising at the University of A Coruña (UDC) and Member of the research group CP2: Persuasive Communication of the University of Vigo, as well as Technical Secretary of XESCOM (International Network for Research in Communication Management). His main lines of research focus on political communication and electoral campaigns, public relations in this field, disinformation, and fact-checking in political debate and electoral debates on television. Along with this, he also highlights his research work in relation to public television and, in particular, about transparency in radio and television broadcasters of this type. Outside the university, he has a wealth of professional experience in the field of public management and communication, A Coruña, Spain.

Digital Communication, Systems and Processes

Absences Predictive Model of for the Outpatient Unit in a Public Hospital

D. M. Rivero-Albarrán[1,3](✉), F. I. Rivas-Echeverría[1,2,3], P. M. Villareal[1], and S. M. Arciniegas[1]

[1] Pontificia Universidad Católica del Ecuador Sede Ibarra, Ibarra, Ecuador
{dmrivero,pmvillarreal,smarciniegas}@pucesi.edu.ec, firivas@inf.utfsm.cl
[2] Universidad Técnica Federico Santa María, Valparaíso, Chile
[3] Universidad de Los Andes, Mérida, Venezuela

Abstract. The quality must be present external in consultation services, either to satisfy the needs of the users and/or to maximize the use of the resources. For this reason, administrators require the necessary information and knowledge to support them in decision-making processes. This paper presents a time series-based model, to predict absenteeism and attendance at the outpatient service. The CRISP-DM methodology, typical of data analytics, was used to explore the models. It was found that the ARIMA model was the one that obtained the lowest absolute and quadratic error. In addition, based on the time series predictions, it was determined that the number of absences to external medicine consultations is around 10% per day. This information can be used to reduce the attention time lost due to absences.

Keywords: Data analytics · Time series · External consultation services

1 Introduction

The quality of health care services is increasingly important, citizens, aware of their rights, demand that health services improve. In other words, they demand a better quality of health services. Quality, as defined by the Royal Spanish Academy (RSA), is seen as a value that is assigned to the set of attributes of a product. In the case of health, some of these attributes are: interpersonal relationship with patients, accessibility to services, equality of care (equity), efficacy of treatment when changing the patient's condition, effectiveness seen as the ability to produce an effect on the patient, economic and technical efficiency [1, 2].

Quality can be evaluated from two perspectives: the quality perceived by the users and the quality of the processes. From the users' point of view, it is measured through the degree of satisfaction that patients have with the care received. That is, for the technical-professional care to solve your health problem, for the treatment received and in general, for the infrastructure of the health institution. If it is wanted to evaluate the quality of health services from the users' perspective, a widely used strategy is to survey these users to measure their degree of satisfaction in different aspects and, based on their

© The Author(s), under exclusive license to Springer Nature Singapore Pte Ltd. 2022
Á. Rocha et al. (Eds.): ICOMTA 2021, SIST 259, pp. 3–12, 2022.
https://doi.org/10.1007/978-981-16-5792-4_1

responses, conclude what the quality of the health service is like [3–5]. Quality, from the perspective of the processes that are carried out, is measured from a set of metrics or indicators, which allow a diagnosis to be made in relation to the operation of the health center. Some of these indicators are: low readmission of patients, decrease in cases of malpractice, optimization in the use of resources, decrease in costs [6–8].

The information obtained from the analysis of the surveys and the indicators are used by the health center administrators to: monitor the performance of the health center, the operation of the institution, make decisions, define policies and strategies to ensure the medium and long-term success and the viability of the health center. Evaluating the performance of an institution is a multi-criteria problem, therefore, for the selection of an adequate model, adequate criteria are needed [9, 10]. Although descriptive and diagnostic studies are useful support tools for managers in their decision-making processes, the information provided by a predictive study, which indicates the behavior of certain variables in the future, is necessary nowadays, having knowledge of what has happened? why it has happened? and what could happen? allows administrators to determine the best course of action to follow, defining strategies that will improve the quality of services.

Among the research works focused on the search for predictive models of absenteeism to outpatient visits are, the work of Salazar et al. [11], in which three algorithms are evaluated to predict a patient's attendance, concluding that decision trees is the algorithm that makes the best predictions. Guinta [12] estimates the absenteeism rate using conditional and marginal logistic regression models. Elvira et al. [13] used gradient boosting algorithms, generalized linear model and deep learning, selecting the boosting gradient as a predictor. Other authors have used classification trees, logistic regression models, and vector support machines to find predictive models of absenteeism [14–16].

This paper presents a descriptive and prescriptive study for the outpatient unit of the Ibarra General Hospital (HGI) in Ecuador. For the descriptive analysis, together with the hospital administrators, a set of graphs was selected to monitor the performance of the unit. For the prescriptive analysis, the behavior over time of attendance and non-attendance at the outpatient service was explored. The prescriptive study will serve to optimize the use of medical resources in the consultation unit, since each absence represents a loss of human resources affecting the costs of care.

The work is organized as follows, in Sect. 2 the methodology used is described and the concepts considered important are presented. Then, in Sect. 3 the results obtained are presented and discussed and finally, in the last section the conclusions and recommendations of this work are given.

2 Materials and Methods

Data analytics has several methodologies to achieve, with a higher probability, project success. In this work, the Cross-Industry Standard Process for Data Mining (CRISP-DM) methodology proposed by IBM [17] was used. The methodology establishes six phases in its life cycle, in this work the first five phases were applied. The sixth will be executed by the management of the external consultation unit, which, using the knowledge acquired through data mining, will define the strategies and modifications necessary to improve and make the best use of the resources of the unit. The first five phases are described below.

2.1 Understanding the Business

In this phase it was determined the main purpose of this study, the objective was defined by the unit administrators, obtaining: 1) Show the behaviors of certain indicators, such as: number of medical care by specialty and year, number of care doctors by place of birth, determination of the most prevalent diagnoses attended in external consultation, Percentage of absenteeism of patients by specialty, among others. that allow a diagnosis of the current situation of the unit; 2) Improve outpatient care, making the best use of medical resources in order to serve the largest number of patients attending the outpatient unit. The second objective will be achieved if 50% of the appointments that remain unattended are used, that is, patients do not attend the consultation.

Regarding the human resources available, the unit's staff participated in the initial meetings (director, doctors) and the information and communications technology (ICT) and statistics staff also have participated. Regarding material resources, all the data stored in the Medical Information System (MIS-AR400) was used, which is used in all services (emergency, hospitalization, outpatient consultation, clinical laboratory, imaging, pathology, among others), the system records the data of the consultations of the patients who attend the consultation and the data of the appointments assigned and the data management services offered by the ICT department of the Hospital.

2.2 Understanding the Data

In this phase, the available tables in the database were analyzed to identify what data could be obtained for each patient (age, sex, appointment date, specialty, among others). After the study, the data needed to meet the objectives were identified. It was identified which data was most relevant to the study, in which tables it was stored, and in which files this data would be stored.

After this, it was agreed to create two files (bd_hgi_ibarra_production, bd_hgi_ibarra_absenteeism), the necessary data to create each file were extracted and the data types of each attribute (numeric, date or categorical) were identified.

The data was analyzed and graphed to observe the behavior of the attributes. Figure 1 shows the histogram generated to observe the frequency of the number of absentee visits per day.

From this graph it was possible to find relationships between the data and identify the probability distribution that some attributes follow. For example, in Fig. 1. it can be seen that the number of absences describes a behavior close to a normal distribution. The graphs of the exploratory analysis also made it possible to identify the presence of outliers.

2.3 Data Transformation

The data files used in the analysis were generated from the MIS-AS400 system data. After selecting the attributes of each file, the observations were generated and the records with more than 50% of the incomplete characteristics were eliminated, the records with less than 50% of missing data were completed by substituting the missing value for

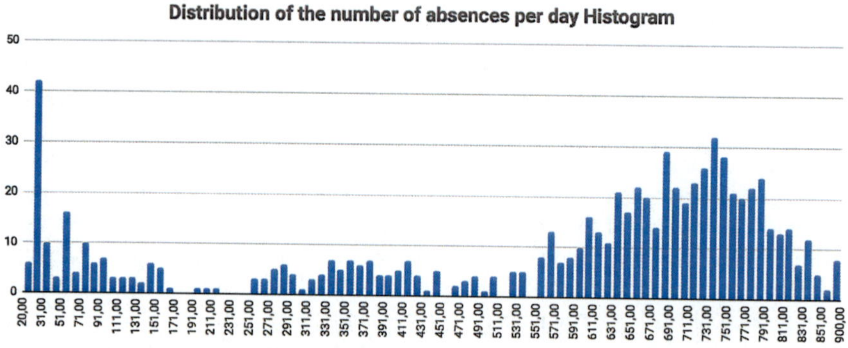

Fig. 1. Distribution of the number of absences per day Histogram

the mode if the data was of categorical type (strings) or the average if the data was of numerical type.

Data that were related to dates were transformed to the date format; it was verified that the registered data belonged to any of the categories established for each attribute. For example, the Attention Status attribute only allows two categories (Attends, Does Not Attend).

In this work, two types of analysis were carried out, one descriptive in which a set of graphs were constructed to show the current situation of the hospital and the other prescriptive, to predict the behavior of the outpatient clinic, in terms of the number of appointments attended (Attends) and not attended (Does Not Attend). For the prescriptive analysis, two additional files were generated containing the data necessary for the exploratory analysis. A table of appointments attended by specialty and another table of appointments not attended was generated.

Figure 2 shows an image of the first 5 records of the table of unattended appointments of the general medicine specialty. As the objective was to predict the number of appointments attended and not attended per day, it was necessary to create a table with the date information and the total number of appointments attended per day. From the initial file, the records by Specialty and Not Attended were selected and the number of appointments they attended per day was calculated. The file was then sorted chronologically and indexed by date. The final file contains 880 observations (323 from the year 2018, 317 from the year 2019, 240 from the year 2020).

	Date	Etareo Group	Code Dep	Sex	Specialty	State	Time Att
0	20180102	08 FROM 50 TO 64 YEARS	36500	F	ENDOCRINOLOGY (CE)	Attended	711.0
1	20180102	09 65 AND OVER	23731	F	GERIATRIA (CE)	Attended	800.0
2	20180102	02 FROM 1 TO 11 months	758391	F	PEDIATRICS (CE)	Unattended	785.0
3	20180102	03 FROM 1 TO 4 YEARS	761412	F	PEDIATRICS (CE)	Attended	20.0
4	20180102	07 FROM 20 TO 49 YEARS	47314	M	CARDIOLOGY (CE)	Attended	924.0

Fig. 2. Records of absences for the General Medicine specialty

From the total of observations, a group of data was used for the adjustment of the model and another group of data for testing, the latter used to calculate the prediction errors of the models found. Errors indicate the difference between the testing and predicted data.

2.4 Modeling

In this phase, for the descriptive analysis, the information that should be presented to the administrators was identified to respond to the information needs that the administrators defined in the first phase, it was indicated what should be viewed: Number of medical cares by specialty and by year, number of outpatient consultations by specialty, most prevalent diagnosis, absenteeism of patients by specialty, among others. Table 1 shows the percentage of absenteeism by specialty.

Table 1. Percentage of absenteeism by specialty

Dependence	Percentage of absenteeism
Odontology	9,56%
General medicine	9,01%
Orthopedic Traumatology	8.05%
Physiatry	7.36%

For the prescriptive analysis, the most suitable algorithms were selected to predict the number of absences to the External Medicine consultation. Time series models were used since they are useful models to find patterns that allow predicting values in future times; they try to identify the nature of the variations in time of the variable under study, they are used to predict demand, number of sales, among others. A time series is represented, generally as:

$$y_1, y_2, \ldots, y_N = (y_t : t = 1, \ldots, N) \textit{ where yt is the observation in time t} \quad (1 \leq t \leq N)$$

Where y can be represented as a vector y = [y1, …, y2, …, yN] t of order 1.

Figure 3 presents the time series of the number of absences during the working days of the year, during the years 2018 and 2019. For the year 2020, we only had the data up to the month of July. It can be seen that the years 2018 and 2019 show a similar seasonal behavior; the variations in the same period of time are similar and therefore can be predictable. However, in 2020, due to the pandemic caused by COVID-19, the behavior changed. This behavior is a sporadic situation that, once the pandemic is over, will not be repeated, therefore, the data from 2020 were not used for the exploratory study.

For the adjustment of the models, it was necessary to establish the values of the parameters p and q, for this the autocorrelation function (ACF) was used to identify the value "q" in the moving average (MA) process and partial autocorrelation (PACF) for identifying the "p" values of the part of the autoregressive process (AR). The ACF indicated that the lag values for "q" were 2, 6, 7. The PACF indicated that the lags for "p" were 1, 5, 6 and 7.

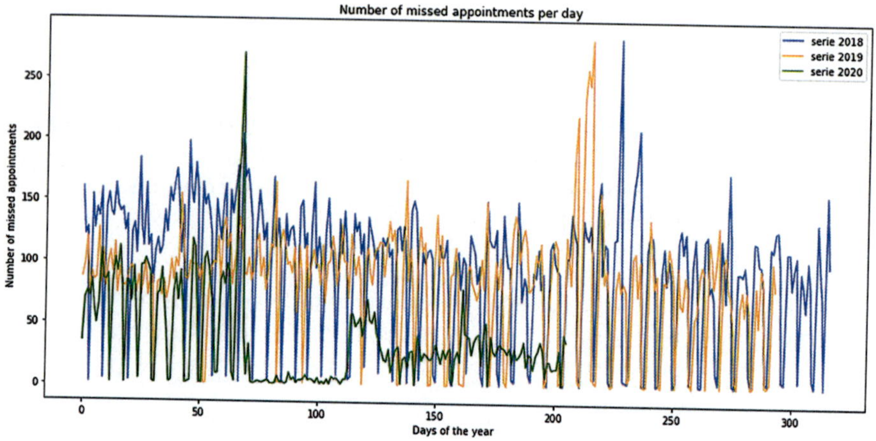

Fig. 3. Number of missed appointments per day (years 2018 to 2020)

In the exploratory analysis, a model was needed to calculate the number of absences per day. Three time series models were selected: AR (p), ARMA (p, q) which is an autoregressive stochastic model of Moving Averages (MA) that identify "p" autoregressive terms and "q" moving terms, combining two polynomials; ARIMA (p, d, q) which is a model for non-stationary time series that after an integration process can be analyzed as stationary. In the model, "p" indicates the number of autoregressive terms, "d" the number of times the series must be differentiated to make it stationery and "q" the number of terms of the invertible moving average [19]. The lag values "p" and "q" identified with the ACF and PACF functions were used to fit the models, as integration values "d" the value 1 was selected.

2.5 Evaluation

For the best model selection, that is, the one that makes the predictions with greater precision, it was necessary to calculate the errors committed by each model, the metrics used were the mean absolute error (MAE), the mean square error (MSE). It was chosen by the model who made the smallest mistake.

3 Discussion of Results

In the descriptive phase, a set of tables were constructed to answer the questions asked by the administrators in phase 1. Table 1 shows the first four data records that were tabulated to show the percentage of absenteeism. This table, together with the specialties with the highest consultation rate (Table 2), were used to select the specialties to be analyzed with the data mining models. If both graphs are observed, it can be deduced that the specialty of general medicine is the second with the highest demand for consultation and number of absenteeism, for this reason, the exploratory analysis was carried out for this specialty.

Table 2. Number of medical care per year.

Dependence	Year				
	2017	2018	2019	2020	Total
Orthopedic Traumatology	19355	15234	13268	4350	53232
General medicine	10791	11013	15238	11894	48936
Gynecology	17568	15004	10718	3075	46365
Endocrinology	14322	12633	12788	4608	44351

The models were adjusted with the values of p and q that were previously identified and the ARMA and ARIMA models with the lowest AIC were selected, the values (p, q) = (6.6) and for ARIMA the values (p, d, q) = (5, 1, 6). Figure 4 shows the predictions made by each model and the time series with the testing data. The AIC of the ARIMA model was 5119.08 and that of the ARMA model was 5130.34. As can be seen, the model with the lowest AIC was the ARIMA model. Finally, Table 3 shows the errors between the predictions and the test data of the selected model (ARIMA) and the AR model.

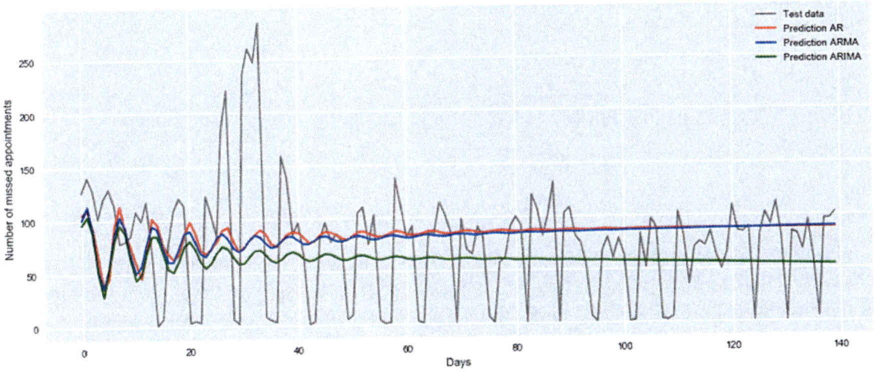

Fig. 4. Testing data and ARIMA and ARMA prediction models

Figure 5 shows the predictions of the AR and ARIMA models (dotted lines). The absenteeism values of the AR Model are between 80 and 90 absences that are close to the data values initially calculated in this study (mean: 77.37; std: 53.381886; mode:

Table 3. RMSE and MAE errors of the ARMA and ARIMA models

Model	MSE	MAE
AR(1)	56.49	40.83
ARIMA(5, 1, 5)	56.22	0.55

87). The absenteeism values for the ARIMA model are between 50 and 55 patients. The results of the predictions for the first 14 days of January are shown in Table 4.

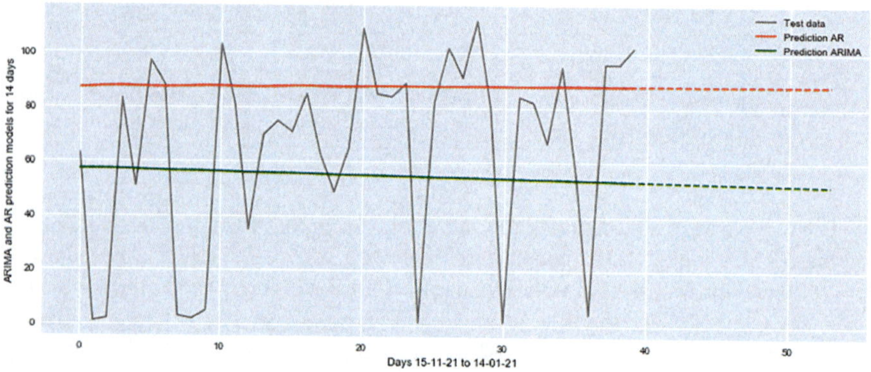

Fig. 5. ARIMA and AR prediction models for 14 days

Table 4. Unattended Appointments Prediction of the ARIMA model for the first fifteen days of the year 2021

Week	1	2	3	4	5	6	7
Jan 1–7	54	53	53	53	53	52	52
Jan 8–14	53	53	52	51	51	51	51

A similar process was carried out to predict the number of "Attended" appointments in the outpatient clinic per day, the best values for "p" and "q" were selected, the models were evaluated and the model with the lowest AIC was selected. As a result, it was obtained that the model that best fit the series was ARIMA with "p" equal to 1, "q" equal to 1 and "d" equal to 2. Table 5. presents the prediction of the ARIMA model (1, 2,1) to predict consultation attendance for the same period of time.

If the data in Tables 4 and 5 are observed, it can be inferred that the number of consultations has a slow growth and that the number of absenteeism also decreases with a very small slope. The percentage of absenteeism is approximately 10%, that is, the personnel assigned to these consultations should be rescheduled in order to maximize the use of resources.

Table 5. Attended appointments Prediction of the ARIMA model for the first fifteen days of the year 2021

Week	1	2	3	4	5	6	7
Jan 1–7	535	536	536	537	537	538	538
Jan 8–14	539	540	540	542	542	542	543

4 Conclusions

Quality of services is one of the main issues in health care services, because it directly affects the society wellness. It is very important to find the appropriate attributes to be considered in health care systems.

One of the most important attributes is the patient's absenteeism, because of its impacts in health, economic and technical conditions and it was the main issue considered in this work.

Different models were analyzed to adjust the time series behavior and, based on them, predict results, AR, ARMA and ARIMA models were used, which are statistical models that work based on seasonal patterns and past trends. ARIMA was found to be the best model for making predictions. A negative trend in absenteeism was observed although its growth is very small. Absenteeism represents 10% of all appointments attended. The work carried out will allow, if the data is updated monthly, to monitor the evolution of absenteeism month by month. The algorithm will incorporate the new data and adjust its predictions.

It will be used other forecast models in order to compare their performance and also it will be studied other of the important attributes in the health care services.

References

1. Hernández, M., Hernández, A., Bringas, N.: El contexto actual de la calidad en salud y sus indicadores. Rev. Mex. Med. Fis. Rehab. **25**(1), 26–33 (2013)
2. Ipinza, M.: Calidad y atención integral de salud. Cuad Med Soc. 5–17
3. Reyes-Morales, H., et al.: Percepción de los usuarios sobre la calidad de la atención ambulatoria en servicios de salud en México. Salud pública de México **55**, 100–105 (2013)
4. Bakan, I., Buyukbese, T., Ersahan, B.: The impact of total quality service (TQS) on healthcare and patient satisfaction: an empirical study of Turkish private and public hospitals. Int. J. Health Plann. Manage. **29**(3), 292–315 (2014)
5. Mosadeghrad, A.M.: Factors influencing healthcare service quality. Int. J. Health Policy Manag. **3**(2), 77 (2014)
6. Saturno-Hernández, P.J., et al.: Implementación de indicadores de calidad de la atención en hospitales públicos de tercer nivel en México. Salud pública de México **59**, 227–235 (2017)
7. García, E.I., Solves, J.M., Mora, M.G., de las Sextas, G.D.T.: Indicadores de eficiencia para contribuir a la sostenibilidad de los servicios de salud en España. Revista de Calidad Asistencial **29**(5), 287–290 (2014)
8. Tsai, H.-Y., Chang, C.-W., Lin, H.-L.: Fuzzy hierarchy sensitive with Delphi method to evaluate hospital organization performance. Expert Syst. Appl. **37**(8), 5533–5541 (2010)

9. Kast, F.E., Rosenzweig, J.E.: Organization and Management: A System Approach. McGraw-Hill Book Co., New York (1974)
10. Laine, J., Linna, M.A.L.: Measuring the productive efficiency and clinical quality of institutional long-term care for the elderly. Health Econ. **14**(3), 245–256 (2005)
11. Salazar, L.H., Fernandez, A., Dazzi, R., Garcia, N., Valderi, R., Leithardt, Q.: Using different models of machine learning to predict attendance at medical appointments. J. Inf. Syst. Eng. Manag. **5**(4), 0122 (2020)
12. Giunta, D.H.: Ausentismo de pacientes a consultas programadas en un sistema de salud: estimación de tasas, identificación de factores asociados, causas y predicción (2019)
13. Elvira, C., Ochoa, A., Gonzalvez, J.C., Mochon, F.: Machine-learning-based no show prediction in outpatient visits. Int. J. Interact. Multimed. Artif. Intell. **29**(4) (2018)
14. Devasahay, S.R., Karpagam, S., Ma, N.L.: Predicting appointment misses in hospitals using data analytics. Mhealth **12**(3) (2017)
15. Huang, Y., Hanauer, D.A.: Patient no-show predictive model development using multiple data sources for an effective overbooking approach. Appl. Clin. Inform. **5**, 836–860 (2014)
16. Huang, Y.-L., Hanauer, D.A.: Time dependent patient no-show predictive modelling development. Int. J. Health Care Qual. Assur. **29**, 475–488 (2016)
17. IBM Knowledge Center - Conceptos básicos de ayuda de CRISP-DM. https://www.ibm.com/support/knowledgecenter/es/SS3RA7_sub/modeler_crispdm_ddita/clementine/crisp_help/crisp_overview.html. Accessed 01 Oct 2020
18. Hamilton, J.D.: Time Series Analysis. Princenton University Press (1994)
19. Nielsen, A.: Practical Time Series Analysis, 1st edn. O'Reilly (2019)

Automatic Data Warehouse Generation Model from BI Requirements in Natural Language

Carlos Andrés Pizarro(✉), Gabriel Novillo(✉), and German Montejano(✉)

Departamento de Informática, Facultad de Ciencias Física Matemáticas y Naturales (FCFMyN), Universidad Nacional de San Luis, San Luis, Argentina
gmonte@unsl.edu.ar

Abstract. The rise of Business Intelligence projects allowed to consolidate and consolidate the existing methodologies for the creation of Data Warehouse. Data Science and Natural Language research provided tools to solve problems that are generated in the different stages of these methodologies. The great dynamics in the management of organizations generate information needs to undergo changes or adaptations in very short periods of time. The processes of creating a Data Warehouse are characterized mainly by being long and expensive. This highlights a problem with respect to the ability of the Data Warehouse to adapt to changes in requirements. This work proposes a conceptual model that allows automating certain stages of the generation process to improve the absorption of changes in requirements.

Keywords: Data warehouse · Business intelligence · Data science · Natural language

1 Introduction

Currently, the large volume of data that is stored in organizations led to the rise of Data WareHouse (DWH) and Data Mining (DM) projects, these methodologies have had a great development in recent years. The important results obtained enhanced its application in different areas, mainly in the area of Business Intelligence (BI) as a basis for obtaining knowledge. In the framework of the organization's domain, obtaining knowledge currently triggers many predictive projects through DM seeking to take advantage of the large volume of data that allows improving decision-making and management of organizations based on the indicators obtained. Thus, it can be seen how these methodologies are achieving a high impact in the execution of these projects. This type of project seeks to have the largest possible volume of data for analysis. The existing methodologies allow us an appropriate design of the data warehouse (DWH) and the definition of the different models to determine knowledge (DM) [1–4, 8].

1.1 Data Quality

Applying data quality concepts has helped solve many problems that arise in the early stages of creating a Data WareHouse. Data quality is a multidimensional concept that

© The Author(s), under exclusive license to Springer Nature Singapore Pte Ltd. 2022
Á. Rocha et al. (Eds.): ICOMTA 2021, SIST 259, pp. 13–21, 2022.
https://doi.org/10.1007/978-981-16-5792-4_2

encompasses different aspects depending on the needs of data consumers or system designers. A set of data quality dimensions serve as a benchmark for measuring data quality. Data Warehousing Institute (TDWI) proposes 6 fundamental dimensions for data quality management (PDF) [4, 15–17]. They would be the following:

- **Accuracy:** The degree to which the data correctly represents the real-world object or event being described is measured.
- **Completeness:** The degree to which the data has the expected value and meets the requirements set. If a piece of information is optional, it should not be considered to achieve 100% completeness.
- **Consistency:** Measures whether the data is free of contradiction and has logical, format or temporal coherence.
- Timeliness: Measures the degree to which data is available when required.
- **Uniqueness:** Each piece of information is unique. With this dimension we seek to correct the unexpected duplication in our dataset.
- **Validity:** Measure whether a value conforms to a business rule or a pre-established standard in terms of format, data type, possible values or specified ranges.

1.2 Data Integration

It is one of the main areas of both research and business, which is responsible for allowing users to access data stored in heterogeneous data sources, presenting a single, unified view of that data [13, 14].

It is the process that allows you to combine heterogeneous data from many different sources in the form and structure of a single application. This makes it easier for different types of information, such as databases, files, and spreadsheets, to be merged with specific processes. Generally, buffers are used where integration takes place and measurable and quality data is generated from which the final DWH is designed and implemented [10–12].

A data integration project generally involves accessing data from all sources and locations whether it is on premises, in the cloud, or a combination of both. Integrating data implies that records in one data source map to records in another. It is a type of data preparation essential for analytics and other applications to be able to use the data successfully.

1.3 Natural Language

Natural Language Processing (NLP) is the field of knowledge of Artificial Intelligence that deals with investigating the way machines communicate with people through the use of natural languages, such as Spanish, English or Chinese. Logically, limitations of economic or practical interest mean that only the most widely spoken or used languages in the digital world have applications in use [8, 18, 19].

1.3.1 Components of Natural Language Processing

Here are some of the components of natural language processing. Not all the type the analysis exist apply to any NLP task, it depends on the purpose of the application.

- **Morphological or lexical analysis.** It consists of the internal analysis of the words that form sentences to extract slogans, inflectional features, and compound lexical units. It is essential for the basic information: syntactic category and lexical meaning.
- **Syntactic analysis.** It consists of analyzing the structure of sentences according to the grammatical model used (logical or statistical).
- **Semantic analysis.** It provides the interpretation of the sentences, once the morphosyntactic ambiguities have been eliminated.
- **Pragmatic analysis.** Incorporate the analysis of the context of use into the final interpretation. This includes the treatment of figurative language (metaphor and irony) as the knowledge of the specific world necessary to understand a specialized text.

1.3.2 How PLN Works

Separate the elementary pieces of language. Generally speaking, NLP tasks divide language into shorter elementary pieces, attempt to understand the relationships between the pieces, and explore how the pieces work together to create meaning. These implicit tasks are often used on higher-level NLP resources, such as content categorization, discovery and modeling of themes, Contextual extraction, sentiment analysis, speech-to-text and text-to-speech conversion, summarization of documents and machine-based translation.

- **Content categorization.** A linguistics-based summary of the document, including search and indexing, content alerts, and duplication detection.
- **Discovery and modeling of themes.** Accurately capture meaning and themes in text collections, and apply advanced analytics to text, such as optimization and forecasting.
- **Contextual extraction.** Automatically extract structured information from text-based sources.
- **Sentiment analysis.** Identification of mood or subjective opinions in large amounts of text, including sentiment mining and average opinions.
- **Speech-to-text and text-to-speech conversion. Transformation of voice commands into written text and vice versa.**
- **Summarization of documents.** Automatic generation of synopses of large bodies of text.
- **Machine-based translation.** Automatic translation of text or speak from one language to another.

This separation of the elementary pieces of the language that the PLN makes, allows us to focus its use in the requirements processing stage. In BI, decision makers constantly carry out their requirements in natural language and with great dynamics. Being able to identify and separate by examples nouns, verbs and types of words of a requirement, would allow us to process it automatically [8, 18, 19].

2 Scope of the Problem

The BI projects strengthened and consolidated the existing methodologies for creating DWH. The increasing emergence of specific tools was the basis for the development of the data science industry. The management level of the organizations determines information objectives that are requirements (input) for the design and implementation of the DWH [5–7]. This triggers a process that is mainly characterized by being long and expensive. It highlights a problem regarding the DWH's ability to adapt to changes in requirements.

The dynamics of organizational management translated into changes in the requirements produces an important impact, since, as a maximum consequence it would imply having to redesign and re-implement the DWH, this lack of adaptability in some opportunities calls into question the execution of these projects.

Making a description as an example, we can mention the impact that the request for new KPIs (Key Performance Indicator) [2, 8, 9] would have by the managers of an organization, which must be validated, that is, verify if they are possible to achieve at Based on the design of the existing DWH, if it can be achieved, the impact is less since it would only require incorporation into the visualization tool and some modification to the data processes. Now what if the new KPIs cannot be derived from the existing DWH design? If the DWH does not contain the data to respond to a new requirement, a process is triggered that among other steps requires, analyze if the data sources or buffers contain the data to respond to the new requirement, if so, analyze the incorporation to the design of the DWH, implement the ETLs to feed the DWH to finally incorporate the new requirement to the data visualization.

The complexity could be increased if the buffers do not have the necessary data to respond to the new requirement, in this situation, the different data sources must be analyzed to verify if it is possible to incorporate the new need, perform the quality analysis of the data and start the entire process until the data is available in the DWH and in the visualization tool. It is clear from this summary description of the problem, the high cost produced by this lack of flexibility of DWH projects, which, in many cases, causes them to be abandoned or limited, this leads to the information responses of the Requirements are processed outside the DWH, which finally gradually becomes limited in its use or limited to a very partial use of it. Being able to give these answers usually requires keeping numerous specialists working for long periods of time assigned to eventual tasks, producing a marked increase in the cost of the projects.

It should be noted that requirements analysis, data quality, ETLs, DWH designers and implementers as well as those in charge of data visualization, are generally part of a large team of qualified specialists that make up large teams of job.

3 Work Hypothesis

Added to the lack of adaptability of DWH to the new requirements is the great dynamics of the management of modern organizations. This is why a model of automatic generation of DWH instances is proposed [2].

For the purposes of obtaining information and trying to minimize the impact on time and costs in the adaptation of the DWH, this hypothesis is based on the maturity reached by the DWH design methodologies and the different IT areas that can be used in the different stages in the generation of data warehouses.

Data Quality and Integration applied in the early stages of construction provide an important basis for achieving consolidated buffers from heterogeneous sources that are the basis for enabling better data warehouse designs.

The use of Natural Language processing in the requirements analysis stage gives us the possibility of treating them automatically, producing the separation into shorter elementary pieces, in order to identify entities and relationships from which to implement managerial indicators.

The lack of flexibility and adaptability of the DWH produces frustration in decision makers since the DWH has little flexibility and adaptability with respect to the dynamism of the organization.

In this framework, combining all these tools, applying each one at the correct stage of the project, would allow us to create an automatic DWH analyzer and generator, which has a greater capacity to absorb changes in management requirements generated in natural language, reducing time and implementation costs. This would allow teams to dynamically incorporate new data into the DWH and its creation in a more agile and efficient way.

4 Proposed Model

The proposed model will allow new requirements to be received and will analyze whether there are data sources in the buffers and, if so, it will automatically generate the DWH design. Thus, it will be possible to have different instances of a DWH in a more agile way and with less effort.

The model will start the process by receiving the new requirements through an interface, expressed in natural language by those responsible for making decisions. Requirements should be expressed, trying to make them express as much as possible the data sources in terms of objects and the desired units of measurements. This will allow for greater efficiency in the identification process. Supported by the PLN algorithms, the words that could potentially be used to evaluate the existence of source data will be identified and selected.

Words that are nouns, verbs and those that express measurement units (amounts, amount, percentages, etc.) will be selected and presented in a list to be analyzed by the DWH designer. Of the nouns, those that, due to their empirical knowledge, already exist in the structure should be discarded. The designer can then start the process of verifying the existence of source data from the intermediate storage that can be selected as a functionality of the interface (Fig. 1).

The verification of the existence of the source data begins with the selection in the interface by the designer of the intermediate storage and then the automatic process begins that will be in charge of the search for entities, relationships, keys and fields that allow the generation of the instance of the DWH. The search is carried out on the intermediate storage where, in a previous process, quality data was obtained. The result of this process is shown to the designer through the interface, where he will determine if the number of entities, relationships and fields found reach the objectives of the requirements and will proceed to the construction of the DWH. The architecture that will have the new design will be a star (Fig. 2).

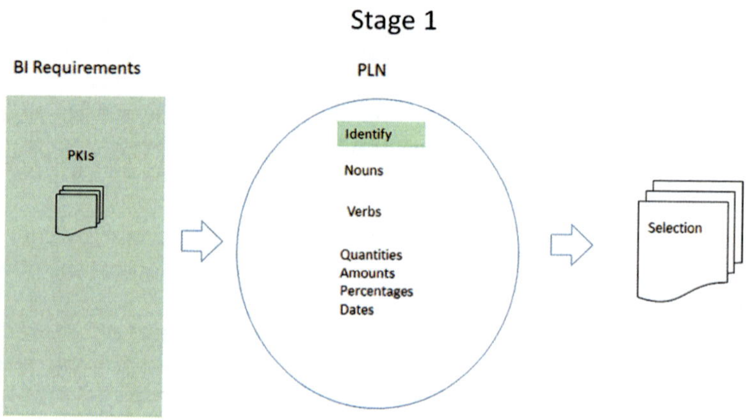

Fig. 1. Stage 1 of the proposed model

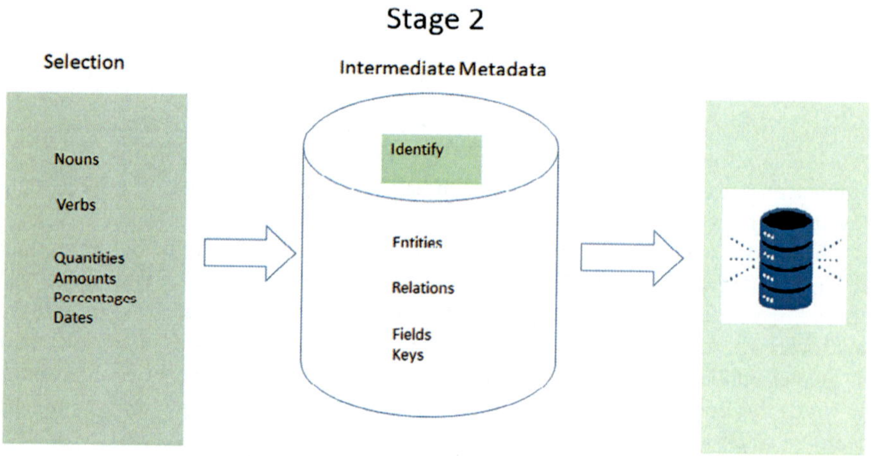

Fig. 2. Stage 2 of the proposed model

Once the creation of the DWH instance is completed, it will be possible to work on the presentation of the data as a final stage to be able to respond to the requirements. According to the visualization tool, the most appropriate type of table or graph will be selected to represent the requested indicators. The DWH will be filled manually by the designer, defining the ETLs and the most convenient update strategies.

In order to finally complete the proposal, we will describe a fundamental stage to achieve the objective of automatic generation of DWH instances. This stage is a prerequisite and will be carried out in the first creation of the DWH and should aim to achieve intermediate storages that are not only limited to supporting the initial requirements, but also allow covering the greatest amount of information possibilities. At this point, it is important to note that it is not intended to have an intermediate repository with a very high volume of data or with information that has a very low probability of use. It should be noted that keeping this repository up-to-date may require a high upgrade effort.

A balance must be found in terms of the amount of metadata to store, as this can impact the performance of ETLs. The update frequency will be here a variable to take into account when designing the strategy for applying the tasks. However, despite the cost of updating, the volume of the intermediate repositories will not impact the performance of the DWH since not only the data that meets the requirements of the instance will be there.

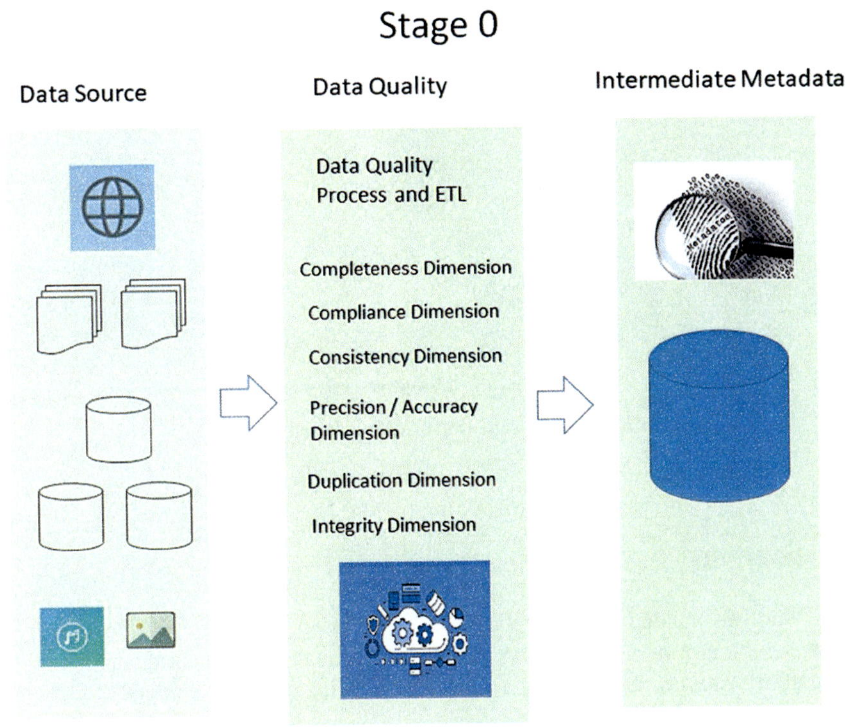

Fig. 3. Stage 0 of the proposed model

As shown in Fig. 3, stage 0 is a complex stage in which the Data Quality and Data Integration lines play a fundamental role in having Quality buffers. We already mentioned the dimensions, the integration of heterogeneous data and the hard work that this stage implies, which will directly impact the possibility of success of the model. The more information on the problem domain exists in the buffers, the more successful results the model will find to automatically respond to the creation of DWH instances to respond to a broad set of requirements.

To achieve greater success in the search for information for each instance and because it is an automatic search and creation, the definition of the nomenclature of the entities and relationships in the buffers takes on a relevant importance. When designing the repositories it will be very valuable keep in mind the keywords of the requirements or possible indicators of the domain. Finally, Fig. 4 shows the complete scheme of the model to generate automatic instances where all the stages can be viewed based on the requirements.

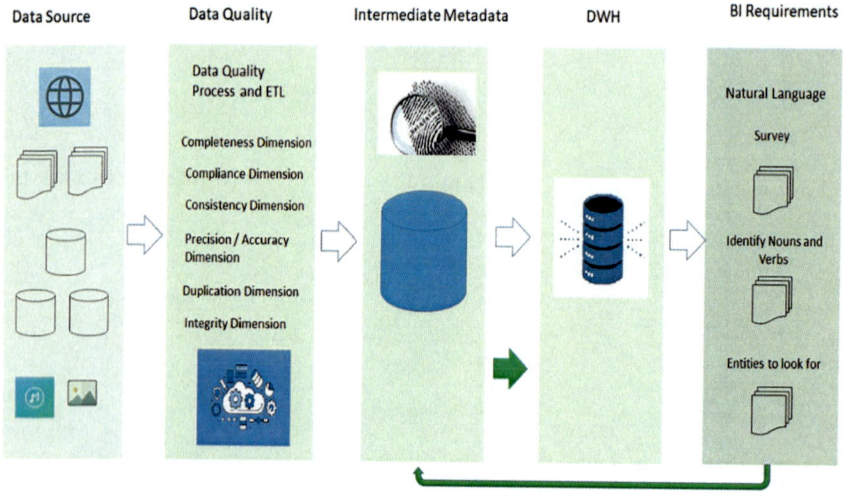

Fig. 4. Representation of the proposed model

5 Validation

To carry out the validation of this model, it is proposed to create a tool that can run the different stages of the model, relying on existing PLN applications and starting from buffers with metadata already achieved, thus being able to specifically verify the generation of automatic instances of DWH.

5.1 Education Domain

The Ministry of Education of the Argentine nation encourages national universities to use the same system for their management. This will allow to unify information and make cross-checks between the information from the different institutions. This is very important because it would be possible to have the same database structure except for some small peculiarities. The generation of a DWH for university management would make it possible to use information from all institutions. This is very important, since if we can carry out the validation of the model in one institution, it could work with small adaptations in all national universities. The dynamics and variability of the requirements of the university system, students, personnel, infrastructure and financial management, presents a good opportunity to validate the proposed model.

5.2 Conclusions and Future Work

In this work, we have presented a model to generate DWH instances from requirements expressed in natural language. This proposal is based on the lack of adaptability of the DWH to new requirements and on the high cost of their redesign processes, which causes underutilization or abandonment of this type of projects. Therefore, in order to achieve the objective of adaptability and provide data analysts or people who make decisions in organizations for a better use of their data warehouses, this model is presented. Automation will allow you to perform tasks with significant time and cost savings and take advantage of the methodological and solution maturity provided by other lines of data science. An interesting research topic is the automatic generation of the filling processes of the instances where the study of update strategies and their variables will be important.

References

1. Piattini Velthuis, M.G., Caballero Muñoz Reja, I., Gómez Carretero, A.I., Gualo Cejudo, F., Merino García, J., Rivas García, B.: Calidad de Datos. Bibiano Rivas Garcia (2018)
2. Cardador Cabello, A.L.: Data warehouse business intelligence (2019)
3. Peter, G.: Big Data Analytics Methods: Modern Analytics Techniques for the 21st Century: The Data Scientist's Manual to Data Mining, Deep Learning & Natural Language Processing (2016)
4. Giráldez, R., Riquelme, Aguilar-Ruiz, J.: Tendencias de la Minería de Datos en España. J. Educ. Data Min. **7**(1) (2015)
5. Corr, L.: Agile Data Warehouse Design: Collaborative Dimensional Modeling, from Whiteboard to Star Schema (2011)
6. Kimball, R., Ross, M.: The Kimball Group Reader: Relentlessly Practical Tools for Data Warehousing and Business Intelligence. Wisley Publishing, Inc. (2010)
7. Inmon, W., Strauss, D., Neushloss, G.: The Architecture for the Next Generation of Data Warehousing (2008)
8. Peter, G.: Big Data Analytics Methods: Modern Analytics Techniques for the 21st Century: The Data Scientist's Manual to Data Mining, Deep Learning & Natural Language Processing (2016)
9. Golfarelli, M., Rizzi, S.: Data Warehouse Design: Modern Principles and Methodologies (2009)
10. Nhung, D.: Developments in Data Extraction, Management, and Analysis (2012)
11. SAS Institute, Inc. SAS Rapid Warehousing Methodology, White Paper (2002)
12. Barroso, V.: Explotación e Integración de Bases de Datos Heterogéneas para la. Universidad de Valladolid (2015)
13. Botello, C.A.: Explotación de bases de datos heterogéneas mediante su integración parcial (2004)
14. Vijay, K., Bala, D.: Ciencia de los datos (2019)
15. Batini, C., Scannapieco, M.: Data Quality: Concepts, Methodologies and Techniques (2006)
16. Naumann, F.: Quality-Driven Query Answering for Integrated Information Systems (2002)
17. Piattini, M., García, F., Caballero, I.: Calidad de Sistemas Informáticos (2006)
18. Indurkhya, N., Damerau, F.J.: Handbook of Natural Language Processing (2010)
19. Allen, J.: Natural Language Understanding. 2nd edn. (2012)

Automation of an Educational Data Mining Model Applying Interpretable Machine Learning and Auto Machine Learning

Gabriel Novillo Rangone[1](✉), Carlos Pizarro[1](✉), and German Montejano[2](✉)

[1] Escuela de Ingeniería y Ciencias Ambientales, Universidad Nacional de Villa Mercedes, Las Heras 383, 5730 Villa Mercedes, San Luis, Argentina
{gnovillo,capizarro}@unvime.edu.ar

[2] Departamento de Informática, Universidad Nacional de San Luis, Ejército de los Andes 950, 5700 San Luis, San Luis, Argentina
gmonte@unsl.edu.ar

http://www.unvime.edu.ar, http://www.unsl.edu.ar

Abstract. Educational Data Mining (EDM) is a discipline related to the development of methods that allow the extraction of knowledge from academic, socioeconomic data, and learning analytics. The information obtained is used in decision-making to improve the indexes of academic performance, educational quality, desertion and student procrastination, among others. The EDM uses techniques of Statistical Analysis, machine learning and data mining within the framework (setting) of a development methodology such as Knowledge Discovery in Databases (KDD), Cross Industry Standard Process for Data Mining (CRISP-DM), and Sample, Explore, Modify, Model, Assess (SEMMA) or variants thereof. A drawback that we have to face mainly in South America is the need to have data scientists who participate in determining stages of a conventional EDM model that applies machine learning. To minimize this inconvenience, a EDM model applied in the university environment is proposed that uses Automated Machine Learning (AutoML) and Machine Learning Interpretability (IML) techniques. These two techniques will allow us to automate stages for data pre-processing, choice of machine learning models, choice of the best hyperparameters for the models, and interpretation of the results and the characteristics that influenced in the results, these last very important from the legal and ethical point of view, because not only must the model classify or predict with a good result, but it must also be able to inform us how it reached the conclusion.

Keywords: Educational data mining · AutoML · Machine learning interpretability

1 Introduction

The 21st century is characterized by knowledge, science, and technology; and within this framework (setting), Educational Institutions play an important role. Following the

© The Author(s), under exclusive license to Springer Nature Singapore Pte Ltd. 2022
Á. Rocha et al. (Eds.): ICOMTA 2021, SIST 259, pp. 22–30, 2022.
https://doi.org/10.1007/978-981-16-5792-4_3

Beijing consensus (2019) when it states "Artificial Intelligence must be at the service of learning and the evaluation of results" and "Ensure an ethical, transparent and verifiable use of education data and algorithms", and adding the lines of research of interest proposed by Romero C. and Ventura [3] on the design of processes or methods that facilitate educators and/or non-expert users in the area of data mining the implementation of knowledge extraction techniques. It is within the framework setting of proposals that this line of research will be carried out using data mining in the university educational environment.

Data Mining (DM) [10, 11], is a field of computer science related to the process of discovering patterns in large volumes of data sets, which brings together many computer research streams, including artificial neural nets, Bayesian learning, decision trees construction, instance-based learning, logic programming, rule induction, and statistical algorithms. It is from the DM that the Educational Data Mining (EDM) [1, 7] began to be developed at the end of the nineties, a field that proposes the use of various techniques, e.g. Statistical Analysis, Machine Learning, and DM to solve educational research problems and understand the environment in which students learn, exploring the unique types of data that come from educational settings [4–6, 12]. Today we could highlight as examples of unique data, the multiple Learning Analytics (LA) from virtual educational environments, academic, pedagogical and sociocultural data, among others.

Data Mining [13] uses methodologies to carry out its projects, of which the best known are CRISP-DM, SEMMA, or KDD, these methodologies fulfill the same role that Traditional or Agile Methodologies do in Software Engineering. The present work has as aims to automate the stages described in these highly complex methodologies in the construction of Educational Data Mining projects, allowing Institutions to carry out projects with professionals with little experience in machine learning (ML), given that the stage where experts are required in data pre-processing, search for ML models, optimal hyperparameter configuration, and interpretability of the obtained models, an attempt will be made to automate [2].

ML has achieved considerable success in virtually every area, from computer vision for face detection, to audio recognition for translation into translated text in hundreds of languages, to detection of complex diseases, cybersecurity anomalies and predictions widely used in the financial field, marketing and scientific research, among others. However, this success depends on ML experts performing the following tasks (preprocess and clean the data, select and build the appropriate features, select a suitable model family, optimize the model hyperparameters, and critically analyze the results obtained). As the complexity of these tasks often outpaces machine learning experts who are in short supply, and added with the rapid growth of machine learning applications, there has been a demand for available machine learning methods that can be used without the need for a data scientist experienced in critical parts of the workflow [2].

Automated machine learning (AutoML) is called the resulting area of research that aims at the progressive automation of machine learning [8].

In this work it is proposed to use AutoML in an educational data mining project in the university environment that allows institutions to improve the decision-making process, with an added Interpretability of the model in an automatic way that allows knowing why the algorithm took a decision, what are the patterns, rules and characteristics that you learned, and what were the characteristics of the data that most influenced the prediction.

This addition is very important because a model must not only provide us with good metrics such as the precision in a classification, but it must also be able to inform us how the result was obtained, so that we can first know if any ethical or legal rule is being violated and second being able to know which were the characteristics that most influenced the results in order to be able to act on the causes of eg academic performance or shelling or desertion.

2 Status of the Issue

Although Educational Data Mining emerged less than 20 years ago, there is a good amount of work available for analysis. Since in 2003, they presented an approach to predict the final grade of students, based on several characteristics extracted from the data recorded in a web-based educational system [14], and regression analysis and decision trees were used to identify the academic satisfaction of students [15], until in 2020 they published on the official website of Educational Data Mining an analysis of student strategies in combined courses using click data [16], numerous investigations have been carried out both for the application of the best data mining methodologies (KDD3, CRISP-DM4, SEMMA5), as well as to solve issues related to the description of the behavior of student populations, student dropouts, analysis/classification of profiles, educational quality and management of virtual classrooms [1, 3, 20], among others using association rules algorithms [17], clustering [18], classification [19].

Educational data mining in the university environment also has a significant number of works that can be summarized as proposed by Panizzi M. in a systematic mapping [21] carried out in 2019, on a methodological search of 112 relevant cases found, the largest amount are in Asia (40%), North America (16%), Europe (14%), Latin America and the Caribbean (4%) and Africa (1%). The topics covered range from academic performance (38%), student profiles (22%), educational quality (17%), university dropouts (11%), followed by student procrastination, cooperative education, student employability, among others. The tools or programming languages used are Weka (37%), Rapid Miner (8%) and Python (5%), and the most frequently named machine learning algorithms are Naive Bayes, J48, decision trees, and the clustering algorithms to a greater extent.

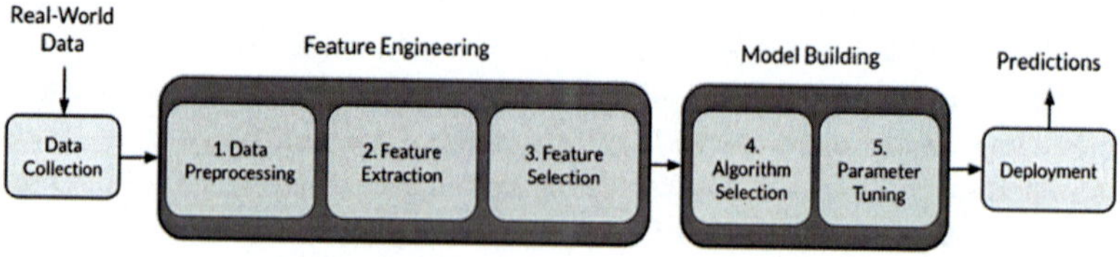

Fig. 1. Machine learning model workflow

The AutoML came from the hand of Thornton C., Hutter F., Hoss H., and Leyton-Brown K., in early 2013 with the Auto-WEKA frame [22]. The intention was to help non-expert users to effectively identify the right machine learning algorithms and hyperparameter settings for their applications, stages 4 and 5 in Fig. 1.

Actually AutoML has been formalized as a Combined Algorithm Selection and Hyperparameter Optimization (CASH) problem [8].

This CASH problem was addressed for the first time by Thornton C. in the Auto-WEKA system [23] using the WEKA machine learning framework (setting) [24] and Bayesian optimization methods based on trees [25], which have better performance in High-dimensional problems versus Bayesian optimization methods based on Gaussian processes that perform better with low-dimensionality problems [26]. Later, other optimization methods were used, such as genetic algorithms, gradient-based optimization, reinforced learning, random and grid search, network map, hyperband, naive evolution, hyperoptsklearn, and Tree-Parzen estimators, among the most important.

From 2014 onwards, the frames and tools to perform automated self-learning both commercial and open source began to arrive (Table 1), which are divided into four large groups (centralized, distributed, in the cloud, and search for neural architecture), most are open source, except for cloud-based frames that are commercial, and the languages in which they are mostly built are python, scala, java and R.

Table 1. Frames and AutoML Tools emerged between 2013 and 2020.

Types of frames	Tools and frames
Centralized	AutoWeka, Hiperopt, Autosklearn, TPOT, Recipe Auto-Meka, SmartML, OBOE, VDS
Distributed	Databriks, D-SmartML, ATMSeer, Rafiki, MLBox, MLBase, ATM
On the cloud	Google AutoML, Azure AutoML, Amazon Sage Maker
NAS	Auto Keras, NNI, NAO, DARTS, enas, Auto Net

Machine Learning Interpretability means giving explanations to end users for a particular decision or process that the model made. "The problem is that a single metric, such as classification accuracy, is an incomplete description of most real-world tasks" [31]. Although the interpretability with simple models and few hyperparameters is not a difficult task, as the models are more complex (random forest, neural networks) and with many hyperparameters, it becomes difficult to understand how a good result was reached. For its approval, it is necessary to know what original or synthetic characteristics were conclusive. Interpretability is important to data scientists, users, legislators, and regulatory entities, all of whom benefit from having an accurate, transparent, reliable, and explainable model [32]. Interpretability can be applied at different stages of an AutoML model development process. The first is in the model inputs, this may include summarizing the main characteristics of your data set, finding representative or critical points in your data set, and finding the relevant characteristics of your data set. The second is in modeling, which can be a white or transparent box or a black or opaque box, a classification that will depend on its simplicity, transparency and explicability, and the third is in a posteriori modeling, which helps us understand the most important features of a model, how those features affect predictions, how each feature contributes to the prediction, and how sensitive your model is to certain features.

The methods used for machine learning interpretability can be classified according to several criteria [33]. Intrinsic or post hoc, specific or independent of the model, local or global, etc. We are interested in understanding the first one, Intrinsic or post hoc? This criterion distinguishes whether interpretability is achieved by restricting the complexity of the machine learning model (intrinsic) or by applying methods that analyze the model after training (post hoc). Intrinsic interpretability refers to machine learning models that are considered interpretable due to their simple structure, such as shallow decision trees or linear or logistic regression models. Post hoc interpretability refers to the application of interpretation methods after model training, this method is model agnostic and allows developers to use any type of machine learning model including intrinsically interpretable models. The desirable aspects of a model-independent explanation system are: Model flexibility, the interpretation method can work with any machine learning model, such as random forests and deep neural networks. Explanation flexibility, you are not limited to a certain form of explanation. In some cases it may be useful to have a linear formula, in other cases a graph with important characteristics. Representation flexibility: The explain system should be able to use a different feature representation than the model being explained. For a text classifier that uses abstract word embed vectors, it may be preferable to use the presence of individual words for explanation. Among the most used methods of an independent explanation system of the model is the partial dependency graph method (PDP), individual conditional expectation (ICE), graph of accumulated local effects ALE), interaction of functions, importance of the permutation characteristic, local surrogate (LIME), scoped rules (anchors), Shapley values, and Shapley additive explanation (SHAP) [9, 33].

The AutoML and its interpretability applied to the university educational environment. Although there are machine learning works applied to the university environment, such as Prediction of academic performance through artificial intelligence techniques [27] or the Model to predict the number of engineering graduates from UTN [28], or a Computer System for the Early Detection of University Student Dropout [29], to name a few, only a single work could be verified applying AutoML techniques and their interpretability in the university environment [30], after an exhaustive search in academic Google, IEEExplorer, ACM and SEDICI.

3 Work Hypothesis

The present work proposes a DEM model, in this case applied to the university environment that can be carried out without the intervention of data scientists in data preprocessing tasks, choice of machine learning models, choice of the best hyperparameters for the models, and interpretation of the results. To achieve this objective, we will take advantage of the corresponding technological advances in MDE, AutoML, and IML, seeking to use the best tools, methods and techniques that adapt to our problem, which is possible from an exhaustive study of the state of the art of the themselves.

Carrying out a study of the available Frames and Tools in Fig. 2, we find that auto sklearn is the most appropriate given that it has been implemented on Scikit Learn, a popular machine learning package that is also written in Python, the most widely used language at the moment and that more libraries have for data science. Both Auto Sklearn, Scikit Learn, and Python are open source, which in this case allows Universities to access and use them in a simpler and less expensive way, since university budgets are not a minor data. To improve generalizability, the latest versions of auto-sklearn create a set of all models tested during the global optimization process, and to speed up the optimization process, auto-sklearn uses meta-learning to identify similar data sets and use the knowledge gathered in the past. These last two characteristics allow them to have better performance both in the expected results and in the time used.

To the results obtained we will add an Interpretability stage to be able to justify and understand the predictions and/or results obtained, applying various methods such as the partial dependency graph (PDP), accumulated local effect graph ALE), interaction of functions, importance of the permutation characteristic, local surrogate, and Shapley's additive explanation (SHAP). In this way, we try to achieve transparency in our development and a clear picture of how our gear works to obtain results. Libraries in Python such as ELI5, PDPBox, and SHAP, among others, will allow us to carry out the Interpretability stage.

4 Proposed Model

The proposed model begins with the description of the educational database that will provide the data for the workflow, followed by the data cleaning tasks, then our Auto ML model will choose a model depending on whether we have decided to classify or perform regression based on the educational problem and you will find the best hyperparameters. To finalize the results, they will go through the Interpretability stage, which will allow us to understand their causes. With the results and their explanation, we will be in a position to answer the proposed educational problem, this can be seen in Fig. 2.

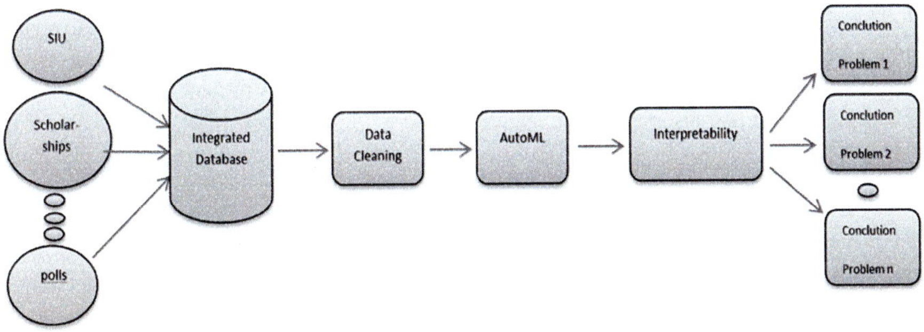

Fig. 2. Proposed model

The conformation of the integrated Database is of vital importance since in a paradigm such as that of machine learning it is "programmed" from the data, that is, the more data we have and of higher quality, the better patterns we can find to solve the educational problems raised. Suppose that our problem is to predict the academic performance of students, we must prepare a Database with the information from the University Information System (SIU), which will provide us with all the academic data, to which we must add the data from the University Information Systems. National and subnational scholarships, data from the teaching, research and extension evaluation systems, and a permanent survey system that contains information concerning the social, family, cultural, sports, occupational, mobility, and connectivity status of the student. The idea with the permanent survey is to have a set of no less than 100 characteristics of the students that, added to the academic ones, allow us to work not only on the problem of predicting academic performance but also on a broad set of problems.

The data cleaning stage will be in charge of the database administrator depending on the proposed problem, although you should know principles and fundamentals of machine learning you do not need to be an expert, database administrators are widely trained for this task.

The AutoML stage will begin with the choice of the data set and will continue with the decision to solve a classification or regression problem. All this in a friendly framework (setting) developed in Python to drive the workflow, which will make available a set of configurations for both classification and regression. From here, the Auto Sklearn library will be used for data pre-processing, the choice of the machine learning model and its hyperparameters. This choice is based on the fact that it is an open source library, it is developed in Python, it takes advantage of the recent advantages in Bayesian optimization, meta-learning and the construction of sets [34], in addition to having good performance in skills such as ChaLearn.

The Interpretability of the results will be given from the choice of the method to be used to interpret the data, whether they are interpretable methods (linear regression, logistic, decision tree, RuleFit, etc.) or independent of the model (PDP, interaction of functions, SHAP, etc.). These Interpretability options will also depend on the configurations chosen in the previous stage, that is, if I choose a configuration option in the AutoML stage with interpretable models in the Interpretability stage, I will also have that option.

The conclusion of the problems should be in charge of a group of multidisciplinary professionals from the educational institution that considers the magnitude of the characteristics (causes) that influenced the result.

5 Conclusion and Future Works

The Educational Data Mining Model presented, has as purpose to allow educational institutions to use techniques and tools from machine learning for the extraction of knowledge in the complex problems of their field, without the need for data scientists to choose the models, their most optimal hyperparameters, and the interpretation of the model results. This is possible due to the inclusion in the process of techniques such as Auto Machine Learning and Interpretable Machine Learning, which democratize the use of Machine Learning. The next step that we have already started is to develop a friendly interface that allows non-expert users to carry out the entire workflow from choosing the dataset or dataset to the results interpretation report.

References

1. Urbina Nájera, A.B., de la Calleja Mora, J.: Brief Review of Educational Applications Using Data Mining and Machine Learning. REDIE (2017)
2. Gimenez, A.: "Data scientists. As attractive as they are scarce". Harvard Deusto Number 121 of Marketing and Sales. http://www.harvarddeusto.com/articulo/Cientificos-de-datos-tan-atractivos-como-escasos. Accessed 05 Mar 2021
3. Romero, C., Ventura, S.: Educational data mining: a review of the state of the art. IEEE Trans. Syst. Man Cybern. Part C (Appl. Rev.) 601–618 (2010)
4. International Educational Data Mining Society (IEDMS). http://www.educationaldatamining.org. Accessed 04 Apr 2021
5. Sanyam, B., Sai, S., Abhay, B.: Applying learning analysis using cluster data mining for analysis of student disposition. Inf. Technol. Educ. **23**, 957 (2018)
6. Amrieh, E., Hamtini, T., Aljarah, I.: Mining educational data to predict student's academic performance using ensemble methods. Int. J. Database Theory Appl. **9**(8), 119–136. https://doi.org/10.14257/ijdta.2016.9.8.13. Accessed 05 May 2021
7. Romero, C., Ventura, S., Pechenizkiy, M., Baker, R.: Handbook of Educational Data Mining. Chapman & Hall/CRC Data Mining and Knowledge Discovery Series. CRC Press, Taylor & Francis Group (2011)
8. Hutter, F., Kotthoff, L., Vanschoren, J.: Automated Machine Learning, Methods Systems and Challenges. The Springer Series on Challenges in Machine Learning. https://doi.org/10.1007/978-3-030-05318-5. Accessed 05 May 2021
9. Molnar, C.: Interpretable Machine Learning, a guide for making black box model explainable. https://christophm.github.io/interpretable-ml-book/index.html. Accessed 05 May 2021
10. SAS.: Data Mining From A to Z: How to Discover Insights and Drive Better Opportunities. https://www.sas.com/content/dam/SAS/en_us/doc/whitepaper1/data-mining-from-a-z-104937.pdf. Accessed 05 May 2021
11. Han, J., Kamber, M., Pei, J.: Data Mining, Concepts and Techniques, 3rd edn. Morgan Kaufmann Publishers is an imprint of Elsevier (2012)
12. Gómez Aguilar, D.A., García-Peñalvo, F.J., Therón, R.: Visual analytics model for educational data. In: Information Systems and Technologies. Proceedings of the 9th Iberian Conference on Information Systems and Technologies, Barcelona, Spain, 18–21 June 2014 (2014)
13. Moine, M., Gordillo, S., Haedo, A.: Análisis comparativo de metodologías para la gestión de proyectos de minería de datos. CACIC 2011. http://sedici.unlp.edu.ar/handle/10915/20034. Accessed 05 May 2021
14. Minaei-Bidgoli, Kashy, Kortemeyer, Punch: Predecir el desempeño de los estudiantes: una aplicación de métodos de minería de datos con un sistema educativo basado en la Web (2003). https://www.ieeexplore.ieee.org/abstract/document/1263284
15. Thomas, E., Galambos, N.: What satisfies students? Mining student opinion data with regression and decision tree. Investigación en educación superior **45**, 251–269. https://doi.org/10.1023/B:RIHE.0000019589.79439. Accessed 05 May 2021
16. Akpinar, N., Ramdas, A., Acar, U.: Analyzing Student Strategies in Blended Courses Using Clickstream Data. Cornell University. https://arxiv.org/abs/2006.00421. Accessed 05 May 2021
17. Yin, X., Han, J.: CPAR: Classification based on Predictive Association Rules. https://epubs.siam.org/doi/10.1137/1.9781611972733.40. Accessed 05 May 2021
18. Chrysostomou, K., Chen, S.Y., Liu, X.: Investigation of users' preferences in interactive multimedia learning systems: a data mining approach. Interact. Learn. Environ. 151–163 (2009)

19. Su, J.M., Tseng, S.S., Lin, H.Y., Chen, C.H.: A personalized learning content adaptation mechanism to meet diverse user needs in mobile learning environments. User Model. User Adapted Interact. 5–49 (2011)
20. Hegazi, M.O., Abugroon, M.A.: The state of the art on educational data mining in higher education. Int. J. Comput. Trends Technol. 46–56 (2016)
21. Panizzi, M.: Establecimiento del estado del arte sobre la Minería de Datos Educacional en el Nivel Superior: Un Estudio de Mapeo Sistemático. Revista de Investigación científica de la Universidad de Morón (2019). https://repositorio.unimoron.edu.ar/bitstream/10.34073/164/1. Accessed 05 May 2021
22. Thornton, C., Hutter, F., Hoss, H., Leyton-Brown, K.: User Guide for Auto-WEKA version 2.6 (2013). http://www.cs.ubc.ca/labs/beta/Projects/autoweka/manual.pdf. Accessed 05 May 2021
23. Thornton, C., Hutter, F., Hoos, H., Leyton-Brown, K.: Auto-WEKA: selección combinada y optimización de hiperparámetros de algoritmos de clasificación, pp. 847–855 (2013). https://dl.acm.org/doi/abs/10.1145/2487575.2487629. Accessed 05 May 2021
24. Hall, M., Frank, E., Holmes, G., Pfahringer, B., Reutemann, P., Witten, I.: The WEKA data mining software: an update. ACM SIGKDD Explor. Newsl. **11**(1) (2009). https://dl.acm.org/doi/abs/10.1145/1656274.1656278. Accessed 05 May 2021
25. Hutter, F., Hoos, H.H., Leyton-Brown, K.: Sequential model-based optimization for general algorithm configuration. In: Coello, C.A.C. (ed.) LION 2011. LNCS, vol. 6683, pp. 507–523. Springer, Heidelberg (2011). https://doi.org/10.1007/978-3-642-25566-3_40. Accessed 05 May 2021
26. Snoek, J., Larochelle, H., Adams, R.: Practical Bayesian optimization of machine learning algorithms. In: NIPS 2012, pp. 2960–2968. Cornell University. https://arxiv.org/abs/1206.2944. Accessed 05 May 2021
27. Castrillon, O., Sarache, W., Ruiz-Herrera, S.: Predicción del rendimiento académico por medio de técnicas de inteligencia artificial. Form. Univ. [online], vol. 13, no. 1, pp. 93–102. ISSN 0718-5006. https://doi.org/10.4067/S0718-50062020000100093. Accessed 05 May 2021
28. Carrizo, C., Saldarini, J., Ribotta, G., Cardona, F., Marotti, J.: Modelo para predecir la cantidad de graduados de Ingeniería de UTN aplicando técnicas de minería de datos (2017). Disponible en http://sedici.unlp.edu.ar/handle/10915/61740. Accessed 05 May 2021
29. Istvan, R., Lasagna, V.: Sistema Informático para la Detección Temprana de Deserción Estudiantil Universitaria. Universidad Tecnológica Nacional, Facultad Regional La Plata Laboratorio de Ingeniería en Sistemas de Información, LINES. https://doi.org/10.24215/26838559e006. Accessed 05 May 2021
30. Bianco, S., Martins, S., Amatriain, H., Merlino, H.: Propuesta de automatización para proyectos de minería de datos educativa, Laboratorio de Investigación y Desarrollo en Ingeniería de Explotación de Información Grupo de Investigación en Sistemas de Información. Universidad Nacional de Lanús. http://sedici.unlp.edu.ar/handle/10915/91015. Accessed 05 May 2021
31. Doshi-Velez, F., Kim, B.: Towards a Rigorous Science of Interpretable Machine Learning. https://arxiv.org/pdf/1702.08608.pdf. Accessed 05 May 2021
32. Kabul, I.: Interpretability is crucial for trusting AI and machine learning, SAS Blogs. https://blogs.sas.com/content/subconsciousmusings/2017/12/18/interpretability-crucial-trusting-ai-machine-learning. Accessed 05 May 2021
33. Ribeiro, M., Singh, S., Guestrin, C.: "Why Should I Trust You?" Explaining the Predictions of Any Classifier. https://arxiv.org/pdf/1602.04938.pdf. Accessed 05 May 2021
34. Feurer, M., Klein, A., Eggensperger, K., Springenberg, J., Blum, M., Hutter, F.: Efficient and Robust Automated Machine Learning. Advances in Neural Information Processing Systems 28 (NIPS 2015). https://aaronkl.github.io/publication/feurer-nips-2015/feurer-nips-2015.pdf. Accessed 05 May 2021

Examining the Tech Stacks of Czech and Slovak Untrustworthy Websites

Jozef Michal Mintal[1,2,3](✉), Anna Macko[2], Marko Paľa[2], Františka Pirosková[2], Pavlo Yakubets[2], Jaroslav Ušiak[1,2], and Karol Fabián[1,2]

[1] Department of Security Studies, Matej Bel University, Banská Bystrica, Slovakia
jozef.mintal@umb.sk
[2] UMB Data & Society Lab, CEKR, Matej Bel University, Banská Bystrica, Slovakia
[3] Center for Media, Data and Society at CEU Democracy Institute, Central European University, Budapest, Hungary

Abstract. The burgeoning of misleading or false information spread by untrustworthy websites has, without doubt, created a dangerous concoction. Thus, it is not a surprise that the threat posed by untrustworthy websites has emerged as a central concern on the public agenda in many countries, including Czechia and Slovakia. However, combating this harmful phenomenon has proven to be difficult, with approaches primarily focusing on tackling consequences instead of prevention, as websites are routinely seen as quasi-sovereign organisms. Websites, however, rely upon a host of service providers, which, in a way, hold substantial power over them. Notwithstanding the apparent power hold by such tech stack layers, scholarship on this topic remains largely limited. This article contributes to this small body of knowledge by providing a first-of-its-kind systematic mapping of the back-end infrastructural support that makes up the tech stacks of Czech and Slovak untrustworthy websites. Our approach is based on collecting and analyzing data on top-level domain operators, domain name Registrars, e-mail providers, web hosting providers, and utilized website tracking technologies of 150 Czech and Slovak untrustworthy websites. Our findings show that the Czech and Slovak untrustworthy website landscape relies on a vast number of back-end services spread across multiple countries, but in key tech stack layers is nevertheless still heavily dominated by locally based companies. Finally, given our findings, we discuss various possible avenues of utilizing the numeral tech stack layers in combating online disinformation.

Keywords: Tech stack · Disinformation · Slovakia · Czechia · Websites · Untrustworthy websites

1 Introduction

The proliferation of misleading or false information in cyberspace has emerged as a significant concern on the public agenda in recent years [1, 2]. Around the globe, a variety of politically and economically motivated actors have been shown to deliberately spread lies online [3]. These actors tend to employ a host of tactics to achieve their desired ends.

© The Author(s), under exclusive license to Springer Nature Singapore Pte Ltd. 2022
Á. Rocha et al. (Eds.): ICOMTA 2021, SIST 259, pp. 31–39, 2022.
https://doi.org/10.1007/978-981-16-5792-4_4

A common technique is the creation of a disinformation ecology consisting of one or multiple websites producing false or misleading content that afterward gets amplified by interconnected social networking service accounts [4]. Such disinformation ecologies can be observed in multiple languages, including Czech and Slovak. Effectively combating this harmful phenomenon has, however, from a governance perspective proven to be difficult.

Policy response tackling the issues of disinformation, as shown by Tenove [2], has usually fallen in three governance sectors: international and national security policies, electoral regulation, and media regulation, with the last garnering much of the public and scholarly attention. Such publicity is likely also fueled by a sizeable distaste aimed at social networking services (SNSs) such as Facebook or Twitter, which have been accused of enacting lax content moderation policies combined with limited or no enforcement. Thus, it might not come as a surprise that the debate about media regulation tends to focus on the 'community standards' of major social networking services or around individual website policies [5]. Even though much important, such a debate approaches content governance from a too narrow a view, missing the overall digital governance ecosystem picture along the way. Social networking services, as well as individual websites, rely upon, and in multiple instances, are directly dependent on a host of service providers, who, in a way, hold substantial power to compel SNSs and websites to adopt more strict content moderation. When approaching the issue of moderating misleading or false information, from such a tech stack perspective, a multitude of additional regulation strategies become apparent. As Donovan [5] has argued, a tech stack approach to content moderation comprises several levels, including domain registrars, cloud services, and internet service providers. Power of tech stacks can be observed in multiple instances, such as EURid's decision to amend its Abuse Prevention and Early Warning System, as to ramp up the blocking of nefarious registration of covid related domain names [6], or Amazon's recent decision to suspend web hosting for an entire SNS called Parler, following its utilization in the 2021 storming of the U.S. Capitol [7].

Notwithstanding the apparent power hold by tech stacks, scholarship on this topic in the context of countering untrustworthy websites remains to a great extend limited [5, 8], with empirical studies being largely confined to one recent paper by Au, Howard and Ainita [8]. Thus, the aim of this article is to (i) provide a mapping of the back-end services used to sustain untrustworthy websites, piloted in Czechia and Slovakia; and (ii) to explore possible avenues of utilizing the identified tech stacks of untrustworthy websites in curbing out the threat of online disinformation. To achieve the above aim, the presented article first offers background information on untrustworthy websites in Czechia and Slovakia. Then, it introduces the methods and results of our empirical study. Finally, based on the findings of our study, we explore in this article some of the possible measures that might help in combating the dangerous phenomenon of online disinformation.

1.1 The Czech and Slovak Untrustworthy Website Landscape

In recent years, untrustworthy websites [9] started burgeoning across many countries around the globe, with Czechia and Slovakia being no exception. As Klingová has noted, the exact number of such websites operating natively in these two countries is difficult to pinpoint, as new websites keep on getting established while some of the old ones cease to exist [10]. Albeit estimates typically range in the couple hundreds, one of the most comprehensive publicly available list of relevant Slovak and Czech untrustworthy websites—konspiratori.sk, which is heavily relied upon by local researchers and policy experts [10, 11], lists 205 websites as of February 2021 [12]. Thematically the websites tracked in the konspiratori.sk list cover a wide range of topics, including, among others, health disinformation, Russian propaganda and the paranormal. Even though some of these untrustworthy websites boast a high number of monthly visitors, with a couple of them even making it into the top 50 most visited websites in their respective countries, transparency wise a sizeable amount of these online outlets remain shrouded in mystery [11, 13, 14]. As Mintal and Rusnak have noted, from an operational and financial perspective, at least in Slovakia, it appears that the untrustworthy website landscape is run by multiple independent entities using various business models to sustain operation[1] [11]. The blend of harmful and potentially also illegal content spread by, in some instances, highly viral untrustworthy websites has, without doubt, created a dangerous concoction. Thus, it might not come as a surprise that the threat posed by untrustworthy websites has emerged as a central concern on the public agenda in both Czechia and Slovakia.

2 Methods

To study the possible tech-stack moderation areas of Czech and Slovak untrustworthy websites, we used a variety of open-source and proprietary tools to collect data and run analyses. Our overall methodology builds on Donovan's [5] concept of a tech stack moderation approach to online content and Au et al.'s empirical study of infrastructural support for controversial covid-19 websites [8]. Stemming from these approaches, in our study, we examined Czech and Slovak untrustworthy websites' (i) top-level domain operators, (ii) domain name registrars, (iii) e-mail providers, (iv) web hosting providers, and utilized (v) website tracking technologies. Data Collection was conducted during the second half of February 2021 and consisted of multiple interlinked steps. First, for our sample size, we used a dataset of 205 untrustworthy websites, taken from the konspiratori.sk database [12]. Inclusion of a website in the database is assessed based on a set of publicly available criteria by a Review Board consisting of, among others, prominent historians, political scientists, medical professionals, journalists and civil society representatives [15]. In utilizing the konspiratori.sk database, we followed best practices used in Czech and Slovak disinformation scholarship [10, 11]. Second, each website in our dataset was manually checked to determine its availability status and primary language. Unavailable websites and websites with a primary language other than Czech or Slovak were discarded. The remaining websites were then manually checked for affiliated social networking service accounts and manually content-coded according to a slightly adapted framework by Mintal and Rusnak [11]. Third, we used two dedicated services to query domain information and DNS records of the websites under investigation [16, 17]. Data collection was in this step focused mainly on identifying the domain registrars, hosting providers and e-mail providers. In addition, we also employed

[1] Popular income sources of untrustworthy websites in Slovakia include tax designation, e-commerce, crowdfunding, and advertising [11].

a bulk domain to IP lookup tool to cross-check the previously collected information on hosting providers [18]. Fourth, to detect web tracking technologies running on the Czech and Slovak untrustworthy websites in our dataset, we used the DMI App Tracker script and cross-checked the data with data obtained from Whatruns [19, 20]. The collected web tracking technology data was then coded according to the DMI Tracker framework [19]. Furthermore, we checked all URLs contained in our untrustworthy websites dataset against the top one-hundred most visited websites in Czechia and Slovakia according to an enterprise-grade web analytics firm [21].

After the data collection phase ended, all generated datasets underwent data cleansing to detect and correct corrupt or inaccurate records; duplicate data was discarded. Subsequently, we calculated basic descriptive statistics for the cleansed datasets and identified the most salient organizations providing infrastructural support to the untrustworthy websites under investigation. Last, we formatted the resultant datasets and visualized the data.

3 Results

Out of our initial sample size of 205 untrustworthy websites, 49 appeared to cease to exist and six were found to be primarily in languages other than Czech or Slovak, and therefore discarded from our dataset. Thus, our final list of untrustworthy websites consisted of 150 websites, out of which 69 were primarily in Slovak and 81 were primarily in Czech. Manual content-coding of the final list, utilizing a modified framework by Mintal and Rusnak [11] showed that the majority of websites under investigation were News-Focused with 72 entries, followed by the Ideological or Supporting Cause category with 49 entries, Health and Lifestyle category with 20 entries, and the Paranormal category with nine entries.

3.1 Top-Level Domain Names and Domain Name Registrars

Querying the tech stack of the websites included in our final list showed that ten of them were hosted on a microblogging or social networking service such as tumblr.com or livejournal.com. To avoid skewed results, in instances where this might have affected the results of our empirical study, such as in mapping the domain registrars or hosting providers, we split the dataset into two—one containing the ten microblogging or social networking service hosted websites and the other dataset containing the rest of the websites under investigation. An analysis of top-level domains (TLDs) and registrars used by the Czech and Slovak untrustworthy websites revealed that the majority of these online outlets tend to use Czech or Slovak TLDs and registrars (see Fig. 1). However, a smaller number of websites use third country services for TLDs and registrars, with some of them utilizing highly privacy and free speech friendly providers in countries such as the United States of America, Panama or the Bahamas.

3.2 Hosting and E-mail Providers

The Czech and Slovak untrustworthy website landscape under investigation utilizes a vast pool of geographically dispersed hosting providers spanning eleven countries. Among

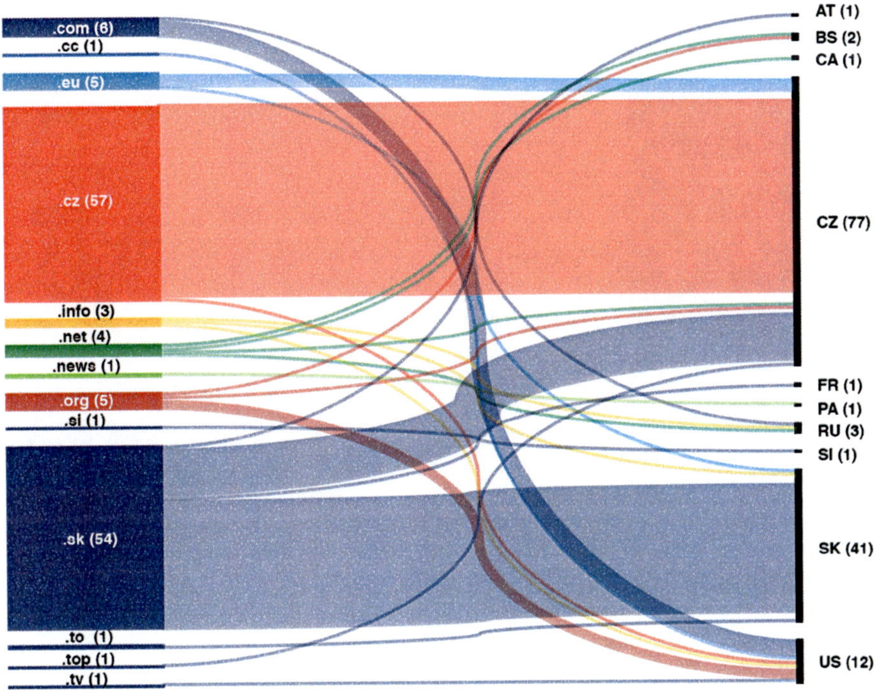

Fig. 1. Top-level domain name suffixes of Czech and Slovak untrustworthy websites by the corresponding country code of the utilized domain name registrar.

these locations, the strongest represented ones are Czechia with 60 entries, followed by Slovakia with 29 entries, the United States of America with 29 entries, and Germany with 14 entries. As for the most utilized hosting providers, two companies are tied for the first place, with each having 13 entries—namely the Czech-based Wedos Internet a.s., and Slovak-based Websupport s. r. o. Apart from the geographical dispersity of the utilized hosting providers, it appears that a sizeable proportion of websites use a content delivery network (CDN), with the most popular being U.S.-based Cloudflare with 13 entries. In regard to e-mail providers, the websites under investigation almost exclusively relied upon an e-mail service provided to them by their hosting provider, with a few exceptions in which websites relied upon a third-party e-mail provider such as Gmail or the privacy-friendly Protonmail.

3.3 Trackers

In our analysis, we detected web tracking technologies on 126 websites under investigation. The most popular trackers present in our dataset were DoubleClick, followed by Google Analytics, and Facebook Connect (see Fig. 2).

In aggregate, we observed 949 trackers with 93 different fingerprints of tracking technologies being represented. Coding of the observed trackers utilizing the DMI

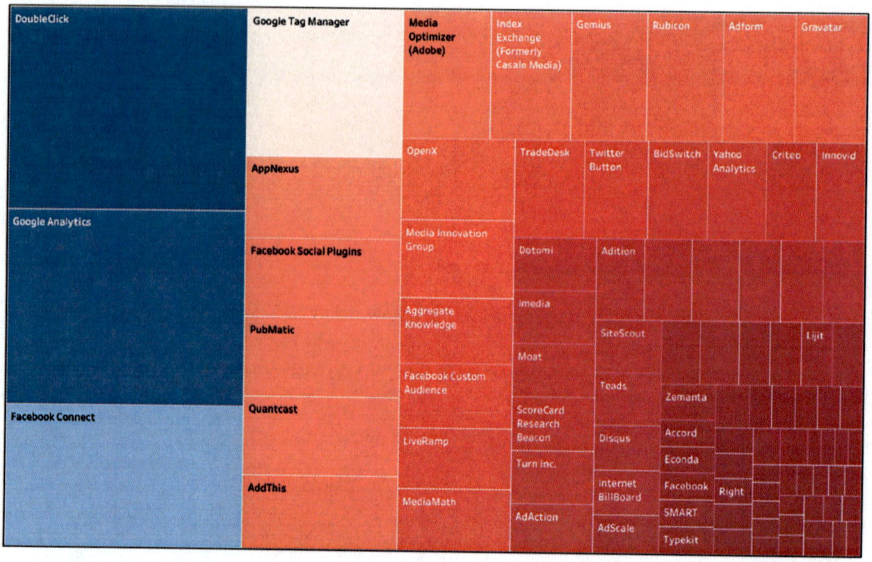

Fig. 2. Treemap of trackers present on Czech and Slovak untrustworthy websites

Tracker framework [19] revealed that 49.10% were advertising elements, 23.07% widget elements, 17.28% analytics elements and 10.53% tracker elements.

4 Discussion

The results described above show that the Czech and Slovak untrustworthy website landscape relies on a vast number of back-end services spread across multiple countries. Even though this geographical diversity is eminent, it can be argued that core layers of these websites' tech stacks, in areas such as TLD operators, domain registrars, and even hosting providers, are nevertheless still heavily dominated by Czech and Slovak based companies.

So, what does this situation mean in terms of utilizing the identified tech stacks of untrustworthy websites to chart possible avenues in combating online disinformation? For the two local governments in question, the reliance of untrustworthy websites on local companies, means among other things, direct jurisdiction over critical areas of the untrustworthy websites' tech stacks. Such control theoretically opens up the possibility of combating the local untrustworthy website landscape through regulation affecting technological intermediaries such as hosting providers or TLD operators. However, an approach like this would likely be seen as highly controversial as, for one, spreading online disinformation might not necessarily be illegal. Besides the fact that not all disinformation can be considered illegal, some critics point out to a supposed nonequivalence between online and offline law, calling for enacting new harmonizing legislative measures. However, ultimately such calls might, among other things, be a red herring. Various legal experts have noted, that generally, behaviour is broadly criminalized to the same extent online as offline [22]; what is, however, oftentimes lacking in regard to the online domain are case law, human and technical capital resources [23] and overall a more active pursue in terms of criminal law enforcement [22]. This line of argument can be illustrated on the Slovak case of the untrustworthy website badatel.net, which, even though has for many years spread disinformation that might be considered illegal, only recently, in 2020, a major legal action has been taken against this website [24]. A somewhat similar situation can be seen in Czechia, where local law enforcement have in the wake of the covid-19 pandemic, more actively engaged in investigating long time disinformation spreading websites such as otevrisvoumysl.cz or ac24.cz [25].

However, governments and law enforcement do not have to be the only driving force behind combating untrustworthy websites. Various key service providers present in the tech stacks of Czech and Slovak untrustworthy websites already have provisions in their Terms of Services that might be used to combat harmful disinformation. A case in point is the action taken by EURid, which is the registry manager of the.eu top-level domain name. As a result of the covid-19 pandemic, EURid has amended its already used Abuse Prevention and Early Warning System, as to ramp up the blocking of nefarious registrations of covid-19 related domain names [6]. However, as a recent report by the Digital Citizens Alliance has found out, multiple major domain Registrars have, in general, done little to prevent the sale of domain names with the potential to spread covid-19 related disinformation [26].

The results of this study, however, bring forth another possible avenue of combating untrustworthy websites. Even though the various layers of a tech stack are from a technical point of view not equally important in keeping a website online, some less critically important services might theoretically wield great indirect power over the actual operational existence of a website. As demonstrated by our data on website tracking technologies present on Czech and Slovak untrustworthy websites, the most widely used tracking elements were directly related to advertising. This finding of heavy reliance on ad serving services is also in line with previous studies exploring the business models of Slovak [11] and Czech [13] untrustworthy websites. Thus, a decision by a major internet ad serving service such as DoubleClick or PubMatic to demonetize untrustworthy websites could have potentially far-reaching implications for the continued existence of such websites and whole disinformation ecologies, thus consequently providing an indirect tool of combating online disinformation. Nevertheless, as with the other in this article discussed avenues of utilizing the power of tech stacks to combat disinformation, the demonetization approach as well, is in some ways vulnerable to the possibility that untrustworthy website owners could create new websites and, in some instances, even shift their already established ones, to rely on tech stack layers based in privacy and free speech friendly jurisdictions. Nonetheless, a demonetization approach might be highly effective at targeting well-established high web traffic untrustworthy websites.

In conclusion, besides providing a first of its kind systematic mapping of the back-end infrastructural support that makes up the tech stacks of Czech and Slovak untrustworthy websites, our article highlighted some of the possible avenues of utilizing the numeral tech stack layers in combating online disinformation. Domain name providers, ad serving services, hosting providers and other various back-end infrastructural services sustaining untrustworthy websites can all play a critical role in creating a safer infosphere. Nevertheless, it must be noted that to achieve such a goal, there is no one silver bullet, instead what appears to be needed is a coordinated approach among various stakeholders, potentially on an international level.

Contributions. J.M.M. designed the study and supervised the research; A.M., M.P., F.P., P.Y. collected the data with input from J.M.M.; J.U. provided the funding; J.M.M. analyzed the data with input from the other authors; J.M.M. wrote the paper with input from the other authors; J.U., K.F. critically reviewed the paper. All authors reviewed the results and approved the final version of the manuscript.

Data Availability. The data that support the findings of this study have been deposited in Zenodo at doi: 10.5281/zenodo.4926213; the data are available upon reasonable request.

Funding and Declaration of Conflicting Interest. This work was supported by Erasmus+ Strategic Partnerships for higher education (grant number 2020-1-IT02-KA203-079902). The authors declared no potential conflicts of interest with respect to the research, authorship, and/or publication of this article.

References

1. Nenadić, I.: Unpacking the "European approach" to tackling challenges of disinformation and political manipulation. Internet Policy Rev. **8** (2019). https://doi.org/10.14763/2019.4.1436
2. Tenove, C.: Protecting democracy from disinformation: normative threats and policy responses. Int. J. Press/Politics **25**, 517–537 (2020). https://doi.org/10.1177/1940161220918740
3. Bennett, W.L., Livingston, S.: The disinformation order: disruptive communication and the decline of democratic institutions. Eur. J. Commun. **33**, 122–139 (2018). https://doi.org/10.1177/0267323118760317
4. Shao, C., et al.: Anatomy of an online misinformation network. PLoS ONE **13**, e0196087 (2018). https://doi.org/10.1371/journal.pone.0196087
5. Donovan, J.: Navigating the Tech Stack: When, Where and How Should We Moderate Content? https://www.cigionline.org/articles/navigating-tech-stack-when-where-and-how-should-we-moderate-content
6. EURid: APEWS. https://eurid.eu/en/register-a-eu-domain/apews/. Accessed 30 Mar 2021
7. Floridi, L.: Trump, parler, and regulating the infosphere as our commons. Philos. Technol. **34**(1), 1–5 (2021). https://doi.org/10.1007/s13347-021-00446-7
8. Au, Y., Howard, P.N., Ainita, P.: Profiting from the Pandemic. Oxford Internet Institute, Oxford (2020)
9. Guess, A.M., Nyhan, B., Reifler, J.: Exposure to untrustworthy websites in the 2016 US election. Nat. Hum. Behav. **4**, 472–480 (2020). https://doi.org/10.1038/s41562-020-0833-x
10. Klingova, K.: What Do We Know About Disinformation Websites in the Czech Republic and Slovakia? https://www.globsec.org/news/what-do-we-know-about-disinformation-websites-in-the-czech-republic-and-slovakia/. Accessed 23 Mar 2021
11. Mintal, J.M.: Slovakia: snake oil spills onto the web. In: The Unbearable Ease of Misinformation. Center for Media, Data and Society at Central European University, Budapest (2020)
12. Konspiratori.sk: List of websites with controversial content. https://www.konspiratori.sk/. Accessed 23 Mar 2021
13. Syrovátka, J., Vinklová, J., Zikmundová, A., Wojtula, L.: Disinformation Business Model. Prague Security Studies Institute, Prague (2020)

14. Krátka Špalková, V.: Výroční Zpráva O Stavu České Dezinformační Scény Za Rok 2019—Kremlin Watch Report. European Values, Prague (2021)
15. Konspiratori.sk: Criteria for including a website in the database. https://www.konspiratori.sk/en/inclusion-criteria.php. Accessed 26 Mar 2021
16. WHOIS Search, Domain Name, Website, and IP Tools - Who.is. https://who.is/. Accessed 23 Mar 2021
17. DNS Lookup - Check DNS All Records. https://dnschecker.org/all-dns-records-of-domain.php. Accessed 23 Mar 2021
18. Domain to IP. Find Location of Websites or Domains. https://www.bulkseotools.com/bulk-domain-to-location.php. Accessed 23 Mar 2021
19. ToolTrackerTracker < Dmi < Foswiki. https://wiki.digitalmethods.net/Dmi/ToolTrackerTracker. Accessed 23 Mar 2021
20. WhatRuns – Discover What Runs a Website. https://www.whatruns.com/. Accessed 23 Mar 2021
21. Research Solution & Data Analysis Tools | Similarweb. https://www.similarweb.com/corp/research/. Accessed 23 Mar 2021
22. Abusive and Offensive Online Communications: A Scoping Report. Law Commission, London (2018)
23. Fabian, K., Mintal, J.M.: Cognitive Analysis of Security Threats on Social Networking Services: Slovakia in Need of Stronger Action (2020)
24. The Slovak Spectator: Health Ministry moves against disinformation website - spectator.sme.sk. https://spectator.sme.sk/c/22486133/health-ministry-moves-against-disinformation-website.html. Accessed 17 Apr 2021
25. Klezl, T.: Dezinformací o vakcíně přibývá. Poplašnou zprávu o mrtvých na Gibraltaru řeší policie | Aktuálně.cz. https://zpravy.aktualne.cz/domaci/dezinformace-vakcina-covid/r~603aecd0647411eb95caac1f6b220ee8/. Accessed 18 Apr 2021
26. Digital Citizens Alliance: Domains of Danger : How website operators and Registrars trade Internet Safety for Profit (2020)

A Prospective Model of a Digital Epidemiological Surveillance 4.0 Based on the Peruvian Public Health System

María Aranguri(✉), Jessie Bravo, Roger Alarcón, Alan Rodriguez, and David Correa

School of Computer and Systems Engineering, Santo Toribio de Mogrovejo Catholic University, Lambayeque, Peru
{maranguri,jbravo,ralarcon,arodriguez,40564392}@usat.edu.pe

Abstract. The health-disease situation of the population and health care delivery services are continuously monitored by epidemiological surveillance systems and health information systems, but since the first cases of COVID-19 appeared in December 2019 and spread globally, each country tried to control the virus by activating their own health protocols, but they became insufficient to face the pandemic and every control attempts seem impossible to all humanity, even more without the support of information technologies, which provides a rapid response for decision-making. Being that the reason why surveillance systems should help mitigate the spread of diseases and, at the same time, plan resources to protect the health status of citizens. Therefore, the aim of this article is to propose a model of a digital epidemiological surveillance 4.0, considering the current technological revolution and the constant evolution of the Internet. This model is divided into 4 phases: situational analysis, planning, execution and evaluation, and supported on 4 key components: logistic support, digital privacy and data protection, communication and technology, and disruptive innovation. A quantitative type of research was applied in a sample of 58 participants, all working as health staff in Chiclayo-Peru, to whom a data collection instrument, based on digital forms and interviews with medical epidemiologists, was applied, that information, which mainly considers the perception and perspectives of the epidemiological surveillance system, served as the basis for the proposed model.

Keywords: Epidemiological surveillance · Information technologies · Public health · Systemic approach

1 Introduction

Epidemiological surveillance [1] is defined as the comparison and interpretation of information obtained from environmental and health monitoring programs, as well as from other sources, to protect human health by detecting fast-growing adverse changes in the health status of populations or the presence of dangerous environmental factors, all in order to offer the necessary information for effective intervention. In the research [2] a comprehensive review of 30 studies was carried out, where the results revealed

© The Author(s), under exclusive license to Springer Nature Singapore Pte Ltd. 2022
Á. Rocha et al. (Eds.): ICOMTA 2021, SIST 259, pp. 40–50, 2022.
https://doi.org/10.1007/978-981-16-5792-4_5

different types of Covid-19 surveillance. The final conclusion was, prompt and correct surveillance data is an essential element for effective Covid-19 interventions. In terms of challenges, the quality of surveillance in developing countries is limited by resources and training, and the main limitations are: the lacking of verification or reporting, lacking of timeliness, and the integrity of surveillance data. The research finally concluded that surveillance is a cornerstone to control the Covid-19 pandemic.

It is also important to highlight the research carried out [3] which describes how digital technologies have been used in public health to deal with COVID-19, providing benefits at a clinical level (such as an improved clinical record of cases, remote care or diagnostic assistance using artificial intelligence), epidemiological (geographic information systems), academic (e-learning) and personal (using mobile apps or searching for information through social networks). Regarding the application of technology in epidemiological surveillance, in a cross-sectional study [4] 52 Covid-19 mobile apps obtained in different app stores with Android and iOS operating systems were reviewed, the study concluded that there are mobile applications on Covid-19 available in most of the countries of the five continents, in the most popular languages of communication, and free of charge; nevertheless, with limited accessibility for people with disabilities. A study [5], in which surveys were conducted to 10,760 participants in the US, and the conclusion was that 21.8% of adults were extremely or very likely to install a mobile app to record symptoms and get recommendations on COVID-19, and a 21.1% reported it was extremely or very likely to use a website to record symptoms, location, and receive recommendations on COVID-19.

The General Directorate of Epidemiology (GDE) of Peru makes available to the general public on its website, graphics and tables related to the pandemic [6], in addition to a section made available by the MINSA (Ministry of Health) called Knowledge Management and Scientific Information - COVID-19, where it shows everything related to COVID-19, classified in 6 important areas: digital innovation, health data and figures, scientific and normative information, scientific research and communication, periodical publications and transmission of knowledge [7]. Regarding the use of technology applied to epidemiological surveillance specifically for COVID - 19 in Peru, there are some solutions developed by regional governments.

From this literature review, the observation is that each country proposes an epidemiological surveillance system that differs from the others and not a standard one that can be applied in any situation of infections or pandemics, such as the one we currently experience, in addition to this we have observed that these surveillance systems do not integrate the support of information technologies as the main axis to achieve the expected results throughout the epidemiological surveillance process. Although in some stages they use computer applications, such as web and mobile applications or IoT solutions, these are isolated and not part of an epidemiological surveillance system such as what it is proposed in this research. In addition, the medical records of the patients are not digitalized and integrated, which, in fact, allows not only better patient care but also the generation of alerts and the ability to take preventive measures immediately, which is exacerbated by not having centralized information from public and private health centers and medical professionals.

Faced with this need, a digital epidemiological surveillance model is proposed, which integrates each and every one of the phases with the support of information technologies, making possible to know the epidemiological reality of the diseases and the current events of the communities.

2 Methods

The type of research according to the purpose is applied and based on the quantitative research method. The population corresponds to the health personnel (508 doctors and 623 nurses) of the city of Chiclayo in December 2019 [8]. To obtain the sample, a confidence level of 90% was considered, with a 10% margin of error, the sample is 58, and the sampling is non-probabilistic. The collection methods were surveys and interviews with health personnel. The surveys were applied to our selected sample and the interview to epidemiologists. The objective of the applied survey is to know the perception and perspectives on the national Epidemiological Surveillance (ES) system in Health Centers (HC) in Peru. A questionnaire of twenty questions categorized into topics such as management and strategy (5), operational Epidemiological Surveillance (ES) (2), infrastructure and support (3), technological tools (3), analysis and evaluation of data (3), information security (1), and communication (3).

Regarding management and strategy, 70.4% are favorable, 14.8% unfavorable, while 14.8% were indifferent to qualify the ES measures applied in health entities; Regarding the rating of the effectiveness of the ES applied by the government, 40.7% think that it was unfavorable; in addition, they rate that the government's participation was unfavorable at 51.8%. Regarding infrastructure and support to face COVID-19 cases, 40.7% consider it as unfavorable while 33.3% consider it as favorable, and 18.5% remain indifferent; regarding technological tools, 66.6% of those surveyed consider the use of mobile and web apps to be favorable and necessary, and also, in approximately 60%, agree that the analysis and exploitation of statistical information would be an important element for the management of the epidemiological situation, in. Regarding the security of information and data of COVID-19 patients, they consider that it is an important element in 48%. Regarding the form and participation of the media in the management of the COVID-19 pandemic, they state that they play an important role in 37.0%.

3 Results

The model developed in this research proposes, in addition to the own processes of epidemiological surveillance, to integrate technological tools in order to obtain the results in a clear and timely manner, to generate indicators to measure the criteria, and to assess continuous improvement. The epidemiological surveillance model is based on the systemic approach, where each phase includes the inputs, the process and the social impact (outputs). Regarding the epidemiological surveillance process, it has been subdivided into 4 phases of continuous feedback: situational analysis, planning, execution and evaluation. In addition, this model is supported by 4 components: Technology and disruptive innovation, digital privacy and data protection, communication and logistical support (See Fig. 1).

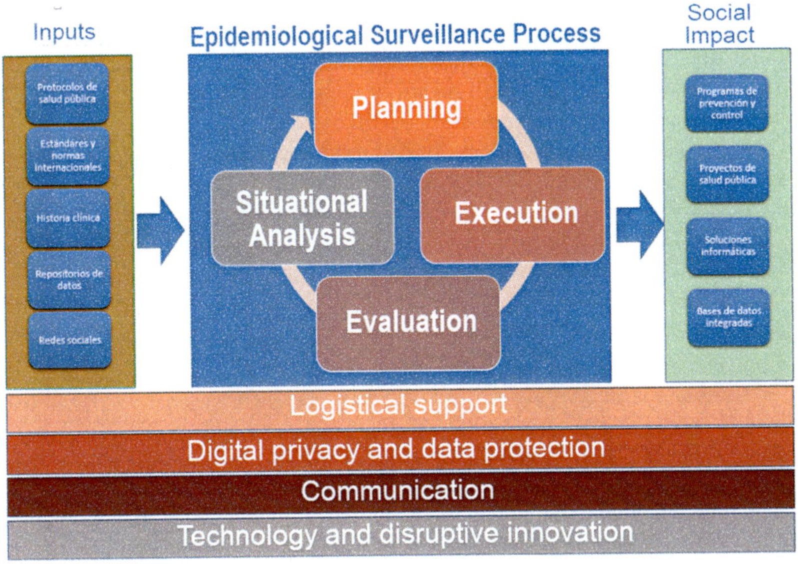

Fig. 1. Digital epidemiological surveillance model

3.1 Model Inputs

Each of the elements that the system may require for its operation are considered in this section, in addition, each phase of the epidemiological surveillance process may require input data that are outputs from other phases.

3.2 Epidemiological Surveillance Process

Analysis Phase

The analysis stage identifies the diseases or events under epidemiological surveillance based on the review of the documents, facts and scenarios of the reality under study and establishes the key requirements according to the various sources of information available. The protocols and standards are applied in a transversal way serving as guidelines, pointing out the guiding thread, facilitating the adoption of strategies, which are arranged according to the context in which it is applied for the continuous improvement process.

To develop this phase we require the following **inputs**: Public health protocols, ISO standards and international norms of processes in public health, constitutional rights, clinical history of the patients, data repositories, information from social networks, research articles, report on the results of the programs and executed projects.

The methodological analysis procedure can be established as follows:

Step 1: Information Gathering: (a) Establish the instruments for information extraction, making use of collaborative online tools that allow the recollection of information from the patient, medical and administrative user, in order to know the status of the epidemiological situation. (b) Review the public health protocols and calibrate the baseline scope level, as well as the gap with regard to the expected conditions. (c) Review the health center's own documentation, forms, request documents, etc.

Step 2: Information Prioritization (Usefulness or relevance): (a) Define the information prioritization criteria. (b) Assess the information based on the established criteria.

Step 3: Information Validation (Reliability): (a) Validate the information based on statistical tools.

Step 4: Statistical Reports Generation: (a) Develop dynamic reports on the epidemiological situation analyzed. (b) Develop reports of projected scenarios, which allow taking preventive actions and reducing health crisis situations.

Step 5: Requirements Definition: (a) Based on the reports generated, establish the requirements according to criteria that allow planning and executing in an orderly and adequate manner. (b) Classify and identify the constraints of the requirements according to their importance.

The **results** of the analysis phase are: Integrated databases, reports based on statistical results by types of indicators, reports of projected scenarios, alert report that allows a quick and timely response for the treatment of the emergency situation, reports of technological resources, economic resources, infrastructure, services, and current and required personnel.

The **Technology and disruptive innovation** component provides support to the entire digital epidemiological surveillance system; in the situational analysis phase, it helps diagnosis through geolocation devices, such as mobile phones; that information is being analyzed through artificial intelligence techniques, data massive (big data), among other techniques. As means of collecting and displaying information, mobile applications (apps), web pages, geographic information systems (GIS) become useful. Regarding self-diagnosis of COVID-19, apps, websites, chatboots, Telegram channels, among others were created, looking to reduce the congestion of primary care. In addition to data processing and generating statistical reports, there are tools such as SPSS, Excel, MegaStat, R, Microsoft Power BI, SAS, Python, Tableau Public, among others.

3.3 Planning Phase

Planning is the process of evaluating public health objectives to create a realistic plan of activities; with action plans according to the strategies that make possible to achieve the established objectives. In planning, it must be taken into account that the strategies would be established for short, medium and long-term periods.

The information required for this phase are: Integrated databases, statistical reports and projected scenarios on the state of public health and patient care services, reports of current and required technological resources, economic resources, infrastructure, services, and personnel, budgets established in the health center or institution in which it is expected to apply the solution, strategic and operational plan of the central government and the health institution under study.

The procedure established in the planning stage must consider:

Step 1: Set Goals: Define the objectives of the health institution to take into account for the preparation of the plan.
Step 2: Identify projects and programs: (a) Define the projects aimed at the epidemiological surveillance, so it will be possible to achieve the specific objectives set out in the previous step. (b) Identify the programs that are required to be executed continuously according to the requirements, which are intended to achieve specific and previously defined objectives to improve the health status of a population.
Step 3: Determine Activities and Resources: (a) Identify the activities required for each identified project and program. (b) Establish the necessary resources in each project and program.
Step 4: Establish evaluation indicators: (a) Identify the priority level of each of the activities for the monitoring, follow-up and control of patients, with development times and delivery milestones. (b) Establish evaluation methods that allow progress to be measured.

The **results** of this phase are: Portfolio of projects / programs to be executed, schedule of activities (Gantt), defining tasks and times, checklist with deliverables by activity at each established milestone.

In the **planning** phase the **Technology and disruptive innovation** component provides support to the entire digital epidemiological surveillance system, following the project life cycle methodology and the use of computer tools that allow its management, such as: Microsoft Project, Wrike, Jira, Trello, Asana, Podio, among others.

3.4 Execution Phase

In this stage, the projects that have been identified, prioritized and valued in the planning phase become operational.

For this stage the required **inputs** are: Portfolio of projects and programs to be executed, reports of current and required technological resources, economic resources, infrastructure, services, and personnel.

The procedure established in the execution phase must consider:

Step 1: Organize project/program resources: Establish the human and material resources of the project/program, in order to be able to assign adequate resources to each task.
Step 2: Develop the products defined in each milestone: The resulting products are elaborated in each milestone of the project/program.
Step 3: Closure of projects/programs: Every project/program must have a closing report that includes completed activities and recommendations that serve as a basis for other projects and programs.

This phase will **result** in the following: Report of projects/programs in execution, report of completed projects/programs, report of projects/programs not completed.

In the **execution** phase the **Technology and disruptive innovation** component provides support to the entire digital epidemiological surveillance system, for monitoring the programs/projects in execution, the mobile or web apps available to use should employ techniques such as the balance score card (table command), generate control dashboards.

Evaluation Phase
The purpose of this stage is to measure the results of projects and programs based on compliance criteria and level of satisfaction, which allow the necessary adjustments to be made. With regard to program evaluation, it is a matter of systematically and objectively determine the structure, process and results of the program. The information required at this stage is Report of projects/programs in execution, completed or not completed, evaluation criteria, current regulations.

To carry out the evaluation of the epidemiological surveillance projects/programs, three aspects are taken into account, which allow a comprehensive evaluation:
Satisfaction level:
To generate the continuous feedback cycle that allows the improvement of the epidemiological surveillance system, the results are evaluated according to the following procedure:

Step 1: Define the satisfaction measurement instruments: (a) The instruments are selected based on the types of patients, taking into consideration the care received and the area of care. (b) Determine the reliability from the statistical approach, to obtain valid information.
Step 2: Apply the measuring instruments: (a) Determine the population and valid sample according to statistical calculations. (b) Identify collaborative online tools. (c) Establish application procedures.
Step 3: Process and get results: (a) Obtain statistical graphical results. (b) Interpretation of results based on the analysis criteria.

Degree of compliance:

Step 1: Evaluation criteria and measurement scales: (a) Based on the established objectives, the evaluation criteria should be determine based on what is going to be evaluated. (b) Determine the measurement scales according to the information obtained.
Step 2: Verification of compliance: Establish the results in a comparative way, to signalize the results obtained.

Health Policy Evaluation
Evaluate the policies, guidelines and health research, based on the functionality, the use of time and the cost of the overall study.

Comprehensive Evaluation
Evaluate comprehensively the satisfaction rates according to the type of user who has received the service, as well as compliance with the established policies and procedures developed. The results will be consolidated to establish risk factors, improvements and recommendations for the execution of future projects.

This evaluation phase generates the following **results**: Efficiency and effectiveness rates of projects/programs, report on risk factors, improvements and recommendations, measurement factors with signalized indicators, comparative analysis between what was planned and what was executed, report on the evaluation of health policies and research.

In the **evaluation** phase the **Technology and disruptive innovation** component provides support to the entire digital epidemiological surveillance system, using analytical tools, KPIs; in addition to determining the level of satisfaction, it is possible to apply surveys (With tools such as Google forms, Survey Monkey, Zoho Survey, among others). It can also be complemented through statistical tools such as SPSS, R, Power BI, Python, Tableau Public, among others.

4 Outputs (Social Impact) of the Model

The Surveillance Model presents the results in a comprehensive manner, generating a social impact on the population through the reduction of events and diseases that are monitored, not only by health centers, but by all related entities, such as: Programs of prevention and control, public health projects, computer solutions and integrated databases.

5 Model Components

As for the four components that support the proposed model, we can detail:

Component 1: Logistics Support
The purpose of the logistical support for public health during a health emergency is to give technical assistance, control in the maintenance and distribution of different materials and supplies, manage transportation, the correct handling of stocks, and the coordination during registered epidemic outbreaks. We must emphasize that the WHO emphasizes that logistical support is essential for detection, diagnosis, care and immunization services, to guarantee available proper equipment and an adequate supply of high-quality materials and supplies at all levels. In the proposed model, this dimension is subdivided into materials and supplies, infrastructure and equipment, support services and human resources.

Component 2: Digital Privacy and Data Protection
This dimension aims to establish the necessary mechanisms for the fulfillment of this fundamental right that affects people who make use of different computer applications and the internet. Privacy and data protection is understood as the fundamental right of everyone to have control of the data that can identify them personally and, specifically, digital privacy refers to the users rights over their information inside computer applications, as well as the right to protect their data on the network and the decision of what information is visible to others. In Peru this is regulated by the Political Constitution of Peru, Law 29733 "Personal Data Protection Law" and its regulations, Supreme Decree No. 003-2013-JUS and the entity in charge of ensuring these rights is the National Authority of Protection of Personal Data. In each country the legislation, regarding this

topic, is different, likewise in some it is not even fully established, as in Peru, which is very important since it would generate confidence in the population and it will improve the acceptance of the users [9]. Thus, the proposed Digital Epidemiological Surveillance Model takes into account the security in the processing of personal data, the information will not be disclosed or transferred to third parties without the user's authorization, and the application's use policies will be explicit, generating trust in users.

Component 3: Communication

The purpose of this component is to establish communication mechanisms in each phase of the epidemiological surveillance system supported by the use of technological resources. Communication is intended to be sufficient, clear and based on the environment in which it is implemented. In addition to providing information to communities, it must raise awareness and mitigate the level of uncertainty in the face of a health crisis.

Technology provides important support where, apart from information and self-assessment websites and applications, there is another series of initiatives to provide useful information to citizens, such as instant messaging apps like WhatsApp and Telegram; another solution is chatbots, automatic conversation systems that interact with people using natural language. Communication is not only vertical but also horizontal, where people can be in contact with their family and friends while also staying informed, the videoconferencing options or the access to social networks, especially Facebook and Twitter, have made possible to cope with confinement, caused by the health crisis.

Finally, communication must be two-way, allowing the community the opportunity to provide recommendations and validate the projects as well as the proposed programs.

Component 4: Technology and Disruptive Innovation

From the beginning of the COVID-19 pandemic, social immobility measures were established around the world, which affected all socio-economic sectors of each country in several ways, generating solutions based on Information and Communication Technologies (ICT).

Regarding solutions to fight the Covid-19 pandemic [10] carried out a study, in which is identified various ICT-based projects that have been collecting large volumes of information through geolocation devices, such as portable phones, which have been analyzed through artificial intelligence techniques, massive data (big data), among other techniques. There are also means of collecting and displaying information such as, mobile applications (apps), web pages, Geographic Information Systems (GIS), Chatboot, specialized communication and information media in Telegram and WhatsApp, as well as traditional media such as landline and cell phone. Regarding COVID-19 assistance, there are numerous applications, in which, the apps developed by the government of Spain and autonomous communities stand out [11, 12].

Based on [13], the mobile apps, which are the most popular computer programs that have been used to help in this pandemic, must meet at least the following criteria: Simple and friendly interface, compatible with iOS and Android, must have security and data privacy, offline capabilities, periodic updates, and should be customizable and interoperable.

Finally, the digital epidemiological surveillance model was validated through expert judgment, obtaining a Kendall coefficient of agreement where the experts agree that the proposal is clear in 64.4% and relevant in 53.2%. In general, the model is acceptable, regarding the evaluation of the phases and components of the model.

6 Conclusions

Mentions in his article [2], it is not enough to identify in a disjointed way each one of the efforts from the point of view of the population, the health system and the state, because it generates limitations of epidemiological surveillance such as the lack of verification or notification, lack of punctuality and integrity of surveillance data, so the proposal model integrates projects and programs with technological support in each of their phases and components with a systemic vision. As analyzed by [4] Digital technology is necessary and must be affordable for all people, which is why the model considers the sector of the population, to whom it is addressed, to be fundamental, in addition to a feedback process based on the level of user satisfaction. Another relevant aspect considered for comprehensive epidemiological surveillance lies in ensuring protocols that preserve the privacy and protection of user data at all levels.

A digital epidemiological surveillance model was developed based on the systemic approach because it includes continuous feedback processes as well as the interrelationships between each of the phases, and it is prospective because considers the analysis of past events and their influence on a current state that allows a better projection in the future, it is made up of phases and components that enables streamline and make epidemiological surveillance more effective.

Finally, the proposed model integrates information technologies in each of the phases and components as a key support for the achievement of the desired objectives.

References

1. García Pérez, C., Aguilar, P.A.: Vigilancia epidemiológica en salud. Revista Archivo Médico de Camagüey **17**(6), 121–128 (2013)
2. Khamis Ibrahim, N.: Epidemiologic surveillance for controlling Covid-19 pandemic: types, challenges and implications. J. Infect. Public Health **13**(1), 1630–1638 (2020)
3. Quispe-Juli, C., Vela-Anton, P., Meza-Rodriguez, M., Moquillaza-Alcántara, V.: COVID-19: a pandemic in the era of digital health, Scielo Pre-print, abril 2020
4. Galindo Neto, N.M., Guarino de Moura Sá, G., Uchôa Barbosa, L., Nunes Pereira, J.d.C., Barros Henriques, A.H., Moreira Barros, L.: COVID-19 and digital technology: mobile app. Available for download in smartphone. Rev. Texto y Contexto de Enfermería **29**(1) (2020)
5. Camacho-Rivera, M., Islam, J.Y., Rivera, A., Christina Vidot, D.: Attitudes toward using COVID-19 mHealth tools among adults with chronic health conditions: secondary data analysis of the COVID-19 impact survey. JMIR mHealth uHealth **8**(12), e24693 (2020)
6. Ministerio de Salud (2021). https://www.dge.gob.pe/salasituacional/. Accessed 20 febrero 2021
7. Datos abiertos Minsa y gestión del conocimiento en COVID-19 (2021). https://www.minsa.gob.pe/datosabiertos. Accessed 21 febrero 2021
8. Ministerio de Salud (2019). https://www.minsa.gob.pe. Accessed 5 noviembre 2020
9. Ministerio de Justicia y Derechos humanos, La Protección de Datos Personales en el Perú. Un proyecto en construcción (2020)

10. Cascón-Katchadourian, J.-D.: Tecnologías para luchar contra la pandemia Covid-19. Profesional de la Información **29**(4) (2020)
11. Servicio web del Gobierno Vasco (2020). https://www.euskadi.eus/coronavirus-app-covid-eus/web01-a2korona/es/. Accessed 25 octubre 2020
12. Comunidad de Madrid (2020). https://coronavirus.comunidad.madrid/. Accessed 29 octubre 2020
13. Fernández Blanco, Y., Fernández Rigondeaux, Y., Sorí Gómez, J.C., Valenciano Rivero, B.L.: Aplic. para dispositivos móviles en el enfrentamiento a la Covid-19. Serie Científica de la Univ. de las Ciencias Informáticas, vol. 13, no. 11 (2020)

The Relevance of Internal Communication in Innovation Processes: The Bosch Case Study

Teresa Ruão, Sandra Marinho, and Sónia Silva(✉)

University of Minho, 4710 Braga, Portugal
{truao,marinho}@ics.uminho.pt, sonia.c.melo.silva@gmail.com

Abstract. Technology, innovation and communication are three interconnected phenomena with great relevance for contemporary companies that caught the attention of Organizational Communication theorists. To expand knowledge on this topic, an action-research was developed in the project management department of a Bosch factory in Portugal. The first phase of the research (diagnosis) is here presented in order to discuss (1st) some of the most frequent communication barriers existing in team work mediated by technological channels and (2nd) the challenges of innovation communication, here related to the introduction of a new digital communication system. Interviews were conducted - with managers and team members – to portray the department's communication system. This diagnosis made it possible to identify significant obstacles to interaction between team members, such as the excess or misuse of channels or the prevalence of a reductionist view of the role of communication in organizations, as a mere support for task information. From the results, guidelines about the future intervention plan are given.

Keywords: Organizational communication · Internal communication · Innovation communication · Action research

1 Introduction

The technology, innovation and communication triangle is an important support of contemporary industries and has been a phenomenon widely studied by Organizational Communication theorists [1–3]. This trend was strengthen at the beginning of the 21st century, when the conviction that technological innovation brings promising and challenging consequences for human and organizational communication grew [4]. Technological innovation is here understood as a creative process depending on a complex network of communication paths that connect the various stages of the innovation practice [5]. And it seems that, as technological innovation is reconfiguring human communication, organizations are (broadly) responding in a positive way, and show interest in the adoption of information and interaction formats that migrate, more and more, to digital environments.

To understand internal communication in the technological innovation processes of contemporary organizations, a study was carried out in a Bosch factory in Portugal.

© The Author(s), under exclusive license to Springer Nature Singapore Pte Ltd. 2022
Á. Rocha et al. (Eds.): ICOMTA 2021, SIST 259, pp. 51–60, 2022.
https://doi.org/10.1007/978-981-16-5792-4_6

This environment was considered relevant as the communication setting of the project management department at the factory – that was the chosen empirical scenery - largely favors digital channels. According to previous studies, the use of these tools has encouraged the democratization of organizational environments, since it promotes bottom-up communication and dialogue between employees and managers, thus simplifying the exchange of ideas, opinion sharing and feedback on tasks status (6–8). However, in the context of this company, the adoption of digital communication platforms over the years also brought some problems to team interaction and efficiency. These problems are currently perceived as disturbing the performance of project teams and, therefore, managers are committed to the development of a new software system to support (in an integrated way) project management processes and to solve some communication issues, such as: content dispersion, interaction obstructions and exceeding information exchange. And this has been a complex internal innovation process.

Thereby, the implementation of this new information and communication platform, has demanded the development of a study on the existing communication system, including the identification of communication barriers that compromise the efficiency of project management and the examination of the needs and expectations of project teams in view of the introduction of this innovative system.

Based on the data collected in this study, we look to discuss (1st) some of the most frequent communication obstacles existing in contemporary team work (especially involving digital channels) and (2nd) the challenges of innovation communication in our globalized and competitive world.

2 Communicating for Innovation

The interest in innovation as a research topic has grown over the 21st century, as organizations and businesses go global and realize how the processes of creating or improving new products or services can impact performance, differentiation and competitiveness, in increasingly volatile markets [9–13].

In the scope of innovation processes, communication is described as a decisive phenomenon. Zerfass [13] states that "(...) an insufficient Innovation Communication is a frequently overlooked reason for this failure of innovation" (p. 4). The relevance of communication is justified to the extent that innovation is a process that results from the interaction between various social actors that bring together creativity and imagination [14].

As so, Innovation Communication scholars argue that organizational members are critical in innovation processes and that communication plays a key role in creative work [1, 10, 12, 13, 15–17]. According to Zerfass [13], internal innovation communication focuses on coordinating actions and clarifying the interests of all those who make up an organization and are involved in the innovation process, such as owners, managers, employees, and others. Communication is essential to define goals for innovation, to take advantage of existing knowledge, to develop shared visions and to help overcome fear of changes [13, 18]. In addition, an innovative organization needs active and motivated members, willing to contribute to the development of innovative ideas, and communication is proven to be a motivational mechanism.

At the Bosch plant, innovation is the watchword of the project management department. This unit is accountable for the constant recreation of industrialization processes [14, 19] and it is led by project managers whose communication skills are essential for the coordination of people and tasks that give life to innovation processes. And it is precisely because of the importance of communication in overcoming the competitive challenges, which the company faces, that the evaluation and restructuration of the information and communication system that supports all stages of innovative project management became urgent.

However, reforms force employees to change their routines and practices, and this context is conducive to distrust, anxiety, or resistance [20–22]. And this is a problem at the Bosch factory. The implementation of a new information system, which will support the project management activity of this unit of the multinational brand, has caused distrust and its full implementation will depend on internal acceptance. Thus, it is important to value everyone's participation in the change process, with emphasis on project managers and team members, who will actively use the new tool.

As stated by Gode et al., [18] and Zerfass and Huck [14], innovation processes must allow the involvement of organizational members that contribute with ideas to the final decisions, while becoming aware of their own responsibilities throughout all stages. In the project management department of the Bosch factory, some efforts had already been made. Project managers presented some of the features of this innovative software to colleagues and members of the project teams. The presentation of the prototype served some relevant functions that have been mentioned by Innovation Communication theorists, namely the identification of anxieties and resistance towards the adoption of the new communication platform, as well as the development of new ideas to be added to the innovative system.

From the point of view of communication, the introduction of the new software system seems to be able to improve the information and interaction processes that are required in the project management department. However, a good implementation supposes a deep knowledge of the department's communicative environment. In this regard, it should be noticed that this research started from the assumption widely proven in the literature that the perceptions of the heads, the project managers and team members would be very important to contextualize the current communicative environment and to inspire the construction of the new platform. Responding to this need for internal knowledge, an action-research was developed and the results of the first phase (diagnosis) are presented below. The Bosch case study was sought to be a good example of the challenges to be overcome in the communication of technological innovation processes.

3 Action Research in an Industrial Company

As an ongoing, systematic and empirically grounded attempt to improve practice, action-research is an interactive methodology that involves the collaborative participation of researchers who seek to solve an identified problem by diagnosing, planning and implementing appropriate action [23, 24]. Improving practices is, therefore, the purpose of action-research.

Within the scope of the commitment to improvement that characterizes action-research, the team of researchers goes through a spiral of steps - which include diagnosis, planning, action, evaluation and readjustment of the action – monitored and adjusted as needed. As shown in Fig. 1, action-research begins with the identification of a problem in its context. Relevant data is collected using appropriate methods that may include interviews, observation, document analysis or other relevant techniques. This collection and subsequent data analysis is carried out to propose solutions to the identified problem, facilitating the appropriate change in the context under study [25].

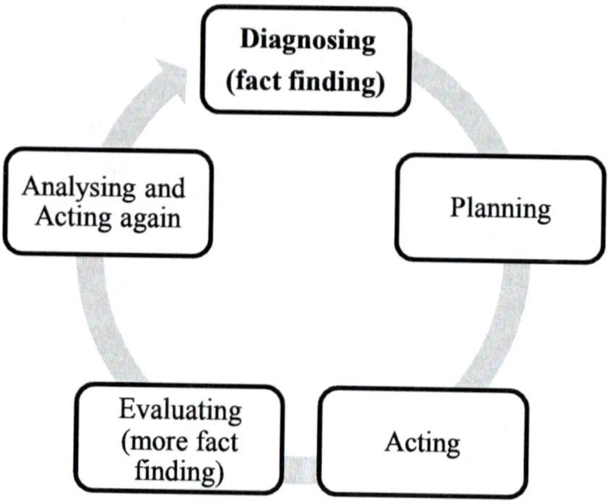

Fig. 1. The action research process

This was, therefore, the methodology used in the Bosch study and this paper presents and discusses the results of the diagnosis phase, in which communication problems existing in the project management department where identified.

Approximately 30 project managers, who are responsible for coordinating the processes of industrialization of new products, operate in this division. However, their performance depends on their relationship with their heads and team members, whose work is developed in different Bosch departments.

A total of 15 interviews were conducted (in May 2020) – including four heads, five project managers and six team members - to characterize the department's communication system. The criterion of theoretical saturation was chosen, according to which data collection can be completed when no new information is provided [26]. In the context of the COVID-19, real-time mediated communication was used, via skype. All interviews were recorded and later transcribed.

The semi-structured interview - complemented by document analysis and non-systematic observation of project meetings - was selected as the most appropriate data collection technique, because it is a useful procedure to apprehend the meanings that are constructed by the individuals that make up the reality under study [26]. The dimensions analyzed were as follows: (1st) the communication system in use in the project management (to identify how individuals understood the communication phenomenon, and its organizational flows and channels); and (2nd) the communication management features (including communication planning practices, communication skills and communication styles of project managers). Questions were constructed from the categories shown in Table 1.

Table 1. Categorization matrix

Thematic	Categories
Communication system	Communication understanding
	Communication flows
	Communication channels
Information and communication system to support project management	Benefits
	Disadvantages

Data analysis was based on categorical content, which implies conducting a descriptive examination through the categorization of interviews in a set of defined themes (Table 1) [26]. The main findings are discussed in the next section.

4 Results and Discussion

4.1 Understanding Communication in Project Management Environment

From the interviews with the leadership figures (heads and project managers) it can be inferred that the importance of communication for project management is acknowledged. Project leaders have no doubt that the management of industrialization projects is dependent on the effectiveness of communication:

> Communication is the most important aspect for project management success. (H1[1])

Nevertheless, the dominant understanding of communication is very basic, since it is reduced to information purposes. All respondents described communication as the process by which messages are transmitted effectively:

> Communication is important to maintain the alignment of activities, to report, to inform and to obtain feedback. (PjM)

This is a view that finds its origin in the positivist tradition of Organizational Communication studies. However, developments in the field have shown that organizations are intersubjective structures of meanings that are produced, reproduced, and transformed through the continuous communicative activities of their members [27]. Therefore, the idea that communication as an information transmission process is quite limited.

[1] Since the identification of the participants is not of interest to the study, the interviewees were identified according to the roles of each one - PjM (project managers), H (from Head, to the heads) and T (from team, for team members).

4.2 Communication Flows and Interaction Difficulties

Data shows that major problems come from vertical communication between project managers and teams. For project managers, the complexity of interacting with people from different departments stands out, as well as the inherent difficulty to articulate tasks and timings between all team members, who work in different divisions and accumulate other functions besides the project. Thus, aligning interests and priorities is a daily challenge:

> Aligning people with diverse ways of thinking is the most difficult challenge. We must try to lead people according to what is best for everyone. (PjM)

For team members, communication problems are different and involve the need to constantly adapt to the different communication and information channels used by each project manager:

> I work with several managers, and each manager works with different tools. There is no standard tool that everyone uses. (T)

Furthermore, teams feel that information is managed inappropriately, since it is either insufficient or excessive and sent without segmentation and channel matching. Team members also mentioned that they receive too many emails with content not targeted to their role in the project, that their tasks are not always fully explained and that delays in the project are not communicated in due time.

Despite these difficulties, informal relationships were described as positive and as good ways to share knowledge and experience among team members.

4.3 Communication Channels: The Dispersion and Replication of Information

The study of communication channels showed that email is the most used communication tool, but paradoxically the one that creates more difficulties. The email misuse and overuse was repeatedly mentioned. Even though it is an important and useful communication platform, as it allows recording and sharing important conversations and documents, the abusive way in which it is used causes significant problems:

> The use of email is absurd. It is a good communication tool, but its use needs to be more thoughtful and thought out. (H)

On the other hand, meetings seem to be valued by everyone. The interviewees would like them to occur more frequently and agree that face-to-face interaction is the best way to get to know teams, to understand the project's objectives, to track task status, and to solve problems or disagreements.

Calling via skype (only with audio) was also referred to as a good way to monitor tasks status and to carry out individual and personalized monitoring. In addition, due to their immediacy, these calls also allow the resolution of urgent problems or the quick clarification of doubts.

Still, the replication of tasks associated with the existence of many communication platforms and the need to complete a lot of documents were mentioned as problems by project managers:

> There are good communication tools. But there is a duplication of the communication tools that make our work very demanding. (PjM)

4.4 Expectations Regarding the Development of a New Communication System

Regarding the development of the new information and communication system, respondents agreed that implementing an integrated platform to support project management and tailored to the company was a good internal measure:

> The ideal was to have a single platform that would allow, in a single place, to talk to everyone and not have to use two or three platforms. (T)

In addition, the interviewees discussed their expectations about the platform and presented a set of ideas. Firstly, the ability to concentrate information from each project was identified as a fundamental feature, as currently information is dispersed, leading to task replication and wasted time. Secondly, the simplification of the monitoring process was referred to as a decisive feature of the platform. Besides, its potential to the teleworking mode was mentioned as useful too, as well as the conception of a mobile application that would facilitate the use of this platform through mobile devices. These two suggestions can be justified by the context of the global pandemic, caused by COVID-19, in which this study was conducted.

Altogether, results show that the innovative project management platform should favor the development of an easy-to-use interface that facilitates information and communication flows. Although, attitudes of distrust and resistance towards the emergence of "another communication platform" were also noticed. There is some fear that the introduction of this information repository and communication channel will further accentuate information dispersion and task duplication.

These attitudes of mistrust seem to be related to the lack of knowledge about the features and potential of the new system. The software is still in its first stage of development and, therefore, the prototype has not yet been fully presented to and discussed with all team members. And this can be a problem. As already mentioned and according to the principles of Innovation Communication, individuals who will be "affected" by innovation must be motivated to participate in the development process and to share ideas and prospects, to establish a position of commitment and trust. As so, this procedure of sharing the software status regularly should be a communication action considered by the company, as the best way to develop a communication system that corresponds to the needs and welcomes the interest of all members who make up project management.

5 Conclusions

Through the diagnosis phase of this action-research study, several common communication issues were identified in the process of developing and implementing a technological innovation. In this final section, we will address the two main concerns of our research: the internal communication obstacles existing in contemporary organizations and the challenges of innovation communication.

Regarding the communication barriers found in organizational work, it should be underlined the reductionist view on the communication phenomenon. At Bosch, as in many other companies, communication is still understood as information diffusion. However, this is an outdated perspective on Human Communication [28] and a narrow vision of Organizational Communication [29] that looks at the phenomenon as a "container" of information that must be managed towards organizational effectiveness - a paradigm that characterized Organizational Communication theory between the 1940s and the 1970s and that remains visible today [27]. Although it was concluded, later, that communication is much more than this "conduct" where information circulates, it is the "glue of the organization" [28] as it allows the general coordination of capacities and the construction of symbolic expressions of its existence. Communication is the organization.

Given this context, how can technological innovation in communication systems be useful to solve communication barriers? On one hand, the adoption of technological solutions that gather documents and enable information exchange, can in fact increase organizational efficiency. But these technologies must also be able to enhance the communicative function, as the support of all organizational activities. This means that it should also allow and promote conversation and dialogue between leaders and team members. This implies including in the technological platforms information archiving and validation systems, but also chats, forums and other interaction mechanisms that complement traditional emailing or meetings.

But placing novelty at the heart of organizational operations is a hard task that must be performed by communication, or innovative communication. As shown in this studied, innovative challenges can be overcome by sharing information with organizational members and hearing them about the changes to be implemented. By doing so, organizations increase creativity and reinforce internal feelings of identity and belonging. Therefore, co-creation seems to be the best model for innovation development and communication, as it increases acceptance, reducing the fear of complexity and uncertainty that characterize the settings of organizational innovation.

These insights became quite strong in this action-research project that gathered data on a particular innovation environment, but that can be useful in broader contexts, bringing inputs for the study of internal communication in current organizations, particularly regarding its relevance to the management of innovation teams. At Bosch, the industrialization innovation teams were themselves involved in an internal communication innovation process, which presents the same challenges as any innovation practice: it involves getting all members to talk about the validity and convenience of changing, so that at the end will be acceptance. Communicating innovation is, therefore, the key to accomplishment.

Acknowledgments. This work is supported by European Structural and Investment Funds in the FEDER component, through the Competitiveness and Internationalization Operational Program (COMPETE 2020) [Project nº 39479; Financing reference: POCI-01-0247-FEDER-39479].

References

1. Kivimaki, M., et al.: Communication as a determinant of organizational innovation. R&D Manag. **30**(1), 33–42 (2000). https://doi.org/10.1111/1467-9310.00155
2. Miller, K.: Organizational Communication: Approaches and Processes. Cengage Learning, Stamford (2015)
3. Taylor, J.R., Flanagin, A.J., Cheney, G., Seibold, D.R.: Organizational communication research: key moments, central concerns, and future challenges. Ann. Int. Commun. Assoc. **1**(24), 99–137 (2001). https://doi.org/10.1080/23808985.2001.11678983
4. Castells, M.: A galáxia da internet: reflexões sobre internet, negócios e sociedade. Fundação Calouste Gulbenkian, Lisbon (2007)
5. Rothwell, R., Robertson, A.B.: The role of communications in technological innovation. Res. Policy **2**(3), 204–225 (1973). https://doi.org/10.1016/0048-7333(73)90003-6
6. Men, L.R.: The internal communication role of the chief executive officer: communication channels, style, and effectiveness. Public Relat. Rev. **41**(4), 461–471 (2015). https://doi.org/10.1016/j.pubrev.2015.06.021
7. Men, L.R.: Strategic internal communication: transformational leadership, communication channels, and employee satisfaction. Manag. Commun. Q. **28**(2), 264–284 (2014). https://doi.org/10.1177/0893318914524536
8. Zyl, A.: The impact of social networking 2.0 on organisations. Electron. Libr. **27**(6), 906–918 (2009). https://doi.org/10.1108/02640470911004020
9. Baregheh, A., Rowley, J., Sambrook, S.: Towards a multidisciplinary definition of innovation. Manag. Decis. **47**(8), 1323–1339 (2009). https://doi.org/10.1108/00251740910984578
10. Malte, A.: The communication of innovation: an empirical analysis of the advancement of innovation. Discussion Papers on Strategy and Innovation, pp. 1–29 (2013)
11. Mast, C., Huck, S., Zerfass, A.: Innovation communication: outline of the concept and empirical findings from Germany. Innov. J. **2**(7), 2–14 (2005)
12. Moenaert, R.K., Caeldries, F., Lievens, A., Wauters, E.: Communication flows in international product innovation teams. J. Prod. Innov. Manag. **17**, 360–377 (2000). https://doi.org/10.1111/1540-5885.1750360
13. Zerfass, A.: Innovation readiness: a framework for enhancing corporations and regions by innovation communication. Innov. J. **2**(8), 1–27 (2005)
14. Zerfass, A., Huck, S.: Innovation, communication, and leadership: new developments in strategic communication. Int. J. Strateg. Commun. **1**(2), 107–122 (2007). https://doi.org/10.1080/15531180701298908
15. Gerhard, D., Brem, A., Bacarella, C., Voigt, K.: Innovation management and marketing in the high-tech sector: a content analysis of advertisements. Int. J. Manag. **28**(1) (2001). https://doi.org/10.2139/ssrn.2433961
16. Gassmann, O., Zedtwitz, M.: Innovation processes in transnational corporations. In: Shavinina, L.V. (eds.) International Handbook on Innovation, pp. 702–714. Oxford: Elsevier Science, Oxford (2003)
17. Suh, J., Harrington, J., Goodman, D.: Understanding the link between organizational communication and innovation: an examination of public, non-profit and for-profit organizations in South Korea. Public Pers. Manag. **13**, 1–28 (2018). https://doi.org/10.1177/0091026018760930
18. Gode, H.E., Johansen, W., Thomsen, C.: Employee engagement in generating ideas on internal social media: a matter of meaningfulness, safety and availability. Corp. Commun. Int. J. **25**(2), 263–280 (2020). https://doi.org/10.1108/CCIJ-03-2019-0024
19. Falkheimer, J., Heide, M.: Strategic Communication: An Introduction. Routledge, Oxon (2018)

20. Ewing, M., Men, L.R., O'Neill, J.: Using social media to engage employees: insights from internal communication managers. Int. J. Strateg. Commun. **13**(2), 532–550 (2019). https://doi.org/10.1080/1553118X.2019.1575830
21. Pan Fagerlin, W., Wang, Y.: Top managers' communication efforts as response to tensions in product innovation: an attention-based view. Baltic J. Manag. (2020). https://doi.org/10.1080/1553118X.2018.1456434
22. Linke, A., Zerfass, A.: Internal communication and innovation culture: developing a change framework. J. Commun. Manag. **15**(4), 332–348 (2011). https://doi.org/10.1108/13632541111183361
23. Baum, F., MacDougall, C., Smith, D.: Participatory action research. J. Epidemiol. Commun. Health **60**, 854–857 (2006). https://doi.org/10.1136/jech.2004.028662
24. Tripp, D.: Pesquisa-ação: uma introdução metodológica*. Educ. Pesqui. **31**(3), 443–466 (2005)
25. Dickens, L., Watkins, K.: Action research: rethinking Lewin. Manag. Learn. **30**(2), 127–140 (1999). https://doi.org/10.1177/1350507699302002
26. Guerra, I.C.: Pesquisa qualitativa e análise de conteúdo. Principia: Cascais (2006)
27. Putnam, L.L., Phillips, N., Chapman, P.: Metaphors of communication and organization. In: Clegg, S.R., Hardy, C., Lawrence, T., Nord, W.R. (eds.) Handbook of Organization Studies, pp. 375–408. Thousand Oaks, Sage (1996)
28. Weick, K.: Sensemaking in Organizations. Sage, Thousand Oaks (1995)
29. Taylor, J.R.: Rethinking the Theory of Organizational Communication: How to Read an Organization. Ablex Publishing Corporation, Norwood (1993)

Model Maturity to Determine Student Profile During COVID-19 Pandemic at Public University

Jessie Bravo(✉), Janet Aquino, Roger Alarcón, and Nilton Germán

School of Computer Engineering and Informatics, Pedro Ruiz Gallo National University, Lambayeque, Peru
{jbravo,jaquino,ralarcong,ngerman}@unprg.edu.pe

Abstract. COVID-19 has accelerated the virtualization of processes in universities, academically, the role played by students. A maturity model was developed to determine the student profile based on digital culture, organizational culture and the psychological aspect, the latter being the most affected during confinement. These aspects were integrated to create a model in which students were classified into five profiles: silent, cooperative, creative, star, and superstar. This will allow us to know what type of student we have and what strategies to implement to achieve that they reach the profile of superstar student and can face the virtual teaching - learning process with success. To validate our model, it was applied to a public university where the level of maturity of the students was evidenced and strategies were established that would allow us to lead students with a superstar profile.

Keywords: COVID-19 · Higher education · Culture · Psychology · Digitization

1 Introduction

University students today belong to a generation that, although it has overcome barriers that previous generations faced, in terms of mastery of technology, they face new challenges that were not contemplated within their plans, the COVID-19 pandemic.

A generation characterized by being digital natives, very diverse socially and culturally, connected and at the same time lonely, immersed in a situation of global crisis that somehow affects their academic performance, now with a new environment for the development of their classes, the virtual.

In a survey applied to university students in the university-case study, it was identified that 45% do not have a computer for the development of their virtual classes and 31% do not have access to the internet service.

In addition to the digital aspect, the organizational aspect, such as their identification with the institution and being a participant in university activities, is also relevant as part of the characterization of the student but due to the current pandemic situation that we are experiencing, the psychological aspect plays a fundamental role as indicated by a

© The Author(s), under exclusive license to Springer Nature Singapore Pte Ltd. 2022
Á. Rocha et al. (Eds.): ICOMTA 2021, SIST 259, pp. 61–70, 2022.
https://doi.org/10.1007/978-981-16-5792-4_7

study carried out in the population and health personnel of China, it was observed that 53.8% had a moderate to severe psychological impact; 16.5% of depressive symptoms, 28.8% of anxiety symptoms and 8.1% of stress, all between moderate and severe [1].

Given this, the purpose of this study is to provide a maturity model focused on three aspects: digital, organizational and psychological, to determine the profile of the student during the COVID-19 pandemic in the public university, in order to allow the generation of strategies in order to have a student with a good academic performance, committed to the development of their institution and capable of overcoming adverse circumstances under the psychological impact of the current global COVID-19 pandemic.

2 State of Art

For the characterization of the student, we have taken into account three aspects: the organizational, the digital and the psychological. Regarding the organizational and digital aspect, we have based ourselves on the research work applied to a public university in which the teacher was characterized taking into account these criteria, both aspects were integrated to create a model in which the teacher was classified in four profiles: anonymous teacher, alpha teacher, beta teacher and gold teacher [2]. In addition, the study carried out by [3] where he examines how university students in developing countries have faced obstacles and yet, despite this, they are still doing everything possible to stay focused on achieving their personal goals. During the pandemic and in the survey of 1,182 people of different age groups from various educational institutes in Delhi – National Capital Region (NCR), India where the possible consequences of the COVID-19 pandemic on the lives of students are being investigated [4].

Regarding the psychological aspect, the psychologist Larrazabal M. indicated: "After the first known effects of the confinement, the specialists warn: COVID will be followed by a "pandemic" of psychological problems, such as phobias, depression or post-traumatic stress syndrome, which can last for three years" [5]. The value of professionals, particularly clinical psychologists, is decisive in mental health, in the different phases of the pandemic [6], furthermore, this can be improved by changing people's behavior and psychology can help explain, prevent and intervene to solve it [7].

There has also been talk about the psychological impact on university students, in research whose objective was to evaluate the levels of anxiety, depression, stress and the perception of the state of health of Mexican university students due to the COVID-19 pandemic [8, 9], in addition, another study investigated the psychological changes in behavior among university students due to the COVID-19 crisis and confinement, based on the Stimulus-Organism-Response (SOR) model [10] and applied research to 2,534 college students from seven US universities in order to assess the psychological impact of COVID-19 where it was concluded that inadequate efforts to recognize and address mental health challenges could have long-term consequences on their health and education [11].

3 Proposal

Public universities as in any organization have been affected by the COVID-19 pandemic, originating a substantial change in their activities, in this case the development of 100%

virtual classes, for this reason our proposal focuses on characterizing the most important actor of the university such as the student, whose situation is affected by confinement and must adapt to the new environment, taking into account their characteristics, we will determine the maturity model to determine their profile.

The type of research for its purpose is applied, according to its quasi-experimental design and according to its approach, it is qualitative. For the characterization of the student, the following methodology has been considered. See Fig. 1.

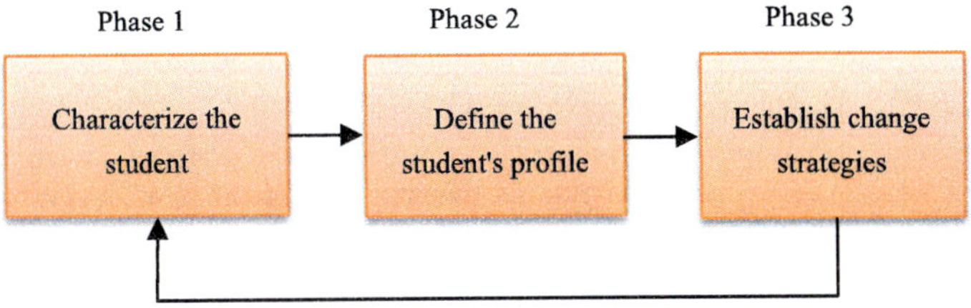

Fig. 1. Methodology

3.1 Phase 1: Characterize the Student

Based on the teacher maturity model [2] where the cultural and organizational aspects are considered now in the study applied to the student, we have also considered the psychological aspect. The tool used is a survey, and the instrument, the questionnaire, which considers the three dimensions: digital, organizational and psychological. Digital culture defines the student's digital profile, which includes the following maturity levels: indifferent, interested, involved and committed, they are defined in Table 1 and in Table 2 the score for each maturity level that consists of 10 questions, where each of them has a rating of 0 to 4 points.

Regarding the organizational culture, it determines the organizational profile of the student, with the maturity levels: indifferent, interested, involved and committed, they are defined in Table 3 and in Table 4 the score for each maturity level that has 13 questions, where each of them has a rating of 0 to 4 points.

Regarding our new dimension, which is the psychological aspect, the maturity levels of the psychological profile are defined: unstable, balanced and resilient, detailed in Table 5, and in Table 6 the score for each maturity level, which includes 7 questions, based on the SISCO SV Academic Stress Questionnaire [12] where each one of them has a valuation of 0 to 4 points.

To determine the level of digital, organizational and psychological maturity, the following formulas are applied:

To calculate the Score in each Dimension:

$$\mathrm{Score}_{\mathrm{Dimension}} = \frac{\sum_{i=1}^{n} \mathrm{Score}_{\mathrm{criteria}}}{n} \quad (1)$$

Table 1. Maturity level of the digital profile

Maturity level of the digital profile	Description
Primitive	Does not handle office tools. Does not use internet. It does not use mobile devices. To communicate, they opt for traditional means such as the telephone. It does not have social networks
Basic	Frequent use of the internet. Office automation domain. Use the internet as a source of information. Use of mobile applications. Frequent use of social networks. He is only a consumer of social networks
Intermediate	He cares about digital security. Make transactions online. Digital self-taught. It is a generator of content on social networks
Advanced	Browse more safely without being a victim of cybercrime. They are fully digital and mobile, multitasking and multiscreen. The mobile phone is the center of your communication and information. They have become, without intending to, influencers in their environment and their family. It is a content generator and remains permanently connected on social networks

Table 2. Score of the maturity level - digital profile

Maturity level of the digital profile	Score model
Primitive	From 0 to 10
Basic	From 11 to 20
Intermediate	From 21 to 30
Advanced	From 31 to 40

For the calculation of the Model Score (digital, organizational and psychological):

$$\mathrm{Score_{Model}} = \frac{\sum_{j=1}^{nd} \mathrm{Score_{Dimension}}}{\mathrm{nd}} \tag{2}$$

$$\mathrm{n} = \text{number of dimension criteria}$$

$$\mathrm{nd} = \text{number of dimensions}$$

3.2 Phase 2: Define the Student's Profile

Our model integrates the dimensions: digital, organizational and psychological of the student of a public university, obtaining a model of 5 profiles, focusing on the most

Table 3. Maturity level of the organizational profile

Maturity level of the organizational profile	Description
Indifferent	He does not know the vision and mission, the statutes and regulations of the university. He is not a participant in the university's strategic plan. He does not maintain permanent communication with the members and authorities of his institution. Does not handle soft skills. He is not interested in university politics
Interested	Know the mission and vision of the university. Know in a basic way the statutes and regulations of the university. Participate only in some of the meetings or events scheduled at the university. He communicates occasionally with the members and authorities of the Institution. Handle some soft skills. He knows about university politics but does not participate actively
Involved	Know the mission and vision, statutes and regulations of the university. Participate only in some of the meetings or events scheduled at the university. Communicates regularly with the members and authorities of the Institution. Manage soft skills at the elementary level. Learn about university politics and actively participate
Engaged	Know and internalize the mission and vision, the statutes and regulations of the university. It identifies with the Institution. He communicates permanently with the members and authorities of the institution. Participate in scheduled meetings and events. Master the relevant soft skills. He leads political groups for the benefit of the university

Table 4. Score of the maturity level - organizational profile

Maturity level of the organizational profile	Score model
Indifferent	From 0 to 13
Interested	From 14 to 26
Involved	From 27 to 39
Engaged	From 40 to 52

important criteria, located on the axis, towards our objective, which we consider as the profile of the ideal student (superstar student), being identified: the superstar student,

Table 5. Maturity level of the psychological profile

Maturity level of the psychological profile	Description
Unstable	It is affected by not having technological resources or means. He lives in an inappropriate environment for the development of his academic activities. In their family environment there are members affected with COVID-19. His mood has been affected by the confinement. He does not feel prepared for the development of his virtual classes. Does not count with family support and not enough time necessary for the development of his academic activities
Balanced	It has the resources or technological means. He lives in an environment suitable for the development of his academic activities. In your family environment, there are or not members affected with COVID-19. His mood has been affected by the confinement. He feels prepared for the development of his virtual classes. He has the family support and the necessary time for the development of his academic activities
Resilient	Look for a way to get hold of resources or technological means. He lives in an inappropriate environment for the development of his academic activities but overcomes this fact. In your family environment, there are or not members affected with COVID-19. His mood has been affected by the confinement. He doesn't feel ready for the development of his virtual classes but still moves on. It has partial family support for its academic development, although it does not have the time for it, but manages it properly

Table 6. Score of the maturity level - psychological profile

Maturity level of the psychological profile	Score model
Unstable	From 0 to 7
Balanced	From 8 to 21
Resilient	From 22 to 28

star, creative, operational and silence, as observed in Fig. 2 and whose characteristics are described in Table 7.

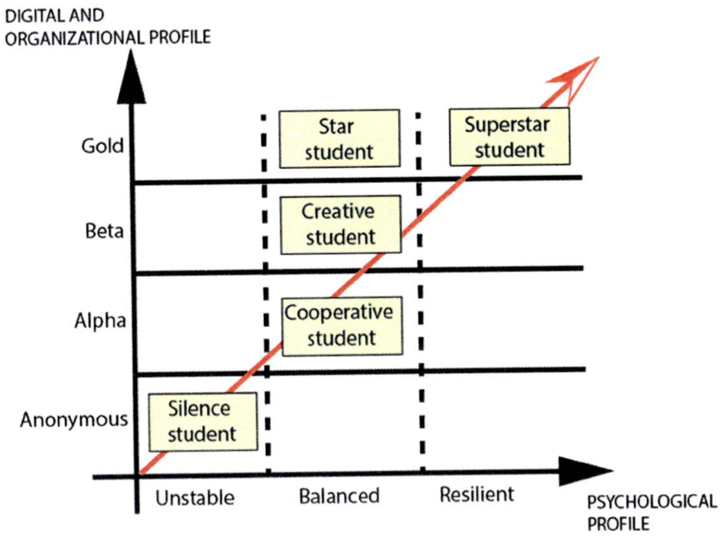

Fig. 2. University student profile

Table 7. University student maturity level

Type of student	Description
Silence	It is the student who is digitally null, does not identify with his institution and is psychologically unstable
Cooperative	It is the student who partially dominates technology, identified with his institution and psychologically balanced
Creative	He is the student who masters technology, partially identified with his institution and psychologically balanced
Star	It is the student who masters technology, identified with his institution and psychologically balanced but does not have the sufficient capacity to overcome obstacles
SuperStar	It is the student who is technological self-taught, identified with his institution and psychologically resilient

3.3 Phase 3: Establish Change Strategies

In this phase, the challenges that the university must take into account to successfully face this situation of the pandemic must be defined.

4 Validation

The present investigation takes as a case study the students of a Peruvian public university, to whom a virtual survey was applied, structured in three aspects: organizational, digital and psychological. The numerical measurement scale was used (0 = never, 1 = rarely, 2 = occasionally, 3 = usually, 4 = always).Our population was 11,998 students, selecting a sample of 631, with a margin of error of 5% and a confidence level of 99%.

4.1 Phase 1: Characterize the Student

The results obtained in each profile after the application of the survey are shown in Tables 8, 9 and 10.

Table 8. Results of the student's digital profile

Maturity level of the digital profile	Amount	%
Primitive	2	0.3%
Basic	163	25.8%
Intermediate	416	65.9%
Advanced	50	7.9%
Total	**631**	**100.0%**

Table 9. Results of the student's organizational profile

Maturity level of the organizational profile	Amount	%
Indifferent	1	0.2%
Interested	25	4.0%
Involved	376	59.6%
Engaged	229	36.3%
Total	**631**	**100.0%**

Table 10. Results of the student's psychological profile

Maturity level of the psychological profile	Amount	%
Unstable	2	0.3%
Balanced	609	96.5%
Resilient	20	3.2%
Total	**631**	**100.0%**

4.2 Phase 2: Define the Student's Profile

In this phase, we can see that the following results have been obtained from the five defined student profiles, highlighting that the star student represents 68.3%, followed by the cooperative student, with 24.4%, but our purpose is to increase the superstar students, currently represent 2.5%, who will be students capable of overcoming obstacles such as the current COVID-19 pandemic (Table 11).

Table 11. Student profile results

Type	Amount	Percentage
Silence student	1	0.2%
Cooperative student	154	24.4%
Creative student	17	2.7%
Star student	431	68.3%
Superstar student	16	2.5%

4.3 Phase 3: Establishing Change Strategies

The change strategies that will allow us to achieve students to overcome, are those listed below:

- Form a team responsible for identifying students affected by the pandemic and high-risk groups.
- Implement a virtual mentoring and counseling plan that supports students in the face of the effects of the pandemic.
- Implement a training plan for teachers and students regarding self-care, resilience and mastery of technological tools.
- Strengthen crisis management procedures in charge of university well-being.
- Define an official communication and advisory channel that provides reliable information on COVID-19.
- Equitably manage technological resources for students.

5 Conclusions

Students were characterized by considering the organizational aspect, digital and especially the psychological aspect, as the most critical in this pandemic COVID-19.

The integration of the three dimensions allowed us to define five types of students: silence, cooperative, creative, star and superstar. Improvement strategies were developed to achieve superstar students who successfully address the consequences of this pandemic.

References

1. Lozano-Vargas, A.: Impacto de la epidemia del Coronavirus (COVID-19) en la salud mental del personal de salud y en la población general de China. Revista de Neuro-Psiquiatría **83**(1), 51–56 (2020)
2. Bravo, J., Aquino, J., Alarcón, R., Germán, N.: Congreso Internacional de Educación y Tecnología en Ciencias, CISETC 2019. In: Maturity Model for Digital Teacher Transformation Based on Digital and Organizational Competencies in Higher Education, Arequipa (2019)
3. Rahiem, M.D.: Remaining motivated despite the limitations: university students' learning propensity during COVID-19 pandemic. Child. Youth Serv. Rev. **120**(1) (2021)
4. Chaturvedi, K., Kumar Vishwakarma, D., Singh, N.: COVID-19 and its impact on education, social life and mental health of students: a survey. Child. Youth Serv. Rev. **121**(1), 1–2 (2021)
5. Rodríguez, S.: 30 abril 2020. www.efe.com. [Online]. https://www.efe.com/efe/espana/destacada/tras-la-covid-19-una-pandemia-de-problemas-psicologicos/10011-4235147. Accessed 15 junio 2020
6. Inchausti, F., García, N.V., Prado, J., Sánchez, S.: La Psicología Clínica ante la Pandemia COVID-19 en España. Clínica y Salud **31**(2), 105–107 (2020)
7. Urzúa, A., Vera, P., Caqueo, A., Polanco, R.: Psychology in the prevention and manag. of COVID-19. Contributions from initial evidence. Terapia psicológica **38**(1), 103–118 (2020)
8. González-Jaimes, N.L., Tejeda-Alcántara, A.A., Espinosa-Méndez, C.M., Ontiveros-Hernández, Z.O.: Psychological impact on Mexican university students due to confinement during Covid-19 pandemic. SciELO - Biblioteca electrónica científica en línea, 11 junio 2020
9. Huarcaya-Victoria, J.: Consideraciones sobre la salud mental en la pandemia de COVID-19. Revista peruana de medicina experimental y salud pública **37**(2), 327–334 (2020)
10. Pandita, S., Govind Mishra, H., Chib, S.: Psychological impact of Covid-19 crises on students through the lens of Stimulus-Organism-Response (SOR) model. Child. Youth Serv. Rev. **120** (2021)
11. Browning, M.H.E.M., et al.: Psychological impacts from COVID-19 among university students: risk factors across seven states in the US. PloS One **16**(1) (2021)
12. Alania Contreras, R.D., Llancari Morales, R.A., de la Cruz, M.R., Ortega Révolo, D.I.D.: Adaptación del cuestionario de estrés académico SISCO SV al contexto de la crisis por COVID-19. Revista Socialium **4**(2), 111–130 (2020)

Political Communication, Technology and Applications

Social Media and Online Political Activism in Protest Communication Strategies: Friends or Foes?

Andreu Casero-Ripollés(✉) and Romina Pepe-Oliva

Universitat Jaume I de Castelló, 12071 Castelló, Spain
{casero,al367984}@uji.es

Abstract. Social media are transforming online political activism. These digital platforms offer opportunities and obstacles for the communicative strategies of social protests. Our aim is to critically analyse the main advantages and risks in this regard. The results allow us to identify three potentialities: the self-mediation of protests, the civic monitoring of the centres of power and the new possibilities in the shaping of the public agenda. We also detected two constraints: the difficulties in capturing mainstream media interest and the structural dependence on commercial social media. These findings demonstrate that social media can reconfigure power relations and favour citizen counter-power, but factors also exist that can limit these transformations.

Keywords: Online political activism · Social media · Political communication · Digital media · Social movements · Protest

1 Introduction: Political Activism, Communication and Democracy in the Context of Social Media[1]

Political activism has found an instrument in the Internet and digital platforms with which to yield greater relevance and social protagonism [1]. This is because they affect the three fundamental dimensions of protest: organisation, mobilisation and communication [2]. Likewise, they encourage the shift from collective to connective action, where interconnected publics network flexibly together with inclusive and personalised action frameworks to defend particular political causes [3].

In this scenario, social media are opening up a process of reshaping power relationships, enabling the emergence of citizen counter-power [4]. The Web 2.0 offers citizens, and with them, political activists, the option of playing a much more active and dynamic role in the political arena.

The links between political activism, communication and democracy are being overhauled in the social media context. On that account, the aim of this chapter is to analyse the extent to which these technologies, which have as their preferred habitat the digital

[1] This chapter is part of the research projects UJI-B2020–14 and GACUJI/2021/04, funded by the Universitat Jaume I of Castelló.

© The Author(s), under exclusive license to Springer Nature Singapore Pte Ltd. 2022
Á. Rocha et al. (Eds.): ICOMTA 2021, SIST 259, pp. 73–81, 2022.
https://doi.org/10.1007/978-981-16-5792-4_8

environment, can enhance the capacity for action of the new social movements from a communicative viewpoint. We will therefore explore the opportunities, on the one hand, and the obstacles, on the other, that these digital platforms present to online political activism.

2 Social Media as an Opportunity for Online Political Activism

2.1 The Self-mediation of Protest

Mediation processes are fundamental to the framing of social reality and, therefore, play a key role in citizens' perceptions of the problems, alternatives and debates which articulate the public sphere. However, in the current context, they are asymmetrical and unequal, since some social actors enjoy appreciably more power and opportunities than other [5]. Political and economic elites, together, with and through the media, have greater chances to speak out and make their voices heard.

For online political activism, having access to communication channels to disseminate its demands and spread its protests is fundamental. However, traditionally, social movements have had serious difficulties in gaining access to mainstream media news coverage [6].

Against this, social media allow political activism to enjoy communicative autonomy. In the web 2.0 environment, users, such as citizen activists, can, through technological platforms such as Facebook, Twitter, YouTube or blogs, produce and broadcast their own messages [7]. For Castells [4], this implies the emergence of a new type of communicative system: mass self-communication. The result is the irruption of user-generated content supposing to be the green shoots of a culture of participation.

In this framework, one of social medias' main contributions to political activism is the capacity to set self-mediated protest actions in motion [8]. The 8M International Women's Movement is an example of how the web 2.0 can contribute significantly to worldwide, collective mobilisation processes [9]. In the digital environment, the monopoly of journalists over news coverage is broken up and new actors are appearing who, from amongst the citizenry, can also access the production and dissemination of content, from individual blogs or profiles on social network sites to alternative media [10]. In this context, political activism can produce and distribute self-representations of its movements and its demands autonomously that can aspire to enter the public agenda and stir up debate in the public sphere, putting its own alternative narratives and counter-frames into circulation [11]. In this way, activists can hope that the media agenda admits their issues and approaches [12, 13].

The capacity to produce their own discursive frameworks that social media grants political activism contributes to the construction of the collective memory of protests, to the expansion and conveyance of its revindications and to the creation of symbolic artefacts of protest through blogs, websites and photo and video sharing platforms [8]. From this point of view, self-mediation possesses great potential.

Despite this, there are some limiting aspects to take into account as well. In consequence, when it comes to content generation, not all Internet using citizens are in a position to create it in effective ways. Socio-demographic variables may form the appearance of a participation gap that means that not all people are able to take advantage of self-mediation to make their voices heard [14]. In fact, when it comes to content creation, some research argues that Web 2.0 users are rather more passive than active [15].

2.2 The Civic Monitoring of Power Centres

Social media provide a second potential for online political activism: the affordance of putting processes for monitoring the actions of the established powers into practice [16]. Thanks to digital technologies and the plethora of communication made possible by the Internet, any citizen can access information or data that might serve to control the actions of those established in power. At the same time, thanks to web 2.0, they have a platform from which to transmit the results of this supervision to the rest of the public, so as to sound the alarm when something is considered wrong. This is something of a novelty, since now the public citizen, through millions of eyes, is transformed into a silent watchdog, playing a new role [17]. This eventuality works not only as an arrangement for citizen empowerment, which implies a strengthening of its political role, but is linked to the concept of "monitory democracy" put forward by John Keane [18].

Monitoring does not appear as a result of the social media; its roots date back to the end of the Second World War. The truly novel aspect that web 2.0 adds to this phenomenon, besides promoting and generalising it, is the recruitment of citizens to keep track. Despite the enormous disparity they can display, four broad ways of civic monitoring can be detected [19]. The first is the extension of the watchdog function, which is based on citizens, individually or in groups, exercising scrutiny by acting as guardians, and protectors, of the public interest in the face of the illegal practices and the inefficiency of the established powers. They complement, or even supplant the journalism which hitherto has enjoyed a monopoly on scrutinising the centres of power. The second is the extraction and leaking of secret or hidden information. This practice, linked to hacktivism [20, 21], has one of its main references in Wikileaks.

The third is the scrutiny alternative journalism bears. The emergence of the latest news actors on the Internet, mainly linked to radical media and citizen journalism, forms the basis of this system. Their reporting pursuits make it possible to publicly disseminate issues excluded from the public agenda, amplifying its voices. This triggers a monitoring process, averting the silencing of news and issues relevant to the public interest. Finally, the fourth is the extension of representation beyond parliaments. It involves the proliferation of un-elected representatives, but who are defenders of specific interests and issues, such as new social movements (Occupy Wall Street, #Yosoy132, 15-M, NuitDebout, V de Vinagre or Plataforma de Afectados por la Hipoteca, among others). These tend to coincide in placing demands for democratic regeneration at the centre of their monitoring actions. Moreover, they frequently connect monitoring with mobilisation. On this basis, online petition sites also belong to this modality, which encourage the channelling of demands by encouraging the public to sign in the form of a digital vote. These include Change.org and Avaaz.org.

The take-off of civic monitoring is especially linked to the strong alienation that citizens experience towards the representative structures, which include the discrediting of the political class, suspicion towards the financial system and distrust towards the media. In Spain, in recent years [22], two cases linked to the 15-M movement stand out.

The first was the initiative "What our representatives do" (http://quehacenlosdiputados.net/). Its objective was to monitor each deputy of parliament's activity in the Congress of Deputies based on the information this public institution provided on its official website. Thus, for each deputy, information was provided on the parliamentary initiatives and interventions each had undertaken (indicating exactly which ones), on their positions in Congress, their political trajectory, their salary and on declaration of assets [22].

The second relevant case of civic monitoring in Spain is the Fundación Civio (http://www.civio.es/). It is a non-profit organisation that fights to promote free access to public data as well as information transparency. It combines the use of technology with journalism, specifically using data journalism. It therefore corresponds to civic monitoring based on alternative journalism [19] and has launched several monitoring actions, starting with the pioneering "Where do my taxes go?" which analyses how much money the Spanish General State Administration spends and how it is spent.

2.3 New Opportunities in Shaping the Public Agenda

Social media, thanks to the possibility they give citizens to autonomously produce and disseminate messages and content, set in motion new dynamics for setting the public agenda. The mainstream media are no longer alone and no longer have a monopoly on news production and distribution [10]. New actors from civil society, linked to the web 2.0 universe, such as bloggers, citizen journalists or content-creating users, now interact with them in a loosely knit environment.

In the web 2.0 environment, citizens and political activists, through the use of social media, can aspire to capture the mainstream medias' attention, provoking them into incorporating their subject-matter and even their discursive frameworks into their agenda [12, 13]. In this way, citizens can determine which stories become news in the mainstream media and become highly visible in society. Acting through social media, the public may be able to influence the selection of news journalists work on.

This potential ability of citizens and political activism to condition the media agenda and thereby affect the creation of the public agenda has been characterised by Sung-Tae and Young-hwan [23] as "reversed agenda-setting". In these cases, it is not the media setting the agenda, but the public. Thus, reversed agenda-setting follows the subsequent scheme: originator (citizen or activist), digital media and mainstream media. A key role in the subject-matter's circulation is played by the information being shared on a massive scale by the users who, through viral communicative processes, increase the radius of its reach and circulation. For the agenda-setting power of social media to be activated, it is essential that the issue is widely shared online. The fact that an issue becomes a trending topic is a fundamental conditioning factor.

To achieve this, some activist collectives have developed and perfected communication management strategies so that, through the use of tags or hashtags, they can trigger off a reversed agenda-setting dynamic. Among the most significant examples are #YoSíTeCreo [24], #Niunamenos [25], #Abortolegal [26] or, particularly, #Metoo [27]. Another significant case that has become global in scope and influence is the School Strike 4 Climate steered by Greta Thunberg to mobilise governments to act on climate change [28].

A relevant case in the Spanish context of reversed agenda-setting was the Plataforma de Afectados por la Hipoteca (PAH). This social movement fighting for the right to decent housing and against evictions, which emerged in Barcelona in 2009 and has spread throughout most of Spain since, managed, through its campaigns and actions, to place its demands first in the media agenda and then in the public agenda [29]. In particular, it placed the issue of dation in payment, or the cancellation of the debt of people affected by evictions by handing over their homes, at the centre of the Spanish public debate.

Some authors argue that, far from being competitors, mainstream media and social media converge symbiotically to broaden the public agenda [30]. However, despite the fact that, in this context, the public agenda is opening up to more actors and sources, the central role of mainstream media in guiding its creation and articulating its content remains unchanged. This shows that, although the Internet offers citizens the option of producing and disseminating information autonomously, doing so is not possible without the mainstream media in order to reach a potentially wide audience and obtain social visibility. This is construed as an uncomfortable reality for political activists who, in spite of their mistrust of the mainstream media, since they consider them defenders of the interests of capitalism, a danger to democracy and a part of the system they are fighting against, are perfectly aware of the extent they are indispensable for the expansion and amplification of their protests [31].

3 Social Media as an Obstacle to Online Political Activism

3.1 Difficulties in Capturing the Interest of Mainstream Media

The mainstream media continue to occupy a central place in shaping the public agenda. Therefore, capturing their attention, making their demands newsworthy, thus attaining social visibility and obtaining favourable news coverage are a priority for political activism when it comes to expanding their protests [12]. However, this task is not easy.

The main reason is to be found in the mainstream medias' lacking inclination towards political activism. This is due to two interconnected factors. The first has to do with the tendency of the legacy media to cover institutional politics and give official sources a high profile [32]. The second has to do with the atmosphere of mutual suspicion that governs the relationship between activists and journalists [33, 34]. The latter either silence the activists' demands, condemning them to social invisibility, or when they report on protests, do so from the paradigm of protest [35], offering adverse coverage and a negative image of the very protests.

To this set of factors, the normalisation of protests should be added [36]. Their occurrence causes protests to become routine and makes capturing the media's attention harder. Likewise, the lack of online political activism adapting to the logic of the media and the criteria used to decide what is newsworthy is also a major handicap [33]. The refusal of new social movements to assume the principles of spectacle and entertainment that dictate media content in their actions often acts as a drawback when it comes to gaining access to news. Paradoxically, when activists choose to apply the logic of damage [36], which involves the destruction of property, the use of violence and large-scale disruption, and thus has a strong spectacularising component, they gain access to media news spaces. Nonetheless, the treatment they receive in these cases is clearly unfavourable and leads to undermined legitimacy [8].

The self-mediation of social-media enabled protest allows new social movements to set up discordant narratives that challenge the hegemonic ones promoted by the political and social elites. Despite this, the influence of these counter-frames is often limited. There are various grounds for this, but the main reasons are twofold. On the one hand, there is a clear inequality between online political activists and political and social elites when it comes to ensuring that their discursive frames gain wide circulation and visibility. On the other hand, counter-frames launched by online political activists often fail to land beyond the boundaries of the activist circle and reach the general public due to selective exposure [37].

3.2 The Structural Dependence on Commercial Social Media

The chief social media, such as Facebook, Twitter or YouTube, are large financial-interest holding business corporations. Their principal activity is primarily directed towards money-making [38]. Moreover, they are highly profitable businesses. Facebook, which went public in May 2012, earned €24 billion in 2020. These platforms, therefore, have a powerful business and market dimension that takes precedence over their potential contribution to improving democracy. In fact, the emergence of web 2.0 originated in the context of the dotcom crisis, which hit technology companies in the early 2000s, and was the result of the search for new business models to attract investors and users with rather than a commitment to the democratisation of communication [38].

This commercial focus can have a significant impact on online political activism. The latter has made social media the centre of its activity in organisational, communicative and mobilising terms [39]. In fact, despite having their own social network sites, such as N-1 or Diaspora*, activists would mostly rather use commercial platforms such as Facebook or Twitter [40]. This even leads to a dynamic of dependence on these digital resources, which have grown vital for many new social movements. This is a risk, as online political activists become structurally dependent on the web 2.0 companies' commercial and corporate interests. These companies can unilaterally close activists' accounts and profiles, delete or censor their content, subject them to surveillance or violate activists' privacy by handing over their data to the authorities, among other actions, for whatever economic or political reasons they deem fit [8]. This leaves online political activists in a position of vulnerability and helplessness in the face of corporate 2.0 interests [41].

This can be a handicap for online political activism and protest. Far from being a hypothetical or unlikely barrier, there is a wealth of evidence that shows the collaboration of social media with governments to cut down on freedoms of expression and reduce the room for manoeuvre of political activists. Thus, in order to favour its economic growth, since January 2012 Twitter has been collaborating with the Thai government to block all those tweets that violate the rules of local Thai law, especially those messages that may be offensive to the monarchy, punishable with up to 20 years in prison. This highlights the potential pitfall for online political activists of relying on commercial social media in certain contexts.

4 Conclusions

Social media provide opportunities for the communicative empowerment of citizens in general and online political activism in particular. Essentially, the enormous potential that digital technologies provide to new social movements from the communicative perspective is threefold: the self-mediation of protests, the civic monitoring of the centres of power and the new possibilities in the construction of the public agenda. The latter are oriented towards reversed agenda-setting, which makes incorporating activist issues and discursive frameworks into the public sphere possible. These courses of action suppose a panorama, in respect to previous outlooks, which is without precedent. They offer political activism new weapons to try to condition public debate in current societies and fight with, in the symbolic and communicative terrain, to defend its demands. This highlights the importance and impact of these digital platforms in the field of political communication. Consequently, it shows that they can act as an ally to activism to spur the communicative strategies of citizen protests.

However, not all that social media contribute to online political activism is positive. These digital platforms also restrict the actions of new social movements, limiting their room for manoeuvre or impairing their normal function in the way they work. The difficulties in capturing the interest of mainstream media and the structural dependence on commercial social media are the basic impediments from the communication perspective. These two problems shape themselves up to be foes that reduce, in part, the optimism regarding the advantages that web 2.0 offers political activism and question its transformative reach.

The existence of opportunities and obstacles reveals that social media can potentially reshape power relations and favour citizen counter-power, but also that there are factors that can limit these transformations. These digital media are introducing important innovations in the communicative side of political activism that can have a significant impact on today's democracy, favouring, among other aspects, pluralism, openness and deliberation. However, they operate in a hybrid scenario, marked by change and continuity, where new possibilities come to the fore, but where old logic and hidden traps endure.

References

1. Caren, N., Andrews, K.T., Lu, T.: Contemporary social movements in a hybrid media environment. Ann. Rev. Sociol. **46** (2020). https://doi.org/10.1146/annurev-soc-121919-054627
2. Casero-Ripollés, A.: Estrategias y prácticas comunicativas del activismo político en las redes sociales en España. Historia y Comunicación Social **20**(2) (2015)
3. Bennett, W.L., Segerberg, A.: The logic of connective action: digital media and the personalization of contentious politics. In: The Logic of Connective Action: Digital Media and the Personalization of Contentious Politics (2012). https://doi.org/10.1017/CBO9781139198752
4. Castells, M.: Communication Power, Oxford (2009)
5. Silverstone, R.: Media and Morality. Polity (ed.), Cambridge (2007)
6. Gamson, W.A., Wolfsfeld, G.: Movements and media as interacting systems. Ann. Am. Acad. Polit. Soc. Sci. **528**(1) (1993). https://doi.org/10.1177/0002716293528001009

7. Jenkins, H.: Convergence Culture: Where Old and New Media Collide. N. Y. N. Press. (ed.) (2006)
8. Cammaerts, B.: The circulation of anti-austerity protest. In: The Circulation of Anti-austerity Protest (2018). https://doi.org/10.1007/978-3-319-70123-3
9. García-González, L.A., Bailey Guedes, O.: La protesta feminista #8M 2020 en México a través de la participación de comentarios en YouTube. Conexión, 14 (2020). https://doi.org/10.18800/conexion.202002.005
10. Chadwick, A.: The Hybrid Media System: Politics and Power, 2nd edn. (2017). https://doi.org/10.1093/oso/9780190696726.001.0001
11. Martínez Avidad, M.: Redes alternativas de comunicación, framing y la construcción del poder político. OBETS. Revista de Ciencias Sociales **6**(2) (2011). https://doi.org/10.14198/obets2011.6.2.05
12. Casero-Ripollés, A., Feenstra, R.A.: The 15-M Movement and the new media: a case study of how new themes were introduced into Spanish political discourse. Media Int. Aust. **144**(1), 68–76 (2012). https://doi.org/10.1177/1329878x1214400111
13. Casas, A., Davesa, F., Congosto Martínez, M.: La cobertura mediática de una acción “conectiva”: la interacción entre el movimiento 15-M y los medios de comunicación. Reis: Revista Española de Investigaciones Sociológicas **155** (2016)
14. Hargittai, E., Hsieh, Y.P.: Digital inequality. In: Dutton, W.H. (ed.) The Oxford Handbook of Internet Studies, pp. 129–150. Oxford (2013)
15. Van Dijck, J.: Users like you? Theorizing agency in user-generated content. Media Cult. Soc. **31**(1) (2009). https://doi.org/10.1177/0163443708098245
16. Alonso-Muñoz, L., Casero-Ripollés, A.: Transparency and political monitoring in the digital environment. Towards a typology of citizen-driven platforms. Revista Latina de Comunicación Social **72** (2017)
17. Feenstra, R.A., Welp, Y.: Sobre demos, cracias y gogias. Reflexiones sobre las democracias. Araucaria **42** (2019). https://doi.org/10.12795/araucaria.2019.i42.25
18. Keane, J.: The Life and Death of Democracy. Simon and Schuster, London (2009)
19. Feenstra, R.A., Casero-Ripollés, A.: Democracy in the digital communication environment: a typology proposal of political monitoring processes. Int. J. Commun. **8**(1) (2014)
20. Lievrouw, L.: Alternative and Activist New Media. Polity, Cambridge (2011)
21. Sampedro, V.: El cuarto poder en red. Icaria, Barcelona (2014)
22. Keane, J., Feenstra, R.: Democracia monitorizada en España. Nuevas formas de participación política en el marco de la era digital. Telos: Cuadernos de Comunicación e Innovación **98** (2014)
23. Sung-Tae, K., Young-hwan, L.: New functions of Internet mediated agenda-setting: agenda-rippling and reversed agenda-setting. Korea J. Rev. **1**(2), 3–29 (2007)
24. Larrondo, A., Morales I Gras, J., Terradillos, J.O.: Feminist hashtag activism in Spain: measuring the degree of politicisation of online discourse on #yosítecreo, #hermanayosítecreo, #cuéntalo y #noestássola. Commun. Soc. **32**(4 Special Issue) (2019). https://doi.org/10.15581/003.32.4.207-221
25. Chenou, J.M., Cepeda-Másmela, C.: #NiUnaMenos: data activism from the global south. Telev. New Media **20**(4) (2019). https://doi.org/10.1177/1527476419828995
26. Laudano, C.: Feministas en la red. Reflexiones en torno a las potencialidades y restricciones de la participación en el ciberespacio. In: R. y L. F. (Comps.) (ed.) Sin feminismos no hay democracia : Género y ciencias sociales (2016)
27. Loney-Howes, R., Mendes, K., Fernández Romero, D., Fileborn, B., Núñez Puente, S.: Digital footprints of #MeToo. Feminist Media Studies (2021). https://doi.org/10.1080/14680777.2021.1886142

28. Boulianne, S., Lalancette, M., Ilkiw, D.: School strike 4 climate": social media and the international youth protest on climate change. Media Commun. 8(2) (2020). https://doi.org/10.17645/mac.v8i2.2768
29. Alonso-Muñoz, L., Casero-Ripollés, A.: La influencia del discurso sobre cambio social en la agenda de los medios. El caso de la Plataforma de Afectados por la Hipoteca. OBETS. Revista de Ciencias Sociales **11**(1), 25 (2016). https://doi.org/10.14198/OBETS2016.11.1.02
30. Mare, A.: A complicated but symbiotic affair: the relationship between mainstream media and social media in the coverage of social protests in southern Africa. Ecquid Novi **34**(1) (2013). https://doi.org/10.1080/02560054.2013.767426
31. Harlow, S., Harp, D.: Alternative media in a digital era: comparing news and information use among activists in the United States and Latin America. Commun. Soc. **26**(4) (2013). https://doi.org/10.15581/003.26.4.25-51
32. Martínez Nicolás, M., Humanes, M.L.: Culturas profesionales del periodismo político en España. El discurso de los periodistas sobre la política y las funciones políticas de los medios. In: Casero-Ripollés, A. (ed.) Periodismo político en España: concepciones, tensiones y elecciones, pp. 47–64. SLCS, Tenerife (2012)
33. Micó, J.L., Casero-Ripollés, A.: Political activism online: organization and media relations in the case of 15-M in Spain. Inf. Commun. Soc. **17**(7), 858–871 (2014)
34. Billard, T.J.: Movement-media relations in the hybrid media system: a case study from the US transgender rights movement. Int. J. Press/Politics **26**(2), 341–361 (2021)
35. Gitlin, T.: The Whole World is Watching: Mass Media in the Making & Unmaking of the New Left. University of California Press, Berkeley (1980)
36. Della, P.D., Diani, M.: Social Movements: An Introduction. Blackwell, Oxford (2006)
37. Stroud, N.J.: Polarization and partisan selective exposure. J. Commun. **60**(3) (2010). https://doi.org/10.1111/j.1460-2466.2010.01497.x
38. Fuchs, C.: Social Media: A Critical Introduction. Sage, London (2014)
39. Gerbaudo, P.: Tweets and the streets: social media and contemporary activism. In: PlutoPress (2012)
40. Fuchs, C.: OccupyMedia! The Occupy Movement and Social Media in Crisis Capitalism. Zero Books, Winchester (2014)
41. Uldam, J.: Social media visibility: challenges to activism. Media Cult. Soc. **40**(1) (2018). https://doi.org/10.1177/0163443717704997

Check for updates

When Memes Become a Serious Business: Memetics as a Political Communication Strategy in the United States and Ecuador

Marco López-Paredes[1](✉), Andrea Carrillo-Andrade[1], and Paulo Carlos López-López[2]

[1] Pontificia Universidad Católica, Ecuador, Quito 1076, Ecuador
{mvlopez,acarrillo745}@puce.edu.ec
[2] Universidad Santiago de Compostela, Santiago de Compostela, Galicia, Spain
paulocarlos.lopez@usc.es

Abstract. The media convergence model refers to a context in which the information is produced by every and anybody, without intermediates or filters. This offers new possibilities for citizens and politicians to interact and frame situations. One way to do so is by memetics. Memes have 3 main characteristics: (1) Diffuse at the micro level but shape the macro structure of society; (2) Use cultural items that people can potentially imitate; (3) Travel through competition and selection. When it comes to political memes, few research has been held. That is why the research question that arises is how memes allow prosumers to interact and opine about politicians? The present investigation based in multimodal analysis compares memes among United States and Ecuador when former Presidents were banned from social networks. It concludes that public discussion memes are the preferred ones for prosumers; they use cultural items to create situational jokes and make fun of politicians. These memes imitate instead of creating new messages, are restricted about the topics and generate polarized meanings.

Keywords: Political communication · Social networks · Memes

1 Introduction

Since 2005, the number of Internet users has been rising. This has been possible thanks to the advancing mobile technology and Internet infrastructure. By 2019, nearly 4 billion users have been registered. Northern American and Southern America have reached the third (90%) of Internet penetration and sixth place (72%) in the global rank, respectively [1]; both regions have shown a sustained growth. Internet users in Latin America had the highest average time spent per day on social media [1]. In Ecuador, 80% of its population uses Internet and most of them prefer to navigate in social networks over getting information from certified sites [2]. The same happens in the United States, where 70% of the population holds a social media account. Then, "these platforms and services have become some of the most popular online activities of the past decades" [3].

© The Author(s), under exclusive license to Springer Nature Singapore Pte Ltd. 2022
Á. Rocha et al. (Eds.): ICOMTA 2021, SIST 259, pp. 82–93, 2022.
https://doi.org/10.1007/978-981-16-5792-4_9

Even if the term "user" is commonly used, for the approximation of this research, it is more exact to talk about "prosumers". This concept was born in 1972 and it proceeds from the fusion of the word's "producer" and "consumer". It modifies the understanding of individuals as passive receptors of information and states that new technology allows people to produce and consume content [4]. In other words, media consumers are not merely passive recipients of content, but they are active participant as they understand and assess it. When it comes to political issues or "politainment", prosumers tend to generate a lot of material. However, this content, in general terms, is characterized by a limited message creation, restriction about the topics and polarized meanings [5].

In the same line of ideas, participatory communication in Ecuador and the United States has similitudes that should be explored: both regions "favor informational models over participatory approaches to communication"; "the weak status of communication as a field of study and practice in development organizations undermine the prospects for expanding the understanding of communication" and there is a limited use of participation thinking [6, 7]. However, even if both nations develop under the model of liberal democracy, freedom of speech in social networks has been questioned in Ecuador during the presidency of Rafael Correa [8]. In the case of United States, visceral, impulsive tweets from @realDonaldTrump ended up being important evidence in lawsuits against him.

With all these cultural, political and communicational and technological comparisons, it is worth to explore how citizen participation is developping by Internet-usage. What is more, the ways of communicating have rapidly spread among both nations. The strongest evidence of this are memes. A meme is a typical internet phenomenon, and it crosses borders. In fact, memes are a worldwide experience. It can present itself as an image or analogy, a catchphrase, widespread behavior or even a challenge [9]. They tend to be ephemeral. That is why their success depends on their replication and stability over time [10]. One of the newer mediums of participatory communication is 'Internet Meme'. Political memes are the center of interest of this research: *how memes allow prosumers to interact and opine about politicians?*

2 The Globalization of Memetics

The media convergence model refers to a context in which the information is produced by every and anybody, without intermediates or filters. According to this model, involvement is easy to reach as people follows and generates content around individual interests [11]. In this context, memetics are born.

The evolutive biologist Richard Dawkins [12] was the first scholar that used the word "meme" to define a "living structure" that propagates by imitation. Dawkins understood a meme as a replicator, and he related it to evolution. The author identified three key elements of a successful meme: copy-fidelity, fecundity and longevity: "copy-fidelity is the ability to replicate accurately; fecundity is its speed of replication; and longevity its stability over time" [10].

Dawkins' conceptualization has been adapted to communication studies. In fact, memes are comparable to dialects: "Just as P. F. Jenkins describes the birth of a new "dialect" in birds, by "change of pitch of a note, repetition of a note, the elision of notes and the combination of parts of other existing songs", memes born as a cultural mutation". However, even if this approach laid the foundation for the study of memetics, it shows some limitations. For instance, "Dawkins conceived memes as ideas, not media forms" [13]. Then, the categories mentioned above do not consider the subsequent uses and appropriations for memes.

In the era of the Web 2.0 and the hipermediations [14], the original concept of Dawkins requires new perspectives. Limor Shifman defines them as "cultural information that passes along from person to person, yet gradually scales into a shared social phenomenon" [13]. Johnson [15] broadens the assertion and determines that memes "can scale into a social phenomenon. and trivial elements of popular culture". Lopez-Paredes and Oñate state that "memes from Internet" consist of the deliberate association of elements (image and text) in the same significant unit. They result from the representation of an idea, concept, opinion or situation [16]. Then, memes allow to register or catch key ideas that are developed in the collective imaginary.

In a digital society with an increasing number of prosumers, memes can be understood as the cultural way to express and generate content; they circulate in social media. Memes are related to the participatory culture of the Internet, characterized by relatively low barriers to artistic expression and civic engagement. Its members believe their contributions matter, and feel some degree of social connection with one another [17].

As it has been stated in lines above, there are different characteristics for memes that can be summered in: first, "memes diffuse at the micro level but shape the macro structure of society; they reproduce by various means of imitation" [13]. According to Berrocal, Campos-Dominguez and Redondo [5] this can be read as a limitation in terms of message creation and topics: prosumers "tend to replay the same message over and over again –the same content but in different versions and formats–, with scarcely any evidence of participative actions as prosumer".

Second, a meme becomes one according to way they travel and reproduce. This is by appropriation, imitation and sharing. It is appropriate to stay that they follow the rules of competitive selection. To do so, it is necessary to generate a "personalized expression via social sharing" [18]. In fact, Bennet and Segerberg relate this attribute to the Logic of Connective Action and politics: "The Logic of Connective Action explains the rise of a personalized digitally networked politics in which diverse individuals address the common problems" [18]. Third, memes travel through competition and selection.

2.1 Memetics and Politics

Until now, we have referred to the creators and replicators of memes as "individuals" and "users", however if we conceive them as citizens, we can broaden the implications of memes in political live. Tay [19] outlined that, in fact, citizen-made political humor memes are an example of engaged citizen discourse. In this context, even we cannot state that this is a new phenomenon—it can be compared to political cartoons—, memes allow amateurs and professionals to create and spread a meaning by "common language" uses.

Shifman [20] clarifies that: "While some political memes are framed in a humorous manner, others are deadly serious. But regardless of their emotional keying, political memes are about making a point—participating in a normative debate about how the world should look and the best way to get there". The author creates a taxonomy to classify them: (1) persuasive memes; (2) grassroots action memes; and (3) public discussion memes. Persuasive memes can be understood as the ones that created with an obvious intention to support a candidate. To do so, they use reason and emotional aspects but also ethical, moral, and ideological appeal. Grassroots action memes are the ones that are related to collective action and networks curated or catalyzed by organizations. Public discussion memes use commonplaces and cultural products. Also, they make joke about political characters [21].

2.2 Ecuador and United States: Globalized Humor and Politics

In the case of Ecuador and the United States, because of the political system, there are some key points in the way citizens involve in political processes. For instance, on one hand, in liberal democracies, the internet affects political processes by lowering the cost of acquiring and producing information. Then, more citizens can express their opinion or generate data in theory without fearing for repression. On the other hand, experience has shown that in this kind of democracies, it is easy to generate polarization among citizens in online discourses [22].

The "user-generated" globalization is a world phenomenon. Shifman, Levy and Thelwall [23] state that Internet does not only provide "equal" technological facilities, but also complex nexus of practices and choices among users. Humor is one of these practices: Internet jokes serve as "powerful (albeit often invisible) agents of globalization".

In this context, Twitter became the main space for politics: it allows to follow in real time an event by filtering hashtags. Besides, the idea of direct communication among citizens and politicians is appealing for prosumers. Twitter for Rafael Correa (@MashiRafael) was not the main channel for his campaign; the former President opened it to communicate from a powerful position [11]. The story is opposite for Donald Trump (@realDonaldTrump) who used Twitter "emotionally" to develop a digital campaign. Trump used fear and patriotic appeals to develop powerful speeches such as "America, people, us" and "Make America Great Again" [24].

Humor-sharing among nations is possible because it tends to "relate to the symbols and stereotypes specific to the place and time of their creation, reflecting norms and aspirations, power structures, and collective fears" [25].

3 Methodology

The research question that guides this investigation is how memes allow prosumers to interact and opine about politicians? To answer it, a case-study, exploratory research is conducted, and it is supported by a multimodal analysis.

In first place, case study allows to examine the empirical world. It is useful for this study to cover the contextual conditions and understand the similarities and differences between memetics in Ecuador and the United States.

In second place, the question should be answered by a qualitative (exploratory) research. Qualitative research allows to look for elements in a "multi-layered and textured social world" [26]. This type of research can generate well-founded cross-contextual generalities.

In third place, Shifman [20] underlines the need to evaluate memes not as isolated units of content, but as a semantic set. This is essential to understand their meanings. Above all because memes are ephemeral, so their value is based on their context. That is why memes in this study are based on Multimodal analysis.

Multimodal analysis is particularly concerned about sources which contain the interaction and integration of two or more semiotic resources—text, static images or moving images (gifs, videos)—or 'modes' of communication" [27, 28]. By using this approximation, we can examine how a text achieves its communicative functions. Multimodality is a central part of this study, and it is based on previous research conducted from the Observatory of Communication (OdeCom) from the Pontifical University of Ecuador (PUCE).

To examine political memes specifically, it is important to summarize their main characteristics and subcategories:

3.1 Units of Analysis

Memes and digital culture seem to fit; that is why everyday more scholars conduct researchers about this topic. However, because of the apparently distance between "politics" (serious business) and memes (mostly humorous content), there is a lack of studies on the universe of online memes and their uses and appropriations in political contexts. That is why an exploratory research is useful as it enables us to understand an early stage of the investigation.

What is more, "in social science exploration is a broad-ranging, purposive, systematic, prearranged undertaking designed to maximize the discovery of generalizations leading to description and understanding of an area of social or psychological life" [29].

After a systematic research based on the quest for similar events in the United States and Ecuadorian political life, a main case was found: the suspension of the accounts of Donald Trump and Rafael Correa. As the aim is to test interactions between politicians and citizens, Twitter was the platform to look for memes by searching for the prominent hashtag. In the case of the United States, the meme was found by using the trend hashtag #TrumpBanned. In this case, hashtag is useful as it can be understood as Unified Political Discourses. Besides, according to Thompson [30], the power relationships can be stablished and sustained by using a symbolic level. Although, for Ecuador the search was different. The meme was obtained through a search over the replies that President Correa received when he published that he was banned from Facebook. This is an advantage (it could not be done for Trump as the Twitter account was closed) as it allows to understand the interactions. However both searches share the same components and are based in a random selection to avoid bias and correlations between explanatory-explained and explanatory-explanatory variables [31].

4 Results

Memes, in the political sphere, can be seen as a way for citizens to express their opinion: "The use of memes tests the horizontal nature of social networks and the relationship

Table 1. Main characteristics of memes and how to analyze them [13, 21]

Characteristic	Analysis for political memes	Definition
1 Diffuse at the micro level but shape the macro structure of society	Persuasive memes, grassroots action memes; and public discussion memes	**Persuasive memes:** Propositional rhetoric and/or pragmatic appeal; Seducing or threatening rhetoric and/or emotional appeal; Ethical and moral rhetoric and/or ideological appeal; Critical rhetoric and/or appeal to the credibility of the source **Grass-roots action memes:** Dynamics of collective or hybrid connective action and networks curated by organizations **Public discussion memes:** Political commonplace; Literary or cultural allusions; Jokes about political characters; Situational jokes
2 Cultural items that people can potentially imitate	Content, form, and stance	**Content:** referencing to both the ideas and the ideologies conveyed by it **Form:** physical message, perceived through our senses **Stance:** when re-creating a text, users can decide to imitate a certain position that they find appealing or use an utterly different discursive orientation
3 Travel through competition and selection	Scope	

between citizens and political actors" [32]. Besides, as they are mostly humorous, they often question the authority, the symbolic power. This is related to the first attribute of memes (Table 1, 1st characteristic). Memes are useful to guide in the meaning of an event that concerns to most citizens.

However, if we investigate the characteristics of memes, to become one, the citizen-prosumer should create material that can be replicated (Table 1, 3rd characteristic). To achieve this, the key is to use humor, cultural empathies or perhaps development a social awareness about political issues that affect a specific group or society [32].

A common dynamic in liberal democracies is to generate memes about the political situation with characters that are easily recognized and with strong positions. This helps citizens to organize information and persuade.

4.1 Making Fun: When the Powerful are Silenced

On January 8, 2021, President Donald J. Trump Tweeted: "The 75,000,000 great American Patriots who voted for me, AMERICA FIRST, and MAKE AMERICA GREAT AGAIN, will have a GIANT VOICE long into the future. They will not be disrespected or treated unfairly in any way, shape or form!!!" [33] Then, the President tweeted: "To all of those who have asked, I will not be going to the Inauguration on January 20th." [33].

That is the evidence that Twitter Inc. included to sustain that the account @realDonaldTrump should be suspended permanently as the messages were a violation of the Glorification of Violence Policy. This happened days after people violently stormed the Capitol on January 6, 2021.

Once the decision was taken, the tendency in Twitter became #TrumpBanned and citizens around the world began to make fun of the former President of the United States (Table 2):

The suspension of the Twitter account is the perfect reason to make some situational jokes: both memes can be classified as "Public discussion" because they present cultural allusions. Meme 1 collects the faces of prominent politicians of USA; most of them Democrats (Hillary Clinton, Barack Obama, Joe Biden, Bill Clinton, Kamala Harris) raising their hands as the text states: "Raise your hand if you still have a Twitter account". However, the last picture is Donald Trump's sad face without raising his hand.

The content is based on the *collage* technique. It is widely available that it is used to compare characters or to put them in the same situation or level. This meme was spread by an American-citizen account. Then, it is evident that the cultural items selected are easily recognized by a young American (it frames the last presidents [1993–2021]).

Meme 2 uses Photoshop technology to create a new meaning from a meme known as "Pablo Escobar waiting". That meme became popular in 2016 after Netflix released the series *Narcos*, based on the life of Pablo Escobar. This meme was posted in an Ecuadorian account, which explains the selection for an original Latin-American item as a main character. This shows new appropriations of the original meme and the circulation of new versions. Besides, it is a case for examining the borders between amateurism and professionalism in contemporary culture because of the use of specialized assembly programs.

The form of both memes is the "basic" one: combination of text and images to generate a new sense for the situation. This allows to juxtapose meanings.

Meme 2 has a stronger political content not only because of the equivalency Trump-Escobar (a criminal) but also because of the use of the #BidenHarrisInauguration, which is a Unified Political Discourse that states support for the current president over the former one. Specially because of the announce of Trump form not going to the Inauguration Day. The aim of Meme 1 is just to make fun of a situation by cultural allusions.

Both memes can be read as an attempt to show a political opinion and they are produced by citizens without political aspirations. They are not calling for a further

Table 2. Memes around #TrumpBanned

Meme 1	Meme 2
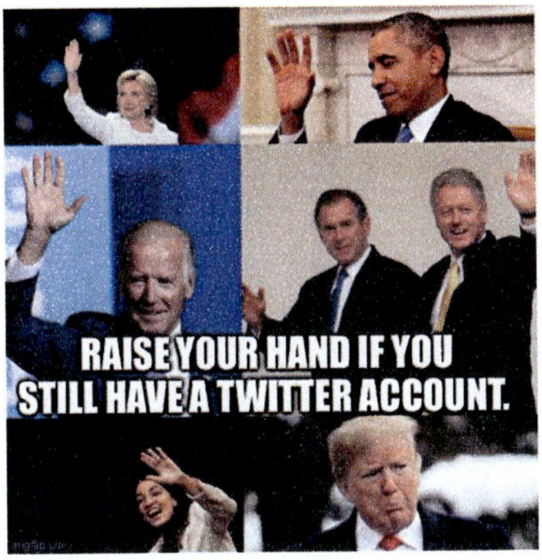	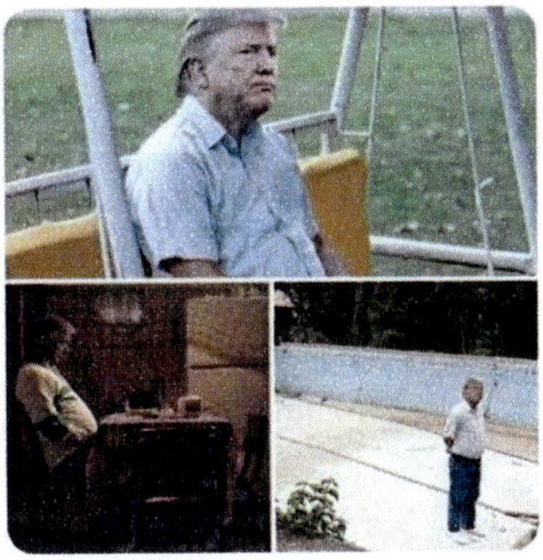
Text (copy): #TrumpBanned	Text (copy): When you have a bad day, but you cannot tweet about it #TrumpBanned #Biden-HarrisInauguration
Classification: Public discussion meme	**Classification: Public discussion meme**
Cultural items: ***Raising hands***: Hillary Clinton, Barack Obama, Joe Biden, George Bush, Bill Clinton, Kamala Harris (prominent politicians of USA). ***No raising hand:*** Donald Trump. Cynical-ironic.	**Cultural items:** Photoshop from the original meme "Pablo Escobar Waiting". Cynical-ironic.
Scope: First results under #TrumpBanned in United States	**Scope:** First results under #TrumpBanned in Ecuador

action and they do not show clues about connective action as they can be read as non-organized individuals that tweet about a specific situation. In the United States, the use of humor from the side of politicians has been historic. In fact, in this country is appreciated a leader with sense of humor. However, the ways of populism imply a new form to relate with citizens. That is why Doubleday states: "Trump's appeal to voters rests less on humor than on the performance of anger" [34].

4.2 Mocking and Flaming: When Freedom of Expression Finds Limitations

On January 7th, 2019, former Ecuadorian President, Rafael Correa used his Twitter account to publish: "And these are the people who talk to us about "freedom of expression"! They not only rob me of the right to express myself. They rob a million and a half people of their right to follow me" (@MashiRafael). He referred to Facebook; the social network suspended his account because it was reported for spreading personal data. Then, Correa decided to open a new fan page, but it was also closed as Facebook do not allow to create new similar pages.

In this case, citizens were able to reply to the tweet. Even though Correa framed the act as a persecution and he related the situation with the INA Papers case, citizens took advantage to insult Correa [35] (Table 3).

Table 3. Memes around Correa's account closure

Meme 1

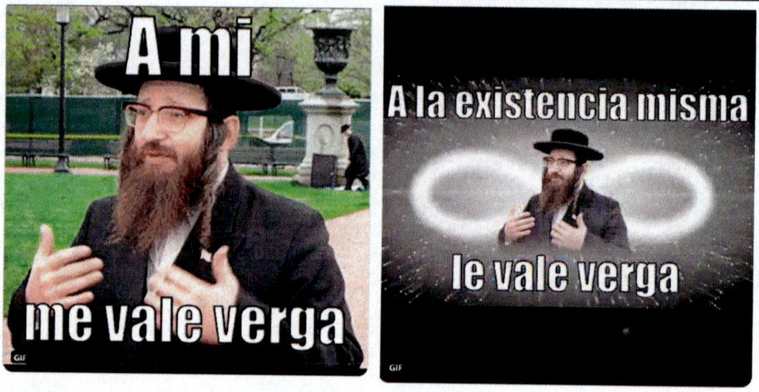
A mi
me vale verga
A la existencia misma
le vale verga

Text (copy): --

Classification: Public discussion meme

Cultural items: The rabbi "is worth my dick"

Scope: Prominent reply

In 2016, the video-meme "The rabbi is worth my dick" became popular. It was originally a video that showed a rabbi "travelling" around different scenarios (small ones such as a park until it arrives to bigger ones such as the Solar system and the universe). The permanent phrase was "is worth my dick". The video can be modified by users, who can add new scenarios or new characters, some of them modified to look like a rabbi.

This meme is a gif, which can be catalogued as a more "evolved meme" in the sense that this format is able to collect and show images like in a silent video. This format has a light weight which allows people to share content easily. Besides, all social networks incorporated the possibility to use this resource by clicking a bottom and searching the content, which is organized by "key words" that can be feelings, characters, or more specific situations. Nowadays, it is also common to find online pages under the classification of "gif generator" or "meme generator" that allow the prosumers to customize famous templates of generate new ones.

In Ecuadorian politics, it is common to read insults and to send offensive messages over the Internet. This phenomenon is called "flaming"; in fact, according to Messina, politicians understand that, through insult, they can "destroy reputations" and "mock their adversaries" [36]. As it can be evidenced in this example, citizens have received this message as an invitation to insult likewise. Although this meme was classified as "prominent" and it included @MashiRafael in the conversation, it did not receive a reply.

In both situations in the two countries, it is important to note that politicians do received support from citizens: Some texted that they disagreed with the decision of the social network and sketched solutions; other called for actions like boycotting the network. However, to show that support, people did not used memes. They preferred flat text. This can be related to the fact that memes are linked to generate humor. Then, as the suspension or closure of the accounts is not a "happy" situation for the supporters, they prefer not to use memes. Also, a possible explanation is the use of bots. By bots, we refer to accounts that are programmed to spread "information" that support or attack certain candidate or to show a strong position over any situation. They use Artificial Intelligence (AI), and they are directly related to the diffusion of fake news of misinformation. For Trump it is common to use them: "19% of all tweets related to the election that year were generated by bots" [37]. In the case of Donald Trump, he had 55 million followers on Twitter. But more than 60% look suspiciously fake [38]. In Ecuador, the circumstances are similar: according to the study "Troops, Trolls and Troublemakers: A Global Inventory of Organized Social Media Manipulation" prepared by the University of Oxford, the country is among the nations whose governments have 'cyber troops' (bots) to manipulate criticism on social networks. For example, Rafael Correa account has 43% of fake followers (spam, bots, propaganda, etc. or because they are no longer active on Twitter) and just 2,25% of high-quality followers, according to SparkToro; which leads to determine that the account has more fake followers than the most [39].

5 Discussion

The media convergence model offers the illusion of connection and transparency among users, who transform into prosumers as they can generate and spread content. This "new" content, as shown in previous works [5], tend to imitate instead of create new messages, are restricted about the topics and generate polarized meanings. That is why public discussion memes are the more popular to interact with politicians.

In first place, imitation is one of the main characteristics of memes. In fact, as they must travel through competition and selection, their adaptability is what will determine their new uses and appropriations. While memes are traveling, their content, form and stance are also manipulated. Political memes appeal to trivial elements of popular culture. This is helpful to register or catch key ideas that are developed in the collective imaginary.

In second place, public discussion memes are limited about their topics because they need that something newsworthy appears to develop situational jokes and have a commonplace to which they can turn. This is part of the "politainment" culture. However, there is a lot of creativity in the selection and adaptation of memes to make fun of politicians. Besides, amateurs and professional prosumers participate in the generation of new images, videos of texts.

In third place, most of memes that were analyzed are "famous" ones. So, it is easy to understand their meaning and to interact from them. But none of them received a reply from the receptor (politician). In the case of Donald Trump, it may be because his account was suspended; for Ecuadorians it can be related to use of bots and fake followers. This, somehow, demystify the speech of horizontal communication and allows people to express themselves and even flame in the digital sphere.

Finally, it calls our attention that even the ban generated positive and negative reactions, memes were created from the side of the opponents. So, memes are used mostly when mocking, while plain text when supporting.

6 Conclusions

Political memes are an example of engaged citizen discourse; from the side of citizens, they allow to create and spread meaning by "common language", but the impact will depend on contextual factors. For instance, public discussion memes are broadly used to referrer to politics and to talk about political characters. However, as this type of memes use commonplaces and cultural products, it is required to share a set of understandings among producers and consumers. They are part of the politainment culture.

From the other side, the politicians commonly do not reply to memes even if they get a huge impact. This may be related to a strategy to manipulate criticism on social networks or to the use of bots. Nonetheless, even if the politicians that inspired the meme do not reply, the conversation among the events continue through citizens prosumers and they can be a strong tool to take part in political life and catch the attention.

References

1. Johson, J.: Internet penetration rate worldwide 2021, by region (2021). https://www.statista.com/statistics/269329/penetration-rate-of-the-internet-by-region/
2. Del Alcázar Ponce, J.P.: Estado Digital Ecuador 2021 – Estadísticas Digitales Actualizadas 2021 (2021). https://blog.formaciongerencial.com/estadodigitalecuador2021/
3. Tankovska, H.: Number of global social network users 2017–2025 (2021). https://www.statista.com/statistics/278414/number-of-worldwide-social-network-users/
4. Islas Carmona, O.: El prosumidor. El actor comunicativo de la Sociedad de la Ubicuidad. Anu. Investig. la Comun. CONEICC **XV**, 323–342 (2008)
5. Berrocal, S., Campos-Domínguez, E., Redondo, M.: Media prosumers in political communication: Politainment on YouTube. Comunicar **22**(43), 65–72 (2014)
6. Waisbord, S.: The institutional challenges of participatory communication in international aid. Soc. Identities **14**(4), 505–522 (2008)
7. Emmerich, G.E., Autónoma, U., México, M.: Democracia y participación en América Latina, no. 3 (1997)
8. P. V.: Libertad De Expresión: La Década Por La Pugna De La Verdad (2017). https://www.planv.com.ec/historias/politica/libertad-expresion-la-decada-la-pugna-la-verdad-1
9. #MuseudeMemes. Codebooks (2018). https://www.museudememes.com.br/codebook/
10. Marwick, A.: Memes. Contexts **12**(4), 12–13 (2013)
11. Navas, A.: Desempeño vs. impacto: un modelo comunicacional aplicado a la política digital. Rafael Correa, Cristina Fernández y Nicolás Maduro. Inteliprix (2021)
12. Dawkins, R.: The Selfish Gene, 2nd edn. Oxford University Press, Oxford (1989)
13. Shifman, L.: Memes in a digital world: reconciling with a conceptual troublemaker. J. Comput. Commun. **18**(3), 362–377 (2013)
14. Scolari, C.: Hipermediaciones: Elementos para una Teoría de la COmunicación Digital Interactiva. Gedisa Editorial, Barcelona (2008)
15. Johnson, D.: Mapping the meme: a geographical approach to materialist rhetorical criticism. Commun. Crit. Stud. **4**(1), 27–50 (2007)

16. López-Paredes, M., Oñate, V.: La memética como lenguaje icónico de nuevas narrativas en las redes sociales. Redes Soc. y Ciudad. no. October, pp. 729–134 (2020)
17. Jenkins, H., Clinton, K., Purushotma, R., Robison, A.J., Weigel, M.: Confronting the Challenges of Participatory Culture: Media Education for the 21st Century (2006)
18. Bennett, W.L., Segerberg, A.: The logic of connective action: digital media and the personalization of contentious politics, no. September (2012)
19. Tay, G.: Embracing LOLitics, pp. 1–236 (2012)
20. Shifman, L.: Memes in a Digital Culture. Cambridge (2013)
21. Chagas, V., Freire, F., Rios, D., Magalhaes, D.: Political memes and the politics of memes: a methodological proposal for content analysis of online political memes. First J. Internet **24**(2) (2019)
22. Tkacheva, O., Schwartz, L.H., Libicki, M.C., Taylor, J.E., Martini, J., Baxter, C.: The internet and political process in different regimes. Internet Free. Polit. Sp. 17–42 (2013)
23. Shifman, L., Levy, H., Thelwall, M.: Internet jokes: the secret agents of globalization? J. Comput. Commun. **19**(4), 727–743 (2014)
24. Stratum Agency: Cómo el marketing llevó a Donald Trump a la Casa Blanca. Stratum, p. 3 (2017)
25. Billig, M.: Laughter and ridicule: Towards a social critique of humor. London (2005)
26. Mason, J.: Qualitative Researching. Sage Publications, London (2002)
27. O'Halloran, K., Smith, B.: Multimodal Studies: Exploring Issues and Domains. Routledge (2014)
28. Jewitt, C., Bezemer, J., O'Halloran, K.: Introducing Multimodality. Routledge, New York (2016)
29. Stebbins, C.R.A.: In the Social Sciences What is Exploration?, no. January 2001, pp. 2–18 (2014)
30. Thompson, J.B.: Ideología y Cultura Moderna. UAM Xochimilco, México (1993)
31. Cariappa, A.G.A.: Randomized Control Trials for Social Science Research, no. January (2020)
32. Investigaci, P.D.E., Ernesto, T., Ch, A.: Los Memes Como Manifestación Satírica De La Opinión Pública En La Política Ecuatoriana: Estudio Del Caso 'Rayo Correizador', pp. 1–135 (2018)
33. T. Inc.: Permanent suspension of @realDonaldTrump (2021). https://blog.twitter.com/en_us/topics/company/2020/suspension.html
34. Doubleday, S.: Are U.S. politics beyond a joke? https://theconversation.com/are-u-s-politics-beyond-a-joke-63096
35. González, J.: Rafael Correa denuncia el cierre de su cuenta en Facebook y advierte que se están abriendo cuentas falsas (2019). https://cnnespanol.cnn.com/2019/04/12/rafael-correa-denuncia-el-cierre-de-su-cuenta-en-facebook-y-advierte-que-se-estan-abriendo-cuentas-falsas/
36. Loaiza, Y.: El insulto político en el Ecuador, su historia y sus abanderados (2019). https://gk.city/2019/08/05/insulto-politico-ecuador/
37. Guglielmi, G.: The next-generation bots interfering with the US election (2020). https://www.nature.com/articles/d41586-020-03034-5
38. Campoy, A.: More than 60% of Donald Trump's Twitter followers look suspiciously fake (2018). https://qz.com/1422395/how-many-of-donald-trumps-twitter-followers-are-fake/
39. SparkToro: Fake Followers Audit for @MashiRafael (2020). https://sparktoro.com/fake-followers/mashirafael

Check for updates

Realities and Challenges of a Democracy in Crisis. Impact of Disinformation and Populism on the Media System

Concha Pérez-Curiel and Rubén Rivas-de Roca(✉)

University of Seville, Avda. Américo Vespucio. S/N, 41092 Seville, Spain
{cperez1,rrivasderoca}@us.es

Abstract. A rescue plan for democracy is urgently needed. In a context of global political disinformation defined by platformization and polarization, electoral contests and vote cleavages are facing an institutional crisis triggered by conspiracy theories and lies. Leaders, instead of governments and parties, stand as the dominant users of the networks and direct shareholders of computational propaganda. At the same time, a radicalized populism emerges, generating levels of fake news never seen before. The media and social platforms have signed a deal against the 'infodemic' in order to obtain public trust. This study examines the causes of the fragmentation of the democratic system in the United States as well as discursive strategies of international populist leaders on Twitter, reflecting upon the reinvention of a new journalistic model that could stop the chaos of fake news. Based on the content analysis of political accounts on Twitter (@realDonaldTrump, @jairbolsonaro, @MLP_officiel, @matteosalvinimi @Santi_ABASCAL), legacy media, international fact-checking initiatives, and the results of public opinion polls (Pew Research Center; CNN; Washington Post-ABC), we confirm the influence of Trump's speech on the rest of leaders. There is a connection between the topics (issue frame) and strategies (game frame) of the right-wing populist discourse, showing electoral effects on their voters. This study also contributes to current discussions on the future of democracy, defining a proposal on a new independent journalism to foster a well-informed public sphere.

Keywords: Disinformation · Populism · Elections

1 Democracy at Stake: Political Leadership and the State of the Public Sphere

The Capitol assault in the US (January 6, 2021) has pointed out the crisis of democracies [28, 32, 44]. This event could be related to the influence of Donald Trump's speech on the voters, through a discursive strategy based on fallacy and propaganda on Twitter [39].

International public opinion barometers [17] have shown the need of a deal between institutions in order to respond to the mistrust of citizens towards politics and the media [5, 50]. The high diffusion of fake news makes public institutions and social platforms to

© The Author(s), under exclusive license to Springer Nature Singapore Pte Ltd. 2022
Á. Rocha et al. (Eds.): ICOMTA 2021, SIST 259, pp. 94–103, 2022.
https://doi.org/10.1007/978-981-16-5792-4_10

act (EU vs Disinfo 2018; European Commission 2018; WHO 2020) [21, 22], identifying disinformation campaigns that tried to influence on the electoral results.

The current state of democracy is the consequence of a wave of populism and far-right movements that pursue geopolitical objectives and interests by promoting chaos and confusion [4]. On the other hand, this trend reinforces a populist leadership style on social networks [6, 20, 48], marked by cyber-rhetoric [29] and the use of lies.

Some studies collect the response of US citizens looking at vote behavior and assessment of the polls [9, 40]. They reveal a rise in turnout, although many citizens criticize the attitude of Donald Trump and the overload of false messages as a widespread problem in the campaign [50]. Moreover, the media have been aligned to the political discourse, spreading messages from the leader without filter or verification [38].

However, the skeptical audience do not trust politicians and journalists. Their news consumption is characterized by making citizen contents popular [24], which causes ignorance of public affairs [27] and a risk for democracy due to the effects of fake news. A public sphere exposed to disinformation requires a media hybridization deal between institutions and digital platforms [8], which builds monitoring systems to evaluate the state of democracies.

2 Populism and Fake News: Looking for Roots

Liberal democracies are in decline as it is endorsed by the increasing support for authoritarian regimes. In addition to this hypothesis, the democratic system is considered as a model that only represents the establishment [23]. In recent years, the mass parties have lost their traditional role. Some of the reasons are the growing individualization of the voter, the ideological changes, or the digital transformation of the media. These conditions have boosted populist policies in which the people face the ruling elite [33]. This means a new model of political leadership [6, 20, 48] that weakens representative democracy.

In a crisis marked by the structural conflict between democracy and capitalism, as well as by mistrust in the institutions, the opportunities for the consolidation of a new populism emerge worldwide. We argue that the socio-political, economic and technological conditions trigger the aforementioned increase in emerging populist policies that legitimize a personalized political leadership (Table 1).

A report published by *The Guardian* [46] on a sample of 40 countries found that the number of populist leaders has doubled in the 21st century. The last elections to the European Parliament (2019) confirmed the success of the extreme right and radical left populism, which got 218 of the 751 seats (29%). The main reasons for the active immersion of populist political parties in European parliaments are founded on the economic recession that boosted left-wing populist politicians in the south of Europe. By contrast, the refugee crisis was a catalyst for right-wing movements and the transformation of non-populist parties into populist ones [51].

The far-right populist parties are achieving great levels of support thanks to disinformation, polarization and political manipulation, based on computational propaganda [52] and cyber-rhetoric [45]. These strategies focus on normal people, using a strong ideological and emotional charge [15]. This approach fits very well into the features of

Table 1. Comparing liberal and populist democracies. Source: [33, 36].

Liberal democracy	Populist democracy
Pluralism and social diversity	Homogeneous society, people vs elite
Well-balanced systems and separation of powers: legislature, executive and judiciary Political independence of the media	Executive preponderance and rule of electoral contests Control of the media
Limited powers	Absolute powers (sovereign)
Checks and balances between the legislature and the judiciary	Full use of sovereignty on behalf of the people (additional powers)
Competitive elections	Permanent and rigged elections
Rational speech	Emotional speech
Diversity of recognized political parties	'We' and 'They' (false confrontation between 'friends' and 'enemies', polarization)
Representative institutions and political parties	Identification between the leader and the general will. Traditional party decline
Politics understood as agreements between parties	Politics understood as the rule of a hegemonic populist project
Fewer popular consultations	Frequent elections and plebiscites

social networks such as Twitter [13]. An emotional storytelling [16] is applied, affecting the whole political and media system. Independent journalism and, therefore, democracy are threatened by this situation [5, 11, 53].

The conflict in the last US elections (2020) and the dissemination of fake news by Donald Trump on Twitter show how this approach is similar to the agenda implemented by other populist leaders [39]. Bolsonaro (Brazil), Le Pen (France), Salvini (Italy) and Abascal (Spain) also represent the charismatic leader that use an illiberal and emotional style. We applied a quantitative and qualitative-discursive content analysis to the tweets of these political leaders posted from 29 September to 8 November 2020, covering the campaign and the days until Joe Biden was proclaimed winner by the legacy media. In total, 1497 tweets were collected through the Twitonomy tool. The codification was carried out manually by the authors, using IBM SPSS Statistics, Version 25, to process the data.

The content analysis focuses on the issue and game frames variables and the propaganda mechanisms. According to our results, the leaders also share the identification with an idealized homeland, as well as a repertoire of actions based on the provocation, polarization and protests [1]. Beyond that, this type of leader respects formal principles of democracy, but promotes anti-pluralist practices [14] and manages public emotions in a dangerous way [3].

As can be seen from Table 2, there is a thematic and strategic convergence of populist politicians with Trump, emphasizing the idea of fraud. The common thematic selection (issue frame) on conspiracy theories, migration, corruption, pandemic, foreign relations, or economic affairs is supported by strategies (game frame) of the emerging pop politics

Table 2. Distribution of messages on Twitter according to issue/game frame (%).

		Donald Trump	Jair Bolsonaro	Marine Le Pen	Matteo Salvini	Santiago Abascal	Total
Issue frame	Conspiracy theories	4.7	1.9	–	2	13.4	2.7
	Migration	3	3.2	39.7	23	10.4	17.9
	Corruption	47.5	2.3	–	0.5	3	8.2
	Gender issues	–	–	1.5	1.2	–	0.8
	COVID-19	5.5	3.7	15.3	15	16.4	12
	Environment	–	3.2	3.1	1.4	–	1.5
	Foreign affairs	0.8	5.1	13	5.4	7.5	5.4
	Economy	0.8	18.5	10.7	7.2	1.5	7.9
Game frame	Horse race	19.9	27.8	2.3	7.2	10.4	11.9
	Personal topics	1.7	1.4	9.9	7.1	7.5	5.7
	Events	5.1	23.1	1.5	7.1	6	8.6
	News management	1.7	5.6	3.1	4	3	3.7
	Others	9.3	4.2	–	18.8	20.9	13.6

[25]. This trend overlaps with the personalization of the political culture [31] as well as on a critical opinion of the mass media.

Interestingly, the most mentioned game frame is the horse race competition, with the exception of Le Pen. This finding underscores the confrontational approach applied by these leaders and preferred over other traditional game frames such as events or news management. Therefore, they clearly aim to identify enemies in their messages on Twitter, using the social network as part of a whole populist political strategy. That tendency is especially detected in Bolsonaro and Abascal, but it is Trump who main develop this sort of horse race frame. Our study empirically tests how the controversial communication of Trump could reduce the quality of the US democracy during the campaign.

However, it also is necessary to reflect upon the use of fallacy mechanisms that feed the political culture of post-truth [10] and endanger the future of consolidated democracies [2]. The reason behind is that fallacy means the principal practice for populist leaders, as it allows to spread false information connected with previous stereotypes among the citizenship. We seek to advance our understanding on this phenomenon through the frequencies of theses mechanisms in the tweets of the sample (Table 3).

Our research provides two inter-related insights to this matter. First, the data obtained offer interesting differences among populist leaders, but they share a common pattern of emotional messages. It thus illustrates the key role of appealing to emotion in their political strategies. The table also indicates that Trump combines in a regular way all the fallacies suggested by the literature [10, 38]. It could be argued that Trump was the first

Table 3. Fallacy mechanisms. Frequencies in tweets (%)

	Donald Trump	Jair Bolsonaro	Marine Le Pen	Matteo Salvini	Santiago Abascal
Appeal to authority	1.7	3.2	3.1	5.2	6
Appeal to emotion	15.2	6.9	49.6	13.2	9
Fallacy against man	0.8	3.2	–	2.2	9
Appeal to force	6.3	0.5	2.3	7	17.9
Appeal to ignorance	4.6	2.8	–	1.2	6
Using other sources	11.8	4.2	–	11.8	–
Opinions as facts	11.8	38.9	0.8	5.9	10.4
News selection	16	6	27.5	7	9

populist leader with global impact, influencing on the political landscape. In this sense, we have to take into account the inherent differences because of the political cultures. Hence, the actions of these leaders are not always homogenous.

Second, and considering the singular strategies on Twitter, our results show the use of opinions as facts by Bolsonaro and the appealing to force in the case of Spain (Abascal). These could be assessed as relevant findings, since Bolsonaro promotes a journalism based on his statements in Brazil, meanwhile Abascal reinforces the link of his party with the military. The examples point to the different applications of a global trend according to national conditions. Future studies may examine the adaption of this pattern with more data.

To summarize, most fallacy mechanisms are present in all leaders with some exceptions once again referring to Le Pen, who clearly prioritizes the appeal to emotion and the news selection. As we previously noted, they belong to the same international populist movement, developing cynical techniques to reach the voters and undermine the opponents.

3 Fact-Checking for Social Media Platforms

Social networks are blamed for a disinformation chaos, although there are many actors involved. In this regard, the confluence of political and media power has contributed more to produce lies than to avoid them. The personalization of political leaders and sensationalism prevail in the media narrative [42]. On the other hand, citizens seem to be highly influenced by social media, acting as spokesmen for fallacies [43, 47].

More specifically, the pandemic and the global crisis have triggered the reaction of institutions and digital platforms, which were until now permissive to political fraud [34, 37]. These authors suggest to develop a culture of security and media literacy that educates critical audiences and restores trust in politicians and the press. Despite the work of the fact-checking platforms [19, 26], we find out a debate on the verifiability due to the news cycle acceleration [12] and its effects on the society through the Internet [55].

There are more than 237 initiatives related to fact-checking around the world. Experts in the verification of political facts such as *Politifact* (www.politifact.com), linked to the Poynter Institute, *Factcheck* (www.factcheck.org) or the fact-checking service of *The Washington Post* (www.washingtonpost.com/news/fact-checker). Other platforms are focused on refuting fallacies of Russian propaganda *(Stop Fake*, www.stopfake.org) or the verification of rumors (*Snopes*, www.snopes.com). Those initiatives are relevant for this study, as they dealt with Trump politics in recent years.

One of the most crucial strategies has probably been the decision of platforms like Twitter to stop the messages of Donald Trump at his last presidential stage. Permanently disabling his account (@realDonaldTrump), and the collaborative work between this social network and several legacy media (@ABC; (@AP); (@CBSNews); @CNN; (@FoxNews; @NBCNews; @Reuters) are the evidence of a change in the media system. Instead of carrying out a journalism based on political statements, the transparency of the media is reinforced. The alarming events in the US have boosted a reaction against fake news that demands the recovery of the journalist's role as verifier of the facts.

According to our compilation (Table 4), the role of journalism and the news management process have a first stage (Code 1. Action) of quick dissemination of fake news [35, 49] and a second stage (Code 2. Reaction) in which quality control systems may rule the news, proposing verification strategies [41] and good practice guides like FACTS [18]. The acronym includes criteria related to the verification of sources, use of antecedents, contextual data and interpretation of the facts, avoiding bias and opinion [30].

To plan future initiatives in the framework of media literacy, we argue that a proper structuration of the current fact-checking journalism is needed. As stated, this could be really helpful in countries in which populist leaders are getting more attention. The central position in their national public spheres is embedded in a context of consolidation of digital technologies for politics. Hence, the response should combine digital and traditional logics.

To check the Journalistic Qualification Level (JQL) of a text, the following equation is applied:

JQL Journalistic Qualification Level= [V1 Presence + V2 Quantity-Diversity of Sources] + [V3 Background-Context +V4 Explanatory-Interpretative-Opinion Data]/JQL Journalistic Qualification Level

The equation has been applied to a sample of news on US elections published on their front pages by *The New York Times* (United States), *O Globo* (Brazil), *Le Monde* (France), *La Repubblica* (Italy), and *El País* (Spain) during the same data collection period as for Twitter. This equation is operationalized through a content analysis that

Table 4. Fact-checking journalism. Source: authors' compilation

Code 1. Action			Code 2. Reaction	
Stage 1 Zimdars, 2016	*Stage 2 Nielsen/Graves, 2017*	*Stage 3 Wardle, 2017*	*Stage 1 Redondo, 2018*	*Stage 2 FACTS standard (El País, 2020)*
Clickbait headlines Rumors Satire. Fake Political News Conspiracy theories Hate speech State propaganda	Soft journalism Sensationalism Lack of accuracy Hyper-partisan content Use of propaganda Use of political lies Sponsorship	Misinformation Parody Provocation Partisanship Advantage Search for political influence	Check authorship Analyze the content (What) Find the date (When) Find the place (Where) Discern Information/Opinion (How) Define the objective (Why)	Filter. Discern Facts/Opinions Avoidance Avoiding fake sites and links Consequence and Context Tests. Showing evidences Sources. Avoiding the use of conflict ones

includes evaluative and formal indicators, and parameters on theme, strategy, and language. The results show how the quality press reproduced the messages of populism and disinformation created for the campaign. There is also an information bias in the coverage of the issues shared on Twitter by the populist leaders.

The JQL should be furthered in future studies, moving forward this line of research. The data from studies on media verification models explain the importance of applying quality control processes compared to other methods proposed by fact-checking platforms, as they do not include an in-depth analysis of these values. In short, ethics and social responsibility has to be the key after times of public mistrust [5, 7]. New identity crises in journalism are looming, which overlaps with new populism and disinformation scenarios.

Some limitations of our analysis are also noted. The data obtained from populist leaders could be compared to other media systems or journalistic cultures. Besides that, we cannot assess the usefulness of the fact-checking parameters, despite some literature highlighting its relevance. More studies are needed to find causal patterns in the use of these practices to fight disinformation.

Finally, we propose that it would be noteworthy to design a world observatory led by specialized journalists to evaluate political, media and digital organizations. The dissemination of non-contrasted news and the appraisal of transparency actions are essential for a democratic society forced to reinvent itself. Beyond the uncertainty about the future of democracy, this work addresses the connection between topics, strategies and fallacies of the right-wing populism on Twitter.

References

1. Arias-Maldonado, M.: La digitalización de la conversación pública: Redes sociales, afectividad política y democracia. Revista de Estudios Políticos **173**(173), 27–54 (2016). https://doi.org/10.18042/cepc/rep.173.01
2. Beck, U.: La sociedad del riesgo global. Siglo XXI, Madrid (2002)
3. Beckett, C., Deuze, M.: On the role of emotion in the future of journalism. Soc. Media + Soc. **2**(3), 1–6 (2016). https://doi.org/10.1177/2056305116662395
4. Bennett, W.L., Livingston, S.: The disinformation order: Disruptive communication and the decline of democratic institutions. Eur. J. Commun. **33**(2), 122–139 (2018). https://doi.org/10.1177/0267323118760317
5. Bennett, W., Pfetsch, B.: Rethinking political communication in a time of disrupted public spheres. J. Commun. **68**(2), 243–253 (2018). https://doi.org/10.1093/joc/jqx01
6. Block, E., Negrine, R.: The populist communication style: toward a critical framework. Int. J. Commun. **11**, 178–197 (2017). https://bit.ly/2zGNG3s
7. Carlson, M.: Fake news as an informational moral panic: the symbolic deviancy of social media during the 2016 US presidential election. Inf. Commun. Soc. **23**(3), 374–388 (2020). https://doi.org/10.1080/1369118X.2018.1505934
8. Chadwick, A.: The Hybrid Media System: Politics and Power. Oxford University Press, Oxford (2017)
9. CNN Exit Polls 2020. https://cnn.it/2NH5phR. Accessed 17 Feb 2021
10. Crilley, R.: International relations in the age of 'post-truth' politics. Int. Aff. **94**(2), 417–425 (2018). https://doi.org/10.1093/ia/iiy038
11. Crilley, R., Gillespie, M.: What to do about social media? Politics, populism and journalism. Journalism **20**(1), 173–176 (2019). https://doi.org/10.1177/1464884918807344
12. Currie-Sivek, S., Bloyd-Peshkin, S.: Where do facts matter? Journal. Pract. **12**(4), 400–421 (2018). https://doi.org/10.1080/17512786.2017.1307694
13. Dader, J.L, Campos-Domínguez, E.: La búsqueda digital del voto. Cibercampañas electorales en España 2015–16. Tirant lo Blanch, Valencia (2017)
14. De-la-Torre, C.: Populist Seduction in Latin America. Ohio University Press, Athens (2010)
15. De-la Torre, C.: Trump's populism: LESSONS from Latin America. Postcol. Stud. **20**(2), 187–198 (2017). https://doi.org/10.1080/13688790.2017.1363846
16. Díez, J.L., Sulca, D.: El storytelling político en Twitter simultáneo a un debate electoral. Una segunda unidad para una segunda pantalla. In: Núñez Gómez, P., de Vicente, D.A.M. (eds.) Aproximación periodística y educomunicativa al fenómeno de las redes sociales, pp. 361–373. McGraw-Hill Interamericana de España, Madrid (2020)
17. Edelman Trust Barometer 2021. https://bit.ly/3qAYFkc. Accessed 18 Feb 2021
18. El País: Fórmulas para no alimentar a la bestia: la batalla europea contra las 'fake news' (2020). https://bit.ly/2LZNaUq
19. Elizabeth, J.: Who are you calling a fact checker? American Press Institute (2014). https://bit.ly/3k0tjB0
20. Enli, G.: New media and politics. Ann. Int. Commun. Assoc. **41**(3–4), 220–227 (2017). https://doi.org/10.1080/23808985.2017.1392251
21. EU vs Disinfo: Understanding the threat and stepping up European response (2018). https://bit.ly/3ude1xQ
22. European Commission: La lucha contra la desinformación en línea: un enfoque europeo. COM(2018) 236 final (2018). https://bit.ly/2NEb9Je
23. Foa, R., Mounk, Y.: The danger of deconsolidation: The democratic disconnect. J. Democracy **27**(3), 5–17 (2016). https://bit.ly/2OK0aOZ

24. Gil de Zúñiga, H., Weeks, B., Ardèvol-Abreu, A.: Effects of the news-finds-me perception in communication: Social media use implications for news seeking and learning about politics. J. Comput.-Mediat. Commun. **22**(3), 105–123 (2017). https://doi.org/10.1111/jcc4.12185
25. Gómez-García, S., Gil-Torres, A., Carrillo-Vera, J.A., Navarro-Sierra, N.: Constructing Donald Trump: Mobile apps in the political discourse about the President of the United States. [Creando a Donald Trump: Las apps en el discurso político sobre el presidente de Estados Unidos]. Comunicar **59**, 49–59 (2019). https://doi.org/10.3916/c59-2019-05
26. Graves, L.: Deciding What's True: The Rise of Political Fact-Checking in American Journalism. Columbia University Press, New York (2016)
27. Lee, S., Xenos, M.: Social distraction? Social media use and political knowledge in two US Presidential elections. Comput. Hum. Behav. **90**, 18–25 (2019). https://doi.org/10.1016/j.chb.2018.08.006
28. Levitsky, S., Ziblatt, D.: How Democracies Die. Broadway Books, New York (2018)
29. López Meri, A.: Twitter-retórica para captar votos en campana electoral. El caso de las elecciones en Cataluña de 2015. Comunicación y Hombre **12**(12), 97–118 (2016). https://doi.org/10.32466/eufv-cyh.2016.12.190.97-118
30. Mantzarlis, A.: Fact-checking 101. In: Ireton C, Posetti J (eds) Journalism, Fake News & Disinformation: Handbook for Journalism Education and Training. Unesco, París, pp. 85–100 (2018)
31. Mazzoleni, G., Sfardini, A.: Política pop. Da 'Porta Porta' a 'L'isola dei famosi'. Il Mulino, Bolonia (2009)
32. Mounk, Y.: The People vs. Democracy. Why Our Freedom Is in Danger and How to Save It. Harvard University Press, Cambridge (2018)
33. Mudde, C., Rovira Kaltwasser, C.: Studying Populism in comparative perspective: reflections on the contemporary and future research agenda. Comp. Pol. Stud. **51**(13), 1667–1693 (2018). https://doi.org/10.1177/0010414018789490
34. Naderi, N., Hirst, G.: Automated fact-checking of claims in argumentative parliamentary debates. In: Proceedings of the First Workshop on Fact Extraction and Verification (FEVER), pp. 60–65 (2018). https://doi.org/10.18653/v1/W18-5509
35. Nielsen, R.K., Graves, S.: News you don´t believe: Audience perspective on fake news. Reuters Institute for the Study of Journalism (2017). https://bit.ly/2LZR2EW
36. Panizza, F. (ed.): Populism and the Mirror of Democracy. Verso, Buenos Aires (2005)
37. Patwari, A., Goldwasser, D., Bagchi, S.: TATHYA. A multi-classifier system for detecting check-worthy statements in political debates. In: Proceedings of the 2017 ACM Conference on Information and Knowledge Management, pp. 2559–2562 (2017). https://doi.org/10.1145/3132847.3133150
38. Pérez-Curiel, C.: Trend towards extreme right-wing populism on Twitter. An analysis of the influence on leaders, media and users. Commun. Soc. **33**(2), 175–192 (2020). https://doi.org/10.15581/003.33.2.175-192
39. Pérez-Curiel, C., Limón Naharro, P.: Influencers de la Política. Estudio de la marca personal de Donald Trump en Twitter y efectos en medios y usuarios. Commun. Soc. **32**(1), 57–76 (2019). https://doi.org/10.15581/003.32.1.57-76
40. Pew Research Center: Sharp Divisions on Vote Counts, as Biden Gets High Marks for His Post-Election Conduct (2020). https://pewrsr.ch/3ayjCa9
41. Redondo, M.: Desinformación: pulsa aquí y te sorprenderá. Cuadernos de Periodistas **36**, 40–56 (2018). https://bit.ly/2NAlupQ
42. Rivas-de-Roca, R., García-Gordillo, M., Bezunartea-Valencia, O.: The far-right's influence on Twitter during the 2018 Andalusian elections: an approach through political leaders. Communication & Society **33**(2), 227–242 (2020). https://doi.org/10.15581/003.33.2.227-242

43. Rodríguez-Ferrándiz, R.: Posverdad y fake news en comunicación política: breve genealogía. El profesional de la información **28**(3) (2018). https://doi.org/10.3145/epi.2019.may.14
44. Runciman, D.: How Democracy Ends. Basic Books, New York (2018)
45. Stromer-Galley, J.: Presidential Campaigning in the Internet Age. Oxford University Press, Oxford (2014)
46. The Guardian: The new populism. Revealed: the rise and rise of populist rhetoric (2019). https://bit.ly/3kcgST7
47. Vosoughi, S., Deb, R., Sinan, A.: The spread of true and false news online. Science **359**(6380), 1146–1151 (2018). https://doi.org/10.1126/science.aap9559
48. Waisbord, S.: Truth is what happens to news: on journalism, fake news, and post-truth. Journal. Stud. **19**(13), 1866–1878 (2018). https://doi.org/10.1080/1461670X.2018.1492881
49. Wardle, C.: Fake news. It's complicated. First Draft (2017). https://bit.ly/3qwylYt
50. Washington Post-ABC: Misinformation dropped dramatically the week after Twitter banned Trump and some allies (2021). https://wapo.st/2NHc5wr
51. Woertz, E., Slocum, J., Colomina, C., Bourekba, M., Owczarek, D.: El populismo en Europa: ¿de síntoma a alternativa? Cidob, Barcelona (2017)
52. Woolley, S.C., Howard, P.N.: Computational propaganda: political parties, politicians, and political manipulation on social media. Oxford Scholarship Online, London. (2018). https://doi.org/10.1093/oso/9780190931407.001.0001
53. World Health Organization-WHO: Munich Security Conference 2020 (2020). https://bit.ly/3s5o0Dn
54. Zimdars, M.: False, misleading, clickbait-y, and satirical "news" sources (2016).
55. Zubiaga, A., Liakata, M., Procter, R., Hoi, G., Wong, S., Tolmie, P.: Analysing how people orient to and spread rumours in social media by looking at conversational threads. PLoS ONE **11**(3), e0150989 (2016). https://doi.org/10.1371/journal.pone.0150989

LatamCovidNewsCheck. Meta-classification of Fact Checking Platforms in Latin America During the Covid-19 Pandemic

Ignacio Balcázar[1], Angel Torres-Toukoumidis[1](✉), and Gabriela Balcazar[2]

[1] Universidad Politécnica Salesiana, Cuenca 010105, Ecuador
ibalcazar@est.ups.edu.ec, atorrest@ups.edu.ec
[2] Universidad de Cuenca, Cuenca 010107, Ecuador
gabriela.balcazar@ucuenca.edu.ec

Abstract. The COVID-19 disease hit the world, especially Latin America, unveiling another equally serious pathology, the virus of fake news, which spreads on a large scale thanks to the Internet, especially social networks, where thousands and millions of Internet users share information lacking scientific support. This work contributes to show and verify a dozen fact-checking agencies in Latin America, their regulations and operation. For this purpose, 12 agencies in Latin America were studied and verified for their review protocols, objectives and categorization of news, in order to establish a fact-checking format. The results obtained from this research show significant data, in terms of formal aspects the tendency was to clarify and verify the news, in the search objectives section, the agencies were linked to controversy, disinformation and public debate, going through their different categorizations or batteries used, the most common of which were true, false, misleading, among others, to end with a fact-checking model for Latin America.

Keywords: Fact-checking · Categorization · Covid-19 · News · Latin America

1 Introduction

During the health emergency, the proliferation of false news and rumors related to the situation produced by the virus has spread in an unprecedented way, so much so that this information intoxication was declared by the World Health Organization as one of the greatest risks produced by the digital communication ecosystem [1]. The viralization of this content through social networks, instant messaging services, among other spaces of virtual interaction is playing a relevant role in the democratic development of nations, compromising the principles of transparency and credibility [2].

This situation has attracted the special attention of the academic community, which has presented alternatives to solve the contingencies, highlighting long-term options such as the promotion of critical skills in citizens [3]; establishing media regulation policies without infringing free speech [4], while in the short term: incorporating campaigns to combat rumors [5]; promoting the dissemination of official spokespersonship [6]; and using fact-checking platforms [7].

© The Author(s), under exclusive license to Springer Nature Singapore Pte Ltd. 2022
Á. Rocha et al. (Eds.): ICOMTA 2021, SIST 259, pp. 104–113, 2022.
https://doi.org/10.1007/978-981-16-5792-4_11

Particularly, the first premise of this research is based on the analysis of fact-checking platforms, known as a journalistic practice dedicated to the verification of true facts to combat the dissemination of false news and thus mitigate its effect on citizens [8], which have been the subject of study during the pandemic. Among the most recognized research is the analysis of the narratives coming from informative disorders demonstrating the response capacity of the verifiers to detect false news [9]; the importance of professional journalism to perform news checks in digital communication [10]; practical recommendations to mitigate disinformation [11]; and linkage between typologies of disinformation with hoaxes intentionality and dissemination channels [12].

The following premise responds to the Latin American context on the use of these platforms during the pandemic, both general and specific case studies are presented. Regarding general studies, there is exclusively the presentation of a quantitative analysis of disinformation through Latam Chequea [13]; review of the degree of informative openness of Latin American governments regarding the coronavirus according to news verifiers in those countries with the highest number of infected people [14]. While referring to specific cases, there is Brazil in which the trends of the content reviewed by the platforms Aos fatos and Agencia Lupa in relation to political decisions are identified [15] and Ecuador performing an analysis of periodicity and sources of Ecuador Chequea to classify the veracity of the information [16].

Although there is extensive scientific literature devoted to the connection between verification platforms and Covid-19, two issues can be glimpsed that justify the innovative nature of this research. The first of these focuses on the symmetry of methodological parameters for classifying hoaxes, i.e., as a premise of this research, a review of procedures and evaluation categories used by news verifiers linked to Covid-19 is prescribed. The second problem is the lack of studies oriented to news verifiers in Latin America. In short, we seek to establish an assessment based on the following questions:

1. What is the purpose of the methodologies used by news verifiers from Latin America?
2. What review protocols do news verifiers from Latin America apply?
3. What type of categorization do Latin American news verifiers include on pandemic-related information?

The incorporation of the "Covid-19 pandemic" case serves the primary purpose of pre-selecting the news sampling, facilitating the localization and reiteration of protocols and categorization in news verifiers due to the over-saturation of the news [17]. Therefore, the following general objective is derived: to examine the methodological symmetry of the news checkers deriving the following specific objectives: to identify the purpose exposed by each Latin American fact-checking; to compare the categories presented by the Latin American fact-checking; and to design a common archetype of news verification on the classifications provided in Latin America.

2 Methodology

This research is prescriptively oriented towards an inductive approach, as it proceeds from a review of particular cases of fact-checking from Latin America to determine a generic perspective towards finality, protocols, and categorization. Regarding the methodological design, content analysis is used. Although content analysis inherently resorts to quantitative studies, the qualitative approach to the subjective interpretation of textual and audiovisual data through the systematic classification process of coding and identification of themes or patterns is also evident [18]. Recognizing this argument, on this occasion, the data are sought from the official web pages attached to the International Fact-Checking Network (IFCN) of the Poynter Institute [19], specifically 12 agencies from Latin America, as shown in Table 1.

Table 1. Fact-checking agencies and country

Fact-checking agency	Country	Website
Agência Lupa	Brazil	https://piaui.folha.uol.com.br/lupa/
Animal Político - El Sabueso	Mexico	https://www.animalpolitico.com/elsabueso-rss/
Aos Fatos	Brazil	https://www.aosfatos.org/
Bolivia Verifica	Bolivia	https://boliviaverifica.bo/
Chequeado	Argentina	https://chequeado.com/
Colombiacheck	Colombia	https://colombiacheck.com/
Cotejo.info	Venezuela	https://cotejo.info/
Ecuador Chequea	Ecuador	http://www.ecuadorchequea.com/
Estadão Verifica	Brazil	https://politica.estadao.com.br/blogs/estadao-verifica/
Silla Vacía	Colombia	www.lasillavacia.com
Agência Pública - Truco	Brazil	https://apublica.org/checagem/
Grupo La Republica Publicaciones SA	Peru	https://larepublica.pe/verificador/

Three phases were established for the methodological procedure of the research. The first is a detailed review of the verification methodologies, protocols and verification exposed by the fact-checking agencies, where the formal characteristics of each website are observed, which can be found mainly on the home page. The second phase, instead, is located as axis the analyzed news about the Covid-19 pandemic limiting from April 2020 to April 2021 obtaining 749 pieces of news that were verified in the mentioned agencies, the purpose of this phase is to recognize the existing proportion on the exposed categories for each of the verification agencies, thus recognizing the implication of the assigned classification. The last phase or third phase of the procedure is to build a singular classification-LatamCovidNewsCheck-which seeks to establish review parameters extracted from the patterns evidenced.

The compiled information was compiled in an Excel document organized by each news verification agency, thus allowing the comparison of the formal aspects as well as the news about the pandemic. As for the coding of qualitative character applied content analysis, the so-called axial coding was used, defined as the determination of connections and relationships between the codes [20], thus arranging the relationship between agencies and news obtained.

3 Results

3.1 Formal Aspects of News Verification Agencies

Regarding the first categorization in terms of the formal aspects of the 12 verification agencies in Latin America, it is evident that the value "mission" tends to clarify and verify political messages, proposals, and freedom of expression, as an example we have Ecuador Chequea with its objective: To lead processes that guarantee the freedoms of expression and association, it should be noted that among the most used words would be: politicians, corruption. As for the value "objectives", the terms most used by the different agencies are polemic, disinformation, public debate, as an example we have Aos Fatos from Brazil: monitor power.

Finally, we have the value "protocols", in this section the news agencies based their protocols of searches and alerts, in social networks, also, the severity, incidence, or "what noise it makes" within the social spectrum, as an example we show the Group La República Publicaciones of Peru: 1-Select a suspicious content of the social networks that are monitored. 2-Find its relevance. 3-Consult, when identifiable, the source. 4-Consult, if identifiable, those involved/affected in the disinformation. 5-Consult the official source. 6-Consult alternative sources. 7-Give context. 8-Confirm or deny the content.

In short, the most reiterated formal aspects are focused on clarification, trends and verification, polemic, disinformation and public debate within news verifiers in Latin America, this implies that verification agencies are aware of trends, debates and above all what is implied in terms of disinformation generated by these two aforementioned elements.

3.2 Categorization of News About Covid-19. *LatamCovidNewsCheck*

Parallel to the formal aspects and recognizing that this is an exploratory analysis focused on the pandemic, 749 verified news items were analyzed, which are organized as follows:

1. Ecuador Chequea: 176 news items.
2. Bolivia Chequea: 169 news items.
3. Chequeado de Argentina: 85 news.
4. Agência Pública - Truco from Brazil: 76 news.
5. Agência Lupa from Brazil: 57 news.
6. La Silla Vacía: 51 news.
7. Cotejo de Venezuela: 48 news.
8. ColombiaCheck: 26 news.
9. Animal Político - El Sabueso de México: 20 news.
10. Aos Fatos from Brazil: 16 news.
11. Grupo La República Publicaciones of Peru: 15 news.

12. Estadão Verifica from Brazil: 10 news.

Based on the number of selected news items linked to the Covid-19 pan-demic and coming from the 12 Latin American verification agencies, the most reiterated categories were reviewed to formalize a classification oriented to this juncture.

In first place is Ecuador Chequea, in which 176 news items related to the pandemic were found, representing 23.4% of the sample, being the verification agency with the highest number of news items reviewed in Latin America on this situation. The news verification is organized in 4 categories:

1. True (8.4%): the statements of political subjects that are accurate.
2. Yes, but (3.9%): the statements are partially truthful data.
3. Unsustainable (3.1%): any expression that does not allow to directly identify the arguments.
4. False (16.4%): a statement that openly contradicts the objective data.

Next, Bolivia Verifica presented 169 articles related to the pandemic, which represents 22.5% of the sample, organized in 5 categories:

1. True (4.8%): contrasted with the most serious and reliable sources and data.
2. False (14.1%): the affirmations lack support and are not coherent.
3. Undoubtedly (2.2%): no explanation is needed.
4. Misleading (1.2%): the statement may partially coincide with certain data, but -intentionally or unintentionally.
5. Explanatory (0.2%): clarification by the person who exposed the news.

On the other hand, Chequeado from Argentina, which has 85 (11.3%) news items, maintains two rating systems, one for the verification of the discourse to leaders, and the other for viral misinformation, in this case, we stick to the second system, obtaining 4 categories:

1. True (3.4%): the entire shared content has proven to be true, by being contrasted with the actors involved and the most serious and reliable sources and data.
2. Deceptive (2.2%): part of the shared content may coincide with certain true data, but -intentionally or not- was manipulated to generate a particular message.
3. False (5.1%): the entire content shared has proven to be false when contrasted with the actors involved and the most serious and reliable sources and data.
4. Unsustainable (0.4%): the claim arises from research with a lack of evidence or serious methodological errors, or is impossible to verify.

The Agência Pública - Truco of Brazil, ranked fourth in terms of the number of news items related to Covid-19 with 10.1%, representing 76 news items. For this, the categories assumed by this checker have been these 7 categories:

1. True (2.9%): analysis of the data and other sources shows that the statement is true. Rounded data are also considered true.

2. No context (0.8%): The statement contains correct information or data, but lacks the context that is important for understanding the facts.
3. Debatable (0.6%): The conclusion about the statement varies according to the methodology adopted.
4. Exaggerated (0.3%): The statement carries inflated data or is an exaggerated statement about a true fact or trend.
5. Understated (1.5%): The statement contains understated data or is an understated statement about a true fact or trend.
6. Unprovable (0.7%): At the time of testing, there are no reliable published data or studies to support this statement.
7. False (3.3%): Analysis of data and other sources shows that the statement is false and does not correspond to reality.

The news checker called Agência Lupa from Brazil gathers a total of 57 articles related to the pandemic, representing 8.1% of the sample, being the fourth agency with the highest amount of news related to the pandemic, evidencing 8 categories of news:

1. True (2.1%): the information has been proven to be correct.
2. True, but (0.7%): The information is correct, but the reader deserves more detail. 3.
3. Still early to say (0.4%): The information may turn out to be true. not true.
4. Exaggerated (0.1%): The information is on the right track, but there was an exaggeration.
5. Contradictory (0.5%): The information contradicts other information.
6. Unsustainable (0.4%): There is no public data to prove the information.
7. False (3.7%): The information is proved incorrect.
8. And of eye (0.2%): Follow-up label.

La Silla Vacía with 51 articles (6.8%) place the articles on the pandemic in the section called lie detector, configured in 8 categories:

1. True (1.3%): reflects recent and reliable information on the issue.
2. True but (0.8%): reflects recent and reliable information on the subject but leaves out a relevant aspect to understand it.
3. Rushed (0.5%): the statement refers to an event that has not yet culminated and therefore anticipates its conclusions.
4. Debatable (0.2%): the statement corresponds to a position of a fact that has solid foundations, but other alternatives also have strong foundations.
5. Exaggerated (0.3%): the statement reflects a true trend or fact but takes it beyond what is shown by the most recent and reliable information on the subject.
6. Misleading (0.5%): the statement is an argument that starts from a true fact to reach an incorrect conclusion.
7. False (2.5%): the information is false in the light of the most recent and reliable information on the subject.
8. Uncheckable (0.7%): the statement cannot be checked either because there is no recent and reliable information on the subject or because it is an opinion.

Cotejo de Venezuela contains 48 verified news items represented by 6.4% of the Covid-19, aligned to 3 categories:

1. truth (2.1%): the evaluated speech or data is true, it is real, it is true.
2. Half-truth (0.7%): the speech or data evaluated is a manipulation of the facts or data presented or an omission of relevant information that does not allow the evaluation to be classified as truth or lie.
3. Lie (3.6%): the evaluated speech or data is false, unreal, uncertain.

Colombiacheck gathers a total of 26 news items, which represents 3.5% of the total number of news items reviewed, occupying the fourth place according to the number of articles related to the pandemic with 5 categories:

1. True (0.8%): when, upon verifying the data of a statement, we find that these correspond exactly with the reality of the facts.
2. True, but (0.5%): the information follows the most recent available data, but leaves out some important part of its context.
3. False (1.3%): the information presented is completely contrary to the reality of the facts.
4. Questionable (0.2%): uses more recently available data, but is used to reach erroneous conclusions, or there is no consensus on what is the correct interpretation.
5. Unchallengeable (0.7%): there is no reliable data to determine its veracity, or that the data corresponds to an opinion.

Animal Político - El Sabueso de México, only 20 news items referring to the pandemic have been found, which is close to 3% of the total number of articles consulted, with 7 categories.

1. Misleading (0.4%): the information shown may be biased.
2. False (1.3%): the information is not true.
3. Inaccurate (0.3%): it maintains a frivolity in its content.
4. Lying with the truth (0.1%): information misrepresented or taken out of context.
5. True (0.6%): real news.
6. Ridiculous (0.2%): focused on sensationalism or sensationalism.
7. Debatable (0.1%): maintains parameters that can be edited for better understanding.

Regarding the number of news items examined for the Aos Fatos Agency of Brazil, 16 news items related to the pandemic were observed, corresponding to 2.1% of the total, which are distributed in 7 categories:

1. False (0.8%): incorrect information is available.
2. True (0.6%): the information is validated with the truth from a reliable source.
3. Contradictory (0.2%): the information is presented in the direction of recurrent information to the refutation.
4. Incorrect (0.2%): has confusing information that is not clarifying.
5. Exaggerated (0.1%): responds to yellowish information.

6. Distorted (0.1%): information with clear signs of inflation of the facts.
7. Unsustainable (0.1%): there is no information to corroborate the news.

On the other hand, Grupo La República Publicaciones S.A. from Peru, with 15 news items (2%), presents 4 categories:

1. False (0.9%): it is oriented to lack of veracity.
2. True (0.6%): implies clarity and reality concerning a statement or event that has occurred.
3. Deceptive (0.2%): it is based on certain elements to support a conclusion that does not coincide with reality.
4. Imprecise (0.3%): the information is unsustainable or there are not enough elements to qualify it as true or false.

Finally, Estadão Verifica from Brazil, represented by articles, is the agency with the lowest number of news items associated with the pandemic, representing only 1.3% of the total sample, in which there are 4 categories.

1. True (0.3%): Real news or statement.
2. False (0.8%): Incorrect news or statement.
3. Misleading (0.1%): News or statement with a degree of fraud or inaccuracy.
4. Out of context (0.1%): News took out of context.

After reviewing and cross-checking the information from the 12 agencies mentioned above, it was determined that an efficient system for discarding and clarifying false news from real news would be to categorize their batteries as follows: 1°true/true, 2°false/lie, 3°misleading, 4°unsubstantiated, 5°true, but, 6°contradictory, 7°unaccurate for pandemic news. In the case of review protocols, it is evident that an optimal fact-checking format would be: 1°monitoring and observation of news, 2°popularity or viralization of social networks, or politicians, 3° search for information (sources, documents, publications) expert analysis, 4°contextualization, 5°classification of the content according to the established categories (Table 2):

Table 2. LatamCovidNewsCheck criteria

Criteria	Points
1°- False/Lie	12 points
2°- True	9 points
3°- Deceptive	4 points
4°- Unsustainable	3 points
5°- True, but	2 points
6°- Contradictory	2 points
7°- Imprecise	2 points

4 Conclusions

After analyzing 12 news verification agencies in Latin America, the need to study and verify the different aspects, both formal and categorical, was reaffirmed to finally establish a fact-checking model.

The first objective was oriented to review the formal aspects of news verification agencies, and three subcategories of analysis emerged: mission, protocols and objectives. Regarding the subcategory called mission, the clarification and verification of political messages, proposals and freedom of expression were observed, followed by the protocols being the tendency to search and alerts in social networks, as well as the seriousness and incidence within the social aspect that generates the different news. As for the objective aspect, the term most used by the different agencies was controversial, disinformation and political debate.

The second objective corresponds to review the categories presented by the 12 agencies studied, of which different positions were found, for example, Bolivia Verifica has different working standards, Chequeado from Argentina has a double categorization system, one of them being the public verification method, and the second the method of verification of speech to leaders. It is worth mentioning that in two verification agencies a specific categorization was not found, I looked for it both on their website and in their social networks.

The third objective was oriented to establish a news verification format after all the information gathered in the two previous objectives, which allowed to establish a format and guide for subsequent journalists or media outlets to take and apply it in their different facets of journalism or information. It should be emphasized that although this categorization comes from an exploratory analysis oriented towards Latin American verification agencies and that at the same time there were limitations referred to the time analyzed, it is intended that future researchers apply the model called LatamCovidNewsCheck to optimize the evaluation and automation in the news review process.

References

1. Sohrabi, C., et al.: World Health Organization declares global emergency: a review of the 2019 novel coronavirus (COVID-19). Int. J. Surg. **76**, 71–76 (2020)
2. Arce, K., Torres-Toukoumidis, A.: Percepción de la educomunicación institucional en Facebook. Caso coronavirus-Ecuador. Servicio Editorial de la Universidad del País Vasco, Spain (2021)
3. Sánchez Tarragó, N.: Desinformación en tiempos de COVID-19: ¿Qué podemos hacer para enfrentarla? Revista Cubana de Información en Ciencias de la Salud **31**(2), (2020).
4. Rodrigues, U.M., Xu, J.: Covid19. Regulation of COVID-19 fake news infodemic in China and India. Media Int. Aust. **177**(1), 125–131 (2020)
5. Campbell, K.M., Doshi, R.: The coronavirus could reshape global order. Foreign Affairs 18 (2020)
6. Zarocostas, J.: How to fight an infodemic. Lancet **395**(10225), 676 (2020)
7. Kim, H., Walker, D.: Leveraging volunteer fact checking to identify misinformation about COVID-19 in social media. Harvard Kennedy School Misinf. Rev. **1**(3) (2020)

8. Vizoso, Á., Vázquez-Herrero, J.: Plataformas de fact-checking en español. Características, organización y método. Commun. Soc. **32**(1), 127–144 (2019)
9. García-Marín, D.: Infodemia global. Desórdenes informativos, narrativas fake y fact-checking en la crisis de la Covid-19//Global infodemic: information disorders, false narratives, and fact checking during the Covid-19 crisis. Profesional de la Información **29**(4) (2020)
10. Torres-Toukoumidis, A., Lagares-Díez, N., Barredo-Ibáñez, D.: Accountability journalism during the emergence of COVID-19: evaluation of transparency in official fact-checking platforms. In: Rocha, Á., Reis, J.L., Peter, M.K., Cayolla, R., Loureiro, S., Bogdanović, Z. (eds.) Marketing and Smart Technologies. SIST, vol. 205, pp. 561–572. Springer, Singapore (2021). https://doi.org/10.1007/978-981-33-4183-8_44
11. Krause, N.M., Freiling, I., Beets, B., Brossard, D.: Fact-checking as risk communication: the multi-layered risk of misinformation in times of COVID-19. J. Risk Res. **23**(7–8), 1052–1059 (2020)
12. Sánchez-Duarte, J.M., Rosa, R.M.: Infodemia y COVID-19. Evolución y viralización de informaciones falsas en España. Revista Española de Comunicación en Salud 31–41 (2020)
13. López-Pujalte, C., Nuño-Moral, M.V.: La "infodemia" en la crisis del coronavirus: Análisis de desinformaciones en España y Latinoamérica. Revista española de Documentación Científica **43**(3), 274–285 (2020)
14. Díez-Garrido, M., Farpón, C.R.: La transparencia institucional y mediática del coronavirus. Un análisis de los portales de datos y de los medios de comunicación digitales en Iberoamérica. Revista Latina de Comunicación Social (78), 393–418 (2020)
15. Ceron, W., de-Lima-Santos, M.F., Quiles, M.G.: Fake news agenda in the era of COVID-19: Identifying trends through fact-checking content. Online Soc. Netw. Media **21**, 100–116 (2020)
16. Bermello, G.L.V.: Inmediatez y fact-checking: análisis del portal Ecuador Chequea. Revista ABRA **40**(61), 63–87 (2020)
17. Orso, D., Federici, N., Copetti, R., Vetrugno, L., Bove, T.: Infodemic and the spread of fake news in the COVID-19-era. Eur. J. Emerg. Med. **27**(5), 327–328 (2020)
18. Hsieh, H.F., Shannon, S.E.: Three approaches to qualitative content analysis. Qual. Health Res. **15**(9), 1277–1288 (2005)
19. Poynter. Code of Principles. EEUU: Commit to transparency. https://ifcncodeofprinciples.poynter.org. Accessed 25 Feb 2021
20. Valdés, G.L.P.: La codificación Axial, innovación metodológica. RECIE. Revista Electrónica Científica de Investigación Educativa, **3**(1), 497–509 (2016)

The Media and the Spanish Monarchy: The Mediating Role of Ideology

Antonio Garrido Rubia(✉), Antonia Martínez Rodríguez, and Alberto Mora Rodríguez

University of Murcia, Avenida Ronda de Levante, 10, 30008 Murcia, Spain
{agarrido,antoniam,alberto.mora}@um.es

Abstract. This article analyses the impact of news coverage of the previous monarch, Juan Carlos I, on the image of the monarchy. To respond to the proposed objectives, a standardised questionnaire was designed and implemented in which 9,420 people from the different autonomous communities in Spain participated, testing a multiple linear regression model and a binomial logistic regression model, in addition to different bivariate techniques of statistical analysis. The study confirms the existence of partisan audiences in the Spanish media system. Finally, the study demonstrates a clear relationship between consumption of certain channels and types of media and the impact of the news on the monarchy, although this relationship is mediated by the ideology of individuals. In this respect, this research provides evidence of the importance of political predispositions in the selection of the information provided by different media, and how this affects the perception of political objects, specifically in this case for the Spanish monarchy.

Keywords: Monarchy · Selective perception · Cognitive dissonance · Mass media · Opinion research

1 Introduction: The Media and Selective Perception

The confidence that individuals have in a country's institutions is influenced by the ideas that the media transmit about those institutions. There is disagreement about the extent to which the media influence or model citizens' attitudes and opinions about political subjects, among other things. The "hypodermic needle" theory, which suggests that the individual is a blank canvas on to which information is projected by the mass media, has been followed by the theory of selective perception. These approaches suggest that individuals follow, or are exposed to, types of information that are consistent with their existing beliefs and that individuals demonstrate the opposite behaviour when faced with information that questions those pre-existing ideas. Consequently, the media play an essential role in reinforcing existing attitudes [6, 13]. These ideas are continued with the theory of cognitive dissonance, developed by Festinger. This approach indicates that the individual aims to achieve consistency. If a person knows various things that are not psychologically consistent with one another, he will try to make them more consistent and his opinions and attitudes will be expressed in ways that are internally coherent [7]. A similar analysis had been previously undertaken by Lazarsfeld and others in their

© The Author(s), under exclusive license to Springer Nature Singapore Pte Ltd. 2022
Á. Rocha et al. (Eds.): ICOMTA 2021, SIST 259, pp. 114–122, 2022.
https://doi.org/10.1007/978-981-16-5792-4_12

studies on political behaviour [16]: "The fact that people select their exposure along the line of their political predispositions is only a special case of a more general law which pervades the whole field of communication research. Exposure is always selective; in other words, a positive relationship exists between people's opinions and what they choose to listen or to read." These analyses gave rise to a focus on the limited effects of the media, which developed in different ways before crystallising into what is known as Klapper's "reinforcement theory" [15]: the media do not change citizen's opinions, they simply reinforce existing beliefs.

From these approaches, different studies in social psychology and communication have been conducted on how individuals experience selective exposure to information in such a way that this idea has become central in the study of communication processes. The question is to what extent the media persuade people to change their opinions and how receptive individuals are to different sources of information. Information campaigns affect above all those who are already convinced. Festinger [7] stresses that issues that go contrary to individuals' opinions create dissonance and the more deeply held the belief or assessment is, the greater the dissonance. Therefore, the individual will tend to follow types of information which are more aligned to their values and opinions and avoid information which goes contrary to their beliefs [20,21].

Different field studies have empirically compared approaches to cognitive dissonance such as Donsbach, as well as survey data from electoral campaigns and studies regarding editorial bias in the press and attitudes to the Iraq War [5]. The idea that individuals select information which conforms to their own beliefs [10] continues to be a very fruitful assessment framework in communication, as is shown by, among other issues, the application of the concept of cognitive bias—with regards to the mental framework for receiving information, particularly ideology—in communicative processes and political campaigns, among others [6].

In the Spanish case, there are few studies which focus on the relationship between selective partisan bias and the media, although previous studies have shown the existence of relationships between voting history and a preference for certain media [11] and the influence of media coverage on electoral behaviour [1]. Equally, the hypothesis of selective exposure [5] has been confirmed and different studies have referenced the fact that political journalism in Spain is characterised by a high level of polarisation and a high degree of ideological alignment [23].

This study will analyse the relationship between the perception of the institution of the monarchy and the media.

2 Monarchy: Trust, Ideology and Selective Perception

One aspect that is of interest to researchers from different fields is the factors affecting citizen trust in democratic institutions. Studies have been published since 2008 about how the economic and political crisis has affected trust in successive governments, parliament and political parties in Spain [19], while analysis of other institutions, such as the monarchy, are almost non-existent, perhaps because of the difficulty in accessing information about the institution, both in Spain and in other parliamentary monarchies [9].

Some researchers have questioned whether citizens use the same criteria to assess all institutions; whether some are more trustworthy than others or whether trust is related to the economy or other social variables [14, 18, 22]. Similarly, other studies have attempted to find a connection between relationships between citizens and the elite and political distrust as well as trust in institutions and emotional polarisation [17]. At these times of economic and political crisis, deepened by the consequences of the Covid pandemic, such issues acquire an importance that goes beyond academic analysis; they receive greater media attention and are present in discussions among politicians and citizens. In this context, the answers are also scrutinised and other relationships are sought, to which this study aims to contribute, based as it is on a specially designed survey.

There has been exhaustive historical research and some legal discussion about the regulation of our head of state, but little analysis of the monarchy by other disciplines [26]. In other contexts, such as the United Kingdom, in addition to traditional approaches based on history and law, from the 1970s onwards, studies of the monarchy began to be published which focused on media influence on people's attitudes, as well as studies of political culture [27] and social representation. In recent times, this research has also included a focus based on political communication, the analysis of discourse, framing [4] and branding, which have conceptualised different monarchies as "corporate heritage brands" [2].

The few studies assessing the king and the monarchy in Spain conclude that: "it has been the most highly valued institution since the beginning of the transition to democracy and this continued support does not appear to be related to changes in how other institutions in the country are viewed" [8]. This approach remained valid until the financial crisis of 2008. After that point, the level of trust that Spaniards placed in the monarchy and other institutions was affected [9]. Despite this, empirical studies on the institution of the monarchy continue to be scarce, making the aim of this article all the more relevant.

3 Objectives, Hypotheses, Method and Variables

This study aims to answer the following question: What is the relationship between the news that people follow about former king Juan Carlos I and the main types of media people use to find out the news? This question was used to create a research hypothesis that the type of media people follow for news and current affairs depends on their ideology and is related to the influence of news about Juan Carlos I. To contrast the research hypothesis a bivariate analysis strategy was conducted, with statistical inference.

In order to conduct this research, an online survey was created and sent to professors at different universities in the country and the sample was configured through snowball sampling and viralisation on social networks. This made it possible to configure a representative sample in terms of age and weighted by autonomous communities to represent Spain as a whole. Given the sensitivity of the research aims to political variables, the sample was weighted by reported voting history. However, it should be highlighted that the aim of this research is to observe and analyse the relationships produced between the key variables, not to conduct a study of societal opinions and attitudes regarding the issue under analysis.

A total of 9,420 people from different autonomous communities in Spain participated in the study. Of these people, 56% were men and 44% women, aged between 18 and 85 years old. Fieldwork was conducted between 31 August and 15 September 2020. A structured, closed survey with few questions was used. It was adjusted to create a model that could be administered to a pre-test of 50 people in order to resolve problems of understanding. The internal consistency of the indicators was also analysed. The study included the following variables, in response to the issues covered in the theoretical framework and the definition of the research hypothesis:

- Exposure to news content: Participants in the study were asked to what extent they watched the news on different media channels with the aim of informing themselves about the monarchy. This made it possible to measure the degree of exposure to television, radio, press and social media. The level of consumption of each type of media was measured on a Likert-type scale from 1 «not at all» to 5 «a great deal». The internal consistency of the indicator ($\alpha = 0.446$) was calculated from the sum and average of the four variables.
- Assessment of Juan Carlos I: Participants were asked to evaluate the emeritus king, Juan Carlos I. A scale of 0–10 was used.
- Ideology: A scale of 1 «left» to 10 «right» was used.
- Main television channel, frequency of radio and press used to follow news and current affairs.
- Knowledge of stories published in the preceding weeks in some media with regards to emeritus king, Juan Carlos I.
- The effect of that news on the participant's view of the Spanish monarchy. This variable was converted to an ordinal value of between 0 "no effect" and 3 "a large effect".

Other categorical variables were also included, such as sex, age, occupation, level of education and voting history in the November 2019 general election.

4 News Monitoring and the Impact of Scandal on the Perception of the Spanish Monarchy

One of the aims of this study is to analyse the relationship between the media and the perception of the Spanish monarchy. In this section, the aim is to confirm whether the hypothesis that the type of media that people follow for news is determined by ideology and the relationship to the influence of news coverage of Juan Carlos I.

As can be seen in Table 1, the ideological self-location of voters who prioritise certain media to inform themselves about politics—in this case, about the November 2019 general elections—shows clear politicisation and reproduces similar dynamics to those seen in the opinion study that was prepared ad-hoc for this article. These findings align with studies that have previously established the existence of partisan audiences in the Spanish media system [12, 13].

For this research, participants were asked if they had heard news published in the preceding weeks about the emeritus king, Juan Carlos I. 97.3% of those interviewed stated they had heard the news. Of those, 49.5% stated that their opinion of the Spanish

Table 1. Data Ideological self-location of voters who follow a specific media outlet (scale of 1–10).

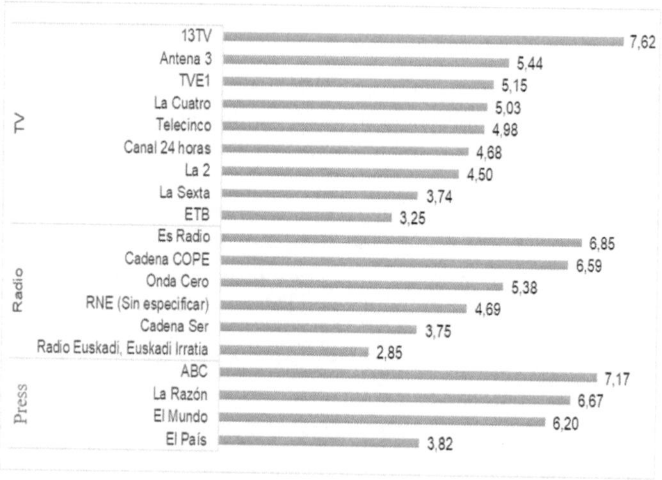

Source: Own elaboration. Post-electoral study of November 2019 general elections (E. Nº 3269) by CIS (Centre for Sociological Research).

monarchy was unchanged, while 25.1% said it was much more negative, 10.4% said that it was rather more negative and 14.4% stated that it was slightly more negative. As noted above, the choice of channels that people use to follow the news is the result of a process that is influenced by political predispositions. Festinger's pioneering study [7] established the tendency for individuals to avoid situations that will produce cognitive dissonance. That is to say, they tend to pay attention to and process information that will not create cognitive disruption and that is consistent with their pre-existing beliefs. The following paragraphs aim to analyse the way participants search for information and investigate whether that is consistent with their political predispositions.

In this section, first we aim to analyse the relationship between ideology and the impact that news about the emeritus king has had on the perception of the Spanish monarchy. As can be observed in Fig. 1, the further to the left that the participants place themselves on the ideological scale, the greater the self-recognised impact of news about Juan Carlos I on their perception of the Spanish monarchy. The ANOVA analysis of a factor between the two variables shows that a statistically significant relationship exists between both questions ($F = 279.33$; $p < 0.001$). Similarly, on conducting a multiple comparison analysis using the Bonferroni method, it is clear there are significant differences in all groups except between those who state that their opinion of the monarchy "is slightly more negative" and those who say it has remained the same.

We then aim to analyse the mean ideological position of participants with regards to the different media they use to follow news on radio, television and in the press, as well as the average perception of the influence of scandals on those preferences. The first issue to mention is that the average differences of the two variables (ideology and the

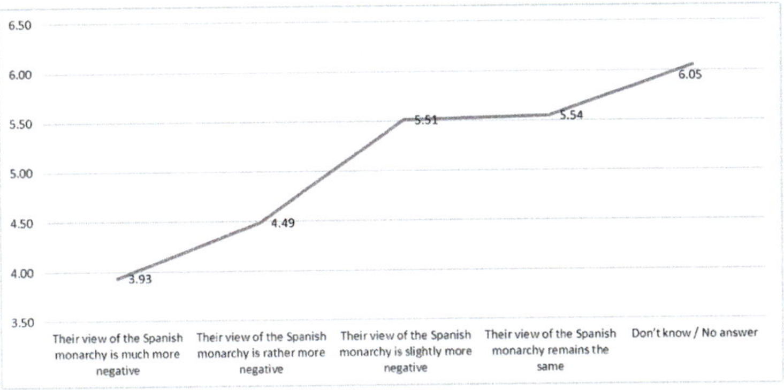

Fig. 1. Ideological self-location and impact of the information on the perception of the Spanish monarchy. Source: Own elaboration.

influence of scandals) are statistically significant in the three types of media that were analysed.

With regards to the press, in Fig. 2, we can see that the ideological profile of the readers of different newspapers varies significantly, with readers of ARA placing themselves further to the left (3.56) and readers of ABC further to the right (7.09). In terms of the two national newspapers with the highest circulation, readers of El País were located at 4.41 on the scale and readers of El Mundo at 6.39. If we consider the perception of the influence of scandals, this was greater in participants who read El Periódico de Catalunya and ARA and lower in readers of ABC and La Razón. The association between the three variables is linear. This linearity is modulated in the case of the Basque newspaper ARA. Although it has the most readers who self-locate on the left of the ideological scale, those readers perceive the influence of scandals as slightly lower than for consumers of the next newspaper on the scale. This dynamic is reproduced in Basque media on the three news channels that were studied: despite having consumers who place themselves further to the left ideologically, the perception of the influence of scandals is not the most extreme.

The radio station whose listeners locate themselves the furthest to the left on the ideological scale is Radio Euskadi (2.92), while esRadio listeners are the furthest to the right in ideological terms (7.21 out of 10). Two leading stations, Cadena SER and La COPE, have listeners who place themselves at 3.73 and 6.79 respectively (Fig. 3). These relationships between ideology and preferred radio stations are consistent with the results of the CIS (Centre for Sociological Research) study, which included these questions[1]. The radio users who felt that the scandals surrounding the emeritus king had most negatively affected their perception of the monarchy were those who listened to Catalunya Radio and Cadena SER listeners, while La COPE and esRadio listeners stated that they had very little effect.

With regards to television channels (Fig. 4), once again, it is the Basque channel ETB which has more followers on the left of the ideological scale, while followers of

[1] For example, in the 2016 and 2019 post-election studies, which asked participants their preferred newspaper, radio station and television channel for following political and electoral news.

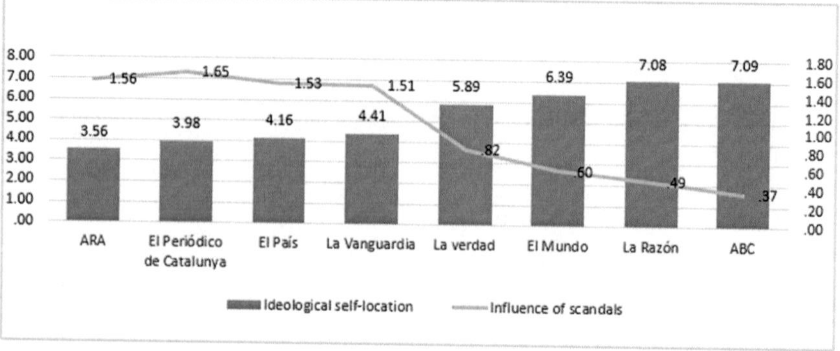

Fig. 2. Printed or digital newspaper most often used to follow news and current affairs. Source: Own elaboration. The range of news has been selected with n > 100

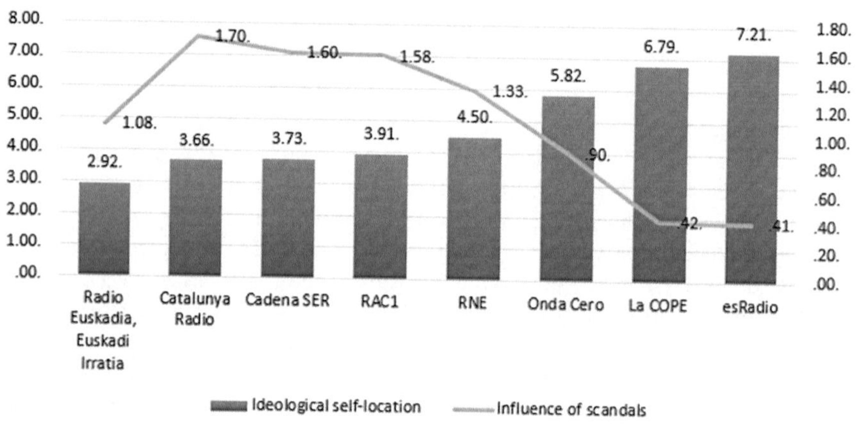

Fig. 3. Preferred radio station for following the news. Source: Own elaboration. The range of news has been selected with n > 100

13TV placed themselves on average at 7.34 out of 10. La 2, TVE1 and Canal 24 horas had the most followers at central positions on the ideological scale (4.17, 4.58 and 5.06 respectively). Viewers who felt that the scandals surrounding the emeritus king had most negatively affected their perception of the monarchy followed news on La Sexta (1.68) and TV3 (1.61), while those who were less affected were viewers of 13TV and Antena 3.

These data corroborate the hypothesis and show that the media that people follow depends on their ideology and is also related to the influence of news coverage of Juan Carlos I. The association between ideology, the influence of news about Juan Carlos I and preferred news outlets reveals an important divide in the attitudes of the different ideological poles, with significantly more moderate behaviour, which was more to the right in ideological terms, of those participants who self-located at central positions on the ideological scale.

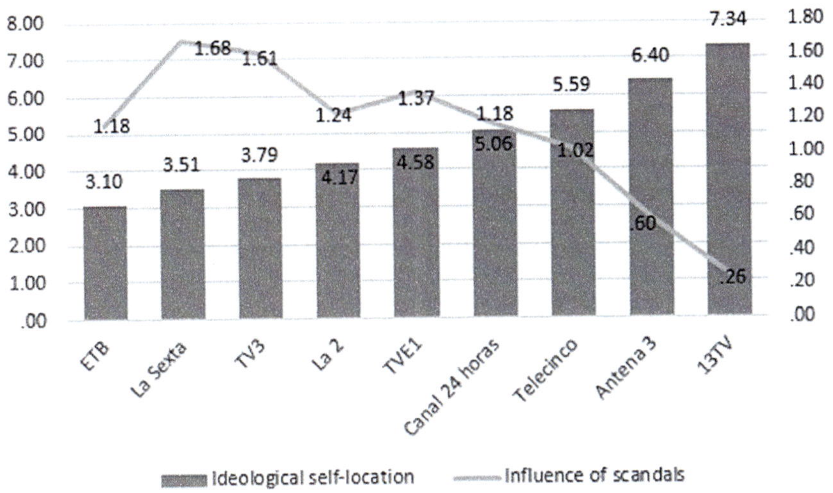

Fig. 4. Preferred television channel for following the news. Source: Own elaboration. The range of news has been selected with n > 100

5 Conclusions

In recent months there has been more intense public debate about the need to reform how Spain is governed. This debate has been affected by different types of information, which have appeared in the media, and which relate to the former Spanish king. There are very few studies available which would allow us to understand Spaniards' views on one of the issues that has been present in public debate to different degrees since the beginning of the political transition, and this is an area to which this study aims to contribute.

The main conclusion aligns with cognitive dissonance and selective perception theories and the role of the media in those processes. In this respect, the data show that the participants follow news about the monarchy, and particularly about scandals surrounding alleged irregularities committed by Juan Carlos I, using media that are more in accordance with their ideology.

References

1. Alcalde Villacampa, J.: Medios de comunicación como intermediarios del voto: la influencia de TVE1 y Antena 3 en las elecciones legislativas de 1993. REIS **104**(3), 145–178 (2003). https://doi.org/10.2307/40184572
2. Balmer, J.M.T., Greyser, S.A., Urde, M.: Monarchies as Corporate Brands. Harvard Business School, Working Paper, 05-002 (2004)
3. Barredo, D.: El tabú Real. La imagen de una monarquía en crisis. Editorial Berenice, Córdoba (2013)
4. Martin LLaguno, M., Berganza, M.R.: Votantes y medios de comunicación en las elecciones nacionales españolas de 1996: ¿exposición selectiva o influencia mediática? Comunicación y sociedad XIV, (1), 51–70 (2001)

5. Best, S.J., Chmielewski, B., Krueger, B.S.: Selective exposure to online foreign news during the conflict with Iraq. Harv. Int. J. Press/Polit. **10**, 52–70 (2005). https://doi.org/10.1177/1081180x05281692
6. D'Adamo, O., García, V., Freidenberg, F.: Medios de comunicación, efectos políticos y opinión pública. Una imagen ¿vale más que mil palabras? Belgrano, Argentina (2000)
7. Festinger, L.: Cognitive dissonance. Sci. Am. **207**(4), 93–102 (1962)
8. García del Soto, A.: Representaciones sociales y fundamentos básicos de la cultura política: opiniones intergeneracionales sobre la Monarquía española [tesis doctoral]. Centro de Estudios Avanzados en Ciencias Sociales del Instituto Juan March de Madrid (1999). https://digital.march.es/fedora/objects/fjm-pub:1106/datastreams/OBJ/content
9. Antonio Garrido, M., Martínez, A., Mora, A.: Monarquía y opinión pública en España durante la crisis: el desempeño de una institución no responsable bajo estrés. Revista Española de Ciencia Política **52**, 121–145 (2020). https://doi.org/10.21308/recp.52.05
10. Gerber, A., Green, D.: Misperceptions about perceptual bias. Annu. Rev. Polit. Sci. **2**, 189–210 (1999). https://doi.org/10.1146/annurev.polisci.2.1.189
11. Gunther, R., Montero, J.R., Wert, J.I.: The media and politics in Spain: from dictatorship to democracy. WP, 176, Institut de Ciencies Polítiques i Socials (1999)
12. Hallin, D.C., Mancini, P.: Comparing Media Systems. Three Models of Media and Politics. Cambridge University Press, Londres (2004)
13. Humanes, M.L.: Exposición selectiva y partidismo de las audiencias en España. El consumo de información política durante las campañas electorales de 2008 y 2011. Palabra Clave **17**(3), 773–802 (2014). https://doi.org/10.5294/pacla.2014.17.3.9
14. Hetherington, M.J., Rudolph, T.J.: Political trust and polarization. In: Uslaner, E. (ed.) The Oxford Handbook of Social and Political Trust. Oxford University Press, Londres (2018). https://doi.org/10.1093/oxfordhb/9780190274801.013.1
15. Klapper, J.T.: The Effects of Mass Communication. Free Press, Mumbai (1960)
16. Lazarsfeld, P.F., Berelson, B., Gaudet, H.: The People's Choice. How the Voter Makes Up His Mind ina Presidential Campaign. Columbia University Press (1944)
17. Listhaug, O., Jakobsen, T.G.: Foundations of political trust. In: Uslaner, E. (ed.) The Oxford Handbook of Social and Political Trust. Oxford University Press (2018). https://doi.org/10.1093/oxfordhb/9780190274801.013.14
18. Rothstein, B., Stolle, D.: The state and social capital: an institutional theory of generalized trust. Comp. Polit. **40**, 441–467 (2008). https://doi.org/10.5129/001041508X12911362383354
19. Rifà, R.: Actitudes políticas en tiempos de crisis. La confianza en las instituciones políticas de España [tesis doctoral]. Universidad Autónoma de Barcelona (2017). https://www.tdx.cat/handle/10803/454992
20. Taber, C.S., Lodge, M.: Motivated skepticism in the evaluation of political beliefs. Am. J. Polit. Sci. **50**, 755–769 (2006). https://doi.org/10.1111/j.1540-5907.2006.00214.x
21. Taber, C.S., Cann, D., Kucsova, S.: The motivated processing of political arguments. Polit. Behav. **31**(2), 137–155 (2009). https://doi.org/10.1007/s11109-008-9075-8
22. Uslaner, E.: The Oxford Handbook of Social and Political Trust. Oxford University Press (2018). https://doi.org/10.1093/oxfordhb/9780190274801.001.0001
23. van Dalen, A., de Vreese, C., Albæk, E.: Different roles, different content? A four-country comparison of the role conceptions and reporting style of political journalists. Journalism **13**(7), 903–922 (2012). https://doi.org/10.1177/1464884911431538

Post-feminism and Post-truth in Reggaeton Video Clips on Youtube

Dámaris Beatriz Alcántara-Segura(✉) and Lorena Teresa Espinoza-Robles(✉)

Universidad Peruana de Ciencias Aplicadas, Lima, Peru
{u201522117,pcavlesp}@upc.edu.pe

Abstract. In the music industry, reggaeton is an urban genre most played on digital platforms such as YouTube. From its beginnings a musical genre that transmitted denigrating messages of women image. Today, these messages have changed due to the incursion of female artists who adopt values associated with the masculine to reinforce an image of empowerment. These artists promote post-feminist messages from the narrative of their songs and music videos, legitimizing representations based on the narrative they propose from fiction. This article analyzes the representation of women in six Karol G reggaeton video clips broadcast on YouTube through a case study with a narrative and gender approach. A content analysis guide was applied to 320 video captures and an interview guide to the art director in charge of Pineapple and Mi cama video clips. The main finding of the research was to show that the narrative and the staging build a post-truth of female empowerment from fiction to show us a convincing story. However, this post-truth legitimizes characters such as the sexual entrepreneur by appealing to the same feminine objectification of the beginnings of the urban genre. Therefore, this study contributes to the existing literature of pervasive communication on social media and post-truth in audiovisual fiction.

Keywords: Post-feminism · Post-truth · Reggaeton

1 Introduction

In the Latin American context, visual content is usually created by reinforcing stereotypes in gender roles [1], the feminine as dependent on the man, housewife, decorative and sexual object [2] and the masculine as defiant, with courage and power [3]. Likewise, there are narratives that use post-truth from fiction, just to show us convincing stories through images [4]. This leads to a symbolic production in digital, cultural and gender studies, which contributes to the deconstruction of the "patriarchal gaze" present in the West through the media and entertainment [5, 6]. In this context, the video clip [7] arises as part of the musical mainstream that is promoted on YouTube and receives thousands of views [8].

However, just as music transmits emotions [9] it also generates spaces for discussion that purify tastes, destroy cultures and diversity [10]. The music video clip as a product integrates the figure of the artist as a brand within its narrative [11, 12] and influences the

© The Author(s), under exclusive license to Springer Nature Singapore Pte Ltd. 2022
Á. Rocha et al. (Eds.): ICOMTA 2021, SIST 259, pp. 123–130, 2022.
https://doi.org/10.1007/978-981-16-5792-4_13

tastes of its target audience. Likewise, the narrative in music video clips is complemented by art direction [13]. In this way the art direction achieves a powerful symbology that generates stereotypes in the mind of the public [14].

1.1 Normalized *Machismo* in Reggaeton Music Videos

In Latin America, reggaeton arises as an underground movement by expressing social denunciations, but over time it has been considered as a hyper-masculine gender whose messages oscillate between phallocentrism and misogyny [15, 16].

Artists such as Daddy Yankee with his most listened hit on Spotify *Gasolina* (2004), and years later Maluma with *Cuatro Babys* (2016) have generated repudiation in society by promoting objectification and presenting different types of violence against women to enhance their masculinity [15, 17].

1.2 New Feminist Proposals in the Reggaeton Industry

For many years, the male gender has dominated this musical category [18, 19]. In this context, Ivy Queen was the first singer who managed to position herself in that scene, focusing her messages on class and gender inequalities [16, 20]. This new empowered woman challenged the ideology of patriarchy and gender discrimination [10, 21, 22].

The post-feminism of these proposals revalued female desire and hispersexuality as a sign of empowerment and of being a sexual subject [23–26]. The female protagonist began to have aggressive behavior in audiovisual formats [23, 25–29]. This provoked a double discourse that evidenced a feminine individualism that displaced women from object to sexual subject [25, 30–33].

However, in the Latin American context, this was new, despite the fact that, for other cultures, Latinas were considered as a sensual and sexual attraction [27]. This generated a change in the production of reggaeton videos and the appearance of female artists such as La Materialista that showed a confident and determined woman in her goals [17, 34]. Then, the figure of the sexual entrepreneur emerges, who plays with the processes of self-objectification, and shows the purchasing power through consumption as a sign of female empowerment [17, 25]. In this scenario, the singer Karol G arises, with a proposal that continues in this way.

2 Methodology

This research applied a qualitative approach under the interpretive paradigm [35, 36]. A case study was designed [37] applied to a sample of six video clips of reggaeton songs performed by the singer Karol G between 2017 and 2019 (see Table 1). The video clips were selected for their scope, as they have more than 150 million views [38–43]. This sample was segmented from the lyrics of the songs and a content analysis was applied to 320 images captured from the six video clips.

The categories of analysis were character construction [44] and staging [45]. In the staging, costumes [13] and scenography with decorations [46] were considered.

Finally, a semi-structured interview [47] was applied to Lucas Spot Flaco, art director of the Colombian audiovisual company 36 Grados. This company made Pineapple and Mi Cama video clips, which are part of the sample of this research.

Table 1. Video clips analyzed

Video clips	Performer, album and release date	Views on Youtube
Ahora me llama (AML)	Karol G, Bad Bunny Unstoppable 26/05/2017	803 M [38]
Pineapple (P)	Karol G Ocean 01/03/2018	205 M [39]
Mi cama (MC)	Karol G Ocean 10/05/2018	661 M [40]
Culpables (C)	Karol G, Anuel AA Ocean 04/04/2019	832 M [41]
Punto G (PG)	Karol G Album: Ocean 04/04/2019	165 M [42]
Tusa (T)	Karol G, Nicki Minaj KG0516 7/11/2019	867 M [43]

2.1 Ethical Considerations

The interview with Lucas Spot Flaco was conducted on September 27, 2020 by a virtual videoconferencing platform in the context of the COVID-19 pandemic. The interviewee was informed of the nature of the investigation and gave his informed consent about the use of his statements.

3 Results and Discussion

3.1 Sexual Agency in the Female Empowerment Narrative

From the analysis proposed to the six videos in the sample (see Table 1), it was evidenced that Karol G's lyrics constantly allude to values such as women's individual freedom, authenticity and success, related to empowerment through sexual agency (see Table 2). In the AML, P and C videos the woman faces a breakup or disappointment in love or an intimate encounter, playing with the feelings or emotions of the opposite sex. Karol G gives agency to her character, desires and also wants to be desired [23].

In this regard, Spot Flaco points out the presence of a movement in Karol G's audio-visual repertoire [48]. Karol G's repertoire, like that of other popular artists, sells us the idea of the independence and autonomy of women, in which they do not need a man [24]. However, this autonomy or liberation is reflected in a sexualized dance, which exploits the female body through flirtatious pelvic and hip movements [27]. The artist becomes

Table 2. Lyrics with sexual agency

Video clips	Lyrics translated (originally in Spanish)
Ahora me llama (AML)	*"I'm single and I do what I want and nobody lifts my skirt... I continue to make fame, later I see that which boy took to my bed"*
Pineapple (P)	*"If I turn off the light, you want to turn it on. That I know that you prefer to touch what you want to see... Ask me everything your body wants"*
Mi cama (MC)	*"Your key no longer fits in my lock. That fever that someone else brings you down... My bed rings and rings"*
Culpables (C)	*"Whenever we do it, we can't avoid the urge that we have... Oh, how delicious, as we give each other. He now calls me saying that he misses me in his bed"*
Punto G (PG)	*"Turn off the light, I prefer it dark. What you want, I already thought about it first"*
Tusa (T)	*"She is hard and abuses, she is tired of being good, now she is the one who uses them... She goes out to the disco and she just wants to dogging"*

hypersexual and exploits the representation of Latin American women in popular culture: short stature, mixed skin, and painted hair.

Karol G constructs the physical dimension of her character based on Latin American beauty, as it was mentioned the conception of femininity as a bodily property. The woman is "sexy" in order to feel powerful in the male gaze. She performs for the camera and for the audience, she frequently shows her lips and thus reveals her sensuality [49]. Close-ups are often used to show the physical attributes of the artist, which is in sync with camera movements and video editing [26]. She positions herself with the idea of a woman who accepts her body, enjoys it and is not perfect. She shows an erotic image like Madonna [23] and Beyoncé [26], but her contents are more inclusive, they move away from the Eurocentric or North American gaze. In MC's video, her character is related to a community in Medellin that is part of the video clip. In PG's video clip she includes Afrodescendants and in P's, overweight people, usually invisible in this type of content.

The artist's messages always go along the lines of female empowerment. However, the hierarchy that is established between the characters within the fiction shows the centrality of Karol G and a dynamic similar to that of the initial video clips of the urban genre, where the dancers were an accompaniment. In the sample it is observed that the dancers are a kind of lackey of Karol G and we see that the values associated with the male figure are now represented by her. Karol G acts under the "male gaze" or a man point of view, thus contributing to the deconstruction of the "patriarchal gaze" that has been present in Latin America for years until today [5]. It is a hybrid of discourses, on the one hand sexual freedom and on the other, oversexualization [17]. As in PG, where she alludes in the lyrics to the erogenous zone of the woman's genital area, reinforcing the oversexualization with pelvic movements in front of the camera. On the other hand, Karol G in the AML and C video clips relates to male artists and shows great complicity and physical and sexual attraction in which she dominates the relationship as a sexual entrepreneur.

From this analysis, it was identified that the narrative of the video clips avoids presenting male domination relationships. On the contrary, a woman is observed sure of herself regarding her corporality and sexuality. However, there are certain characteristics of the artist that through her fictional characters, seeks to create a new image of women's bodies and behavior in order to deconstruct the "patriarchal gaze".

3.2 Female Empowerment from the Art Direction

The company 36 Grados arrived at Karol G at the time of "romantiqueo", a stage of the urban genre where a new aesthetic began to be proposed in reggaeton videos, based on new proposals in the action of the artists, singers and dancers that change the mood of the stories [48]. From the art direction, strong symbologies are proposed in the public mind and at the same time in the generation of stereotypes [14]. In the video clips analyzed, worlds that are far from reality are planned from recording studios and decorated with very little props, as in the case of AML, which present the artist as distant and unattainable. In the studio scenes Karol G projects power as in AML or T. In T she is shown in unreal spaces as when she appears with two white horses that allude to the pegasi of Greek mythology. In these "beauty shots" there is no narrative thread in relation to the story, but rather they are moments that are enhanced from the scenography, through the art direction [48].

The narrative in Karol G's stories sometimes breaks in those scenes of the video where there is no narrative arc with the sole purpose of highlighting the star, however Spot Flaco refers that the artist always proposes a common thread, with beginning, middle and end, despite these narrative breaks [48]. In those cases, the story continues to be told from elements of color, props, styling, scenery, decorations that contribute to reinforcing the empowerment of women in fiction, but with elements that are usually associated with the male domination of the urban genre. The use of gold jewelry, high-value alcoholic beverages, clothing from recognized brands and the latest model cars consolidate the image of the sexual entrepreneur in fiction, drawing on the values promoted by male singers at the beginning of the urban genre. The figure of a vintage-style upholstered sofa in her video shows the artist in the center of the image on a kind of throne, pretending to be a "queen of sensuality". The woman becomes the center from her beauty, as in T where we see diamonds in the female characters, as well as fine household items, associating the value of wealth and the exclusive to the feminine. In another case, the use of water to highlight her voluptuous figure with a translucent and soaked wardrobe. Or when she collects religious references, as in the case of P, with the serpent that refers to the myth of Adam and Eve, where Eve eats the forbidden fruit [48].

Finally, the color palette determines the mood of the video clip. White and black or sepia are tones that are used to reflect memories, dreams, thoughts or sadness [48], as in the betrayal of the characters in C. Color is used to lead the user through a proposal full of sensoriality centered on the impressive image of the artist. In P, neon colors are shown that reflect the dream that Karol G had with a pineapple. In T, when representing the goddess that refers to Greek mythology, pastel colors are shown. In MC, the vibrant colors highlight the warmth of the artist's visit to a community that celebrates Christmas in Medellin. While in AML and PG cold tones are shown as colors ranging from green to blue, to make the artist cooler. The scenography as well as the color proposal contribute to create a staging that highlights the centrality of the artist at any time. A centrality that plays with the change of image or makeover [33] where the character created by the artist in fiction goes back and forth from post-feminist values to the traditionality of certain values of male domination where the woman is associated with the beauty, the elegant and the sexy.

4 Conclusions

We conclude that videoclips analyzed evidence a post-feminist construction in the physical, social and psychological dimensions of the character and art direction. However, despite the fact that the artist seeks to break gender stereotypes, in many scenes she moves in a constant game of meanings that show a devalued view of women. Post-feminist reggaeton presents a dual message, on one hand it empowers and on the other hand it objectifies. To that extent, we conclude that the video clips of the artist on YouTube selected by her scope show the handling of a post-truth of female empowerment from fiction. The staged narratives associated with entertainment in an intrinsic way possess and viralize values of the society that houses them, however, narrative content legitimized by these messages is not questioned as they are fictional products. This research has been conducted in the field of critical studies applied on audiovisual formats of musical genres employing data from videoclips viralized on social media to promote a Latin American reggaeton star, which have become an important media phenomenon on Youtube. Therefore, this study contributes to the existing literature of pervasive communication on social media and post-truth in audiovisual fiction.

Aknowledgements. This study has been supported by the Universidad Peruana de Ciencias Aplicadas (UPC) through the UPC Research Incentive Fund (2021).

References

1. Vaca, B., Carpio, L., Barrazueta, P., Ordóñez, K.: Los estereotipos y la representación de género en la publicidad ecuatoriana. RISTI - Rev. Iber. Sist. e Tecnol. Inf. E26, 335–348 (2020)
2. Bittner, V., Mensa, M.: Portraits of women: Mexican and chilean stereotypes in digital advertising. Commun. Soc. **33**, 63–78 (2020). https://doi.org/10.15581/003.33.1.63-78
3. Kang, J.A., Hubbard, G.T., Hong, S.: Gender and credibility in branded storytelling. Gend. Manag. **34**, 702–714 (2019). https://doi.org/10.1108/GM-02-2019-0015
4. Keyes, R.: The post-truth era (2011)
5. Marzal-Felici, J.: Propuestas para el estudio de las imágenes en la era de la posverdad. El Prof. la Inf. 1–18 (2021). https://doi.org/10.3145/epi.2021.mar.01
6. Gabelas, J., Marta-Lazo, C.: Los influencers, oráculos del liderazgo, chamanes en las redes sociales. In: Aparici, R. and García Marín, D. (eds.) La Posverdad. Una cartografía de los medios, las redes y la política. p. 201. Gedisa (2019)

7. Roncallo, S., Uribe-Jongbloed, E.: La estética de los videoclips: Propuesta metodológica para la caracterización de los productos audiovisuales musicales. Cuad. Music. Artes Vis. y Artes Escenicas. **12**, 79–109 (2017). https://doi.org/10.11144/Javeriana.mavae12-1.evpm
8. Guarinos, V., Sedeño-valdellós, A.: El videoclip social . Análisis de su narrativa y estética Social music video. Narrative and aesthetic análisis. methaodos. Rev. ciencias Soc. **8**, 120–129 (2020)
9. Sánchez-Olmos, C.: Formatos y sectores en el branded content musical: videoclip y moda, pop stars de la musicidad. Rev. Mediterránea Comun. J. Commun. **9**, 1–16 (2018). https://doi.org/10.14198/medcom2018.9.2.5
10. Bicudo, A.: Women's representations in advertisements: conceptual explorations/As representações das mulheres em propagandas: explorações conceptuais. Rev. Estud. Da Ling. **28**, 747–776 (2020). https://doi.org/10.17851/2237-2083.28.2.747-776
11. Sánchez, C., Segarra, J., Hidalgo, M.: Brand placement in billboard hot 100 music videos: brand integration or imposition? Tripodos **44**, 63–81 (2019)
12. Villalustre, L., Del Moral, E.: Digital storytelling: Una nueva estrategia para narrar historias y adquirir competencias por parte de los futuros maestros. Rev. Complut. Educ. **25**, 115–132 (2014). https://doi.org/10.5209/rev_RCED.2014.v25.n1.41237
13. Bordwell, D., Thompson, K.: Arte cinematográfico (2003)
14. Vegas, F.: Cine, videoclip americano y videoclip japonés: la dirección de arte como hilo conductor. El caso de Not Another Teen Movie. Fotocinema. Rev. científica cine y Fotogr. **11**, 235–260 (2015)
15. Arévalo, K., Chellew, E., Figueroa-Cofré, I., Arancibia, A., Schmied, S.: Ni pobre diabla, ni candy: Violencia de género del reggaetón. Rev. Sociol. **33**, 7–23 (2018). https://doi.org/10.5354/0719-529X.2018.51797
16. Goldman, D.E.: Walk like a woman, talk like a man: Ivy Queen's troubling of gender. Lat. Stud. **15**, 439–457 (2017). https://doi.org/10.1057/s41276-017-0088-5
17. Dávila, V.: Acelerando la femenidad en el reggaetón: La chapa que vibran de La Materialista. In: Nadal-Ramos, V. and Smith Silva, D. (eds.) Perspectives on Reggaeton. pp. 59–66. University of Puerto Rico (2016)
18. Carballo, P.: Reggaeton e identidad masculina. Cuad. Inter.c.a.mbio sobre Centroamérica y el Caribe **3**, 87–101 (2006)
19. de Toro, X.: Métele con candela pa' que todas las gatas se muevan. Identidades de género, cuerpo y sexualidad en el reggaetón. Rev. Punto Género. 81–102 (2011). https://doi.org/10.5354/0719-0417.2011.16824
20. Báez, J.M.: "En mi imperio": Competing discourses of agency in Ivy Queen's reggaetón. Cent. J. **18**, 62–81 (2006)
21. Kang, J.A., Hubbard, G.T., Hong, S.: Gender and credibility in branded storytelling. Gend. Manag. Int. J. **34**, 702–714 (2019). https://doi.org/10.1108/GM-02-2019-0015
22. Erazo, M., Jiménez, M., López, C.: Empoderamiento y liderazgo femenino; su papel en la autogestión comunitaria en el corregimiento El Hormiguero-Valle Del Cauca. Av. en Psicol. Latinoam. **32**, 149–157 (2014). https://doi.org/10.12804/apl32.1.2014.10
23. Tortajada, I., Araüna, N.: Mujeres, violencia y posfeminismo en los videos de Madonna. Área Abierta **14**, 24–40 (2014). https://doi.org/10.5209/rev
24. Araüna, N., Tortajada, I., Figueras-Maz, M.: Feminist reggaeton in Spain: young women subverting machismo through 'Perreo.' Young **28**, 1–18 (2020). https://doi.org/10.1177/1103308819831473
25. Gill, R.: Empowerment/Sexism: figuring female sexual agency in contemporary advertising. Fem. Psychol. **18**, 35–60 (2008). https://doi.org/10.1177/0959353507084950
26. Hansen, K.A.: Empowered or objectified ? personal narrative and audiovisual aesthetics in beyoncé' s partition. Pop. Music Soc. **7766**, 0–17 (2015). https://doi.org/10.1080/03007766.2015.1104906

27. Arrizón, A.: Latina subjectivity, sexuality and sensuality. Women Perform. **18**, 189–198 (2008). https://doi.org/10.1080/07407700802495928
28. Lindsay, S., Lyons, A.C.: "Pour it up, drink it up, live it up, give it up": masculinity and alcohol in pop music videos. Men Masc. **21**, 1–21 (2018). https://doi.org/10.1177/1097184X17696189
29. Tortajada, I., Araüna, N., Willem, C.: From bullfighter's lover to female matador: the evolution of madonna's gender displays in her music videos. Catalan J. Commun. Cult. Stud. **9**, 237–248 (2017). https://doi.org/10.1386/cjcs.9.2.237_1
30. McRobbie, A.: Post - feminism and popular culture. Fem. Media Stud. **4**, 255–264 (2004). https://doi.org/10.1080/1468077042000309937
31. McRobbie, A.: The aftermath of feminism. Gender, Culture and Social Change. Nouv. Quest. Fem. **28**, 14–34 (2009). https://doi.org/10.3917/nqf.281.0014
32. Gill, R.: Postfeminist media culture: Elements of a sensibility. Eur. J. Cult. Stud. **10**, 147–166 (2007). https://doi.org/10.1177/1367549407075898
33. Giraldo, I.: Posfeminismo / Genealogía, geografía y contornos de un concepto. Debate Fem. 59, 1–30 (2019). https://doi.org/10.22201/cieg.2594066xe.2020.59.01
34. Benavides, C.: Los estereotipos femeninos en los videos musicales del género reggaeton: una cuestión de género. Rev. Estud. 187–200 (2007)
35. Creswell, J.W.: Qualitative Inquiry and Research Design. SAGE, Los Angeles (2013)
36. Given, L.M. (ed.): The Sage Encyclopedia of Qualitative Research Methods (2008)
37. Daymon, C., Holloway, I.: Qualitative Research Methods in Public Relations and Marketing Communications. Routledge (2011)
38. Karol, G.: Karol G, Bad Bunny - Ahora Me Llama (Official Video). https://www.youtube.com/watch?v=4NNRy_Wz16k
39. Karol, G.: Karol G - Pineapple (Official Video). https://www.youtube.com/watch?v=8q1NFlE17qs
40. Karol, G.: Karol G - Mi Cama (Official Video). https://www.youtube.com/watch?v=8-mloCL49vs
41. Karol, G.: Karol G, Anuel AA - Culpables (Official Video). https://www.youtube.com/watch?v=xfdG6vwIGGU
42. Karol, G.: Karol G - Punto G (Official Video). https://www.youtube.com/watch?v=sgBZVLr91ug
43. Karol, G.: Karol G, Nicki Minaj - Tusa (Official Video). https://www.youtube.com/watch?v=tbneQDc2H3I
44. McKee, R.: El guión story: sustancia, estructura, estilo y principios de la escritura de guiones. Alba Editorial, Barcelona (2016)
45. Casetti, F., Di Chio, F.: Cómo analizar un film (2007)
46. León, L.: Un acercamiento a la dirección de arte en el videoclip colombiano desde el recorrido de "Aterciopelados" (2011)
47. Mason, J.: Qualitative Researching. SAGE Publications (2002)
48. Spot Flaco, L.: Interview to Lucas Spot Flaco by Dámaris Alcántara (2020)
49. Railton, D., Watson, P.: Music video and the politics of representation (2011)

Check for updates

Twitter and Politics: An Analysis of the Account of Former Peruvian President @MartinVizcarraC Before and During the Pandemic

Francisco Arbaiza[1] (✉), Tomás Atarama-Rojas[2], and Ricardo Atarama-Rojas[3]

[1] Universidad Peruana de Ciencias Aplicadas, Lima, Peru
francisco.arbaiza@upc.edu.pe
[2] Universidad de Piura, Piura, Peru
[3] Posavi Group, Piura, Peru

Abstract. This research addresses the dynamics that developed on the official Twitter account of Peru's former president, Martín Vizcarra, before and during the Covid-19 pandemic. In the analysis, four trends crucial to political activity via Twitter are explored. These are the predominance of the emotional and affective component, the growing influence of fake news, deepening polarization that prevents dialogue, and the use of the platform as an information window. Results show that the pandemic effected a change in the account's dynamics and audience participation: posting frequency on the @MartinVizcarraC account decreased, but Twitter users' engagement more than doubled compared with the pre-pandemic period. In addition, the account strongly tended toward predominance of the emotional and affective component and informative value was the second most relevant topic for Vizcarra's account. The communication of @MartinVizcarraC was unidirectional, focusing on the dissemination of content and avoiding conversation.

Keywords: Twitter · Politics · Affectivity · Fake news · Polarization · Information · Peru

1 Introduction and Literature Review

As social networks have increased the communicative power of citizens and their possibilities to access information (p. 473) [2], political communication faces these networks' omnipresence to reach and connect with audiences. Twitter has emerged as the preferred channel for political communication since it avoids journalistic and traditional media intermediation. The platform allows authorities or political leaders to propose the desired frame to reach the audience directly [14]. Twitter's success "is due to the possibility of real-time access to information, that is, the possibility it offers its users to launch or collect direct and immediate testimonies" (p. 1278) [3].

The characteristics of this social network allow it to be considered a propitious platform for developing a form of participatory democratic commitment [13], increasingly

© The Author(s), under exclusive license to Springer Nature Singapore Pte Ltd. 2022
Á. Rocha et al. (Eds.): ICOMTA 2021, SIST 259, pp. 131–139, 2022.
https://doi.org/10.1007/978-981-16-5792-4_14

turning into "a substitute communication channel for the traditional press release, more laborious and less universal in scope" (p. 69) [5]. Twitter has become an option for following and participating in political news, as it is an open network where information flow is available to any user [16].

In this context, this study focuses on the exploration of a specific case in relation to four trends used for political communication via Twitter. The account of the former president of Peru, @MartinVizcarraC, is studied to recognize if emotional and affective messages predominate; if fake news are disseminated, corrected, or clarified; if it falls into a dynamic of polarization; and if the platform is used as an information window.

The dynamics of the predominance of the emotional component on Twitter enable the formation of digital communities as result of affective construction [7], where expressive use and emotional bonding prevail [1]. This affective bond is recognized in the use of the platform and highlights that gratification of social needs plays an important role in sustaining its use (p. 467) [10], as political communication responds to a predominantly emotional discourse [18]. Hansen et al. [11] found that communication with positive feelings favors content virality when there is an affinity with that community.

These digital communities are formed via the circulation of affection that brings together some users with certain groups but not with others [7]. The social network's algorithm shows the messages to those who are more related to the ideas that are expressed in a certain space. In effect, the transfer of politics to the digital environment produces a sentimental effect on public conversation and representative democracy [1] because it facilitates more direct and closer citizen participation in public affairs [3].

Cabezuelo Lorenzo and Manfredi (p. 272) [2] showed that fake news are part of post-truth, which "can be a lie assumed as truth or even a lie reinforced as a belief or as a fact shared in a society through the different digital tools that exist." In the absence of control or immediate verification mechanisms, Twitter becomes a platform where large groups of followers can be misinformed instantly; when many share content, it begins to be considered true. This is sustained by Twitter's nature, which favors discourses that are simple, impulsive, and politically incorrect [17].

In the post-truth context, "objective facts influence less the formation of public opinion than appeals to emotion and personal belief" (p. 472) [2]. In this sense, the framing a politician uses for a message can generate disinformation even if it is based on fact. The activity of content creation that is potentially valuable to the public and based on facts, but contains traces of fiction, is called creating pseudo-events. Caro [4] explained that the new media ecosystem has favored incorporation of pseudo-events into the dynamics of social networks with a clear promotional component but not an informative one.

Importantly, fake news are often distributed in the Twitter environment to harm a politician; however, such actions could lead those affected to deny such fake news and reveal the intention to deceive and confuse [12].

Polarization is a phenomenon that has always been present in politics and that has intensified with the advent of social networks. Twitter does not necessarily facilitate constructive dialogue [6] and tends to push discussions toward peak controversy [9]. This dynamic is related to Twitter's affective nature, since people experience feelings of community, adhere to a specific moral tribe and develop the consequent antagonism toward perceived rival social groups [1].

Thus, the establishment of an antagonist against whom a political identity is built is an important factor in Twitter dynamics [6], where the discussion acquires polarized forms that are based on the support for some and the opposition to others [9] Social networks, particularly Twitter, "have become a fundamental pillar for the dissemination of messages and slogans and, above all, for social mobilization and the creation of a certain state of opinion" (p. 67) [5]. This link to a slogan or a movement usually brings about the confrontation with opponents of that slogan or the social movement's objective.

Twitter has become a window to spread quickly and without intermediaries any type of message [15]. More than a platform that encourages dialogue, Twitter is a window to give greater scope to information dissemination [16]. This brings politicians closer to their audience, as they express their ideas, thoughts, and emotions directly to their followers. Therefore, Twitter is a space to generate a political narrative that favors personalization [8]. Consequently, information acquires the legitimacy and authority of the politician who manifests herself or himself and takes advantage of the characteristics of immediacy and scope to increase message dissemination [3]. In the current media ecosystem, Twitter becomes a window of exposure that supplants the media's traditional role, which even takes politician's tweets as news sources.

With this review, the four trends in Twitter use for political communication have been briefly explained. Next, the research material and methodology are detailed to explore how former president Martín Vizcarra has used his official account before and during the pandemic that triggered a health and social crisis.

2 Material and Methodology

The research explores the use and interaction dynamics generated by the tweets of the official account of Peru's former president, Martín Vizcarra, during two equally long periods before and during the Covid-19 pandemic. Twitter was selected because it offers greater potential for interaction related to political life, as Ghai Bajaj [8] highlighted. In Peru, the political dynamic is especially strong on Twitter and authorities are very active. In addition, Twitter, unlike other networks, allows interaction with accounts outside a user's personal network. Finally, the character limit for a tweet favors relatively homogeneous content, ideal for analysis and comparison.

Overall, 70 tweets were analyzed, of which 40 correspond to the first analysis period—from July 9, 2019 to March 13, 2020—and 30 to the second, from March 14 to November 17, 2020. Both periods combined cover 496 days, meaning in each period tweets from 248 days were studied. On March 14 pandemic-related mobility restrictions were announced in Peru, representing a turning point to study Vizcarra's behavior on Twitter. On November 17, Francisco Sagasti assumed the presidency, following political instability marked by protests after Vizcarra left office.

The methodology includes two levels of analysis. The first level is quantitative and develops a metric analysis of Vizcarra's account, @MartinVizcarraC, during the two study periods. This allows exploring how the former president used Twitter during an ordinary period of political development and during a period of health crisis and social uncertainty. The data collected and compared is presented in Table 1.

Table 1. Data collected and compared in the metric analysis.

Account analyzed	Data
@MartinVizcarraC	Number of tweets
	Frequency of publication
	Average number of Likes
	Average number of Retweets
	Average Likes + Retweets
	Likes/Retweets Ratio

The second level applies qualitative content analysis, following the approach of Ghai Bajaj [8]. This study considers the periods and the level of interaction generated by each tweet as a criterion for analysis and focuses on the categories of topic, affect, fake news, polarization, and informational purpose. The analysis categories and descriptions appear in Table 2.

Table 2. Analysis categories and descriptions.

Category	Description
Topic	Analysis of a tweet's topic to explore if there is any area in which the audience interacts more
Affect	Analysis of whether the tweet predominates or is appealing to an emotion, that is, if the tweet has an affective orientation
Fake News	Analyzing if the tweet seeks to correct, clarify, or specify any false information that is circulating on social networks
Polarization	Analyzing if the tweet directly aims to replicate or answer any expression of another political figure
Informative	Analyzing if the tweet provides information on some circumstantial event or of relevance to citizens

The 70 tweets were studied manually and simultaneously by the researchers to guarantee a neutral analysis. After the observation, the researchers validated the results and cross-checked with the level of interaction generated by each tweet. For the research, tweets that more clearly represented the trends found in the sample were collected to accompany the results and reflect on these examples.

3 Analysis of Results

The metric analysis of @MartinVizcarraC revealed that the frequency of publication was approximately one tweet every six days in the first period and approximately one tweet every eight days in the second period. Vizcarra reduced the dissemination of messages through Twitter during a more turbulent, uncertain, and crisis period. This could be related to higher visibility attained through live press conferences Vizcarra provided almost daily on television during the first weeks of the quarantine, as the lowest number of tweets corresponds precisely to April 2020. Table 3 presents the detailed results of the metric analysis.

Table 3. Results of the metric analysis of @MartinVizcarraC.

	Period 1	Period 2	Change (%)
Number of tweets	40	30	−25.00
Publication Frequency	0.16	0.12	−25.00
Average number of Likes	7,721.75	29,898.43	+287.20
Average number of Retweets	1,193.68	4,020.30	+236.80
Average Likes + Retweets	8,915.43	33,918.73	+280.45
Likes/Retweets Ratio	7.22	7.44	+2.97

Although the number of tweets and publication frequency decreased in Period 2 compared to Period 1, audience activity and level of participation increased considerably. Especially the increase of 287.20% in the average number of Likes and the increase of 236.80% in the average number of Retweets stand out. These data reveal user participation rose as the pandemic emerged, more than doubling activity in relation to the previous period.

Thus, a first dynamic can be observed in the behavior of political communication on Twitter: Activity on the @MartinVizcarraC account decreased by 25%, but audience participation increased by 280.45% (average number of Likes + Retweets). Also, the Likes/Retweets ratio increased only slightly at 2.97%, meaning the proportion among these two activities did not vary significantly and the audience largely maintained the level of Like/Retweet activity.

The first result of qualitative content analysis is the confirmation of a trend that emerged with the political use of Twitter: the predominance of the emotional and affective component. Of the 70 tweets, 56 included a clear predominance of the affective component where Vizcarra used phrases that appealed to the audience's emotions. Another relevant point is that during the two periods under analysis, the tweet respectively generating most interaction was an affective tweet. During Period 1, it was a greeting to journalists on a special journalists' day, and the tweet during Period 2 related to Vizcarra's dismissal as president. Table 4 shows these tweets and interaction levels.

Both tweets contain a clear affective component—the search to generate emotions among the audience predominates—to empathize with it through phrases that express ideals, desires, and recognition. Interestingly, the farewell message of November 10, 2020 reached the highest interaction among the entire sample. One reason to explain this level of audience participation is the political context in which the message was given and the narrative it generated. Vizcarra left office due to a rapidly developing process

Table 4. Tweets with the highest level of interaction in each period under analysis.

Period	Tweet	Likes	Retweets
Period 1	[01 Oct 2019] On # DíaDelPeriodista, I express my appreciation to the women and men of the press, whose work is essential to strengthen freedom of press and expression, fundamental pillars of our democracy. Happy day!	36,229	4,940
Period 2	[Nov 10, 2020] Dear Peruvian people: During these two years and eight months of government, you have been my greatest support and strength. Together we built this path, despite adversity. I leave with a clear conscience, my head held high and my duty accomplished. Until another chance	126,730	15,821

that enabled him to present himself as a victim, generating empathy among the audience. This shows that interaction on Twitter can often respond to the external situation, with a relation between events of political life and activity on this social network. Future research could explore the correlation between these two variables.

Tweets with a predominant affective and emotional tone address various topics. In the period before the pandemic, messages of encouragement stood out, including gratitude to sports institutions, congratulations to athletes who won medals in the Pan American Games, or condolences regarding the death of a beloved public figure or greetings on important dates like Christmas. But during the pandemic period, messages with greatest interaction addressed issues such as condolences to and solidarity with families, affirming support for international authorities, Vizcarra's personal life, gratitude to health personnel working on the pandemic front line, and daily protection measures to defeat the virus.

The topics were diverse, a content creation line is not observed, but Vizcarra takes temporary events and issues messages that present him close and attentive to and concerned about the problems the population is confronting. During the pandemic, the tenor of his messages did not change, but shifted to address conjunctural issues with the same affective approach. Thus, the fight against the pandemic manifested itself in the messages with greatest interaction as a romantic slogan where the Peruvian people were the protagonists of a battle they had to fight together and with perseverance. The topics serve as input to develop an emotional discourse that appeals more to a fan of the digital community than a citizen (p. 1038) [18].

The @MartinVizcarraC account issued only one message aimed at clarifying rumors stemming from fake news. The tweet appeared on March 15 and explains that the measures to stop the pandemic did not include the closure of some businesses:

> These measures will in no way contemplate the closure of commercial establishments of basic necessities, pharmacies or banks, which will remain permanently supplied and working. It is time to show responsibility and love for our Peru. (@MartinVizcarraC, March 15, 2020)

And although polarization emerged as an increasingly relevant trend on Twitter [2], evidence for it could not be found on Vizcarra's account proper, but it was prevalent in some users' (so-called trolls) responses to tweets. After analyzing the tweets, only two were found that could be read as a confrontation with an idea in the political context.

The first tweet related to a corruption case. Vizcarra highlighted his fight against corruption, weakening any link with a case that had been revealed. And in the second case, Vizcarra urged the Constitutional Court to rule on the unconstitutionality of the measure Congress applied to oust him, which was a controversial measure under which two extremes formed. In these cases, the phenomenon of adversarial discussion is observed, where the president stands on one side as "us" and the opponent on the other as "them," promoting polarization (p. 872) [9].

Informative value was the second most relevant topic for Vizcarra's account. Vizcarra expressed frequently informative content with an affective tenor, so his Twitter communication style stood out for having a component that appealed to emotion, even when addressing informational issues. A tweet in which he informed about the start of infrastructure works serves as example:

> The decontamination of Titicaca, the highest navigable lake in the world, was a historical aspiration. Today we are taking a fundamental step to achieve this with the delivery of the contract for the construction of 10 wastewater treatment plants. Arriba Puno and Arriba Peru! https://t.co/DsDjzKfBVP (@MartinVizcarraC, November 15, 2019).

Several other tweets also involve an emotional frame while communicating data, news, or relevant information. This confirms the trend that political communication on Twitter has a high affective component and that Vizcarra tried to frame events with a component that appealed to the feelings of his audience, because in the political context the perception of truth is mediated by emotional projection of the political leader.

Finally, it was found that Vizcarra did not respond even to the most prominent comments under his tweets, confirming findings by Carrasco Polaino et al. [5] that Twitter is used as a broadcast channel rather than a conversation channel. Political actors have joined the new environment of social interaction, but beyond adapting their communicative logics, they only use it to achieve a greater scope of their messages [16].

4 Conclusions

Results show that the pandemic led to a change in the dynamics of the account studied and of the audience's participation. Posting frequency on the @MartinVizcarraC account decreased, but Twitter users' engagement more than doubled compared with the pre-pandemic period. This dynamic can be explained with the activity of some relevant users who receive information and contribute to its dissemination throughout the network (Caldevilla et al., 2019), in addition to greater exposure of the audience to screens and generally higher activity on social networks during the quarantine.

In addition, the predominance of the emotional and affective component stood out. Twitter works as a persuasion and propaganda tool in political contexts [5]. It is not a neutral environment because users seek support from their followers and want opinion affirmation. Hence, the emotional and affective character of the messages influences the creation of a close relationship and transmits concern for the audience.

Appealing to the emotional aspect via social networks makes it possible to highlight connections and create communities based on a desire to interact with persons that explore the same affect [10]. Emotional speech is linked to polarization since it appeals to a person's sentimental part and not to reflective reasoning. In this sense, the finding of Kušen & Strembeck [12] is relevant. They showed that politicians who prioritized a sentimental component in their messages tended to polarize within the framework of the general discourse. The polarization developed, in the case of Vizcarra's account, at the level of replies but not in the main messages issued.

Polarization in social networks should lead to the reflection and attention of researchers and professionals, because increasingly extreme polarization, anchored in othering mechanisms, is counterproductive and harmful for the construction of a citizen dialogue, as the search for the common good does not predominate, but the defeat of the opposition [6].

This research confirms the finding of Mauricio and Rubio [16] regarding the predominantly unidirectional nature of political communication on Twitter. The communication of @MartinVizcarraC was unidirectional, focusing on the dissemination of content and avoiding conversation. In the research sample, the development of bidirectionality in political discourse on the Internet was not observed. This represents an area for improvement and development to favor a context of political dialogue on Twitter.

References

1. Arias Maldonado, M.: La digitalización de la conversación pública: redes sociales, afectividad política y democracia. Revista de Estudios Políticos **173**, 27–54 (2016). https://doi.org/10.18042/cepc/rep.173.01
2. Cabezuelo Lorenzo, F., Manfredi, J.L.: Postverdad, fake-news y agenda política en el discurso de Trump en Twitter. Historia y Comunicación Soc. **24**(2), 471–483 (2019). https://doi.org/10.5209/hics.66291
3. Caldevilla, D., Rodríguez, J., Barrientos, A.: El malestar social a través de las nuevas tecnologías: Twitter como herramienta política. Rev. Lat. Comun. Soc. **74**, 1264–1290 (2019). https://doi.org/10.4185/RLCS-2019-1383-66
4. Caro, L.: La transformación del pseudoevento en las redes sociales. El caso de #LaHoraMágica en Twitter. Revista Internacional de Relaciones Públicas **VI**(12), 209–230 (2016). https://doi.org/10.5783/RIRP-12-2016-12-209-230
5. Carrasco Polaino, R., Villar Cirujano, E., Tejedor Fuentes, L.: Twitter como herramienta de comunicación política en el contexto del referéndum independentista catalán: asociaciones ciudadanas frente a instituciones públicas. Icono **16**(1), 64–85 (2018). https://doi.org/10.7195/RI14.V16I1.1134
6. Corona, A.: Mecanismos de otrificación entre la oposición política en Twitter durante las elecciones estatales de 2017 en México. adComunica. Revista Científica de Estrategias, Tendencias e Innovación en Comunicación **16**, 45–70 (2018). https://doi.org/10.6035/2174-0992.2018.16.4
7. Flowers, J. C.: The affective politics of Twitter. In: Wittkower, D. (Ed.) 2019 Computer Ethics - Philosophical Enquiry (CEPE) Proceedings, vol. 2019, p. 16. Digital Commons (2019). https://doi.org/10.25884/thbh-z535

8. Ghai Bajaj, S.: The use of Twitter during the 2014 Indian general elections: framing, agenda-setting, and the personalization of politics. Asian Surv. **57**(2), 249–270 (2017). https://doi.org/10.1525/AS.2017.57.2.249
9. Guimarães, A., Wang, L., Weikum, G.: Us and them: adversarial politics on twitter. In IEEE International Conference on Data Mining Workshops, ICDMW, November, pp. 872–877. IEEE (2017). https://doi.org/10.1109/ICDMW.2017.119
10. Han, S., Min, J., Lee, H.: Antecedents of social presence and gratification of social connection needs in SNS: a study of Twitter users and their mobile and non-mobile usage. Int. J. Inf. Manag. **35**(4), 459–471 (2015). https://doi.org/10.1016/j.ijinfomgt.2015.04.004
11. Hansen, L.K., Arvidsson, A., Nielsen, F.A., Colleoni, E., Etter, M.: Good friends, bad news - affect and virality in Twitter. In: Park, J.J., Yang, L.T., Lee, C. (eds.) FutureTech 2011. CCIS, vol. 185, pp. 34–43. Springer, Heidelberg (2011). https://doi.org/10.1007/978-3-642-22309-9_5
12. Kušen, E., Strembeck, M.: Politics, sentiments, and misinformation: an analysis of the Twitter discussion on the 2016 Austrian presidential elections. Online Soc. Netw. Media **5**, 37–50 (2018). https://doi.org/10.1016/j.osnem.2017.12.002
13. Lewis, J., Pond, P., Cameron, R., Lewis, B.: Social cohesion, Twitter and far-right politics in Australia: diversity in the democratic mediasphere. Eur. J. Cult. Stud. **22**(5–6), 958–978 (2019). https://doi.org/10.1177/1367549419833035
14. Manfredi-Sánchez, J.-L., Amado-Suárez, A., Waisbord, S.: Presidential Twitter in the face of COVID-19: Between populism and pop politics. Comunicar **XXIX**(66), 79–90 (2021). https://doi.org/10.3916/C66-2021-07
15. Marcos-García, S., Alonso-Muñoz, L., López-Meri.: Electoral campaigns and Twitter. The dissemination of media content in the digital environment. Cuadernos.info (48), 27–47 (2021). https://doi.org/10.7764/cdi.48.27679
16. Mauricio, L., Rubio, C.: El uso de Twitter por los partidos políticos durante la campaña del 20D. Sphera Publica **I**(17), 111–131 (2017)
17. Ott, B.L.: The age of Twitter: Donald J. Trump and the politics of debasement. Crit. Stud. Media Commun. **34**(1), 59–68 (2017). https://doi.org/10.1080/15295036.2016.1266686
18. Pérez-Curiel, C., García-Gordillo, M.: Política de influencia y tendencia fake en Twitter. Efectos postelectorales (21D) en el marco del Procés en Cataluña. El Profesional de la Información, **27**(5), 1030–1040 (2018). https://doi.org/10.3145/epi.2018.sep.07

Framing and Immigration: New Frames in Media and Social Networks

Andrés Tirado-Espín[1,2](✉), Ubaldo Cuesta[1], Luz Martínez-Martínez[1], and Diego Almeida-Galárraga[3]

[1] Universidad Complutense de Madrid, 28040 Madrid, Madrid, Spain
{ctirad01,ucuestac,luzmar03}@ucm.es
[2] School of Mathematical and Computational Sciences, Yachay Tech University, Hacienda San José s/n, San Miguel de Urcuquí 100119, Ecuador
ctirado@yachaytech.edu.ec
[3] School of Biological Sciences and Engineering, Yachay Tech University, Hacienda San José s/n, San Miguel de Urcuquí 100119, Ecuador
dalmeida@yachaytech.edu.ec

Abstract. Spain continues to be an attractive destination for the migration of people from all over the world. The presence of immigrants implies an interaction with local people, being able to modify social, cultural and political dynamics; and provoke conflict. The Theory of framing and agenda-setting shows how the way in which news about immigration is presented and its repetition influence the creation of stereotypes and prejudices. The objective of this work is to identify the news frames that predominate in the Spanish media on immigration and the frequency with which the subject appears. A descriptive content analysis was carried out in the media TVE, Telecinco, El País and ABC and social networks Twitter and Facebook, during the 12 months of 2018. A total of 307 news items were coded and analyzed. The results show that immigration is approached as an irregular event, causing feelings of rejection and xenophobia.

Keywords: Agenda-setting · Framing · Immigration · Media · Social networks

1 Introduction

The phenomenon of migration in Spain is an issue that causes diverse opinions and responses in different sectors of society: citizens, politicians, institutions and the media. Hate speeches are one of the many manifestations in this regard, which translate into racism and xenophobia [1]. This premise is based on the way in which the information generated from this fact has been approached by the media, being a fairly prominent field of research trajectory [2].

Currently, the Spanish population registers 47,329,981 inhabitants, of which 5,235,375 are foreigners, equivalent to 11%. Of this figure, the nationalities that registered an increase stand out, Colombian (62,355 more), Venezuelan (53,288) and Moroccan (47,346) [3].

© The Author(s), under exclusive license to Springer Nature Singapore Pte Ltd. 2022
Á. Rocha et al. (Eds.): ICOMTA 2021, SIST 259, pp. 140–152, 2022.
https://doi.org/10.1007/978-981-16-5792-4_15

The data show how Spain continues to be an attractive destination for the migration of people from different regions of the world. The mobility of these individuals is not always framed in regularity. The social, political, economic conditions, wars and persecutions, among others; are some of the causes of their mobility. In 2018, there were 70 million people who had to travel in search of new destinations. A figure that UNHCR records as the highest in the last 70 years. The migration crisis has generated massive flows of people trying to enter Europe. In 2019, it is estimated that around 63,311 people arrived, of which an estimated 1,028 lost their lives in the attempt [4].

In 2018, the European Union Agency for Fundamental Rights (FRA), shows in the "Report on Fundamental Rights 2019" that there are still several Member States of the European Union that have not yet incorporated into their framework political legislation on racism and xenophobia. On the other hand, in 2018, only 15 Member States had action plans and strategies to combat ethnic discrimination and racism [5]. A year earlier, the European Union Agency for Human Rights (2017) developed the "Second Survey of Minorities and Discrimination of the European Union", which produced among many data the following: immigrants have been victims of harassment motivated by hate, 90%. It also indicates that 88% of foreigners were discriminated against because of their ethnic origin [6].

This migratory process generates several tensions with the inhabitants of the host societies. The presence of immigrants implies an interaction with local people, which causes social, cultural and political dynamics to change. This situation gives rise to limited views of this reality, suppressing characteristics of the members of the outgroup and associating them with epithets that provoke fear about the presence of the "other", that is, the formation of prejudices is understood [7].

Faced with this political and social situation, the media fix their lenses on this phenomenon, giving rise to the construction of their agendas. On the other hand, the way the news is framed will have a degree of influence on the perception of Spanish citizens towards this group of people [8]. Due to the above, the studies that have been carried out are quantitative cohort, analyzing the frequency with which the media have covered the topic. And there are also qualitative ones, focused on critical discourse analysis.

This research has been developed under an empirical-conceptual approach. The starting points are the theories of framing and agenda-setting, which give rise to a double objective: 1) to identify the news frames of the messages of the media and social networks that address the issue of immigration; 2) analyze the frequency with which news about the migratory phenomenon in Spain is published. Therefore, this research is focused to answer the following research questions:

- **RQ1:** What are the main sources that publish information about immigration in Spain in the media and social networks?
- **RQ2:** What are the main news frames that predominate in the construction of messages from the media and social networks regarding migration in Spain?

On the other hand, a Boolean algorithm [9–11] has been designed defining specific descriptors on the subject, which allowed a more exact search in the Google Scholar Advanced, Scopus and Web of Science databases; in order to identify relevant and updated literature on the subject of study.

2 Related Work

2.1 Framing Theory

The media make reality known to their audiences from different approaches, which are determined by a frame that is both "a frame and a scheme" [9, p. 145], in the first the context of reality is designated, while in the other objective external data is incorporated; respectively. The frames are not final, but are subject to continuous review as reality changes.

To better understand the previous section, the phenomenon of migration is analyzed. Audiences perceive this social event according to how the media has framed the information. People generate an interpretation scheme of the event that they are trying to understand from the frame, which feeds on culture and manifests itself in all types of social discourse.

Ardèvol-Abreu (2015) points out that the image of an immigrant in conflict situations such as detention, activates a framework of understanding in which immigration is linked to crime [13]. Perceptions and social constructs are a cognitive process that is carried out through attributions based on automated deductions. When people process information, they do not consider that they construct meanings and that their expectations, stereotypes, goals and desires influence the way they see reality. So, the readings that the people of this group make based on the messages of the media will be of fear, phobia and irrationality, mainly.

There is a wide debate about the effects that occur around framing. One of them is cognitive, the frames can influence the content of people's thoughts and channel the way the subjects reflect on the issues covered in the news. However, another effect is the influence on emotional responses or reactions, which, according to the way the news is described, will induce different emotions towards the object narrated in it, that is, this is of an attitudinal type [14].

The objective of the study of framing is "to know the meanings of reality disseminated from the media and its repercussion on the meanings of that same reality for audiences" (p. 161) [9]. However, McCombs (2006) points out that framing does not have a clear conceptualization, he argues that framing is equivalent to the second level of agenda-setting theory, a natural extension of the agenda model [15].

In the research Inmigracionalismo 2 on the messages related to immigrants in the media, it is highlighted that the frames are conditioned by sensationalism and stereotypes. In the notes of the different Spanish media, the nationality of a person appears if they star in a negative or criminal act. Likewise, immigration and crime are associated, scaremongering about migration is encouraged, information is reduced to numerical terms and there is an excess of dramatization [16]. For the construction of the opinions and perceptions of the audiences, the media have played a decisive role contributing to the rejection of immigration and the maintenance of prejudices towards immigrants, offering a distorted and biased vision of the phenomenon and its contributions to society [17].

2.2 Agenda-Setting Theory

McCombs, Shaw and Weaver (2014) affirm that the studies carried out regarding the agenda-setting theory agree that the media have the ability to create reality for society [18]. The formation of public opinion is a consequence of the role of the media, since they are in charge of selecting and ordering the issues that are considered the most important [19]. The conformation of the agenda is subject to a thematic order of media information in a superposition of several layers of influence, referring to the "onion layers" model [18]. Based on this model, three types of agendas are defined, the same ones that are related to each other. Each of them has its own characteristics, allowing them to be linked in their individual and collective part. These are media agenda-setting, public agenda-setting, and political agenda-setting [20].

The media agenda-setting is directly related to the media and the information they present. Analyze its content taking into account different variables such as the topics covered, number of headlines, printed pages, position of the notes in the middle, time zone, etc. Several studies have been carried out regarding the conformation of the agendas of the Spanish media, determining the frequency with which the issue of immigration is broadcast, disseminated or publicized [21–23]. On the other hand, the conformation of the agenda in social networks and digital media has also been analyzed, generating spaces for the exchange of opinions and ideas of its readers, allowing communication to be democratized. However, it is identified that the anonymity of users represents a niche to spread hate speech that translates into racism [24, 25].

The public agenda-setting is built from the problems that arise in a certain place. It is proposed in the "Most Important Problem" (PMI), through which the country or the policy that is generated is studied [26]. This idea coincides with Alzate and Romo [19], who establish that the objective of this agenda is to determine what are the public problems or issues that citizens demand. Once identified and having the certainty that they are of general interest, they are transferred to the government, through strategies and public policies for their attention [19].

The political agenda-setting is the result of the unification of the other two agendas, in response to the PMI. It has been proven that, through the relevance of empirical facts, they can influence the political agenda, which is why political groups will do everything possible to control or, in some way, influence the media agenda [27].

The definitions presented of the three agendas show that the media have the ability to raise issues with citizens, giving rise to what will be called the public agenda, which in turn will be the origin of the issues on the political agenda. These three agendas maintain a close relationship and codependency [18, 19, 20].

2.3 Stereotypes and Prejudices of the Immigrant Population in Spain

The analysis of how the media treat or address issues related to immigration has a wide research trajectory in recent years [1]. In the European context, the migratory flow generates tensions with the host society, as it modifies social, cultural and political dynamics [25]. Complex multicultural realities are created, since different human groups must coexist in the same geographical space [28]. This situation causes prejudices and stereotypes to emerge on the part of host societies, giving rise to a limited vision of their reality, suppressing some attributes and highlighting or associating them with others [7].

Stereotypes are popular beliefs about the particularities that characterize a social class and on which there is a definite agreement. This idea agrees with Furrer (2013) who assures that they are socially agreed beliefs and accepted by a group of people. Gender, ethnicity, status, among others; are some of the conditions that mark the differences between social groups [29].

In recent years there has been a change in the news frames, a better treatment of the informative notes about immigrants is carried out. However, the truth is that there is still information that reinforces prejudices and stereotypes about these individuals. The media make use of rhetorical figures and metaphors to refer to immigrants. In Spain the most used metaphor is "problem". Although, also, military-type expressions are used such as "invaders", "gangs", "illegal", "clandestine", "traffickers", "assailants"; and other epithets that provoke fear about the presence of the "other" (p. 32) [7]. The effect sought by the media is to act on the collective imagination, associating the immigrant as dangerous, avoiding their entry and looking for ways to expel them.

For van Dijk (2011), the press articulates a discourse that integrates two elements on racism and the disqualification of the immigrant. The first refers to a discourse of the elites, where the prejudices of the wealthiest sectors of society take shape. While, the other component highlights the speeches of the popular classes, which have the same violent intention as the previous ones, although they are less exclusive [1]. The media reveal what is called "negative identities", where racism seeks the exclusion of cultural groups.

Immigration perceived as a problem generates rejection and biases with the endogroup. This is due to the large amount of information to which people are exposed and the limited capacity of the cognitive system to process it [30]. The Stereotype Content Model (SCM) identifies that those individuals with less capabilities will be relegated to the lowest rungs of the occupational pyramid [31]. These mental constructs are reinforced through the transmission of informative notes and audiovisual products from the media. As a consequence of this phenomenon, different investigations have focused on studying the construction of prejudiced and stereotyped discourses and audiovisual content, referring to immigrants in the media [29] on manifestations of violent discourses on social networks and digital media [25, 32], violent attitudes on the part of the in-group towards the out-group [33] or racism towards Muslims and other ethnic groups, in general [2].

3 Research Method

A descriptive content analysis was carried out, through which it is possible to interpret the media and social networks based on quantitative and qualitative measurement techniques [34, 35]; in a final sample of 307 news, 250 in the media and 57 in social networks.

To carry out this research, a systematic random sample was taken, during 2018, from January to December. The week of January was randomized, resulting in the second, from this process a sample of successive weeks was taken in the following months. In addition, seven days a week are considered, starting on Monday and ending on Sunday.

The news was searched on the media websites, using Google's advanced search tools, and the "CISION" monitoring software, with the keywords: «migration», «immigrants», «migrants», « refugees "," Mediterranean "," patera "," Morocco "," Africa "," Aquarius "," Open Arms "during the established periods of time. In TVE, El País and ABC, the search engine of the web pages was investigated directly with the keywords. In the case of Telecinco, it was decided to use the advanced Google search, due to the incipient search engine on the website of that channel. In the case of TVE, initially TVE1 and TVE2 were selected, but the channel 24 Horas, which belongs to TVE, was also included to broaden the range of results. The media selected for monitoring were two of the newspapers with the largest circulation nationwide, ABC and El País, a conservative and Catholic medium, and another progressive and secular; respectively. Therefore, the ideological differences that separate both media and the "model of society" that one and the other defend [34] are taken into account. Regarding the television channels, the Spanish public television TVE and Telecinco were considered, for this selection the editorial line and the ideological-political tendency of the medium are considered. The public media opt for less impressive, contrasted and objective pictures; while private channels seek to show images with striking frames at a visual and sound level, they opt for sensationalist models [23].

For social media monitoring, media headlines were analyzed. The most used terms were established, both by television channels and by the press, to analyze their impact on the Internet, using the Google Trends tool. Once the most used ones were verified, it was possible to identify the following hashtags on social networks, with the following time periods as a maximum: #Refugees (June); #Migrants (June); # Immigrants (June and July); #Patera (July and August); #Aquarius (July and August). These terms when setting trends, do not necessarily appear as hashtag, but are included in social media posts. 57 units of analysis were identified from the total sample, on Twitter (n = 23) and on Facebook (n = 34). The former has been playing an extremely relevant role in journalism, since both communication professionals and the media themselves use this network to learn about current world events. While, the second provides alternative spaces for the socialization of information that does not fit on the pages of newspapers or on TV programming [24]. In addition, they point out that trending topics provide visibility at the moment of events, breaking up to one hundred points with the agenda-setting theory.

To record the information, a code book was created which groups variables obtained from both an inductive and deductive process, by analyzing the press releases of the media's web pages and, also, the messages of the pages and profiles of social networks. This implies "a construction of a measurement model, which must necessarily be corroborated by empirical evidence" (p. 158) [21]. Taking as reference these previous studies [20, 34, 36–38]. The codebook was organized around four dimensions: 1) Basic identification data for the media and social networks, 2) Importance index, 3) Information source and 4) Index of immigration news frames.

4 Results

Of the two television channels, 20% (n = 50) of the sample taken were obtained from TVE and 20.40% (n = 51) from Telecinco. Regarding the press, El País obtained 34.40%

(n = 86), while ABC 25.20% (n = 63). On the other hand, in social networks, publications on Facebook are 59.60% (n = 34), while on Twitter the figure is around 40.40% (n = 23).

The analysis of the frequency with which information regarding immigration in Spain is transmitted in audiovisual media shows that the mid-day news programs are the most abundant on the subject, with 46% for TVE and 51% for Telecinco (Table 1). The highest number of informative notes were obtained in the case of TVE, of the Telediario with 62% and, in the other case, of Informativos Telecinco with 92.20%.

Table 1. Frequency of immigration notes.

Time zone	TVE		Telecinco	
	Frequency	Percentage	Frequency	Percentage
Morning	15	30%	16	31,40%
Noon	23	46%	26	51%
Night	12	24%	9	17,60%

In social networks, the profiles, pages or groups that generate the most content about immigrants provoke interest in users. Audiences react to posts by "I like you" and also by joining their profiles as "followers". From these two categories, the accounts with the highest number of "likes" are identified, in the Facebook posts and the Twitter accounts with the most "followers" (Table 2). We see the highest values for the profiles of Podemos, VOX and Doctors without Borders Spain on Facebook and those of Santiago Abascal, Doctors without Borders and Vox on Twitter.

Table 2. Most recurring profiles, pages and groups in generating content about the migration.

Facebook	Likes	Twitter	Followers
Podemos	1,337,258	Santiago Abascal	86,6 mil
VOX	426,351	Médicos sin Fronteras España	430,2 mil
Médicos sin Fronteras España	238,257	VOX	416,6 mil
España no se rompe	182,790	UNICEF España	281,9 mil
CEAR	56,359	Comité español ACNUR	174 mil
SOS Refugiados	34,739	Open Arms	170 mil

In relation to the index of informative importance, some aspects of the construction of news in the media and in publications on social networks are identified. From the selected sample, an average is obtained for the following categories: duration of the informative notes in audiovisual media, 4:04 min in TVE and; 1:24 min on Telecinco. As for the characters of the written media, it is detailed that, for El País, there are 5,334; while for the ABC they are 2775. While, for the social networks it is determined in Twitter there are 17.6 thousand followers in the profiles and; for Facebook 15.9 thousand likes in the post. Finally, it is analyzed whether the press releases and social media posts have images to accompany the text. It is found that without exception the images are present.

Information sources are one of the most important components that determine the media agenda. In response to RQ1, it is important to comply with the maxim of journalism, which establishes that all communication must have a source [37]. For this reason, in this work a classification is carried out, with the public authorities; foreign dependence; NGO; state institutions; political actors. However, for social networks, two categories are incorporated: media or journalist; Nonprofit organizations. The reason responds to the fact that the publications generally refer to complaints by people or institutions that protect the rights of the immigrant group. Figure 1 shows a great deal of activity by NGOs as sources of news or immigration publications, this is maintained in the different channels (especially in TVE, El País and Twitter). Also, public authorities generate communications, although their actions are more limited to audiovisual media (television and digital newspapers). For the third place we find certain differences depending on the medium. In the case of television networks, there is a considerable number of news offered by state institutions, especially in Telecinco, where we also find news about immigrants, unlike TVE. In the case of newspapers, in addition to state institutions, they are the media where we find more news of foreign dependency. Different sources appear in social networks that are not found in other channels such as political actors.

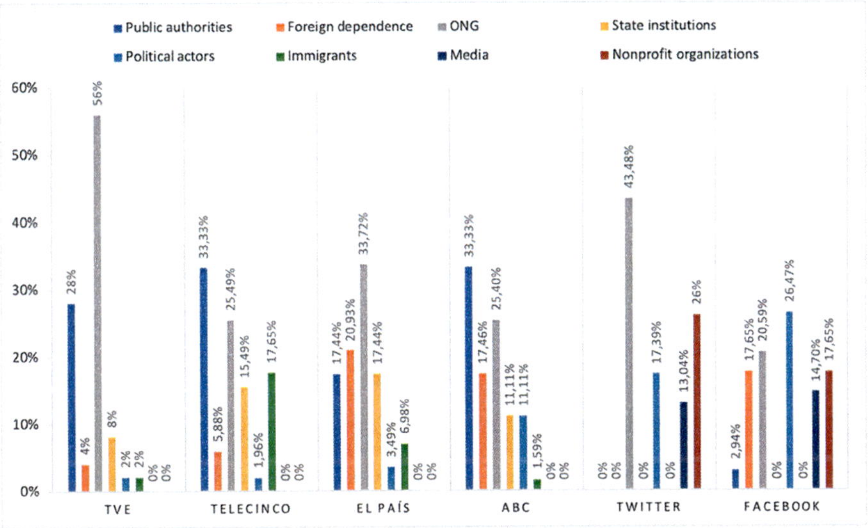

Fig. 1. Most recurring sources for the preparation of news and publications.

In response to RQ2, ten have been detected as the main news frames referring to immigration in Spain, which predominate both in the media and on social networks

(Fig. 2). The most prominent among all is "irregular immigration", since the construction of the news focuses on showing immigrants trying to enter Europe. In relation to the previous framing, two frames that originate as a consequence are highlighted, "administration of the European Union" and "xenophobia". The first tries to solve the phenomenon of migration between all member countries. However, it is evident that their policies are not enough and border control is constantly circumvented. Faced with this challenge, citizens become restless and hate speeches [1] arise, which are translated into prejudices and stereotypes [32]. In addition, these moments have been taken advantage of by right and far right political groups that blame immigrants for all the ills of Spain, transferring this issue to the political debate [39].

Regarding social networks, it is emphasized that the profiles and/or pages denounce the "violation of human rights", of this group at risk. As well as the inability of the European Union to manage the massive influx of people fleeing armed conflicts from their countries of origin. These communication channels are an alternative form of expression by citizens. This event gives rise to an analysis that takes immediacy as its starting point. Audiences have the ability to transmit all information at any time, reaching a considerable number of people. As a consequence, the grid that the traditional media have determined is called into question, according to the agenda-setting [24].

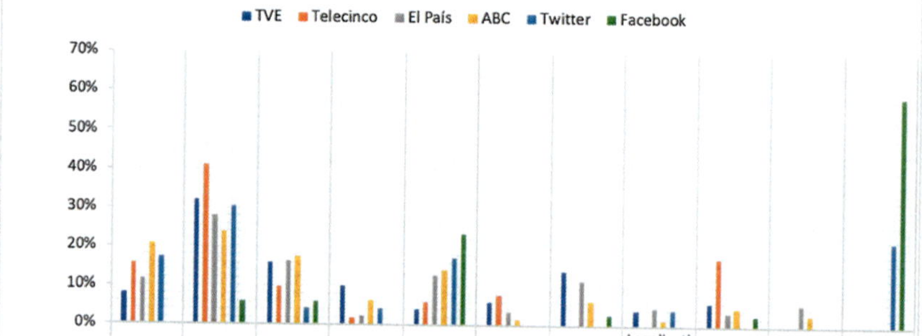

	Political debate	Irregular immigration	Adm. UE	Solidarity acts	Xenophobia	Human trafficking	Protection measures	Legalization of documents	Criminal acts	Expulsion /repatriation	Violation of Human Rights
TVE	8%	32%	16%	10%	4%	6%	14%	4%	6%	0%	0%
Telecinco	15,69%	41,18%	9,80%	1,96%	5,88%	7,84%	0%	0%	17,65%	0%	0%
El País	11,63%	27,91%	16,28%	2,32%	12,79%	3,49%	11,63%	4,65%	3,49%	5,81%	0%
ABC	20,63%	23,81%	17,46%	6,35%	14,29%	1,59%	6,35%	1,59%	4,76%	3,17%	0%
Twitter	17,39%	30,43%	4,35%	4,35%	17,39%	0%	0%	4,35%	0%	0%	21,74%
Facebook	0%	5,88%	5,88%	0%	23,53%	0%	2,94%	0%	2,94%	0%	58,82%

Fig. 2. New frames of the media and social networks, in the context of immigration.

Sánchez and Zarauza pointed out that private media build sensational news frames [23]. In Fig. 2, it is observed that the frames "criminal acts" and "human trafficking" are addressed by the Telecinco channel. A fact that agrees when observing the absence of notes with frame "protection measures", at the same time that there is a low production in "solidarity acts".

5 Discussion and Conclusion

The mass media frame the information of the migration like a crude fact, where the people who try to enter Europe are not civilized [13]. The images and editorials show men, women and children aboard small boats known as pateras or cayucos, which in their desperate attempt are shipwrecked [35]. NGO lifeboats are sent in relief response and in cooperation with European governments they are rescued. Then, another dilemma arises which country allows the arrival of lifeboats on its shores. Such is the case that, in 2018, the Aquarios ship was stranded [38]. In this research, also, all these events are corroborated through the content analysis (qualitative) of a (quantitative) sample of news and publications related to the migratory event.

Depending on the medium (audiovisual, written and social networks) the information is treated differently. The public media present a more humane and democratic approach, proposing an inclusive society model. However, the private media opt for sensationalist information, protected by their political ideologies [23]. Many of them with the firm conviction of promoting a discourse where it is clearly identified that the immigrant is an "enemy" [38]. A discourse where there is no room for "others", because there is only room for "us" [7]. The CEAR report points out that the information transmitted by the media is framed by prejudice. However, he also points out that in recent years there has been a change in the news frames, a better treatment of the informative notes about immigrants is carried out [40].

In the previous investigations, in their majority, an analysis of the content of newspapers, television and radio is carried out. However, there is not much literature on the messages that are transmitted on social networks. This study analyzes the correlation between sources and news frames, such is the case that both the media and social networks coincide in three frames that have been the product of the same sources [20, 24]. Among the most recurrent sources, "foreign agencies", "state institutions" and "political actors" stand out; which in turn give rise to the frames "administration in the European Union", "irregular immigration" and "xenophobia" [36].

From the explanation indicated, the objective of the agenda is fulfilled, which is to determine which are the PMIs demanded by citizens [26, 27]. Once identified, they are transferred to the government through strategies and public policies for their attention. Then, it follows that the most common frames are related to negative connotations about immigration (Fig. 2), which will influence a problematic conception of it, affecting the perception of the population. The reason lies in the large amount of information to which people are exposed and the limited cognitive capacity [30].

Migration is a fact that captures everyone's attention, giving rise to both good and ill-intentioned reasoning. Thus, the profiles and accounts on Facebook and Twitter with the highest "number of followers" and "I like you" are opposed in their values, ideology and political tendency. On the one hand, there is the Podemos account (left), framing its messages through empathy. While, on the other hand, there is the Vox profile (far right), with hate messages that incite the outgroup to commit violent acts against the in-group [33]. In the same vein, racism towards Muslims and other ethnic groups, in general, is explained [2].

References

1. van Dijk, T.: Discurso y Poder. Editorial, Barcelona (2011)
2. Casáus Arzú, M.E.: El racismo y su proyección actual: ¿un fenómeno nuevo o un problema sin resolver? Cuad. Trab. Soc. **31**(1), 121–137 (2018). https://doi.org/10.5209/CUTS.55732
3. Instituto Nacional de Estadística: Flujo de inmigración procedente del extranjero por semestre, país de origen y nacionalidad (española/extranjera) (2020). https://www.ine.es/jaxiT3/Tabla.htm?t=24394. Accessed 15 Apr 2020
4. La Agencia de la ONU para los refugiados: Situación en Europa. Emergencias (2019). https://www.acnur.org/emergencia-en-europa.html#:~:text=1.028&text=Un. estimado de 362.000 refugiados,y migrantes ingresaron a Europa
5. European Union Agency for Fundamental rights: Informe sobre los derechos fundamentales 2019. Dictamen de la FRA, pp. 1–24 (2019). https://fra.europa.eu/sites/default/files/fra_uploads/fra-2019-fundamental-rights-report-2019-opinions_es.pdf
6. Agencia de la Unión Europea de Derechos Humanos: Agencia de la Unión Europea de Derechos Humanos (2017). https://fra.europa.eu/en/news/2017/fight-against-discrimination-and-hate-towards-minorities-still-fails-deliver-nearly-10. Accessed 01 June 2020
7. Sar, A.: La construcción mediática de los inmigrantes en Iberoamérica. Rev. Int. Comun. y Desarro. **1**(3), 25–39 (2016).https://doi.org/10.15304/ricd.1.3.2946
8. Martínez, L., Cambra, U., Espín, C.: Las noticias de inmigración en redes sociales y sus efectos sobre los jóvenes.: análisis descriptivo de las investigaciones en revistas científicas desde 2012 a 2017. In: Salinas, A.I.A., Sastre, G.V., Trujillo, T.A.N. (eds.) Comunicación, paz y conflictos, pp. 173–182. Dykinson (2018). https://doi.org/10.2307/j.ctv9hvtdx.19
9. Almeida-Galárraga, D., Ros-Felip, A., Álvarez-Sánchez, V., Marco-Martinez, F., Serrano-Mateo, L.: Kinematics based physical modelling and experimental analysis of the shoulder joint complex. Ing. e Investig. **37**(3), 115–123 (2017). https://doi.org/10.15446/ing.investig.v37n3.63144
10. Almeida-Galárraga, D.A., Ros Felip, A., Marco Martínez, F., Serrano-Mateo, L.: Photoelastic analysis of shoulder arthroplasty: current descriptive analysis of research in scientific journals. In: Lhotska, L., Sukupova, L., Lacković, I., Ibbott, G. (eds.) World Congress on Medical Physics and Biomedical Engineering 2018, vol. 68/2, pp. 713–717. Springer, Singapore (2019). https://doi.org/10.1007/978-981-10-9038-7_132
11. Aguiar Salazar, E.D., et al.: Design of a glove controlled by electromyographic signals for the rehabilitation of patients with rheumatoid arthritis. In: Rodriguez Morales, G., Fonseca C., E.R., Salgado, J.P., Pérez-Gosende, P., Orellana Cordero, M., Berrezueta, S. (eds.) TICEC 2020. CCIS, vol. 1307, pp. 3–11. Springer, Cham (2020). https://doi.org/10.1007/978-3-030-62833-8_1
12. Sádaba, T.: Origen, aplicación y límites de la, "teoría del encuadre" (framing) en comunicación, vol. 14, no. 2 (2001). https://doi.org/10.15581/003.14.2.143-175
13. Ardèvol-Abreu, A.: Framing o teoría del encuadre en comunicación. Orígenes, desarrollo y panorama actual en España, La Laguna, Tenerife, July 2015. https://doi.org/10.4185/RLCS-2015-1053
14. Igartua, J., Moral-Toranzo, F., Fernández, I.: Cognitive, attitudinal, and emotional effects of news frame and group cues, on processing news about immigration. J. Media Psychol. **23**(4), 174–185 (2011). https://doi.org/10.1027/1864-1105/a000050
15. McCombs, M.E.: Estableciendo la agenda. El impacto de los medios en la opinión pública y en el conocimiento. Paidós Comunicación, Barcelona (2006)
16. Red Acoge: Inmigracionalismo 2. Madrid, p. 31 (2015)
17. Igartua, J., Muñiz, C., Otero, J.A., de la Fuente Juan, M.: El tratamiento informativo en los medios de comunicación españoles. Un análisis de contenido desde la Teoría del Framing.

Estud. sobre el Mensaje Periodístico, vol. 1, no. ISSN: 1134-1629, pp. 91–110 (2007). https://s3.amazonaws.com/academia.edu.documents/33116187/Igartua_et_al._EMP_2007.pdf?response-content-disposition=inline%3Bfilename%3DEl_tratamiento_informativo_de_la_inmigra.pdf&X-Amz-Algorithm=AWS4-HMAC-SHA256&X-Amz-Credential=ASIATUSBJ6BAC4CBSWUX%2F20
18. McCombs, M.E., Shaw, D.L., Weaver, D.H.: New directions in agenda-setting theory and research. Mass Commun. Soc. **17**(6), 781–802 (2014). https://doi.org/10.1080/15205436.2014.964871
19. Alzate Zuluaga, M.L., Romo Morales, G.: La agenda pública en sus teorías y aproximaciones metodológicas. Una clasificación alternativa. Rev. Enfoques Cienc. Política y Adm. Pública, vol. XV, no. 26, pp. 13–35 (2017). http://www.revistaenfoques.cl/index.php/revista-uno/article/view/448
20. Tirado-Espín, A., Cuesta, U., Martínez-Martínez, L., Almeida-Galárraga, D.: Agenda-setting e inmigración: análisis crítico del discurso y frecuencia en los medios : Estudio descriptivo de investigaciones en revistas científicas desde 2015 a 2020. Rev. Ibérica Sist. y Tecnol. Inf. **E35**, 289–302 (2020)
21. Aruguete, N.: El efecto entre las agendas política, mediática y pública: herramientas para su medición y análisis. Más Pod. local, vol. 26, pp. 34–35 (2016). http://maspoderlocal.es/files/articulos/244-F569a35272441452946727-articulo-1.pdf
22. Martín Rodríguez, E., Príncipe Hermoso, S.: Crisis Migratoria y su proyección en prensa: ambigüedad de conceptos y disfunciones informativas. In: Bermúdez Vázquez, M., Macho Reyes, R.D. (eds.) Análisis del discurso mediático: un enfoque multidisciplinar, 1st ed., pp. 146–153. Egregius, Sevilla (2017)
23. Sánchez Castillo, S., Zarauza Valero, T.: El desplazamiento de los refugiados ante las cámaras de los informativos de TVE. Tonos Digit. vol. 38, pp. 1–26 (2020). http://www.tonosdigital.es/ojs/index.php/tonos/article/view/2386/1146
24. Corral, A., Fernández, C.: Las agendas de lo araboislámico en Twitter y El País. In: Sabés, F., Verón, J.J. (eds.) Innovación y cambio en la comunicación postindustrial, Asociación de Periodistas de Aragón, pp. 13–27 (2015)
25. Ferré Pavia, C., Simelio Solá, N.: Comentarios sobre inmigración en tres periódicos en línea españoles: Aproximación a un discurso racista enmascarado. Rev. Q. **10**(20), 137–156 (2016). https://doi.org/10.18566/revistaq.v10n20.a06
26. Rodríguez Díaz, R.: Teoría de la Agenda-Setting aplicación a la enseñanza universitaria. Observatorio Europeo de Tendencias Sociales, Alicante (2004)
27. Hopmann, D., Elmelund-Præstekær, C., Albæk, E., Vliegenthart, R., de Vreese, C.: Party media agenda-setting. Party Polit. **18**(2), 173–191 (2012). https://doi.org/10.1177/1354068810380097
28. Romero-Rodríguez, L.M., De-Casas-Moreno, P., Maraver-López, P., Pérez-Rodríguez, M.A.: Representaciones y estereotipos latinoamericanos en las series españolas de prime time (2014–2017). Converg. Rev. Ciencias Soc. **93** (2018). https://doi.org/10.29101/crcs.v25i78.9162
29. Mancha Castro, J.C.: Prejuicios, estereotipos y xenofobia en comentarios de lectores de prensa digital. El caso de una niña musulmana en el diario El País. Altern. Cuad. Trab. Soc. **25**, 9–31 (2018). https://doi.org/10.14198/ALTERN2018.25.01
30. Herrero, C., Villar, A., Guillén, Á.S.: Las facetas del bienestar: una aproximación multidimensional a la calidad de vida en España y sus comunidades autónomas (2006–2015) Fundacion (2018)
31. Fiske, S.T., Cuddy, A.J.C., Glick, P., Xu, J.: A model of (often mixed) stereotype content: competence and warmth respectively follow from perceived status and competition. J. Pers. Soc. Psychol. **82**(6), 878–902 (2002). https://doi.org/10.1037/0022-3514.82.6.878

32. Correa, F., Calvo, P.: Posverdad, redes sociales e islamofobia en Europa. Un estudio de caso: el incendio de Notre Dame. Revista de la Asociación Española de Investigación de la Comunicación **6**(12), 35–57 (2019). https://doi.org/10.24137/raeic.6.12.8
33. Igartua, J., Frutos, F.J.: Socio-Cognitivos De Películas Sobre Inmigración. El Papel Moderador Del Prejuicio Hacia Inmigrantes. Migraciones **40**(2016), 33–61 (2016). https://doi.org/10.14422/mig.i40.y2016.009
34. Barbero, C., Sánchez-García, P.: Islamofobia en la prensa escrita: de la sección de opinión a la opinión pública. Historia y Comunicación Social **23**(2), 509–528 (2018). https://doi.org/10.5209/HICS.62271
35. Zuloaga Lojo, L.: La concepción securita de la inmigración en el caso español. Athenea Digit. **16**(2), 215–244 (2016)
36. Cheng, L., Igartua, J., Palacios, E., Acosta, T., Otero, J.A., Frutos, F.J.: noticiosos sobre inmigración en la prensa regional de Castilla y León. Zer **14**(26), 35–57 (2009)
37. Santillán Buelna, J.R.: Imágenes de México en la 'La Vanguardia' y 'El Periódico de Catalunya' (2013–2016). Index. Comun. Rev. científica en el ámbito la Comun. Apl. vol. 8, no. 1, pp. 101–121 (2018). https://journals.sfu.ca/indexcomunicacion/index.php/indexcomunicacion/article/view/365
38. Galvañ, A., Ortega-Giménez, C.: Discurso del odio en radio: análisis de los editoriales de las cadenas COPE y SER tras la llegada del Aquarius a España. Miguel Hernández Communication J. **11**, 117–138 (2020). https://doi.org/10.21134/mhcj.v11i0.317
39. Cartón, N.P., Seró, C.S.: El ascenso de García Albiol. Politización del discurso migratorio y aplicación de la teoría del «agenda setting» en las elecciones locales de 2011. Papers. Revista de Sociologia **101**(2), 137 (2016). https://doi.org/10.5565/rev/papers.2140
40. Díaz, N., Díez, Á., Muñiz, R., Senante, A.: Discriminación y persecución por orientación sexual e identidad de género: El camino hacia una vida digna. Madrid (2015.)

Posting to Belong: Instagram Features Enhance Marketed Goods Used as Conduits to Leverage Group Affiliation

Lizardo Vargas-Bianchi(✉)

Graduate School, Universidad de Lima, Av Javier Prado 4600, Lima 15023, Perú
lvargas@ulima.edu.pe

Abstract. Belonging Conduits are resources available in the market (such as products, services, or brands) that people use as a means to favor their affiliation to a group. The conduits are a construct of the belongingness-oriented consumption model, which explains the process that subjects follow when their consumption patterns favor their affiliation to a group. This study aims to examine how young consumers are using the social media platform Instagram to produce content using Belonging Conduits to promote their group affiliation. A qualitative research with a deductive approach was conducted among young Instagram users. Data were collected through interviews, using the mobile instant messaging interview (MIMI) technique. The information was analyzed using structural coding and thematic analysis. The findings confirm that young people use consumer goods as vehicles to favor their belonging. In addition, it becomes clear that participants recognize Instagram as an functional outlet for exhibiting Belonging Conduits. Furthermore, Instagram's features allow to add additional layers of information to these conduits, particularly music, and to increase the reach of content oriented to favor group affiliation.

Keywords: Belonging · Brands · Consumer behavior · Instagram · Belonging conduits

1 Introduction

Several authors argue that the need for acceptance by others and group affiliation are factors that influence our purchasing decisions [1–3]. Studies by Griskevicius and Kenrick [4], and Ahuvia [5] agree that the need to belong influences the products we choose. This phenomenon is observed in the purchase of products such as clothing, entertainment venues, or vacation travel. Studies show that certain consumer behaviors can operate as a means to create and maintain close interpersonal relationships. Social networks are not exempt from this phenomenon, and a major motivator to use social networking sites is the need to belong [1, 2].

The use of brands, products, and consumption practices as a means to achieve affiliation is an understudied area [6]. Arias & Otnes [7, 8] propose an initial theoretical framework to explain how individuals conduct their consumption behavior to satisfy

© The Author(s), under exclusive license to Springer Nature Singapore Pte Ltd. 2022
Á. Rocha et al. (Eds.): ICOMTA 2021, SIST 259, pp. 153–163, 2022.
https://doi.org/10.1007/978-981-16-5792-4_16

their need to belong. Vargas-Bianchi [9] confirmed the model transferability and polished it for improvement. The model is composed of different constructs, one of which is Belonging Conduits, which are the resources available on the market (such as products or brands) that consumers use as instruments to favor their affiliation to a group. Information on how young cohorts select and use the conduits in social networks is still limited and preliminary [9]. Moreover, little is known about the use of social networks to display conduits. The aim of this research is to analyze the use of Instagram as a channel to display Belonging Conduits, when the creation and distribution of content through the social network aims at favoring belonging in a group.

2 Literature Background

2.1 The Need to Belong to a Group

Studies on belonging define it as the human need to know oneself is part of a group and to be accepted and treated positively by the members of that group. Belonging is manifested as an articulated experience, in which the person perceives acceptance, attention, and support from other members [10, 11]. In their extensive review of the literature, Baumeister and Leary [12] put forward a belongingness hypothesis that has been relevant to studies in this field. The authors assert that two criteria are required to satisfy the drive to belong: First, there is a need for frequent affectively pleasant interactions with a few people, and, second, these interactions must take place in the context of a temporally stable and enduring framework of affective concern for each other's welfare. Although the Need to Belong (NTB) theoretical proposal describes different dimensions and behaviors of the person, Baumeister and Leary [12] do not mention a relationship between consumption and belonging, although they argue that the NTB is a fundamental human motivation. The link between consumption, social relationships, and group affiliation has been examined in consumer behavior studies. For example, Griskevicius et al. [13] argue that the desire to belong influences purchase decisions, especially of products such as consumer electronics, and that these products help people maintain their social relationships. Their observations are consistent with the study by De Gregorio and Sung [14], who found that adult consumers' placement-related attitudes and behaviors are always subject to the influence of circles of friends and acquaintances.

Wattanasuwan [15] argues that the purchase of goods expresses not only our individual sense of identity but also our sense of belonging to a group and the collective identity of that group. The relationship between the use of goods and social relationships has been covered in the literature by other authors, who have shown that the bond we have with things is not composed of only two elements (person–things), but involves three elements: person–things–person [16]. On the other hand, Ahuvia [5] analyzes the social bonds underlying different consumption practices, in which there is a sense of affiliation or belonging to certain groups. This author refers to the use of consumption as a means to create and maintain close interpersonal relationships. A common example in the literature referring to this phenomenon are brand communities, where a specific brand (such as Harley-Davidson motorcycles or products of the Star Wars saga) is established as the axis that generates interpersonal closeness, and based on which relationships and the sense of belonging in the community are structured [17–22].

2.2 Belonging-Oriented Consumption and Belonging Conduits

A very small number of papers have analyzed consumption behaviors used to satisfy the need for affiliation [6]. Arias and Otnes [7, 8] put forward a preliminary model on this phenomenon. Vargas-Bianchi [9] conducted a review of the theoretical model, based on which its transferability was confirmed, in addition to refining the model, thus contributing to its development. The model is shown in Fig. 1.

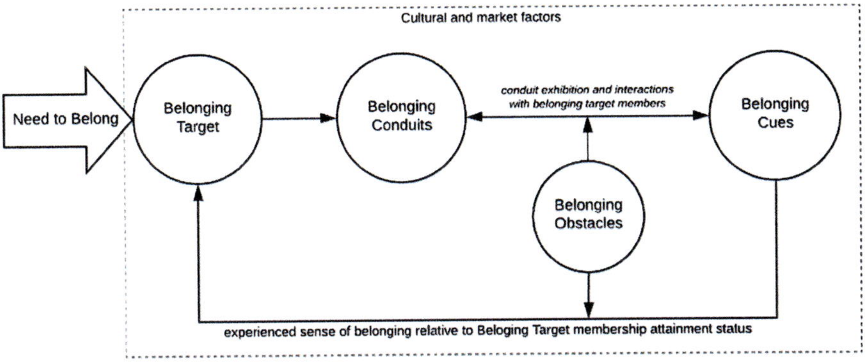

Fig. 1. Belonging-oriented consumption model.

In the belonging-oriented consumption model, Belonging Conduits are the resources available in the marketplace, which consumers use to promote their affiliation to a group. Conduits serve as a vehicle for signaling group affiliation to others. Conduits can be brands, products, or services, to which the subject has access, whose symbolic and operational properties make them suitable to serve as instruments to promote affiliation. For example, brands of sneakers among the members of a group that practice a specific sport. Similarly, sports equipment or food products among members of a healthy lifestyle group. The way in which a product or service is consumed can also serve as a conduit. For example, eating at restaurants of a certain type of cuisine and price, or choosing to attend specific entertainment events or tourist destinations. Vargas-Bianchi [9] showed that elements such as the geographic location of an establishment, such as a restaurant or gym, can be used as part of the Belonging Conduit. The author also argues that conduits not only respond to the cultural context of the individuals, but also to the market in which they are located. In addition, subjects may have access to markets other than the one in which they live, for example if they travel to other markets and purchase products or brands to use as Belonging Conduits.

2.3 Instagram and the Search for Belonging

In the last decade, social networks have become important spaces in people's lives, and are considered one of the main dissemination channels in brand communication strategies. These media satisfy consumers' desire to interact with those brands they wish to associate with, fostering a connection with their customers and a sense of belonging among them [1, 2, 23]. Instagram is a social network that allows users to take photos, apply filters, and share the photos with followers who can click "Like" and comment on these posts [24]. Instagram also allows posting "stories" -one or more videos of a few seconds that remain in the user's content history for a limited time- in addition to live streaming. This has contributed to Instagram receiving more average interactions per post than other social networks [25]. Sheldon and Bryant [26] and Ilich and Hardley [27] observed that the use of Instagram "To follow my friends" and 'to see what other people share" were the preponderant motivations, oriented to peer-to-peer recognition and validation. On the other hand, Wong, Amon & Keep [3] found that a greater desire to belong positively predicted frequency of Instagram use in a significant way. The study aimed at exploring how frequency of online interactions can be affected by a sense of belonging and perceived potential social support.

3 Methods

The study followed a deductive method, using the belonging-oriented consumption model as a basis. For the research, the experiences reported by young consumers regarding their way of using conduits on the social network site Instagram were analyzed. To that end, the following research questions were posed:

- **RQ1:** In what ways do young people use Instagram to develop content that showcases Belonging Conduits intended to promote their group affiliation?
- **RQ2:** What are the Instagram features used by young people when generating content using convenient Belonging Conduits to favor their group affiliation?

The study followed a qualitative research method and two data analysis techniques, an initial structural coding [28] and, subsequently, a thematic analysis technique [29, 30].

3.1 Sample

Participants were selected by purposive sampling [31, 32] based on the belonging-oriented consumption model. The case participants were 17 young people who acknowledged having posted content on social network with the primary objective of favoring their belonging to a group. Several studies argue that adolescents and young people show greater sensitivity to their social relationships linked to their group belonging and in accordance with their peers [33, 34]. The following inclusion criteria were established for selection: (i) being between 19 and 23 years old, (ii) actively using the Instagram account by checking it at least once a day, (iii) being in the habit of generating content for the Instagram account, both in feed posts and in the stories feature. The mean age of participants was 21.7 (median = 22; mode = 22; SD = 1.95). Out of the total, 65% of participants were female, and 35% were male. All participants belonged to a Western living environment, and to a Latin American social and cultural framework, and were immersed in a metropolitan urban life typical of an emerging economy.

To contact the participants, the researcher asked professors from a university to provide a list of students and their e-mail addresses. They were contacted by e-mail and were offered to participate in the study. Those who responded positively were sent a digital questionnaire to identify whether they met the inclusion criteria, and, if applicable, to continue their participation.

3.2 Data Collection

The mobile instant messaging interview (MIMI) technique was used. Through this technique, a mobile messaging application is used as a tool to obtain information from participants, while they are in the different circumstances of their everyday life [35, 36]. The process reported by Kaufmann and Peil [35] was followed, and the WhatsApp messaging application was used due to its widespread adoption among case participants. MIMI provides a means to prompt the self-documentation process, which in turn allows for the inclusion of photographic, audiovisual, and documentary material, during a real-time dialogue [35]. For the interviews through MIMI, a guide was developed, structured in three themes consistent with the goal of the study: (i) the type of branded or consumer information they use to foster belonging, (ii) the Instagram features they use and value to project the Belonging Conduit, and (iii) the influence of social distancing, caused by the SARSCovid-19 pandemic, on the use of Belonging Conduits on Instagram. Each theme had semi-structured questions that were raised in conversation with the participants. To collect the data, each participant was contacted at random times between 8 am and 9 pm, so that they could not prepare answers, nor deliberately choose specific activities about their Instagram use. The procedure was carried out simultaneously with the participants, and the average duration of each interview was two days. If there was no response after each message during the interview, they were contacted again in the following two hours. Informants were encouraged to use the full range of WhatsApp multimedia features, such as sending photos, videos, and screenshots. Interviews were conducted via a WhatsApp account used exclusively for this study. Once the conversations were completed, the texts were extracted from the application and exported to separate digital documents in text format.

Regarding the ethical aspects of the research, participants agreed to be involved on a voluntary basis and were asked to sign an informed consent form before conducting the interviews. Anonymity and confidentiality of participant information was maintained by assigning letter codes. The confidentiality of the individuals included in the publications that the participants might share was also maintained. No participant declined to continue with the study or required withdrawal of the information provided.

3.3 Analysis Procedure

A first cycle of analysis was carried out using a structural coding technique with the texts of the conversations and material sent by the participants. Structural coding applies the concepts that represent the research topic to the data set of a study [28]. The topics for this coding were: resources available in the market, interaction and search for belonging, generating content on Instagram, and posting on Instagram. Once the codes were obtained, the analysis continued with thematic coding, in order to identify themes or patterns in the set of codes obtained. Thematic analysis allows to identify, analyze, and report on the phenomenon studied based on the data [29], by recognizing patterns, revealing consistencies and basic meanings, within the study data, in which emerging themes become the categories for analysis [30]. The multi-phase procedure proposed by Braun & Clarke [29] was followed. Nvivo 13 was used for both analysis cycles.

4 Results

The participants mentioned different ways of using Instagram in connection with their relationship with other people. Specially, with the friends who are among their account followers, in contrast with the people the participants follow in their network accounts. The contents to favor the relationship and group belonging are as varied as the formats for content creation offered by Instagram, and the available features to enrich contents in the social network. After the analysis, three themes were identified. It is possible to observe these themes transversally, which, in the experience of the participants, all the content they produce and consume on Instagram, has a component related to relationship and belonging.

4.1 Theme 1: Use of Resources Traded in the Market

This theme refers to participants' recognition and use of resources available that are traded in a marketplace, which, due to their associated meanings, are functional vehicles to further their affiliation to a group. Participants include these resources- brands, products, or services-in their Instagram posts. This theme is consistent with preceding studies on product display as a means of satisfying group affiliation.

One participant states that in their posts they can include many types of resources: *"[by including music in stories] it can be evidenced that I use Spotify, that I drink beer of a specific brand, that I smoke cigarettes, that I dress in such a way, or that I use a computer of a certain brand"* (Participant H, male). Another participant narrates her experience: *"In my highlight stories, I appear with a Corona brand beer. Other brands that appear when I make virtual meetings with my friends are Samsung and Apple"* (Participant P, female).

This example highlights the use of brands, clothing of a specific style or characteristics (regardless of the specific brand), as well as product consumption practices. Another interviewee shares a similar experience, with greater emphasis on certain brands: *"people, when documenting their day-to-day lives in stories, indirectly tend to show products such as clothing, accessories, or electronic devices as part of their daily lives. I would highlight brands like Nike, Calvin Klein, or Apple"* (Participant D, male). The same participant argues that the brand is functional as a vehicle to promote group affiliation *"because you know that among your acquaintances [that brand] has some kind of cultural weight"* (Participant D, male).

Among the consumption practices that the participants commented on to evidence their affiliation or effort to be linked to a group, are restaurants and entertainment services.

An interviewee in the study stated that she sometimes shares what she consumes on her social network profile: *"when eating at a restaurant, or going to a place. For example, when I went to the theatre I would post a story on Instagram indicating the place and the play"* (Participant Y, woman).

As mentioned at the beginning of the study, this analysis was conducted during the initial months of the Covid-19 pandemic. The interviewees were in a circumstance of limited mobilization following a strict quarantine. This context had an effect on some publications aimed at encouraging them to belong to groups: *"Now it's harder to show your clothes (...). Although you can take photos in your room, living room, or rooftop (...) You don't have enough space to take a photo where the entire body can be seen or make poses that help you show your clothes" (Participant U, male).* Another participant shares her experience referring to posts of this nature: *"I have noticed that there is less 'shareable' content (...) [before the pandemic] most of it was about travel or group outings or going to interesting places"* (Participant V, female).

4.2 Theme 2: Instagram Extends the Belonging Conduit

This theme refers to Instagram features that allow participants to create and enhance content appropriate to promote group affiliation. Youth interviewees find that Instagram's features allow them to (i) incorporate resources available in the marketplace into their posts and (ii) add layers of additional information to that content, information that enhances the display of the Belonging Conduit in the post. This reality is what the title of the theme points to, to the fact that the social network allows extending the strength of a conduit by annexing additional data about that consumption. The most mentioned Instagram features are the following:

- Post location. "*In the 'add location' option I always tag the place where I was. I think I do all this to evidence that I did something interesting*" (Participant I, female); "*On Instagram you can post the place where you are, even who you are with. Those options can help someone external to notice the groups I belong to*" (Participant Y, female).
- Text. "*Slyly, you want [the brand] to be seen in the photo or short video. This is always accompanied by text at the very least*" (Participant D, male).
- Hashtags. "*You can accompany those photos with a hashtag, like #family or similar from the group*" (Participant G, male).
- Gifs. "*I usually tend to use a combination of filters, gifs, music, and shapes*" (Participant U, male).
- Tagging other Instagram users. "*When it is a closed group, like the ones at the gym*" (Participant V, female); "*well, I see myself included in the publications or stories they make, plus they also tag me so you can see that it is my profile*" (Participant C, female).

4.3 Theme 3: Music Amplifies the Belonging Conduit

The theme encompasses the incorporation of musical backgrounds as part of the content of Instagram posts, as a resource that enables participants to add an additional information layer to the content. The selection of the song or artist amplifies the Belonging Conduit selected for the post. The use of music emerged with distinction among the other resources available on Instagram, thus it is considered a separate theme from the preceding one. This feature is enabled for the social network's "stories" format, which is preferred by the study participants.

The choice of the music track seems to have different motivations. For example, one interviewee expresses that *when someone makes a story with their friends, they can use a song whose lyrics mentions friendship"* (Participant G, male). Another young woman argues that *"when [it is] something more artistic, you add music to it to make it interesting"* (Participant V, female). In general, they seem to choose music that goes with the content or emotions they want to convey: *"Because it is related to the story"* (Participant K, male), or in the words of another interviewee *"the day I finished college I uploaded a story with the song We are the champions"* (Participant E, female). The interviewees stated that songs allow them to express emotions when they share them in a story, and also to add an additional tone or style to their posts.

5 Discussion

This study looks at the use of Instagram as a medium to showcase Belonging Conduits. Specifically, identifying content development practices among young people in this social network, when their goal is to promote their affiliation to a group. The findings obtained from the interviews show that the participants view Instagram as a useful channel to display the conduits, due to the possibility of including consumer goods in photographs and videos that can be shared on the social network. A relevant finding is that Instagram features allow you to add layers of additional information to the conduits, which increases their reach and information quality. This observation is consistent with previous studies on consumer behavior and group affiliation, whose theoretical model proposes that people use all the resources that are available in the market to instrumentalize them in favor of their group affiliation [7–9]. The findings contribute to the knowledge and details of the belonging-oriented consumption model, in particular regarding its construct, Belonging Conduits.

The conduits usually used by young people are brands and products that are easy to display and recognize, such as clothing, sneakers or bags, and electronic devices like cell phones or a smart watch. As for Instagram, it does not specifically showcase its use or brand, but it is used as a channel to distribute the chosen conduits. However, Instagram is equally a brand as well as a service available on the market, thus it is also included in the definition of Belonging Conduits. The use of two or more conduits simultaneously does not contradict the definition, and is a regular practice. For example, when a subject posts photos of himself/herself in a chain of coffee shops valued by the group, using a laptop whose brand is also appreciated by its members. However, in a strict sense, the use of Instagram is not showcased, it operates as a channel that allows information layers to be added to the main object of the conduct.

Instagram's geolocation feature is a good example. It allows people to report the specific area where the person is consuming something, or the location of a particular store. These data are important and valued by members of the group to which the individual seeks to belong. The same is true of other features, such as adding text to posts or animated graphic elements. Identifying that Instagram is a conduit, just like a product or a brand, shows that Belonging Conduits can be composed of resources that complement each other in different dimensions. According to the previous examples, a person can post a photo drinking coffee in a well-known coffee shop chain and inform the location of the place. In this case, it can be affirmed that the coffee brand is the primary object of the conduit, and that the location data complements its quality as a vehicle. The incorporation of musical backgrounds is also an additional dimension to the conduit used in Instagram. The selection of a song or artist amplifies the conduit's communication possibilities when it is posted. The use of music emerged prominently among the Instagram features available, affirming that participants value the tool to enrich their content on the social network.

An observation shared by one of the young participants is that posting content on Instagram generates the perception of being part of a group. In their words, *"when you post content related to these topics, you feel like you belong more to those groups."* While it may take group members to confirm your affiliation status, for example, through likes or comments, making your content visible to others creates an experience of belonging or being part of a community. This observation is consistent with preceding studies examining the social motivation behind Instagram use [37], that gratification originating from social interaction positively impacts users' intention to continue using Instagram [38]. Both studies analyze motivations in the use of social networks, in the framework of the uses and gratifications theory [24, 26]. Social network use motivated by the social gratification of experiencing group affiliation is consistent with the theoretical model. Future studies are needed to further explore the relationships of this phenomenon and the theory.

A limitation of the study is that the information analyzed is obtained by participants' self-report, and it may be that the intention to post content on Instagram to favor group affiliation is not always a conscious act. Future research may use different data collection techniques to bridge the limitation and continue to delve deeper into this phenomenon. Another limitation is that the data were obtained during partial quarantines due to the Covid-19 pandemic, which reduced access to commercial venues, restaurants, or gyms. Participants did not stop displaying products or services as conduits on their Instagram accounts, however, the opportunities were reduced. Future research could continue to explore the use of musical resources in social media posts aimed at promoting group affiliation. There is an opportunity whether music bands or their creations are commercial resources available in the market, and therefore considered as Belonging Conduits. The same question could be raised regarding thought stances, such as environmental protection or minority rights, when brands take a stance on these issues and use them in their communications strategies. It is worth examining whether in that case the thought stance becomes a dimension of the Belonging Conduit, as an effect of the use by a brand.

References

1. Nadkarni, A., Hofmann, S.G.: Why do people use facebook? Pers. Individ. Dif. **52**, 243–249 (2012)
2. Seidman, G.: Self-presentation and belonging on Facebook: how personality influences social media use and motivations. Pers. Individ. Dif. **54**, 402–407 (2013)

3. Wong, D., Amon, K.L., Keep, M.: Desire to belong affects Instagram behavior and perceived social support. Cyberpsychol. Behav. Soc. Netw. **22**, 465–471 (2019)
4. Griskevicius, V., Kenrick, D.T.: Fundamental motives: how evolutionary needs influence consumer behavior. J. Consum. Psychol. **23**, 372–386 (2013)
5. Ahuvia, A.C.: Nothing matters more to people than people: brand meaning and social relationships, pp. 121–149 (2015). https://doi.org/10.1108/S1548-643520150000012005
6. Mead, N.L., Baumeister, R.F., Stillman, T.F., Rawn, C.D., Vohs, K.D.: Social exclusion causes people to spend and consume strategically in the service of affiliation. J. Consum. Res. **37**, 902–919 (2011)
7. Arias, R., Otnes, C.: The belonging process: elements and enactment within a consumption context. In: Gneezy, A., Griskevicius, V., Williams, P. (eds.) NA - Advances in Consumer Research, vol. 45, pp. 500–502. Association for Consumer Research (2017)
8. Arias, R.: Toward a conceptual understanding of belonging in consumer research. Adv. Consum. Res. **33**, 212–217 (2016)
9. Vargas-Bianchi, L.: Shopping to belong: qualitative testing and advancement of a theoretical framework on consumer behavior aimed to promote belonging. Preprint SocArxiv, pp. 1–25 (2020). https://doi.org/10.13140/RG.2.2.14120.93448
10. Mellor, D., Stokes, M., Firth, L., Hayashi, Y., Cummins, R.: Need for belonging, relationship satisfaction, loneliness, and life satisfaction (2008). https://doi.org/10.1016/j.paid.2008.03.020
11. Pickett, C.L., Gardner, W.L., Knowles, M.: Getting a cue: the need to belong and enhanced sensitivity to social cues. Pers. Soc. Psychol. Bull. **30**, 1095–1107 (2004)
12. Baumeister, R.F., Leary, M.R.: The need to belong: desire for interpersonal attachments as a fundamental human motivation. Psychol. Bull. (1995). https://doi.org/10.1037/0033-2909.117.3.497
13. Griskevicius, V., et al.: Blatant benevolence and conspicuous consumption: when romantic motives elicit strategic costly signals. J. Pers. Soc. Psychol. **93**, 85–102 (2007)
14. De Gregorio, F., Sung, Y.: Understanding attitudes toward and behaviors in response to product placement. J. Advert. **39**, 83–96 (2010)
15. Elliott, R., Wattanasuwan, K.: Brands as symbolic resources for the construction of identity. Int. J. Advert. **17**, 131–144 (1998)
16. Belk, R.W.: Possessions and the extended self. J. Consum. Res. **15**, 139–168 (1988)
17. Algesheimer, R., Dholakia, U.M., Herrmann, A.: The social influence of brand community: evidence from european car clubs. J. Mark. **69**, 19–34 (2005)
18. Muniz, A.M., O'Guinn, T.C.: Brand community. J. Consum. Res. **27**, 412–432 (2001)
19. Ahuvia, A.C.: Beyond the extended self: loved objects and consumers' identity narratives. J. Consum. Res. **32**, 171–184 (2005)
20. Berger, J., Heath, C.: Where consumers diverge from others: identity signaling and product domains. J. Consum. Res. **34**, 121–134 (2007)
21. Bettman, J.R., Escalas, J.E.: Reference groups, and brand meaning. J. Consum. Res. **32**, 1–10 (2005)
22. Goulding, C., Shankar, A., Canniford, R.: Learning to be tribal: facilitating the formation of consumer tribes. Eur. J. Mark. **47**, 813–832 (2013)
23. Enginkaya, E., Yılmaz, H.: What drives consumers to interact with brands through social media? a motivation scale development study. Procedia - Soc. Behav. Sci. **148**, 219–226 (2014)
24. Alhabash, S., Ma, M.: A tale of four platforms: motivations and uses of Facebook, Twitter, Instagram, and Snapchat among college students? Soc. Media + Soc. **3**, 205630511769154 (2017)

25. Casaló, L.V., Flavián, C., Ibáñez-Sánchez, S.: Be creative, my friend! engaging users on Instagram by promoting positive emotions. J. Bus. Res. (2020). https://doi.org/10.1016/j.jbusres.2020.02.014
26. Sheldon, P., Bryant, K.: Instagram: motives for its use and relationship to narcissism and contextual age. Comput. Human Behav. **58**, 89–97 (2016)
27. Ilich, K.L., Hardey, M.: 'It's all about the packaging': investigation of the motivations, intentions, and marketing implications of sharing photographs of secondary packaging on Instagram. Inf. Commun. Soc. **23**, 1–19 (2020)
28. Saldana, J.: The Coding Manual for Qualitative Researchers. Sage (2013)
29. Braun, V., Clarke, V.: Thematic analysis. In: Cooper, H., et al. (eds.) APA Handbooks in Psychology®. APA Handbook of Research Methods in Psychology. Research designs: Quantitative, Qualitative, Neuropsychological, and Biological, vol. 2, pp. 57–71. American Psychological Association (2012)
30. Buetow, S.: Thematic analysis and its reconceptualization as 'saliency analysis.' J. Health Serv. Res. Policy **15**, 123–125 (2010)
31. Coyne, I.: Sampling in qualitative research. Purposeful and theoretical sampling; merging or clear boundaries? J. Adv. Nurs. **26**, 623–630 (1997)
32. Gentles, S.J., Charles, S.J., Ploeg, C., Mckibbon, J.A.: Sampling in qualitative research: insights from an overview of the methods literature. Qual. Rep. **20**, 1772 (2015)
33. Hornsey, M.J., Jetten, J.: The individual within the group: balancing the need to belong with the need to be different. Pers. Soc. Psychol. Rev. **8**, 248–264 (2004)
34. Oishi, S., Diener, E., Suh, E., Lucas, R.E.: Value as a moderator in subjective well-being. J. Pers. **67**, 157–184 (1999)
35. Kaufmann, K., Peil, C.: The mobile instant messaging interview (MIMI): using WhatsApp to enhance self-reporting and explore media usage in situ. Mob. Media Commun. **8**, 229–246 (2020)
36. Kaye, L.K., Monk, R.L., Hamlin, I.: "Feeling appy?" Using app-based methodology to explore contextual effects on real-time cognitions, affect and behaviours. In: Costa, C., Condie, J. (eds.) Doing Research in and on the Digital. Research Methods Across Fields of Enquiry, pp. 11–29. Routledge (2018)
37. Lee, E., Lee, J.A., Moon, J.H., Sung, Y.: Pictures speak louder than words: motivations for using Instagram. Cyberpsychol. Behav. Soc. Netw. **18**, 552–556 (2015)
38. Hwang, H.S., Cho, J.: Why Instagram? Intention to continue using instagram among Korean college students. Soc. Behav. Pers. **46**, 1305–1315 (2018)

Check for updates

Is Facebook a Tool to Achieve True Friendship? A Study from an Ascetic Perspective

Juan Gabriel García-Huertas[1](✉), Pablo Garrido-Pintado[2], and Pável Sidorenko-Bautista[1]

[1] Universidad Francisco de Vitoria, Madrid, Spain
{jg.garcia.prof,pavel.sidorenko}@ufv.es
[2] Universidad Complutense, Madrid, Spain
pablo.garrido@ucm.es

Abstract. With the rise of social media networks, young people have found a channel of communication where they can create and maintain their personal relationships. But, among the wide range of possible relationships we should determine the role of true friendship as a vital element in the full development of one's personality. Although many point out that Facebook is losing followers, it is still the leading social network with 2.8 billion users, 65 percent of whom are under the age of 35. Thus, based on the study of the ascetics of friendship by Pedro Laín Entralgo, we will analyse the way in which Facebook enables this through a study conducted with university students 18 to 22 years of age. The results will allow us to conclude that social networks do not provide the tools necessary to pass from fellowship, camaraderie and sympathy towards the experience of true and fulfilling friendship.

Keywords: Facebook · Friendship · Social media

1 Introduction

Social media has revolutionised communication, both in business and interpersonal relationships. For Vallor [13] "in of the greatest attractions is its capacity to facilitate gratifying reciprocal exchanges". In the case of Facebook, this exchange begins with the request for friendship which, once accepted, continues with the posting of pictures and video on the page, labelling friends, playing with them of gaming platforms or contributing to social causes. This process, far from diminishing, has only increased with the acquisition by Facebook of Instagram [4]) a social media platform focussed on the exchange of images and the instant messaging service Whatsapp [5].

Facebook, despite growing competition, has maintained its leading position. According to recent statistics, the social network accounts for 59% of all social media users [6]. Facebook data [7] shows that the platform has 2,800 million users, of whom, 1,840 million connect to the platform daily. Although it is commonly believed that the popularity of Facebook has fallen among young people, data from Statista [12] reveal the contrary; some 65 percent of Facebook users are under the age of 35.

© The Author(s), under exclusive license to Springer Nature Singapore Pte Ltd. 2022
Á. Rocha et al. (Eds.): ICOMTA 2021, SIST 259, pp. 164–172, 2022.
https://doi.org/10.1007/978-981-16-5792-4_17

Adolescents spend more time interacting online via social media networks than any other traditional medium [8]. These are digital natives who have grown up in a world saturated with technology and are the group most engaged with these types of platforms [3]. Young people attach a great deal of importance to their online presence and are fully aware of the messages they send and receive via social media. Of particular importance within this process, is the experience of friendship, a phenomenon which requires continuous communication and which, among this segment of the population, are conditioned by the use of various types of technologies.

This process is not without norms and rules. Youth and adolescence are very important life stages and the experience of true friendship is an "ethical good which elevates the individual and which should be a part of every aspect of life and the world of communication is no exception" (p.4) [2].

A number of studies have found that online friendships are an important element in the life of social media users. Research by Marder, Joinson and Shanker [9] has shown that, among university students, Facebook friends have diverse social back-grounds, and include online and off relationships including friends, siblings, friends of friends, colleagues or casual social acquaintances.

However, the path toward the experience of true friendship is not an easy one and may lead to confusion with other types of relationships. Thus, the present study will analyse the necessary factors for a relationship to develop into true friendship within the technological context provided by Facebook.

We are immersed in a true digital revolution. We have moved from an atom-based to a bit-based culture [1]. The implications are huge, especially since digital technology removes the need to be in the same place at the same time to meet for whatever purposes. Space-time coordinates were, until recently, the frame of reference for any human activity [2].

2 Literature Review

The principal aim of this study was to determine if the relationship between Facebook contacts can develop into a true friendship. Our hypothesis is the following: Facebook constitutes a valid communication tool to progress from certain types of relationships towards true friendship. To identify the types of relationships practiced on social media we take as a reference the work "On Friendship" by the doctor and philosopher Pedro Laín Entralgo [10]. Of the various dimensions studied, we will focus on relationships of proximity, camaraderie and sympathy, linked to ascetics. Furthermore, we will analyse the influence of the gender of social media users on the validity of our main hypothesis.

The term ascetic is derived from the Greek verb askeô meaning "to be active in something, to achieve by means of its exercise a certain habit [...] thus, the ascetics of friendship is the One may ask, how does followship become friendship? For Contreras, "fellowship is proximity and closeness, leading to an endless array of possible relationships". The four pillars of fellowship are benevolence, beneficence, confidence and equality. Benevolence, by definition, is something positive found in a friend. Without this benevolence, the condition of friend disappears [1]. Two people acting with mutual benevolence enhance their relationship, raise it through love and seek from the other to deserve rather than receive. To evaluate whether benevolence is present in the relationships established through Facebook it is necessary to determine if actions or posts in relation to others truly seeks the benefit of others. We have therefore established five levels, from the lowest, indicating that no actions taken by the user seek the benefit of another, to the highest, that all actions on Facebook seek the benefit of another.

According to Kant, friendship is a bond between two people based on reciprocal love and respect. For Vallor (p. 188) [13] "reciprocity is a primitive biological impulse which acts as the seed of human sociability and characteristic of all forms of friendship". This reciprocity must also be understood as including beneficence. No doubt Kant was drawing on Aristotle when he affirmed "friendship requires several activities other than mutual contemplation: shared hours together, joint projects, mutual beneficence" (p. 235) [15]. A priori, beneficence may seem a virtue of those professing it rather than those receiving it, but this is a virtue with leads to friendship when it is reciprocal, the giver and receiver can reverse their roles. As noted by Rivadulla [11], "while a benefactor is concerned with the happiness of others, the friend s also happy when their fellows are well" (p. 219). With this understanding of beneficence, we asked participants if, among their Facebook contacts, they had done or given something in a disinterested way to benefit another. This does not refer necessarily to a material benefit but something performed through the communication channels provided by social media.

Another pillar of fellowship is confidence. For Visentini [14] this is an essential aspect of friendship, conditioned by a prior and careful selection of the friend, "given that nothing can do more harm to a person than a false friend with whom they share everything, trusting the other without truly knowing them" (p. 215). This refers to the ability to count on another as if counting on oneself. Knowing that a friend does not judge but accompanies in this confidence and provides help if ever necessary. Based on these premises, we asked the participants if, using Facebook as the medium, they share important confidences with their contacts. As with the rest of the questionnaire, the responses were ranked on a scale of 1 to 5, with 1 meaning participants never shared confidences on social media and 5 meaning that all their actions are oriented towards being shared. Finally, dentro de la fellowship, we must understand the notion of equality, that is, a proportionality in what one gives and receives, for the mutual satisfaction of both persons.

Furthermore, camaraderie involves a number of characteristics which, when present, may lead to true friendship. For Laín Entralgo [10], the first ingredient must be a disposition not based on fanaticism but a balance between expression and treatment. Secondly, it must be a relationship based on current reality since nostalgia or speculations on the future do not truly reveal the genuine personality of the comrade. Finally, a third necessity is that the comrade is not regarded as merely a means to an end but as an end in themselves.

According to Laín Entralgo [10], sympathy or friendliness is defined as a natural virtue of the individual, as opposed to, for example, the more profound attitude of fellowship. A sympathetic person may share the joy or sadness or another but in a largely superficial manner, either as part of their nature or as social etiquette. Being sympathetic is not necessarily loving but merely friendly. A sympathetic person may feel comfortable with this condition and not necessarily seek to deepen the relationship to the level of true friendship. Thus, friendship requires, in addition to benevolence, beneficence and confidence, a willingness on both sides to be open, that is, the open character of the two people allows the step towards the possible experience of true friendship.

To quantify the experience of friendship, we designed a questionnaire, verified with a test group of 20 individuals in order to validate the concepts being studied. As these concepts are proper to the world of ascetics, it was necessary to confirm the degree of understanding prior to administering the questionnaire to the selected sample. The universe comprehends the audio visual communication university students who study in Comunidad de Madrid, which represents a total of 2550 students. After the validation fase, the cuestionary was presented to 300 subjects, young university students, between 18 and 25 years old who study in public and private universities of Comunidad de Madrid (España), specifically, students of Universidad Complutense de Madrid and Francisco de vitoria University. It's about a non-probabilistic intencional or convenience sample due to the presented characteristics. Given the size of the population (2850) and the sample (300), with a confidence level of a 95%, the margin of error is of a 5,35%. Each questions was quantified from 1 to 5, where the responses 4 and 5 are considered affirmative. Analysing the results will allow us to determine, not only if the relationships may lead to a true friendship but also, where this is not the case, the characteristics that are lacking. The results are presented as a percentage and in order to evaluate the degree of approach to true friendship it is necessary that all the evaluated aspects of the relation have a high percentage of responses in the 4 to 5 range on the scale. Once the basic statistics have been obtained, a Mann-Whitney U-test is conducted using the SPSS analysis software. This is a non-parametric test which will allow us to determine the effect of gender on the results.

To contribute to this literature and to further understand the advantages and disadvantages of the use of ICTs in education, this study explores the perceptions of Spanish students during the first months of the COVID-19 pandemic in Spain. From March to June 2020, due to the lockdown, Spanish universities were forced to move their teaching from the physical to the online space. What were the perceptions of students about the online teaching that took place during this exceptional moment? As such, this study presents a series of specific characteristics. First, the adaptation to the online methodology was carried out in a forced and unnatural way, with limited time. Moreover, the change was abrupt. This means that students and teachers could not be previously trained in the use of the technology necessary to implement the online teaching. To this must be added an extraordinary social situation, characterized by the concerns with the social and health consequences of the pandemic and with home isolation. All this has caused online teaching to not be as accurate as it should. This offers a good opportunity to explore this process in motion and to highlight current needs in terms of online and face-to-face educommunication.

3 Results

The results of the questionnaire are presented below, showing the statistic obtained for the subdimensions of fellowship (benevolence, beneficence, confidence and equality), camaraderie (non-fanatical and balanced disposition, based on the current reality and with the person as the end) and sympathy (open contacts, open person and actions of benevolence, beneficence and confidence).

3.1 Fellowship

Benevolence. The results show that only some 13% of participants sought to perform actions of benevolence on social media, compared to over 86% who reported they did not or rarely had such intentions.

A Mann-Whitney U-test produced a value of $p > 0.05$, indicating there are no significant differences in the results according to the gender of participants.

Beneficence. Some 70% of participants reported they did not perform actions seeking the good of others through Facebook. A mere 11.67% claimed they often or always take actions of this type. The result of a Mann-Whitney U-test was $p = 0.568$ ($p > 0.05$), indicating there were no significant differences between male and female participants.

Confidence. The results of the questionnaire show that only slightly more than 10% of participants always or often share confidences on Facebook. The result of the Mann-Whitney U-test was $p = 0.09$ ($p > 0.05$). Thus, as was the case with benevolence and beneficence, there were no significant differences according to the gender of the participants.

Equality. 50% of participants reported that all their actions on social media are based on a relationship of equality with others. For this aspect, a necessary condition of true friendship, a Mann-Whitney U-test was also conducted, producing a value of $p = 0.688$ ($p > 0.05$). This indicates that, as with the other aspects, no significant differences were found in terms of gender.

The results for the variable fellowship are presented in the table below (Tables 1 and 2):

Table 1. Results for Fellowship.

Response	Benevolence	Beneficence	Confidence	Equality
1	45,00%	27,33%	22,67%	03,00%
2	25,00%	42,67%	51,00%	06,67%
3	16,67%	18,33%	16,00%	16,67%
4	09,00%	09,00%	07,33%	23,33%
5	04,33%	02,67%	03,00%	50,33%

Table 2. Results of the Mann-Whitney U-test for Fellowship.

Benevolence	Beneficence	Confidence	Equality
P = 0,075	P = 0,568	P = 0,090	P = 0,688

3.2 Camaraderie

Non-fanatical, balanced disposition. Only 8% of participants reported their contacts always have a non-fanatical, balanced disposition, while 70% reported that their contacts never or almost never show non-fanatical or balanced behaviour or that this is generally habitual.

The result of the Mann-Whitney U-test was $p = 0.29$ indicating there are no significant differences in the non-fanatical and balanced disposition of contacts according to gender.

Disposition towards current reality. Some 24% of participants reported that they often or always deal with current reality. 70% reported this was occasionally the case while only 5% never address issues related to current reality. The result of the non-parametric test was $p = 0.657$. Here again, the p value was greater than 0.05, indicating no significant differences in terms of gender in dealing with current reality.

Person as an end in itself. 55% of participants reported they rarely or never consider their contacts a means to an end. By contrast, some 7% regard their contacts as a means to an end, while 7.67% report they habitually use their contacts to achieve a specific end. The non-parametric test produced a p value greater than 0.05, again indicating that there are no significant differences in the results in terms of gender.

The results for camaraderie are presented in the table below (Tables 3 and 4):

Table 3. Results for Camaraderie.

Response	Balanced character	Current time	User as a means
1	04,00%	05,00%	07,00%
2	20,00%	30,00%	07,67%
3	47,67%	40,33%	23,33%
4	20,33%	18,33%	23,67%
5	09,00%	06,33%	38,33%

Table 4. Results of the Mann-Whitney U-test for Camaraderie.

Balanced charater	Current time	User as a means
P = 0,290	P = 0,657	P = 0,505

3.3 Sympathy

Contact with an open disposition. The results on a scale of 1 to 5 are as follows: Some 20.33% of participants reported that their contacts never indicate an openness towards being known in greater depth. 28.33% report that some of their contacts are open to being known in greater depth while 24% indicated that their contacts habitually show themselves to be open. 17% reported this was frequently the case and 10% reported this was normal among their contacts.

The result of the Mann Whitney U-test was $p = 0.398$ indicating that there were no significant differences in this aspect in terms of gender.

User with an open disposition. For this aspect, 20.33% of participants reported they are never open and approachable with their contacts while 28.33% report that they are so with some of their contacts. 24% of participants reported they habitually act and present themselves as open and approachable. Some 17.33% reported they often act in this way while 10% claimed to be open and approachable always, willing to reveal themselves without fear. The Mann Whitney U-test produced a value of $p = 0.414$, again indicating that gender had no significant influence on the results for this aspect.

Actions from a disposition of benevolence, beneficence and confidence. Regarding these types of actions, some 10% of participants reported they believe neither they nor their contacts would ever act in this way. 40.33% reported they or their contacts had acted in this way on some occasions. 25.33% reported this to be habitual while 20% claimed this was very often the case. 4.33% of participants reported they and their contacts always acted in this way.

The results obtained for this variable are presented in the table below (Tables 5 and 6):

Table 5. Results for sympathy

Response	Contacts with an open disposition	User with an open disposition	Actions
1	20,33%	27,33%	10,00%
2	28,33%	42,67%	40,33%
3	24,00%	18,33%	25,33%
4	17,00%	09,00%	20,00%
5	10,00%	02,67%	04,33%

Table 6. Results of the Mann-Whitney U-test for Sympathy

Contacts with an open disposition	User with an open disposition	Actions
P = 0,398	P = 0,414	P = 0,156

4 Conclusions

Evaluating the results of the questionnaire we can conclude that it is unlikely that relationships of fellowship and camaraderie with Facebook contacts further develop into true friendship. Considering that responses in the 4 to 5 range indicate a significant presence of the parameters being analysed, the results are not sufficiently decisive to suggest that deeper relationships are possible. The results also show that gender has no influence on the possibility of experiencing true friendship.

A closer analysis shows that the possibilities are remote of passing from fellowship to true friendship in terms of benevolence, given that a mere 13% of participants reported they acted in this way to any significant degree on Facebook. Beneficence and confidence show similar results. The data reported by the participants does not indicate relationships of confidence between social media users. However, regarding equality, we can conclude that almost three quarters of participants report their interactions with their contacts are always or almost always from a position of equality.

Regarding the step from camaraderie to true friendship, the results indicate this is also highly unlikely. Only 28.33% of participants report their contacts always or almost always demonstrate a balanced character. Similar results were found for the second item referring to dealing with current reality. Finally, for the third item, regarding treating contacts as an end in themselves rather than instrumentally we find that some 50% of participants rarely or never use their contacts to achieve personal objectives.

Finally, the third aspect of the ascetics of friendship, the step from sympathy to friendship, again does not support the hypothesis. The survey results for the three items necessary appear insufficient to affirm that this step is possible.

When asked about the open disposition of their contacts, almost 50% of participants reported this was only occasionally or never the case. Regarding the open disposition of the user towards their contacts, only 27.3% described themselves as often or always open and approachable.

The results of the questionnaire regarding actions based on benevolence, beneficence and confidence, both given and received, similarly do not uphold the hypothesis. Only 24.33% of participants responded in a manner necessary for any approach towards true friendship.

For the three aspects of friendship analysed in the survey, the Mann Whitney U-tests indicate that gender has no influence on the results.

We can therefore affirm, from the perspective of ascetics, Facebook does not provide the conditions or tools which facilitate the development of true friendship from a relationship of fellowship, camaraderie and sympathy. Thus, the supposed friendships on social media do not go beyond that of mere contacts with negligible possibilities for a deeper relationship by means of mediated social media platforms. Social media platforms employ the notion of friendship in an instrumental way, far removed from the conditions necessary for the building of true friendships. Within the context of social media, friendship is a symbolic projection, a false myth, which in the majority of cases leads to poor, superficial and generally unequal relationships which are far from a truly fulfilling experience of friendship.

References

1. Cicerón, M.T.: De la Amistad, Aguilar, Madrid (1963)
2. Díaz del Campo, J.: La enseñanza de la ética y de la deontología de la comunicación y el riesgo de adoctrinamiento, Visión Libros (2013)
3. Dingli, A., Seychell, D.: The New Digital Natives Cutting the Chord. Springer, Heidelberg (2015). https://doi.org/10.1007/978-3-662-46590-5
4. Elmundo.es: Facebook compra Instagram por 1000 millones de dólares. https://www.elmundo.es/elmundo/2012/04/09/navegante/1333991473.html. Accessed 15 May 2021
5. Europapress: Facebook compra Whatsapp por cerca de 22.000 millones de dólares. https://www.europapress.es/internacional/noticia-facebook-compra-whatsapp-cerca-22000-millones-dolares-20141007004852.html. Accessed 26 Feb 2021
6. Emarketer: Social Networks will experience a pandemic driven boost in 2020 but no equally. https://www.emarketer.com/content/social-networks-experienced-pandemic-driven-boost-2020. Accessed 28 Feb 2021
7. Facebook Investor Relations. https://investor.fb.com/investor-news/press-release-de-tails/2021/Facebook-Reports-Fourth-Quarter-and-Full-Year-2020-Results/default.aspx. Accessed 20 Mar 2021
8. Gentina, E., Chen, R., Yang, Z.: Development of theory of mind on online social networks: evidence from Facebook, Twitter, Instagram and Snapchat. J. Bus. Res. **124**, 652–666 (2021). https://doi.org/10.1016/j.jbusres.2020.03.001
9. Marder, B.M., Joinson, A.N., Shanker, A.: Every post you make, every pic you take, I'll be watching you: behind social spheres on Facebook. In: Proceedings of 45th Hawaii International Conference on Systems Science (HICSS 12), pp. 859–868 (2012)
10. Laín, P.: Sobre la Amistad. Espasa Calpe, Madrid (1985)
11. Rivadulla, A.: Amistad, sumo bien y Sociedad civil en Kant. Revista de estudios kantianos **5**(1), 210–218 (2020)
12. Statista: Facebook uses by age and gender, January 2021. https://www.statista.com/statis-tics/376128/facebook-global-user-age-distribution/. Accessed 26 Mar 2021
13. Vallor, S.: Flourishing on Facebook: virtue friendship & new social media. Ethics Inf. Technol. **14**(3), 185–199
14. Visentini, C.: De la Amistad. Un tema universal en el medievo español. Cuadernos de Humanidades, **13**, 213–225 (2002)
15. Veltman, A.: Aristotle and kant on self-disclosure in friendship. J. Value Inquiry. **38**, 225–239 (2004)

Check for updates

Fact-Checking on COVID-19 After a Year of Global Infodemic. Analysis of Digital Misinformation in Spain, Portugal and Latin America

Pedro-Luis Pérez-Díaz(✉) and Lourdes Albert-Botella

Catholic University of San Antonio (UCAM), 30107 Murcia, Spain
plperez@ucam.edu, lalbert2@alu.ucam.edu

Abstract. Based on a theoretical framework on the role of journalism in combating contemporary information disorders, this research aims to determine the characteristics of digital misinformation about COVID-19, explore how it circulated across nations, and address the possible correlation between the demand for information on the disease and the frequency of related news stories that required to be verified. For that purpose, content analysis is performed on the fact-checks conducted by 35 fact-checking organizations based in Spain, Portugal, and Latin America during the year after the declaration of global emergency ($n = 2{,}868$ fact-checks). Among the conclusions, we found that the vast majority of fact-checked information was rated as false or misleading and was spread primarily in textual format. The predominance of fact-checks of viral content shared through social media and messaging apps—mainly Facebook and WhatsApp—is also confirmed, as well as that of misinformation about treatments and cures. Our study demonstrates the high permeability with which fake news spread between the countries studied, given that false content had a rate of transnational mobility four times higher than true stories. Finally, we corroborate the positive and very strong correlation existing in the first months of the pandemic between the number of fact-checks conducted and the global searches on the keyword "COVID-19" that Google Trends registered.

Keywords: Fact-checking · COVID-19 · Misinformation · Fake news · Infodemic

1 Introduction

In the digital age, news stories are shaped by a multitude of actors who gather factual information in an interactive and participatory way, although the rise of post-truth imposes obstacles to distinguish the facts [1]. As Waisbord argues, post-truth threatens the normative conception of the journalistic profession as the guarantor of a democratic public life based on facts and rationality [2]. On the Internet, fake news is disseminated and consumed at a greater speed and scale, a circumstance catalyzed by the "digital proliferation of opportunities for public expression and identity communities with different epistemologies in their engagement with news and information" [2].

© The Author(s), under exclusive license to Springer Nature Singapore Pte Ltd. 2022
Á. Rocha et al. (Eds.): ICOMTA 2021, SIST 259, pp. 173–183, 2022.
https://doi.org/10.1007/978-981-16-5792-4_18

In this context, the search for truth as a common and collective effort faces a complex reassignment of roles and spaces for all the agents that must be coordinated for an effective debunking of deceptions: governments and legislators, big tech companies such as Google or Facebook, the media, and an active and vigilant citizenry [3]. In recent years, an epistemology based on emotional bias has tried to legitimize this way of reorganizing events; something possible at a time of persistent undermining of science and crisis of industrial media structures, aggravated by the rise of digital platforms that allow the massive dissemination of unvetted information [4]. All these "information disorders" have in common their intentionality and interest in sowing doubt, fear, or controversy with the aim of altering the cognitive perception of broad social groups and thus, obtain economic or ideological returns [4].

1.1 Fact-Checking as a Reaction to Information Disorders

The global fact-checking movement has experienced its greatest development within the information ecosystem in parallel with the rise of the aforementioned disorders. From the occupational point of view, this movement has its origin in the questioning of political claims in the United States, from where it begins to be welcomed globally by a wide variety of political and journalistic cultures [5]. As already argued in our previous work [6], fact-checking narratives involve a Lippmannian and elitist logic that vindicates journalistic expertise and authority of journalists to act as arbiters of the truth. Their practices tend to open up and rely on external non-professional players [5], who collaborate in processes of monitoring, verification, or dissemination of results [7].

Fact-checking organizations are essentially reactive in their daily operations but they take the initiative when it comes to promoting a certain media literacy. Many of these fact-checkers consider that the public service they provide by informing citizens, even having a limited impact, constitutes a way to correct the inefficiencies of the legacy media [7]. Despite the fact that in each country fact-checking initiatives adopt different morphologies from the organizational and practical point of view, two organization models stand out: the newsroom model, with fact-checkers based out of established news outlets and the NGO model, in that independent fact-checkers partner with other news organizations [8].

The emergence of the global COVID-19 pandemic at the beginning of 2020 forced governments around the world to adopt restrictions and communicate them to educate the population in combating the rapid spread of infections, while the scientific community implemented an unusual speed in the process of reviewing and publishing research concerning the disease, freely available in open repositories. Consequently, the fact-checking organizations needed to verify statements about the governmental management of this health crisis, frequently supported by fallacious political speeches [9] that generated polarization, but also tried to stop the confusions and social panics derived from the fragile and changing scientific knowledge about the new coronavirus [10].

The patent ineffectiveness of the big tech firms to control these flows of misinformation on social media and messaging apps has made the work of fact-checkers even more difficult, revitalizing the concept of 'infodemic' that was coined during the SARS outbreak of 2003. This term is a portmanteau that has been used by the WHO [11] to describe the rapid and wide scope of information about the new coronavirus—both precise and imprecise—that saturates global society.

1.2 Fact-Checkers in a Global Infodemic Scenario

In a global crisis of this magnitude, the dissemination and demand for large volumes of information converge in a context that favors the spread of misinformation. Thus, between January and March 2020, a growth of up to 900% was registered in the number of English-language fact-checks [12]. Similarly, on the Spanish-language Internet, this higher incidence of misinformation occurred in parallel with the development of the health crisis [13]. Searches for information on the disease and its associated keywords experienced growths that were closely related to media coverage [14], and were two weeks ahead of the peak of new cases [15]. Likewise, the interest in fake news was correlated with the rise of the death toll [16].

In the early stages of the health emergency, most hoaxes circulated on WhatsApp and Twitter [17], a circumstance of great relevance considering that the segment of the population with a low level of education in countries such as Spain or Argentina relied more on social media platforms and messaging apps for news than on news outlets [18]. In general, most fact-checked contents implied some type of distortion of existing information, such as actions taken by public authorities and institutions [12]. Precisely, this type of misinformation, which transforms or disfigures previous information, is more difficult to verify than the less prevalent contents that constitute complete fabrications [19]. Consulting different sources of information (including official ones and those that had been supplanted) was one of the most common verification strategies, ahead of some methods or specialized tools such as reverse search engines [20].

Public figures such as politicians or celebrities who spread misleading statements were certainly a minority, but their posts concentrated most of the engagement on social media [12]. Evidence was also found that, although the deceptive or imprecise tweets were numerous, those that brought false information to light were much more retweeted [21]. In this sense, refuted claims about COVID-19 rose as the contents that drove the most engagement on the Twitter profiles of 8 relevant fact-checking organizations that operated in Spain and Latin America between March and June 2020 [22]. Initial studies on fact-checks in Spanish and Portuguese-speaking countries detected a high frequency of hoaxes related to infections and prevention measures, as well as the difficulty in identifying the source of these contents [13]. To delve into these matters, this study seeks answers to the following research questions:

RQ1: What were the characteristics of the fact-checked misinformation in the first year of the pandemic?
RQ2: How did the misinformation circulate across the different countries in that period?
RQ3: Was there any type of correlation between the number of fact-checks conducted and the worldwide interest in COVID-19 represented by the number of web search queries on Google?

2 Method

Ibero-America (usually known as Latin America) is made up of the American territories where Iberian Romance languages are spoken because in the past they were viceroyalties and provinces administered by the crowns of Spain and Portugal. This common history is translated into cultural ties and constant migratory flows for political and economic reasons, facilitated by the mutual intelligibility of the Spanish and Portuguese languages. It is, therefore, one of the largest and most cohesive language and cultural communities on the planet. Spain and the Spanish-speaking countries of America host 468 of the 489 million people who speak this language natively [23], just as Portugal and Brazil account for the majority of Portuguese speakers. It is a huge market of readers to which many news organizations of panhispanic ambition or that are oriented to the lusophone world have not given up, especially due to the information porosity on both sides of the Atlantic. The circulation of digital misinformation in the Latin American sphere would be a priori favored by affinity and linguistic kinship, consolidated by the relevance of Spanish as the third most used language on the Internet [23].

Since the beginning of the pandemic, an alliance of 35 fact-checking organizations located in the aforementioned countries collected their fact-checks in a database called LatamChequea [24], which has served journalists, curious and researchers as an instrument to curb the spread of rumors and false information. The result of this collaborative effort makes it possible to share the verifications, which is of interest in view of the fact that "the misinformation that circulates in many cases is the same in different countries and being able to count on the work of others helps to refute falsehoods more quickly and prevent their spread" [24]. The initiative is coordinated by the Argentine-based website Chequeado.com with the support of Google and is inspired by the equivalent English-language database created by the International Fact-Checking Network (IFCN).

Our study period runs from January 31, 2020, the date on which the WHO declared the international health emergency, until the same day in 2021, one year later. The data collection work consisted of extracting and selecting the fact-checks conducted in that period from LatamChequea ($n = 2{,}868$), after which we performed a meticulous cleaning and data transformation of the raw data gathered by this initiative. Consequently, the data collected were recoded into variables and categories of interest for a content analysis that would allow us to answer our two initial research questions, as reflected in the coding sheet shown in Table 1. For the last research question, it was necessary to obtain the Google Search Volume Index (GSVI) offered by Google Trends for worldwide searches of the keyword "COVID-19" during each of the weeks of the year studied. The data obtained were treated using the statistical software SPSS 24 and their most relevant results are presented through interactive visualizations created with Flourish.

Table 1. Content analysis coding sheet.

	Variable	Values/Categories
Identification	1. Title	*String variable: contains a title that synthesizes the fact-checked content*
	2. Description	*String variable: contains a description of the fact-checked content*
	3. Publication date	*Values:* From 29/01/20 to 29/01/21
	4. Type of piece	*Categories:* • Explainer • Fact-check of statements by public figures • Fact-check of stories published by media outlets • Fact-check of viral content
Fact-checker	5. Organization	*Categories:* • #NoComaCuento (La Nación) • AFP • Agência Lupa • Agencia Ocote • Animal Político • Aos Fatos • Bolivia Verifica • Chequeado • ColombiaCheck • Convoca • Cotejo.info • Ecuador Chequea • EFE Verifica • Efecto Cocuyo • El Surtidor • EsPaja.com • Estadão Verifica • Gato Encerrado (Despacho 505) • GK • La Silla Vacía • La Voz Chequea (La Voz de Guanacaste) • LaLupa.press • Mala Espina Check • Maldita.es • Newtral.es • OjoPúblico • Periodismo de Barrio and El Toque • PolétikaRD • Polígrafo • Salud con lupa • Spondeo Media • Verificado • Verificador (La República)
	6. Country	*Categories:* • Argentina • Bolivia • Brazil • Chile • Colombia • Costa Rica • Cuba • Dominican Republic • Ecuador • Guatemala • Mexico • Nicaragua • Paraguay • Peru • Portugal • Spain • Uruguay • Venezuela
Content	7. Format	*Categories [multiple choice]:* • Text • Image • Audio • Video • Others
	8. Topic	*Categories [multiple choice]:* • Cases and situation of a territory • Characteristics of the coronavirus disease • Cures and treatments • Diagnostic tests • Government responses and measures • Infections • Origins of the coronavirus • Predictions • Prevention • Symptoms • Others
	9. Actors involved	*Categories:* • Business leaders and companies • Celebrities • Health workers and centers • Journalists and media outlets • Politicians, officials, and public institutions • Scientists and scientific institutions • Members and institutions of civil society • Social media users • Unidentified • Others
	10. Rating	*Categories:* • False • Misleading • Questionable • True • Humorous • Multiple fact-check • Unverifiable • Not applicable

(*continued*)

Table 1. *(continued)*

	Variable	Values/Categories
Spread	11. Source	*Categories [multiple choice]:* • Media outlets • E-mail • Facebook • YouTube • Twitter • WhatsApp • Instagram • Others
	12. International circulation	*Categories:* • To Spain, Portugal or Latin American countries • To Africa • To other American countries • To Asia • To other European countries • To Oceania • Global spread

3 Results

3.1 Characteristics of the Fact-Checked Misinformation

Distribution of Verifications by Countries and Organizations. Spain was the country with the most fact-checks (27%), followed by Argentina (16.6%), Colombia (13.8%), Brazil (9.6%), and Mexico (8.2%). Together, these five nations contribute three-quarters of the study units. By organizations, those that contributed the highest volume of verifications were Maldita.es (Spain), which was responsible for almost one in five of the pieces studied (19.3%), Chequeado (Argentina, 15.7%), ColombiaCheck (Colombia, 8.1%), Agência Lupa (Brazil, 7.6%), Newtral.es (Spain, 5.7%), Animal Político (Mexico, 5.7%) and La Silla Vacía (Colombia, 5.7%).

Topics Present in the Information that was Fact-Checked. Leaving aside miscellaneous topics, which appear in 22% of the sample, cures and treatments (22.6%) were the leading topic that required the highest number of verifications. It is followed by fact-checks about government responses and measures (13.6%), prevention (12.6%), cases and situation of a territory (12.3%), infections (9.5%), and origins of the coronavirus (6.5%). The least frequent verifications were those related to characteristics of the coronavirus disease (2.8%), diagnostic tests (1.8%), symptoms (1.4%), and predictions (1%). The streamgraph represented in Fig. 1 shows the chronological evolution of these topics throughout the year analyzed, and reveals that the highest volume of verifications occurred between March and July (73%). Cures and treatments was the most persistent topic throughout the study period, in contrast to the progressive decline of the rest of the subjects. The late appearance of fact-checks regarding diagnostic tests can also be discerned, which did not begin to become visible until June 2020.

Ratings. Explainers aside, the organizations studied concluded that the bulk of the fact-checked misinformation was false (83.7%) or misleading (9.3%). A smaller set of units of analysis were rated as questionable (2%), required multiple fact-checking (0.8%), turned out to be unverifiable (0.8%), or had a humorous intent (0.1%). Only 3.3% of the verified stories turned out to be true.

Types of Fact-Checking Pieces. Most of the published pieces were fact-checks of viral content (69%) that circulated through social media and messaging apps. Explainers that

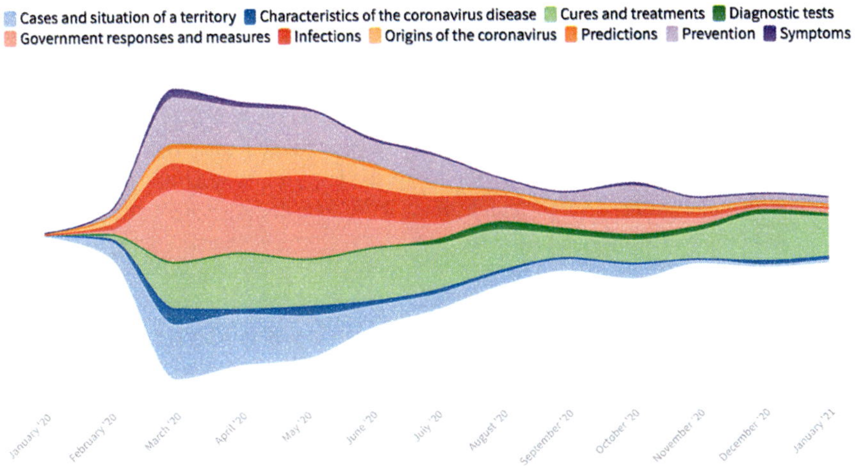

Fig. 1. Evolution of fact-checked topics related to COVID-19. Source: Our interactive visualization from the data gathered by LatamChequea. Available at: https://public.flourish.studio/visualisation/5894492/

tried to simplify complex aspects of the pandemic also gained prominence, supposing one in five pieces in the sample. In addition, fact-checks of statements by public Figs. (6.3%) were slightly higher than fact-checks of stories published by media outlets (4.2%). Practically one out of every four fact-checks of viral content was related to treatments and cures (24.6%, $\chi^2 = 20.08$, $p < 0.05$), while one out of every three fact-checks of public figures took place in connection with the situation of a territory (33.3%, $\chi^2 = 115.11$, $p < 0.05$). Likewise, the explainers focused on clarifying facets related to treatments and cures (19.1%, $\chi^2 = 20.08$, $p < 0.05$), and prevention (17.6%, $\chi^2 = 29.82$, $p < 0.05$). They constituted a genre that was especially cultivated in this first year of the global pandemic by two organizations studied, Maldita.es and Chequeado, which jointly produced 72.3% of this type of pieces.

Sources and Format of the Information that was Fact-Checked. Explainers aside, among the digital spaces in which factually dubious content was spread, Facebook (42%) and WhatsApp (26.5%) stood out. In the second instance, Twitter (11.5%) and the media outlets (9.6%) conveyed a notable number of stories that required fact-checking. Finally, the information that would end up being verified circulated less frequently through YouTube (3.6%), Instagram (0.9%), e-mail (0.6%), and Telegram (0.3%). When grouping these sources according to their nature as platforms, it is concluded that the unvetted information circulated on social media in 71.8% of cases, while it was distributed through messaging apps in 26.8% of the time. Regarding the format of the content that had to be verified, 58.7% was textual, 22.4% was image-based, 20.5% was video-based, 4.1% was audio-based, and 4.4% was presented in other formats.

Actors Involved in the Information that was Fact-Checked. Explainers aside, concerning the actors who originated or to whom the factually dubious content was attributed, the vast majority remained unidentified (78.5%). Of those that it was possible to identify, journalists and media outlets are credited with the dissemination of a significant amount of the information that ended up being reviewed (36.6%), practically on a par with politicians, officials, and public institutions (35.6%). Health workers and centers (7.4%), social media users (5.8%), and members and institutions of civil society (5.5%) were less frequently implicated. Finally, the least relevant actors were scientists and scientific institutions (3.5%), celebrities (2.9%), business leaders and companies (1.5%), and others (1.1%).

3.2 International Circulation of the Information that Was Fact-Checked

The organizations studied were only able to confirm transnational dissemination in 14% of the cases that compose the total sample. Of these 504 pieces of information that did manage to cross borders, the majority circulated bi-directionally between the Iberian Peninsula (Spain and Portugal) and the Latin American countries (36.5%) or between the Latin American countries themselves (25%). To a lesser extent, information of global scope was found (7.1%), as was the case with information that circulated from or to Asia (7%), or from or to Oceania (2.4%), and from or to Africa (1%). Stories rated as false underwent international mobility four times higher than those that ended up being true (18.1% vs. 4.3%, $\chi^2 = 217{,}39$, $p < 0.05$). As can be seen in Fig. 2, Spain, Colombia, Mexico, Argentina, and the United States make up the group of nations to which these contents were most widely disseminated.

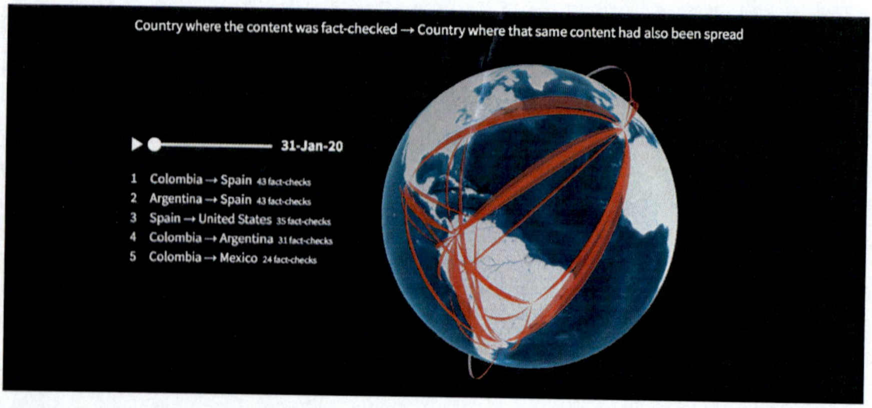

Fig. 2. International circulation of digital misinformation related to COVID-19. Source: Our interactive visualization from the data gathered by LatamChequea. Available at: https://public.flourish.studio/visualisation/5893414/

3.3 Correlation Between Web Search Queries and Publication of Fact-Checks

The weekly values of the GSVI web search queries of the term "COVID-19" were correlated with the number of fact-checks conducted with that periodicity by all the organizations analyzed. The GSVI is based on the number of searches on a given keyword in relation to all searches conducted for all keywords during the specified period, so it takes a value between 0 and 100. Given that the values of both metric variables followed a non-normal distribution, we used the nonparametric Spearman's rank correlation coefficient (ρ), which measures this degree of association resulting in values between 1 and -1. During the onset of the pandemic until May 25, the correlation between the intensity of web searches about the disease and the number of verifications conducted was positive and very strong ($\rho = 0.902$, $p < 0.01$). In the following months until the last week of September, when the nations of Latin America were still trying to overcome their first wave, the correlation became only moderate ($\rho = 0.543$, $p < 0.05$). The last four-month period of the year studied, which coincided with the second wave in Spain and other European countries, did not show a significant correlation.

4 Discussion and Conclusions

Regarding our first research question, the data obtained after analyzing 2,868 fact-checks allow us to outline the main characteristics of the fact-checking journalism on COVID-19 developed in Spain, Portugal, and Latin America during the first year of the global infodemic. Our findings give relevance to three geographic regions from which most of the stories were verified: organizations based in Spain, Argentina, and Colombia contributed most of the fact-checks and, among them, the abundant pieces produced by Maldita.es and Chequeado prevailed.

The fact-checks of viral content demanded most of the efforts of the organizations studied since they accounted for up to 69% of the published pieces. Those stories were generally shared through social media and mobile messaging apps such as Facebook and WhatsApp, platforms that concentrated the dissemination of more than two-thirds of all the contents examined. The leading topic by frequency and persistence over time was related to cures and treatments, that is, the solutions that brought hope to people became the main focus of confusion, rumors, and lies. This flow of misinformation was also in tune with the current news at the time: hoaxes about diagnostic tests only became relevant in June, after the generalization of the rapid antigen tests used for the detection of SARS-CoV-2. 93% of the verifications concluded that the questioned information was false or misleading and, although the authorship of the vast majority of misinformation remained anonymous, 72% of what it was possible to identify was disseminated by the media or the political sphere. In line with what was referred to in the previous literature [19, 20], misinformation through texts was predominant compared to that which took the form of audios or images.

This research also shows the importance of shared language and cultures in the transnational circulation of misinformation, which facilitated an intense permeability between the Iberian Peninsula and Latin American countries (36.5%) and between the Latin American countries themselves (25%). Although this reciprocity was already pointed out in previous studies [13], in light of our data, the disputed news stories about COVID-19 that crossed borders presented a relevant bias: those that turned out to be false were four times as many as the true ones, which is consistent with the idea that falsehood spreads broader than truth online [25].

The culturally and regionally delimited diffusion already described contrasts with the unquestionable global nature of the ravages caused by the virus, which is also evident in the scale of the information disorders that affect the news ecosystem. Based on our results, we can confirm that the first months of the year gave rise to an almost perfect proportionality between the demand for information on COVID-19 (through web searches on Google) and the need to verify it (i.e., fact-checks conducted), which grew in parallel in that initial period. As the months progressed, that association weakened until it ceased to exist, which highlights questions about the passage of time as a significant factor that should be properly explored in future research.

References

1. Martin, N.: Journalism, the pressures of verification and notions of post-truth in civil society. Cosmop. Civ. Soc.: Interdisc. J. **9**(2), 41–55 (2017)
2. Waisbord, S.: Truth is what happens to news. Journal. Stud. **19**(13), 1866–1878 (2018)
3. Magallón Rosa, R.: Unfaking News. Cómo combatir la desinformación. Pirámide, Madrid (2019)
4. Del-Fresno-García, M.: Desórdenes informativos: sobreexpuestos e infrainformados en la era de la posverdad. El profesional de la información **28**(3), 1–11 (2019)
5. Graves, L.: Boundaries not drawn: mapping the institutional roots of the global fact-checking movement. Journal. Stud. **19**(5), 613–631 (2018)
6. Pérez-Díaz, P.L.: El impacto de la participación ciudadana en el periodismo digital: un estudio multidimensional en cibermedios españoles. Universidad Católica San Antonio de Murcia (2019)
7. Singer, J.B.: Border patrol: the rise and role of fact-checkers and their challenge to journalists' normative boundaries. Journalism. Advance Online Publication (2020)
8. Graves, L., Cherubini, F.: The rise of fact-checking sites in Europe. Reuters Institute for the Study of Journalism, Oxford (2016)
9. Pérez-Curiel, C., Molpeceres, A.: Impacto del discurso político en la difusión de bulos sobre Covid-19. Influencia de la desinformación en públicos y medios. Revista Latina de Comunicación Social **78**, 65–97 (2020)
10. Aleixandre-Benavent, R., Castelló-Cogollos, L., Valderrama-Zurián, J.C.: Información y comunicación durante los primeros meses de Covid-19. Infodemia, desinformación y papel de los profesionales de la información. Profesional de la información **29**(4), 1–20 (2020)
11. Adhanom-Ghebreyesus, T., Ng, A.: Desinformación frente a medicina: hagamos frente a la 'infodemia' (2020). https://elpais.com/sociedad/2020/02/18/actualidad/1582053544_191857.html
12. Brennen, J.S., Simon, F., Howard, P.N., Nielsen, R.K.: Types, sources, and claims of COVID-19 Misinformation. Oxford, Reuters Institute for the Study of Journalism (2020)
13. Sánchez-Duarte, J.M., Magallón Rosa, R.: Infodemia y COVID-19. Evolución y viralización de informaciones falsas en España. Revista Española de Comunicación en Salud Supplement **1**, 31–41 (2020)
14. Sousa-Pinto, B., Anto, A., Czarlewski, W., Anto, J.M., Almeida Fonseca, J., Bousquet, J.: Assessment of the impact of media coverage on COVID-19–related google trends data: infodemiology study. J. Med. Internet Res. **22**(8), 1–12 (2020)
15. Strzelecki, A.: The second worldwide wave of interest in coronavirus since the COVID-19 outbreaks in South Korea, Italy and Iran: a Google trends study. Brain Behav. Immun. **88**, 950–951 (2020)

16. Villa Gracia, A.D., Cerdán Martínez, V.: Bulos durante la pandemia del Covid-19 en España: un estudio a través de Google Trends. Rev. Lat. Comun. Soc. **78**, 169–182 (2020)
17. Salaverría, R., Buslón, N., López-Pan, F., León, B., López-Goñi, I., Erviti, M.C.: Desinformación en tiempos de pandemia: tipología de los bulos sobre la Covid-19. Profesional de la información **29**(3), 1–15 (2020)
18. Nielsen, R.K., Fletcher, R., Newman, N., Brennen, J.S., Howard, P.N.: Navigating the 'infodemic': how people in six countries access and rate news and information about coronavirus. Oxford, Reuters Institute for the Study of Journalism (2020)
19. García-Marín, D.: Infodemia global. Desórdenes informativos, narrativas fake y fact-checking en la crisis de la Covid-19. Profesional de la información **29**(4), 1–20 (2020)
20. Aguado-Guadalupe, G., Bernaola-Serrano, I.: Verificación en la infodemia de la Covid-19. El caso Newtral. Revista Latina **78**, 289–308 (2020)
21. Pulido, C., Villarejo-Carballido, B., Redondo-Sama, G., Gómez, A.: COVID-19 infodemic: More retweets for science-based information on coronavirus than for false information. Int. Sociol. **35**(4), 377–392 (2020)
22. Ramon-Vegas, X., Mauri-Ríos, M., Rodríguez-Martínez, R.: Redes sociales y plataformas de fact-checking contra la desinformación sobre la COVID-19. Hipertext.net **21**, 79–92 (2020)
23. Instituto Cervantes: El español: una lengua viva. Informe 2020. Instituto Cervantes (2020)
24. LatamChequea. https://chequeado.com/latamcoronavirus/. Accessed 18 Apr 2021
25. Vosoughi, S., Roy, D., Aral, S.: The spread of true and false news online. Science **359**(6380), 1146–1151 (2018)

Post-truth of Female Empowerment in the Fake News of Peruvian Reality Shows

Lorena Teresa Espinoza-Robles[1](✉) and Oscar Alfredo Aybar-Cabezudo[2]

[1] Universidad Peruana de Ciencias Aplicadas, Lima, Peru
pcavlesp@upc.edu.pe
[2] Universidad de Lima, Lima, Peru
oaybar@ulima.edu.pe

Abstract. This study investigates the fake news generated from the content of the reality television format in Peru. This format, by mixing informational or reality elements with fictional elements, contributes to misinformation from the inexhaustible generation of news that, despite being real, falls into the category of fake news. They are considered fake news, not because of their content, but because of the unusual informative relevance assigned on digital social networks. In this way, the reality TV narrative becomes part of the Peruvian imaginary and contributes to misinformation from a news proposal that appeals to post-feminism to actually justify a macho and misogynistic gaze through news that permanently devalues the value of women. Therefore, a qualitative methodology was applied that includes a content analysis of the news related to characters from the reality show Esto es Guerra (Peru), who are considered media figures of mainstream culture, and which have been published in the official Facebook page of the TV program and then in the news portal America Noticias. The composition and visual meanings of the message have been analyzed from a gender perspective. This study opens new lines of research on the study of fake news in the entertainment genre and promotes media literacy in the mass public that consumes the products of this genre.

Keywords: Post-feminism · Post-truth · Reality show

1 Introduction

The largest number of articles and investigations on misinformation derived from fake news refer to clearly journalistic issues situated in the political order and how these news affect the discernment of users to detect their veracity [1–3]. They point out that people's prior beliefs influence this discernment about what is real and what is not [1]. That is why information bubbles are created in digital communities where everyone believes that there is a trend that leads public opinion, when in reality the algorithm of digital social networks makes us live the post-truth of our digital community populated of homogeneous truths [4, 5]. In this context, the creator of the content does not always have an intention to misinform. Content creators in journalistic work face economic,

© The Author(s), under exclusive license to Springer Nature Singapore Pte Ltd. 2022
Á. Rocha et al. (Eds.): ICOMTA 2021, SIST 259, pp. 184–192, 2022.
https://doi.org/10.1007/978-981-16-5792-4_19

technological and political factors [6]. Along these lines, the digitization of news provides a space for "non-journalists" to reach a massive audience; citizen journalism, vloggers or users in general create content through their social media accounts [3]. In response to this, the Peruvian media ecosystem welcomes some types of fake news mentioned as, for example, political satire, news parodies, press releases, political propaganda, and photo manipulation [3]. In the Peruvian case, this manipulation occurs from the mass media, in a time of post-truths and areas of ethical gloom [7].

1.1 The Peruvian Media Ecosystem and Women Sexualized Representation

At the time of Alberto Fujimori, the first scandalous case of fake news was presented in Peru with the *chicha* newspapers [8]. A series of yellow tabloids were dedicated to inventing news of political enemies of the government of the day. However, the first case in which entertainment was clearly mixed with these practices was with Laura Bozzo's program, the most famous talk show in Peru worldwide. It could be the first fake show in Peruvian history for its armed cases, for promoting stereotypes of what Peruvians are like and for supporting a government from its contents [9, 10]. Although those times seem distant, today a business group manages more than 80% of the written press in Peru, as well as the television channel with the most tuning and a long list of companies associated with information [11]. In this context, there are news items derived from the most successful reality show program of this group, which have a place on the news agenda and present a devalued vision of women [12].

Since the beginning of television in Peru, the representation of women has been related to the exploitation of physical beauty. This is the case of the naked starlets used on the covers of tabloid newspapers in the 80's to generate news [13]. Nowadays, that void left by starlets has been filled by the participants of reality shows [12]. The reality show is a popular format due to its low production cost [14]. A hybrid television show that takes elements from news and fiction [15–19]. Physical, verbal or relational violence is often used in its episodes [14, 20]. Furthermore, these reality programs follow a global pattern of gender stereotypes in operation [12, 21].

Espinoza-Robles et al. (2020) mention a count of various international reality shows that legitimize heteronormative and patriarchal stereotypes based on their narrative. An emblematic case is that of Donald Trump, for example, who managed to consolidate his media image in a reality show called The Apprentice, where he was an almighty who gave his opinion, decided who won and, by a narrative condition of the same format television, did not give explanations to anyone of those decisions [22, 23]. Reality show formats mix elements of reality and fiction and that is why they turn out to be so dangerous, insofar as the audience believes what the characters say and positively validates it in their imaginary [24].

In Peru, reality shows have replaced education, many children and young people take their participants as references without questioning their discourse [25]. In this context, this research affects the representation of female participants in reality shows at a time when popular culture has revalued feminism from a post-feminist perspective. In other words, women go from being an object to a sexual subject, but this is linked to capitalism and the neoliberal ethos [26].

Feminism is used by the mainstream as branding or femvertising [27]. Faludi [28] mentions many cases of television fiction products that were presented in favor of women, with female protagonists, but that nevertheless highlighted images of single women always behind a man. All these ideas continue to be legitimized in television fictions from different parts of the globe, since gender stereotypes are a global phenomenon [17, 21, 29–33]. On the other hand, news in this format is used to spread stereotypes [12], however, until now there has been no impact on studying its quality as fake news, not because of its level of factuality, but because of the unusual informative relevance it raises.

According to this, being the reality show a hybrid format that takes elements from news and fiction, it is not only relevant to enter into its analysis as a television entertainment genre that culturally constructs the sex/gender system [34–36], but from a journalistic approach that affects the fake news that is generated daily from their narratives on digital social networks such as Facebook. Therefore, the present investigation answers the research question, how can we deconstruct the message of fake news on Facebook derived from the stories generated by Peruvian reality shows from a gender perspective?

2 Methodology

This research has been carried out from a qualitative approach under the interpretive paradigm [37, 38]. The design is a case study and the technique used is the content analysis applied to the text, image and video that make up the news posted on networks following the methodology of Rose [39] in visual studies. A sample of 20 news (see Table 1) was taken from 3 Facebook accounts related to the Peruvian open signal television channel América Televisión: Esto es Guerra Perú (EEG Peru), América Televisión (AT) and América Espectáculos (AE). The selection criteria applied were to include news that had been published with the hashtag #EEGElOrigen, that in the story included in a woman in a leading role and that all the news disseminated on social networks had a development in the news portal América Noticias (AN).

The categories of analysis are the composition of the message and the visual meanings [39]. The composition of the message includes the content, color, spatial organization, montage, sound, light and expressive content. Visual meanings are those associated with economic, social, and political relationships, institutions, and practices that surround the message. In a first stage of the research, the composition of the message will be analyzed, in this case, the headlines, the photo and the text displayed in the post published on Facebook and in a second stage the visual meanings of the audiovisual material that accompanies the journalistic note in the post (see Table 1).

2.1 Ethical Considerations

For reasons of anonymity and confidentiality, the names of the characters have been replaced by alphanumeric codes to analyze the characteristics of their media behavior. Only information referring to their public exposure in the media is handled.

3 Results and Discussion

On the home page of "América Noticias" (AN) web portal of April 18, 2021, next to the news of the Peruvian Nobel Prize winner Mario Vargas Llosa in favor of the candidacy of Keiko Fujimori in the second round of the 2021 Presidential Elections in Peru, a story that comes from the narrative of the reality show Esto es Guerra is covered in equal proportions.

This story has a reality girl as the protagonist in her role as a couple. The headline specifies the statements of a former partner of this reality girl. The concept of reality girl or boy refers to the participants of the most watched reality show in Peru, Esto es Guerra. The program is characterized by confronting two groups of participants who call themselves the "warriors" (guerreros) and the "combatants" (combatientes). The program is part of the entertainment proposal of the most tuned open signal TV channel in Peru.

3.1 The Use of Fake News with a Level of Facticity

There is information derived from the program that is placed in the informative offer of the news portal América Noticias. These news are generated from the same narrative of the EEG program and are contents that contribute more to the branding [27] of the EEG brand than to the information. The events usually involve the activities or moods of the female participants as protagonists and as the hook of the story (see Table 1).

The analyzed news enter as entertainment news, but in reality the informative relevance is null. None is in the public interest, since their context can only be understood by those who follow the program. They are news that become news because they have in their favor all the machinery of the business group that welcomes them. Then, they are considered false news not because of their level of facticity, but because of their null informative relevance.

They are news that correspond more to a gossip portal. Some of the published notes are even related to content that the participants make on their personal Tik Tok [40] or Instagram [41] accounts.

Table 1. Analyzed Facebook posts

Posted	Character code	Fact	Facebook account	News AN
19/02/2021	A8	Woman shocks with her movements	EEGPerú	[42]
25/02/2021	A3/A9	Women compete in Tik Tok challenge	AT	[43]
16/03/2021	A6	"Negrita" woman makes participant nervous	AE	[44]

(continued)

Table 1. (*continued*)

Posted	Character code	Fact	Facebook account	News AN
17/03/2021	A1	Woman becomes former television personality	EEGPerú	[45]
31/03/2021	A6/A1	Woman does photoshoot with mischief	EEGPerú	[46]
5/04/2021	A1/A2	Women hosts faced each other	EEGPerú	[47]
6/04/2021	A6/A7	"Negrita" woman gets upset with another participant	EEGPerú	[48]
6/04/2021	A1/A2	Female hosts face off in competition	EEGPerú	[49]
7/04/2021	A1	Female host is bothered by attention to another host	EEGPerú	[50]
9/04/2021	A6	Woman is excited by her partner's successes	EEGPerú	[51]
9/04/2021	A6	Woman cries for hard moment	EEGPerú	[52]
9/04/2021	A5	Woman cries for not being in first places	EEGPerú	[53]
9/04/2021	A4/A5	Woman beats her former rival	EEGPerú	[54]
12/04/2021	A7/A10	Woman almost gave in to another participant	EEGPerú	[55]
12/04/2021	A6	Woman stumbles	EEGPerú	[56]
12/04/2021	A3	Woman cries from helplessness and lack of support	EEGPerú	[57]
12/04/2021	A1	Woman has unexpected reaction	EEGPerú	[58]
14/04/2021	A3	Woman falls to the ground in extreme game	EEGPerú	[59]
15/04/2021	A4	Woman surprises her mother with a gift	EEGPerú	[41]
15/04/2021	A4	Women unite in choreography	EEGPerú	[40]

3.2 Post-truth of Female Empowerment

On the other hand, these "false news" present in their narrative a post-truth of female empowerment. The concept of the program that is associated with the participants is related to the struggle for a goal, however, in the name of that value, the participants are forced to go through situations that test their physical and emotional resistance by the rating. It is women who constantly break down [52, 57]. On the one hand, the concept of struggle is sold above all else, however, the female participants are valued for qualities associated with female stereotypes. Women appear romanticized, overwhelmed or vulnerated. The Facebook accounts related to the America Television channel compete in the local media eco-system with communities such as fan clubs, haters, trolls and messages such as memes, viral videos, edits, reactions, news, rumors, etc. In this context, they adopt practices from this digital ecosystem. For example, the use of non-inclusive language is standardized. In the posts about A6, the only afrodescendant female participant, she is called "negrita".

Likewise, the images of the posts highlight the female figure, the suggestive poses, the tight suits and a handling of the photographs that shows the woman always sexy and voluptuous, so it welcomes gender stereotypes [17, 21, 29–33, 60]. It is a false post-feminist gaze, since the news positions the reality girl not as a sexual subject, but as an objectified woman. In the program, the male captains are the ones who put order and establish a clear relationship of power with the opposite sex, as was done since the beginning of Peruvian television [13]. In this scenario, the characters change, but the same practices remain. The way in that messages were posted on Facebook is organized always creating photographic collages where the shape of the female body is highlighted as the central image, they can be gestures of surprise, annoyance or dance poses.

The visual meanings of these publications are associated with an homogenizing culture where heteronormativity prevails [21]. All the participants feed a narrative line linked to romance and as a rule none of these characters have any political opinion. They are flat characters that follow the narrative conditions of the format. In a country like Peru, one would have to wonder who should maintain these practices. The scenario is quite auspicious for those who pull the strings of popular taste from their position of power, owners of social networks, owners of traditional media, governments, businessmen and various figures of power in the current media ecosystem.

4 Conclusions

We conclude that the posts and the news analyzed show a post-truth of female empowerment. The analyzed material allows us to show how news content is positioned as branding of the EEG brand. The brand's narrative implies a post-truth of female empowerment that is presented in the form of fake news that usually have a woman in a protagonic role. Fake news is configured by its null informative relevance. This particular strategy to position the contents of the program shows the information crisis in Peru due to the concentration of media that allows and validates these practices. The inclusion of fake news from the mass media opens up new lines of research related to the use of entertainment as the instigator of a homogenizing thought. Hybrid products that mix elements of fiction and reality such as the reality show have in their intrinsic nature a high viralization value that is used to position messages that contribute to building a viewer and at the same time a citizen. Therefore, the study opens new lines of research on fake news in the entertainment genre and promotes media literacy in the mass public that consumes the products of this genre. Finally, it contributes to the existing literature on gender studies applied to the news and entertainment genre, as well as post-truth studies in the media.

Aknowledgements. This study has been supported by the Universidad Peruana de Ciencias Aplicadas (UPC) through the IX UPC Research Incentive Contest (2021).

References

1. Michael, R.B., Breaux, B.O.: The relationship between political affiliation and beliefs about sources of "fake news". Cogn. Res. Princ. Implic. **6** (2021). https://doi.org/10.1186/s41235-021-00278-1
2. Tandoc, E.C., Lim, Z.W., Ling, R.: Defining "fake news": a typology of scholarly definitions. Digit. Journal. **6**, 137–153 (2018). https://doi.org/10.1080/21670811.2017.1360143
3. Tandoc, E.C., Jenkins, J., Craft, S.: Fake news as a critical incident in journalism. Journal. Pract. 2786 (2018). https://doi.org/10.1080/17512786.2018.1562958
4. Pariser, E.: The filter bubble (2011)
5. Flaxman, S., Goel, S., Rao, J.M.: Filter bubbles, echo chambers, and online news consumption. Public Opin. Q. **80**, 298–320 (2016). https://doi.org/10.1093/poq/nfw006
6. Molina, M.D., Sundar, S.S., Le, T., Lee, D.: "Fake news" is not simply false information: a concept explication and taxonomy of online content. Am. Behav. Sci. **65**, 180–212 (2021). https://doi.org/10.1177/0002764219878224
7. Keyes, R.: The post-truth era (2011)
8. Cappelini, M.: La prensa "Chicha" en Perú. Chasqui. Rev. Latinoam. Comun. 32–37 (2004)
9. Antebi, S.: The talk show uploaded: YouTube and the technicity of the body. Soc. Identities **15**, 297–311 (2009). https://doi.org/10.1080/13504630902899036
10. Arriarán, G.: Laura Bozzo y la Fuente del Placer. Anthropol. Dep. Ciencias Soc. **18**, 252–269 (2000)
11. Maldonado, P.: Grupo El Comercio: un pulpo de los medios de comunicación. Ideele (2013)
12. Espinoza-Robles, L., Aybar-Cabezudo, O., Gallardo-Echenique, E.: Gender stereotypes in the intrinsic narrative of the peruvian competition-based reality shows. In: INTED2020 Proceedings, vol. 1, pp.7060–7069 (2020). https://doi.org/10.21125/inted.2020.1870
13. Cáceres Sztorc, Á.C.: Perspectiva de los roles de género y sus representaciones en la televisión peruana. Análisis de casos emblemáticos desde 1980 hasta 2010. Cambios Permanencias **9**, 232–263 (2018)
14. Glascock, J., Preston-Schreck, C.: Verbal aggression, race, and sex on reality TV: is this really the way it is? J. Broadcast. Electron. Media **62**, 427–444 (2018). https://doi.org/10.1080/08838151.2018.1451859
15. Barbón, O., Romero, A., Rodríguez, J., De Lucas, L., Gil, R.: Los valores en la era de los "concursos de talento" (Got Talent). Rev. Dilemas Contemp. Educ. Política Valores. **VI**, 1–20 (2019)
16. Coiro-Moraes, A.L., Lisbôa Filho, F.F.: Character types in Brazilian reality shows: cultural manifestation of a media protagonist syndrome. Lat. Am. Res. Rev. **52**, 446–455 (2017). https://doi.org/10.25222/larr.35
17. Galán Fajardo, E.: Personajes, estereotipos y representaciones sociales. Una propuesta de estudio y análisis de la ficción televisiva. ECO-PÓS **9**, 58–81 (2006)
18. Imbert, G.: El zoo visual. Editorial Gedisa, Barcelona (2003)
19. Salo, G.: ¿Qué es eso del formato? Gedisa Editorial S A (2003)
20. Coyne, S.M., Robinson, S.L., Nelson, D.A.: Does reality backbite? Physical, verbal, and relational aggression in reality television programs. J. Broadcast. Electron. Media **54**, 282–298 (2010). https://doi.org/10.1080/08838151003737931
21. Matthes, J., Prieler, M., Adam, K.: Gender-role portrayals in television advertising across the globe. Sex Roles **75**(7–8), 314–327 (2016). https://doi.org/10.1007/s11199-016-0617-y

22. Cheung, C., Sung, M.: Language and gender in a US reality TV show: An analysis of leadership discourse in single-sex interactions. NJES Nord. J. English Stud. **12**, 25–51 (2013)
23. Kinnick, K.N., Parton, S.R.: Workplace communication: what the apprentice teaches about communication skills. Bus. Commun. Q. **68**, 429–456 (2005). https://doi.org/10.1177/1080569905282099
24. Kaplan, D., Kupper, Y.: Toward an interaction-centered approach to media events: mediated public intimacy on the reality TV show big brother. J. Commun. **67**, 758–780 (2017). https://doi.org/10.1111/jcom.12322
25. El Comercio: El 52,8% de niños aspira a ser como los "chicos reality" | Lima | El Comercio Perú. https://elcomercio.pe/lima/52-8-ninos-aspira-chicos-reality-273293
26. Giraldo, I.: Posfeminismo/Genealogía, geografía y contornos de un concepto. Debate Fem. **59**, 1–30 (2019). https://doi.org/10.22201/cieg.2594066xe.2020.59.01
27. Fernández Hernández, L.: El feminismo como producto mediático: la paradoja de Beyoncé. Investig. Fem. **8** (2017). https://doi.org/10.5209/infe.54975
28. Faludi, S.: Backlash: The Undeclared War Against American Women (Three Rivers Press, 1991, 2006) (1991)
29. Galán, E.: Construcción de género y ficción televisiva en España. Rev. Científica Comun. Educ. **28** (2007)
30. Smit, A.: Reading South African bridal television: consumption. Fantasy Judge. Commun. **42**, 63–78 (2016). https://doi.org/10.1080/02500167.2016.1252781
31. Belmonte, J., Guillamón, S.: Co-educar la mirada contra los estereotipos de género en TV. Comunicar. **15**, 115–120 (2008). https://doi.org/10.3916/c31-2008-01-014
32. Masanet, M.-J.: Pervivencia de los estereotipos de género en los hábitos de consumo mediático de los adolescentes: drama para las chicas y humor para los chicos. Cuadernos. Info 39–53 (2016). https://doi.org/10.7764/cdi.39.1027
33. Alarcón, L.: Estereotipos de la mujer andina en los programas de humor de la TV peruana. Concortv, Lima (2015)
34. García Rubio, I.: Las mujeres y el trabajo en las series de ficción. Cambio social y narraciones televisivas. In: Fidalgo, A., Serra, J.P. (eds.) Ciências da Comunicação em Congresso na Covilhã (CCCC) actas do III Sopcom, VI Lusocom, II Ibérico. Universidade da Beira Interior (UBI), Labcom - Laboratório de Comunicação e Conteúdos Online, Covilhã (2004)
35. Mulvey, L.: Afterword: some reflections on the engagement of feminism with film from the 1970s to the present day. Mov. Image Rev. Art J. **7**, 82–90 (2018). https://doi.org/10.1386/miraj.7.1.82_1
36. Nasehi, E., Kara, N.: Buttressing strategy: a theory to understand the neopatriarchal unconscious of iranian society/cinema. Rev. Cercet. si Interv. Soc. **60**, 157–173 (2018)
37. Given, L.M. (ed.): The Sage Encyclopedia of Qualitative Research Methods, vol. 1 and 2. SAGE, Los Angeles (2008)
38. Creswell, J.W.: Qualitative Inquiry and Research Design. SAGE, Los Angeles (2013)
39. Rose, G.: Visual Methodologies. SAGE Publications, Great Britain (2016)
40. América Noticias: Yahaira Plasencia y Angie Arizaga sorprendieron con espectacular baile de TikTok. https://www.americatv.com.pe/esto-es-guerra/yahaira-plasencia-y-angie-arizaga-sorprendieron-espectacular-baile-tiktok-noticia-127572?hootPostID=7baa708fb8d116b024efa1cb81b8805f4cf233c548ea6cbebc6fb3b8435e7891%0A
41. América Noticias: Yahaira Plasencia sorprende a su madre con detalle de cumpleaños (2021)
42. América Noticias: EEG: Paloma Fiuza venció a Gino Assereto tras retarlo en "Tiktokers: Los rivales" (2021). https://www.americatv.com.pe/noticias/espectaculos/eeg-paloma-fiuza-vencio-gino-assereto-retarlo-tiktokers-rivales-n434602
43. América Noticias: EEG: Luciana Fuster defendió su título en duelo de TikTok con Michela Elías. https://www.americatv.com.pe/noticias/espectaculos/eeg-luciana-fuster-defendio-su-titulo-duelo-tiktok-michela-elias-n434988%0A

44. América Noticias: EEG: La reacción de Jota Benz luego de que Fabio Su llegara a retar a Angie Arizaga. https://www.americatv.com.pe/noticias/espectaculos/eeg-ximena-peralta-afronto-tenso-momento-angie-arizaga-plantear-reclamo-n437416
45. América Noticias: EEG: Johanna San Miguel revivió a "Queca" en medio de imperdible tiktok. https://www.americatv.com.pe/noticias/espectaculos/eeg-johanna-san-miguel-revivio-queca-medio-imperdible-tiktok-n436303%0A
46. América Noticias: Angie Arizaga derrochó toda su sensualidad en pleno programa ¿Y Jota Benz se puso celoso?. https://www.americatv.com.pe/noticias/espectaculos/angie-arizaga-derrocho-toda-su-sensualidad-pleno-programa-y-jota-benz-se-puso-celoso-n436993
47. América Noticias: EEG: María Pía Copello ingresó al reality como dupla de Johanna San Miguel. https://www.americatv.com.pe/noticias/espectaculos/eeg-maria-pia-copello-ingreso-como-dupla-johanna-san-miguel-n437413
48. América Noticias: EEG: Ximena Peralta afrontó tenso momento con Angie Arizaga tras plantear reclamo. https://www.americatv.com.pe/noticias/espectaculos/eeg-ximena-peralta-afronto-tenso-momento-angie-arizaga-plantear-reclamo-n437416%0A
49. América Noticias: EEG: María Pía Copello ganó reto a Johanna San Miguel en "Desafío de conductoras". https://www.americatv.com.pe/noticias/espectaculos/eeg-maria-pia-copello-gano-reto-johanna-san-miguel-desafio-conductoras-n437488
50. América Noticias: Johanna San Miguel le dedica unas "chiquitas" a María Pía Copello. https://www.americatv.com.pe/noticias/espectaculos/johanna-san-miguel-le-dedica-unas-chiquitas-maria-pia-copello-n437525%0A
51. América Noticias: Angie Arizaga se emociona así por los éxitos de Jota Benz. https://www.americatv.com.pe/noticias/espectaculos/angie-arizaga-se-emociona-asi-exitos-jota-benz-n437663%0A
52. América Noticias: EEG: Angie Arizaga terminó llorando al hablar de este duro momento en competencia. https://www.americatv.com.pe/noticias/espectaculos/eeg-angie-arizaga-termino-llorando-al-hablar-este-duro-momento-competencia-n437699%0A
53. América Noticias: EEG: Rosángela se quebró al expresar su "frustración" y sorprendió con pedido de pase a los Guerreros (2021)
54. América Noticias: Yahaira Plasencia tras primer triunfo en EEG: "La actitud tiene mucho que ver". https://www.americatv.com.pe/noticias/espectaculos/yahaira-plasencia-primer-triunfo-eeg-actitud-tiene-mucho-que-ver-n437676
55. América Noticias: EEG: Ximena Peralta ganó reto tras angustiantes momentos en competencia con Melissa Loza (2021)
56. América Noticias: Jota Benz apoyó a Angie Arizaga tras sufrir fuerte caída durante competencia. https://www.americatv.com.pe/esto-es-guerra/jota-benz-apoyo-angie-arizaga-sufrir-fuerte-caida-durante-competencia-noticia-127529?hootPostID=be9fc4b9f7e51ea41d4e478d275834762bc2e4b3a8707c7618899503934af164%0A
57. América Noticias: EEG: Michela Elías cuestionó el apoyo de su equipo y Luciana Fuster salió en su defensa. https://www.americatv.com.pe/noticias/espectaculos/eeg-michela-elias-cuestiono-apoyo-su-equipo-y-luciana-fuster-salio-su-defensa-n437701%0A
58. América Noticias: Gian Piero Díaz regresó a EEG y recibió esta noticia por parte del tribunal (2021)
59. América Noticias: EEG: Michela Elías sufrió fuerte lesión durante competencia con Paloma Fiuza. https://www.americatv.com.pe/noticias/espectaculos/eeg-michela-elias-sufrio-fuerte-lesion-durante-competencia-paloma-fiuza-n437888%0A
60. Fedele, M., Masanet, M.-J., Ventura, R.: Negotiating love and gender stereotypes among young people: prevalence of "Amor Ludens" and television preferences rooted in hegemonic masculinity. Masculinities Soc. Chang. **8**(1) (2019). https://doi.org/10.17583/mcs.2019.3742

YouTuber and Instagrammer Phenomenon in the Andean Community

Rebeca Córdova-Tapia[1(✉)], Diana Rivera-Rogel[2], Eduardo Loaiza Lima[3], and Andrea Velásquez-Benavides[2]

[1] Becaria de Investigación en Universidad Técnica Particular de Loja, 11-01-608, Loja, Ecuador
racordova7@utpl.edu.ec

[2] Docente de la Universidad Técnica Particular de Loja, 11-01-608, Loja, Ecuador
{derivera,avvelasquez}@utpl.edu.ec

[3] Alumni de la Universidad Técnica Particular de Loja, 11-01-608, Loja, Ecuador
evloaiza@utpl.edu.ec

Abstract. The impact of social media has increased significantly in the last decade, thus proliferating the number of users on these platforms and with it the emergence of influencers in different digital environments, mainly on YouTube and Instagram. This study aims to expose the most popular figures of young YouTubers and Instagrammers in the Andean Community, presenting a ranking of content creators based on the reach of their accounts. The methodology employed combines quantitative and qualitative techniques for the collection and analysis of information. Datasheets were used to extract general data on the profile of the influencers and, at a second level, the content published on their accounts was analyzed, with emphasis on the topics addressed and the language used in the publications. The results show the top 10 YouTubers and the top 10 Instagrammers of the Andean Community, where gender equity is observed among the outstanding profiles. As a result of the analysis carried out on these accounts, it is determined that the language most used by the influencers of both platforms is expressive, a finding that coincides with one of the objectives of the influencers, which is to connect with their audience. In terms of topics, the content preferred by YouTubers is entertainment, while on Instagram influencers prefer to focus on fashion and trends.

Keywords: YouTuber · Instagrammer · Andean community · Social media · Influencer

1 Introduction

Social networks are means of communication with an immense capacity to influence people's lives. In Latin America, several social sectors do not have basic services, but their members are permanent users of social networks. "Amid the 21st century, the ubiquity that our Smartphones and Iphones provide us, thanks to the Internet and mobile applications (Apps), allows us to be constantly connected" (p. 188) [17].

© The Author(s), under exclusive license to Springer Nature Singapore Pte Ltd. 2022
Á. Rocha et al. (Eds.): ICOMTA 2021, SIST 259, pp. 193–202, 2022.
https://doi.org/10.1007/978-981-16-5792-4_20

Nowadays, YouTube and Instagram are platforms without limits. In the case of YouTube, it ceased to be a simple video search engine, since its benefits allowed innovating and turning unknown characters into popular YouTubers, who have had a great impact on society, becoming a trend in a very short time. Their boom is not only in the publication of videos but also in the form of participation through social networks such as Facebook and Twitter, by sharing their videos and spreading them until virilizing them [22]. As far as Instagram is concerned, this social network is boosted by the fact that photography becomes the main element to capture audiences. Instagrammers are people who have a significant number of followers on this social network and thus obtain a relevant number of interactions, which allows them to be considered in advertising and marketing campaigns, due to the influence they exert on their followers (p. 206) [21]. Influencers since their emergence have become the best option to support the growth of a brand and position it in the market. Consumers currently search for products on the Internet and due to the great growth of social media, companies are adapting to new communication models, which is where the real dimension of those who use YouTube and Instagram to influence consumer behavior appears (p. 102–103) [8].

This study aims to gather information on the most recognized influencers on platforms such as YouTube and Instagram at the level of the Andean Community, a region that currently consists of Bolivia, Colombia, Ecuador, and Peru, countries that, united by the same past, varied geography and a great cultural and natural diversity, continue to strive for common objectives and goals [24]. In the Andean Community, there are no official rankings of YouTubers, only statistics of the most influential characters in this social network can be accessed through specific sources up to country level, in most cases. A similar situation exists for Instagrammers, as rankings can be found through measurement tools, but only at the country level. It should be noted that two publications present a general map of these influencers, separated by social network. The research presented by Rivera & Córdova [6, 21] offers a first approach to content creators in the Andean Community.

1.1 Social Media in the Andean Community

Due to the development of the Internet and therefore of social media in the world, it is important to address its growth and introduction in the countries of the Andean Community. But it is important to mention that it is not possible to point out an exact date of the emergence of social media in the world; however, these digital platforms are consolidated and popularized in the last decade. Ávila-Toscano [3] rightly refers to social media as a universal system under permanent construction, whose main actor is the social component due to the dynamic nature of content exchange.

YouTube platform was created in 2005, its name is based on the culture of self: broadcast yourself, its success was so great that it soon became the main site on the Internet to review videos with original features [10]. While Instagram appeared in 2010 and has more than one billion registered users [11]. It is a digital scenario with a lot of visual strength, capable of transmitting various sensations and narrating stories through images [9]. According to GlobalWebIndex [11, 26], 43% of the population under study admitted logging in for longer during the pandemic, highlighting the increase in the creation and publication of videos during this season, an activity that is led by generation

Z (16–23 years old), increasing 8% points between April and June. This phenomenon was also experienced in the Andean Community, where Facebook, YouTube, and Instagram are the most used social networks.

1.2 Phenomenal YouTuber and Instagrammer

According to Aran-Ramspott et al. [2], YouTubers are a fundamental part of teen culture, able to influence large groups to motivate in the consumption of products designed and targeted for young people. One of the main characteristics of content creators on Instagram is the use of images to show their day-to-day life. Instagrammers are able to position brands in a target audience, thanks to the influence they have on their profile. That is why these influencers turned their activity into a paid profession to which they dedicate much of their time and sacrifice, which also demands constant preparation and dedication to content creation. Studies developed on these theories show that Instagrammers, participate in large advertising campaigns and have commercial agreements with large companies [1].

In order to group the content creators according to the subject matter they deal with, the approaches of two authors are taken as a reference. In the case of YouTube, the platform offers fifteen categories to organize the channels and videos published on this site, of which the two that are related to the content handled by YouTubers in the Andean Community are detailed: Entertainment (channels with a diversity of content, who address the classic format of videoblogs, where the YouTuber shows himself in front of the camera and connects with his followers) and Games (accounts where reviews or user experiences in games, mainly video games, are presented) [19]. While, for the Instagram platform, we present the distinction proposed by Díaz [7], taking into consideration three of the seven groups identified by this author: Fashion and trends (influencers who show fashion tips in their publications, where the aesthetic prevails), Beauty (accounts dedicated to makeup and hairstyle topics, they are known as beauty bloggers) and Entertainment and humor (content creators who are governed by Internet trends) [23]. These classifications will be key to the categorization of influencers in this study.

2 Design and Materials

This research used quantitative and qualitative methods, considering the mixed methodology as the most appropriate to collect all the information regarding YouTube and Instagram influencers. Let us remember that this methodological combination enhances "the possibility of understanding the phenomena under study, especially if they refer to complex fields where human beings and their diversity are involved" [20]. This statement corresponds to the objective of this study as it analyzes the profile of the content creators and the scope of their accounts and, in turn, the language used in their publications.

The present research arises after the research presented by Rivera and Córdova in 2020 and 2021 [6, 21], who show a general map of content creators at the level of the Andean Community. To determine the corpus of the present study, the following criteria were established: the age of the selected influencers should range between 0 and 25 years

-focusing on the young population- and their nationality should correspond to one of the four countries under study -Bolivia, Colombia, Ecuador, and Peru-, in addition to contemplating only the so-called social media influencers, according to the classification of Díaz [7], and those who had self-created content. Data were collected in February and March 2021.

The first approach was made through measurement tools such as Social Blade and StarNgage, which offer rankings by country of the best-rated profiles based on certain variables: Social Blade (YouTube) number of videos published, subscribers, and views, adding an icon that classifies each channel according to the predominant theme of their videos. StarNgage (Instagram) number of followers, adding the possibility of filtering accounts by theme.

At this point, it is worth mentioning that the information found in the two aforementioned tools was not 100% reliable, so it was contrasted with the profiles or channels of each influencer, and inconsistencies were found in the number of followers, country of nationality, or theme of the account.

Within YouTube, the number of videos, followers, and views of each channel was checked, in addition to corroborating the subject matter of each account. Likewise, the "channels" section was reviewed to identify the suggested profiles offered by each influencer, finding some YouTubers that were not included in the SocialBlade ranking and that met the parameters previously determined. As for Instagram, each profile was entered to check the number of followers, the theme of the account, and the nationality of the character. The similar accounts recommended by the application (30 for each profile) were manually registered, listing the users that met the parameters set in this study.

The design used corresponds to a mixed method with equal status (CUAN → CUAL), where quantitative methods are applied in a first phase for the selection of profiles and ranking of influencers and, subsequently, qualitative methods are used to analyze the content they publish in social media; however, the data obtained are evaluated with equal relevance in the study. The design used corresponds to a mixed method with equal status [14].

The quantitative methodology made it possible to evaluate influencers based on the impact of their accounts, taking into consideration the number of subscribers/followers as the main figure to obtain two rankings at the Andean Community level, one top 10 for each platform (YouTube and Instagram). From these top 20 influencers, quantitative files were prepared to analyze the profiles found, taking into consideration the following data: subject matter, number of subscribers/followers, and gender. Subsequently, qualitative files were prepared to analyze the language used by the creators in their videos/publications, a technique defined by Krippendorff [15] as "a research technique for making replicable and valid inferences from texts (or other meaningful matter) to the contexts of their use" (p. 18).

It should be noted that for the analysis of content within YouTube, two videos were selected from each channel (the first and last video published), ending with a sample of twenty videos; while on the Instagram platform, one photograph and one video were analyzed for each account (selecting the most recently published ones), with a total of ten photographs and ten videos examined. Within Instagram, neither reels material nor

IGTV was considered, since these formats require specific analysis due to their different reach, dissemination, and duration compared to a regular video in the feed.

Once this information was obtained, a comparison was made between the rankings of the two platforms studied, to find those influencers that were popular in both lists. The data of the corresponding profiles were compared to determine the relationship between the year of creation of the account and its reach, results that will be presented below.

3 Results

As the first result of this research, we present the rankings of the most popular young influencers in the Andean Community, both on the YouTube platform (Table 1) and Instagram (Table 2). These listings are ranked based on the number of subscribers/followers.

Table 1. Top 10 YouTubers of the Andean community.

	Channel name	Subscribers	Country
1	Lulu99	11.2M	Colombia
2	RaptorGamer	8.71M	Ecuador
3	Sofia Castro	8.63M	Colombia
4	Amara Que Linda	8.37M	Colombia
5	Calle y Poché	7.56M	Colombia
6	MrStiven TC	7.2M	Colombia
7	MIS PEQUEÑOS ACTORES	6.49M	Ecuador
8	William Vladimir Show Kids TV	6.45M	Perú
9	Flex Vega	5.95M	Colombia
10	JeanCarlo León	5.16M	Colombia

For the ten most popular young YouTubers in the Andean Community, we observe that Colombia occupies most of the positions within the ranking (seven YouTubers), a situation that corresponds to the research conducted by Córdova & Rivera [6], who report the existing dominance of Colombian content creators on the YouTube platform, something that is maintained in the current sample. Ecuador is present in two places in the table (positions two and seven), while Peru is located in the eighth position, with the channel William Vladimir Show Kids TV. With this quick reading of the table, it is evident that Bolivia does not have any YouTuber in this ranking, since the Bolivian channel with the highest number of subscribers reaches only 1.9 million subscribers.

Table 2 shows the ten most popular young Instagrammers in the Andean Community, where Colombian influencers are the most popular since nine of the ten boxes are occupied by Colombian Instagrammers. Only in the number six position is an Ecuadorian content creator (kevlexd), who with 4.6 million followers, is positioned within the ranking of this region. In this list, there are no representatives from Bolivia or Peru, which shows the poor reception received by Instagrammers from these countries, compared to influencers from Colombia and, to a lesser extent, Ecuador.

Table 2. Top 10 Instagrammers of the Andean community.

	User name	Followers	Country
1	sofiaalcastro	7M	Colombia
2	jashlem	6.7M	Colombia
3	la_liendraa	5.5M	Colombia
4	calleypoche	5.2M	Colombia
5	amara.aa	4.6M	Colombia
6	kevlexd	4.6M	Ecuador
7	poche	4.4M	Colombia
8	carlosferiag	4.3M	Colombia
9	luisa_castro1585	4.4M	Colombia
10	danielaacallee	3.7M	Colombia

Another aspect to highlight is the repetitive presence of Colombian influencers María José Garzón (@poche) and Daniela Calle (@danielaacalle), who, in addition to appearing in the ranking with their personal accounts, are positioned, and with the largest number of followers, at number four on the list, with a joint account (@calleypoche).

3.1 Influencer Profile and Language

About YouTubers, equal participation between men and women is observed, taking into account the rationale raised by the Association of Women Filmmakers and Audiovisual Media CIMA [4], who consider an equal distribution when there is a participation of women lower or higher than 50%, with an interval of 10% points, i.e. between 40% and 60%. The ranking shows five channels of male content creators therein (RaptorGamer, MrStiven TC, William Vladimir Show Kids TV, Flex Vega, and JeanCarlos León), four profiles of female YouTubers (Lulu99, Sofia Castro, Amara Que Linda, Calle and Poché, the latter made up of two people, both women) and a mixed channel (MIS PEQUEÑOS ACTORES) with the participation of twelve members, eleven children and one adult, of which seven are male and five are female.

As for the top young Instagrammers, there is a balance between men and women, with the presence of six female influencers (sofiaalcastro, calleypoche, amara.aa, poche, luisa_castro1585, and danielaacalle) and four male content creators (jashlem, la_liendraa, kevlexd and carlosfergiag). The existence of gender equity in the rankings of YouTubers and Instagrammers in the Andean Community demonstrates an equal acceptance by the audience, which contrasts with what happened in countries such as Spain (considered a leader in digital platforms for Spanish-speaking countries), where nine of the ten most popular YouTubers are male [5].

About the themes of the YouTubers, there is a preference for content classified as entertainment, six of the ten channels deal with this type of content (Lulu99, Sofia Castro, Amara Que Linda, Calle y Poché, MIS PEQUEÑOS ACTORES, and Jean-Carlo León). This category encompasses a diversity of themes, in the words of Murolo and Lacorte [19] "the audiovisuals on these channels usually deal with every day and domestic issues" (p. 19). Another topic that is well received by YouTubers and their communities is gaming, in the ranking of the Andean Community we observed three gamers' channels (RaptorGamer, MrStiven TC, and Flex Vega) and a fourth that is dedicated to documenting the experience of a child with his toys (William Vladimir Show Kids TV), thus confirming that the gaming category is one of the preferred by the audience. In figures from YouTube, in 2020 users watched more than 100 billion hours of game-related audiovisual material [26]. Analyzing the content topics addressed by the Instagrammers of the Andean Community, there is a close relationship with the trends presented on YouTube, since the existing categories within the ranking are: fashion and trends; entertainment and humor; and beauty. Five of the ten influencers dedicate their publications to fashion and trends (sofiaalcastro, jashlem, calleypoche, amara.aa, and kevlexd), through images that project their daily lives, with the classic #ootd (outfit of the day), or videos that add to the viral content on the network. According to the study published by Socialbakers [25], fashion is the leading industry in interaction within the Instagram platform (24.7%), which corresponds with the preference of users for this content and the reception received by influencers from the Andean Community who belong to this category. As the second popular theme is entertainment and humor, with three accounts that address mixed content (la_liendraa, carlosferiag, and luisa_castro1585), mostly related to Internet trends or challenges, but from a comical perspective. Finally, two profiles deal with beauty-related content (poche and danielaacalle), mainly through makeup posts. It should be emphasized that on Instagram users do not radically categorize their content, as their feed has very varied content, mainly dedicated to showing their lifestyle and being part of the trends of the moment.

Another crucial aspect when analyzing the content of influencers in social media is the language, remember that Márquez & Ardèvol [18] emphasize that YouTube favors oral narrative by the audiovisual condition of its contents, therein lies the reason why YouTubers resort to the use of colloquial language that causes identification in the young audience that follows them and favors the creation of a link between the YouTuber and his followers. This situation extrapolates to content creators on Instagram, since let us remember that this social network allows capturing, modifying, publishing, discovering, and interacting through photographs and videos, through a single device [16]. Likewise, thanks to the functions implemented in recent years, this application greatly favors interaction and allows maintaining daily contact with followers. Such is the impact of this social network that, according to the indaHash report [12], 85% of influencers choose it as their trusted application.

Taking into consideration Jakobson's [13] classification of language, the dominance of the expressive function in the contents of the most prominent influencers of the Andean Community was determined because twenty of the forty materials analyzed made use of this function of language when transmitting a message, this in their attempt to connect with the audience that follows them, expressing their feelings or moods openly. The second most used language in the contents of the sample is referential, with fifteen videos or photographs where the content creator transmits a message as close to reality as possible. This classification included gamers' videos, where this language function is used to narrate what the YouTuber observes in his environment within the video game, trying to describe as faithfully as possible the reality presented therein. Finally, five contents were found that used the conative function, transmitting messages that sought to motivate the audience to perform a certain action.

As the last result of this article, the table of convergence between the two social networks (YouTube and Instagram) is presented, detailing those profiles that appear in both rankings (Table 3).

Table 3. Convergence of YouTubers and Instagrammers in the Andean community.

Influencer	YouTube		Instagram	
	Subscribers	Year of creation	Followers	Year of creation
Sofia Castro	8.63M	2014	7M	2014
Amara Leguízamon	8.37M	2014	4.6M	2013
Daniela Calle and María José Garzón	7.56M	2015	5.2M	2016
Jean Carlo León	5.16M	2014	6.7M	2013

It can be observed that the content creator Sofía Castro, leads the table with a total of 15.63 million followers between the two social networks; however, it is worth mentioning that the number does not represent the number of people who follow the influencer because the same user can follow her on YouTube and Instagram. It is also worth noting that, except for Jean Carlo León, the platform on which content creators accumulate the largest number of followers is YouTube, which corresponds to the number of users this network has, compared to Instagram (2 billion vs. 1.22 billion).

It should also be noted that the date of creation of the profiles on these platforms is between 2013 and 2016, but this does not represent a determining factor with the number of followers, as Amara Leguízamon created her Instagram account in 2013; however, she has fewer followers than the profile of Calle y Poché, which was created three years later (2016). On YouTube, we have the example of Jean Carlo León, who creates his channel the same year as Sofía Castro and Amara Leguízamon (2014) but has approximately three million followers less than the YouTubers mentioned. Finally, we name once again influencer Sofía Castro, who is the only one to create both profiles in the same year, which could explain part of her success in building a community simultaneously on these two platforms.

4 By Way of Conclusion

The culture of participation and user-generated content have awakened new digital communication channels, thus consolidating the figures of YouTubers and Instagrammers also present in the Andean Community where they play an important role, on YouTube aimed at entertainment content and on Instagram at fashion and trends.

Through the data presented, we have an approach to the influencers of the Andean Community. When consolidating the rankings, it is observed that Colombia is the country with the highest participation in both platforms, in addition to highlighting the difference between the reach that these influencers receive compared to the other countries under study, calling into question the non-existence of borders in social media. Next is Ecuador, with representatives in both rankings, then Peru, a country that has only one representative in the top of Instagrammers, and finally Bolivia, which does not appear in the total results of this study, but at the time of the exploration it was found a low reception of Bolivian influencers about their peers. This finding merits an in-depth investigation to determine the specific reasons for this phenomenon. It can be inferred that there is a marked digital divide, both in terms of access to the network and bandwidth available in Bolivia, reasons that could be related to the low impact received by content creators in this country.

Influencers in the Andean Community, men, and women have equal conditions in terms of the number of followers and preferences. The most used language is expressive, that is, messages that convey emotions, directly related to the intention of influencers to create a community that identifies with them, creating closeness and loyalty to their followers.

For future lines of research, the analysis of audiovisual narratives and the implementation of transmedia and cross-media by content creators in this region should be further explored.

References

1. Aponte, M., Riaño, D., Velásquez, L.: Monetary income generation for instagramers. Fundación Universitaria del Área Andina (2018)
2. Aran-Ramspott, S., Fedele, M., Tarragó, A.: Social functions of YouTubers and their influence on preadolescence. Comunicar **57**, 71–80 (2018). https://doi.org/10.3916/C57-2018-07
3. Ávila-Toscano, J.: Social networks and network analysis: applications in community and virtual contexts. 1st edn. Corporación Universitaria Reformada, Barranquilla (2012)
4. Asociación de Mujeres Cineastas y de Medios Audiovisuales (CIMA): CIMA Report 2018: The representativeness of women in the Spanish film industry (2018)
5. Conde, M., Forteza-Martínez, A., Andrade-Martínez, C.: Analysis of the leadership skills and charisma of the main Spanish YouTubers. 3C TIC. Cuadernos desarrollo aplicados a las TIC **9**(3), 17–41 (2020). https://doi.org/10.17993/3ctic.2020.93.17-41
6. Córdova, R., Rivera-Rogel, D.: Una mirada a los YouTubers de la Comunidad Andina. Rev. Ibérica Sist. Tecnol. Inform. **35**, 377–389 (2020)
7. Díaz, L.: Soy Marca: Quiero trabajar con influencers, 1st edn. Profit editorial, Barcelona (2017)
8. Espejo, A., Yaguachi, J.: Influencing strategy in Ecuador: the view of the main agencies in Guayaquil and Quito. Strategic Commun. Collect. **2020**, 102–105 (2020)
9. González-Carrión, E., Aguaded, I.: Engagement and evolution of Spanish-speaking fashion instagramers. RLCS Rev. Latina Comun. Soc. **77**, 231–252 (2020). https://doi.org/10.4185/RLCS-2020-1456

10. González, M., Carrión-Salinas, G., Velásquez, A., Rivera-Rogel, D.: Youtubers, a phenomenon also in Latin America. Rev. Iberoamericana (Electron.) Sist. Cibern. Inform. RISCI, 209–214 (2021)
11. Hootsuite, We Are Social: Digital 2021 Global Overview Report (2019)
12. IndaHash.: The new normal: how social media will change in 2020? (2020)
13. Jakobson, R.: Ensayos de lingüística general. Ariel, Barcelona (1984)
14. Johnson, R., Christensen, L.: Educational Research: Quantitative, Qualitative, and Mixed Approaches, 5th edn. SAGE Publications, Los Angeles (2014)
15. Krippendorff, K.: Content Analysis: An Introduction to Its Methodology, 2nd edn. SAGE Publications, Beverly Hills (2004)
16. Manovich, L.: Instagram and Contemporary Image. 1st edn. (2017)
17. Marinas, L.: Instagram: where millennials, generation Z, Mcluhan and Bolter intersect. CIC: Cuadernos Inform. Comun. **24**, 187–201 (2019)
18. Márquez, I., Ardèvol, E.: Hegemony and counterhegemony in the YouTuber phenomenon. Highlights. Rev. Ciencias Soc. (56), 34–49 (2018). https://doi.org/10.29340/56.1876
19. Murolo, N., Lacorte, N.: From bloopers to YouTubers. Ten years of YouTube in digital culture. Question **45**(1), 15–29 (2015)
20. Pereira, Z.: Mixed method designs in educational research: a concrete experience. Educare Electron. J. **15**(1), 15–29 (2011). https://doi.org/10.15359/ree.15-1.2
21. Rivera-Rogel, D., Córdova-Tapia, R.: Most influential Instagrammers in the Andean community. Rev. Ibérica Sist. Tecnol. Inform. **E40**, 205–217 (2021). http://www.risti.xyz/issues/ristie40.pdf
22. Rivera-Rogel, D., Velásquez, A., B-Flandoli, A.: Youtubers from Ecuador and Colombia and their contribution to education. In: III International Congress on Media Competencies (2018)
23. Sanz, P., Pérez, C., Velasco, A.: Hacia un cambio en el sector de moda y lujo. Del dominio del influencer a la marca: Gucci, Loewe y Margiela. Rev. Comun. **19**(2), 263–284 (2020). https://doi.org/10.26441/RC19.2-2020-A15
24. Servicio Nacional de Aduana del Ecuador, Comunidad Andina (CAN): Historical review. https://bit.ly/3bQ1Nnn. Accessed 18 Apr 2021
25. Socialbakers.: Social media trends report: key insights from Q3 2020 (2020)
26. Wyatt, R.: 2020 is YouTube Gaming's biggest year, ever: 100B watch time hours. Head of Global Gaming (2020)

Intellectual Disability in Media and Political Agendas and Its Status as a Social Minority

Carmen Carretón-Ballester(✉)

Universidad de Alicante, Alicante, Spain
mc.carreton@ua.es

Abstract. The presence of intellectual disability and its treatment in the media, with the generation of news in its proactive contribution to the social reality of this collective, reflects the media's role in the formation of public opinion through responsible communication. Moreover, the behaviour of the political agenda concerning public service in terms of intellectual disability is manifested through the parliamentary initiatives implemented from its legislative, control, and policy orientation functions. Methods: Reference is made to 2016, the year in which the assessment report of the Action Plan of the Spanish Disability Strategy (2014–2020) was published, and the time interval from 2016 to present, for the content analysis of the dimensions defined for the study of news on intellectual disability in the El País and El Mundo newspapers (media agenda) and the parliamentary initiatives related to intellectual disability (political agenda). In a cross-sectional analysis between the agendas and this Strategic Plan, we sought to determine the relationships of the attitudes and behaviours achieved by the different social agents. Results: The analysis contributes to the consideration of intellectual disability as a minority issue in political and media agendas. Discussion and Conclusions: The exiguous implication of responsibility in the media agenda and the lack of commitment in the political agenda prevent the construction of the real situation of intellectual disability (public agenda) derived from its consequences.

Keywords: Intellectual disability · Media agenda · Minorities · Political agenda · Public agenda · Public relations · Responsibility

1 Introduction

The World Health Organisation (WHO) defines disability as "a complex phenomenon, reflecting the interaction between features of a person's body and features of the society in which they live (...) that encompasses impairments, activity limitations, and participation restrictions"[1] [20–22]. Consequently, disability should be addressed from the social model that understands that disability arises in a society that has not known how to ensure compliance with the rights of this collective and that focuses on support to improve its quality of life [16].

[1] https://www.who.int/topics/disabilities/es/.

© The Author(s), under exclusive license to Springer Nature Singapore Pte Ltd. 2022
Á. Rocha et al. (Eds.): ICOMTA 2021, SIST 259, pp. 203–215, 2022.
https://doi.org/10.1007/978-981-16-5792-4_21

From this model, according to Schalock [28], intellectual disability (henceforth ID) should be understood from the limitations that an individual has in order to carry out everyday activities and participation in its social context. In 2018, the UN Commission's report on the rights of persons with disabilities stated that "in the Spanish educational system there is no generalised recognition of the human rights model of disability and there is a lack of access to inclusive and quality education for people with disabilities" (p. 16). "(…) insufficient measures have been adopted to promote inclusive education for people with disabilities, and the poor predictability of the system for the promotion and protection of the rights of people with disabilities…" (p. 17), violating Article 24 on Education of the International Convention on the Rights of Persons with Disabilities (CRPD). However, the Spanish government expressed its disagreement with these conclusions [15].

The reality of disability in Spain affects almost 4 million people[2] who are significantly impacted by the report, given its scarce media impact, coinciding with the opinion of Cortés and Correyero [5] who exposed the gap that exists between the media's treatment of people with disabilities and the demographic statistics they represent.

The most active behaviour is exhibited by the collective committed to ID which, consistent with the social issues of its reality and from the social model, shows the scarce knowledge of the actors of the political and media agendas.

This study analyses the treatment of ID, a type of disability that has a greater variability due to the interaction between health problems, personal, and environmental factors. Analysing the presence of ID and its treatment in different agendas allows us to know the media's role in forming public opinion, as well as the role of political actors in the generation of measures and initiatives on ID. The control of the agenda as "the ability to limit the possible actions of other actors, selecting the social problems that attract the attention of political and media institutions is, therefore, a "true exercise of power" (p. 25) [26].

2 The Social Issues of Intellectual Disability

As Suriá, Bueno, and Rosser (pp. 875–876) [30] establish on the collective of young people with disabilities, "the barriers, obstacles, and difficulty in accessing the labour market, as well as exposure to certain risk situations, position them as social groups that are especially vulnerable to exclusion".

In Public Relations, the intellectually disabled (hereinafter, ID) are considered to represent a minority of the disability. Among the problems that arise from this collective (discrimination, exclusion, absence of affirmative actions…), minorities surface who seek to project their problems on the media agenda and get their objectives to be considered on the political agenda.

The social problems affect a significantly considerable number of people in ways that are harmful and which can be corrected by collective social action [7]. However, Blumer [2] adds the need to legitimise the problem by all of society's actors in order for

[2] In this normative context, the latest study conducted in our country by the Ministry of Health, Consumer Affairs, and Social Welfare (2016) concluded that 3,378,622 people are "considered disabled", of which 1,686,563 are men and 1,692,019 are women.

it to be defined as a social problem. Nevertheless, for an issue to be perceived as a social problem, there must be continuous interaction between the actors that intervene in that problem [13], and it must be interpreted, defined, and explained by the actors based on the knowledge they receive from the people it affects [18]. The construction of the public problem is the consequence of this relationship between the actors. These actors come together to debate and propose initiatives, and include the issue in the political agenda [1]; the agenda being the social issues selected and ranked by the different institutions [10].

In this way, interaction between the agendas is needed to provide access for social issues, in particular issues of interest to minorities, and to institutional and social agencies to achieve their objectives. However, the media's coverage of ID issues is not sufficient; the commitment of all social actors with affirmative actions and responsible behaviour is required to form a favourable public opinion [3].

The following relations with minorities and objectives that extend beyond non-discrimination [11], adapted to ID are listed below: 1. Propose affirmative actions, 2. Determine issues of particular interest for the ID collective, and 3. Investigate the opinion of the actors in the communities or the leaders of the ID collective. In consequence, the media has the social role of broadcasting, reporting, and publicising issues on ID, and the political agents and competent bodies have the public role of complying with the rules and regulations that ensure non-discrimination of the ID and promote affirmative actions that benefit the collective.

3 The Agendas' Role

3.1 The Media Agenda: A Social Role for Intellectual Disability

The media agenda fulfils a proactive role in the social sphere [17], forming cognitions in people, but also attending to the role they play in the construction of its agenda. In its role as the backbone, influencer, and director of currents of public opinions, the media, on the one hand, is an instrument used to spread messages and positive images [27] and, on the other, it is an active agent in the commitment to act in the face of social problems [9].

In the context of disability, the media's role at the service of the society described by Mac Bride [14] – to inform, socialise, motivate, discuss, educate, culturally advance, entertain, and integrate –, hinges on its social responsibility with the issues of ID collectives to make them visible and generate public opinion to promote social inclusion and reduce discrimination.

Fernández, Chipre and Vidal (p. 29) [6] maintain that "the media has the capacity to make disability familiar and thus neutralise all the social constructions with stereotypes that exist around it". For this, it is necessary to expand the knowledge, modify the attitudes or languages of communication professionals for the correct treatment of disability [6] and contribute to reducing stigma, therefore "the nominalisation of adjectives such as deficient, disabled, or handicapped is discouraged, and even more so, the use of others in the full and inappropriately negative meaning of the word, such as invalid" (p.29) [4].

However, as channels for a proper formation of public opinion and attending to the levels of social responsibility of the media in their behaviour with minorities [3], the following levels are established for ID:

- **Level 1 (LR1):** The media serves to make the ID collective visible and generate public opinion: dissemination and visibility.
- **Level 2 (LR2):** The media is actively involved in the *issues* or needs of the ID collectives: commitment and active role.
- **Level 3 (LR0):** The journalist cares about knowing and inquiring about the ID collectives and uses a proper treatment of the terms.

3.2 The Political Agenda: A Public Role for Intellectual Disability

In the Spanish parliamentary system, the first function is legislative, which includes the approval of laws and the approval of the State's general budgets.[3] The control function refers to the fact that the political management of the Government is subject to the control of the bicameral legislative chambers (*Cortes Generales*) throughout its execution.[4] This control may be exercised through inquiries, oral questions, written questions, appearances, or requests for reports. Furthermore, from the policy orientation function, parliamentary groups can submit non-legislative proposals, motions, or plans and programmes.

The people who dedicate themselves to politics are public servants with political responsibility, administrative responsibility, and civil responsibility in the exercise of their functions. For a social issue to access the political agenda, it requires the definition of the problem in order to demand actions from the public powers, proposals to solve it, and a favourable attitude of all political actors towards the problem [26].

The Government of Spain has the 2014–2020 Action Plan of the Spanish Disability Strategy to develop the Spanish Disability Strategy framed in the Convention of the United Nations (UN) on the Rights of People with Disabilities, in the guidelines of the 2010–2020 European Disability Strategy, in the 2020 European Strategy and the provisions of the Spanish Disability Strategy. On the other hand, the General Law on the Rights of People with Disabilities and their Social Inclusion constitutes the legal reference and principles on which the aforementioned Plan was inspired [19]: Respect for inherent dignity, individual autonomy, including the freedom to make one's own decisions, and personal independence; Independent living Non-discrimination; Respect for difference and acceptance of people with disabilities as a part of diversity and the human condition; Equal opportunities; Equality between women and men; Normalisation; Universal accessibility; Universal design or design accessible to all people; Full and effective participation and inclusion in society; and Civil dialogue. "Public policies for persons with disabilities, as well as legislative reforms provide coverage with the aim of building an inclusive society" (p. 219) [8]. In this framework, the analysis of the political agenda's issues of interest with parliamentary initiatives from their different functions portrays political behaviour in terms of public service in the context of the ID.

[3] https://www.congreso.es/web/guest/cem/fleg.

[4] https://www.congreso.es/web/guest/cem/fcontrol.

4 Objectives and Methodology

To achieve the objectives of: 1. Determine the presence and treatment of ID in media and political agendas; 2. Know the level of responsibility in the relationship between the media, the political sphere, and the ID collective (3 agendas) and 3. Determine the presence of the Principles from the 2014–2020 Action Plan of the Spanish Disability Strategy with respect to ID in the different agendas, all the news about DI (123) from the two Spanish newspapers with the highest coverage are selected, *El País and El Mundo* (FACTIVA Database) and the existing parliamentary initiatives on ID (24) from the control and policy orientation functions from the last four legislatures were selected (period: 2016-present). The content analysis method was chosen [23, 29] for which the study dimensions of the news (Table 1) and political initiatives (Table 2) on ID were defined. Both analyses were crossed with the principles, objectives, and measures described in the results report of the first phase (2014–2016) of the 2014–2020 Action Plan of the Spanish Disability Strategy on ID. The statistical programme SPSS Statistics, V.22 was used for data processing.

Table 1. Variables and units of analysis of the news

Issue	1. Disease; 2. Drama; 3. Problem; 4. Educational needs/problems of the collective; 5. Labour needs/problems of the collective; 6. News/case/testimony; 7. Awareness. World and/or National Days; 8. Sexist violence/School violence
Treatment	1. Person with intellectual disability; 2. Disabled;
Responsibility	1. Level 1 (LR1); 2. Level 2 (LR2); 3. Level 3 (LR0)
Principles of the Action Plan of the Spanish Disability Strategy	

Table 2. Variables and units of analysis of policy initiatives

Source	1. Government; 2. Parliamentary Group; 3. Pressure groups/lobbies
Actions/Issues	1. Labour market: increase employment opportunities for people with intellectual disabilities; 2. Education: reduce the school failure rate; 3. Social inclusion: reduce the number of people below the poverty line; 4. ID rights
Conduct	1. Presentation of plans/Specific actions (attitude, intention); 2. Development/implementation of plans and/or actions (manifest conduct in development); 3. Approval of regulations. Law proposals (overt behaviour-public policies); 4. No overt behaviour (passive)

5 Results

5.1 The Political Agenda

There are two important legislative advances in relation to the disabled: in October 2017, the proposal of an Organic Law amending Organic Law 5/1995 [24], of 22 May, of the Jury, to guarantee the participation of people with disabilities without the exclusions indicated in its Article 8.5: "People with disabilities may not be excluded from serving on a jury on the basis of their disability, and the Justice administration must provide the necessary support as well as make reasonable adjustments…" and Organic Law 2/2018 [12, 25], of 5 December, for the modification of Organic Law 5/1985, of 19 June, of the General Electoral Regime to guarantee the right to vote of all people with disabilities that dedicates Article 3.2 to people with ID, "Any person may exercise his or her right to vote actively, consciously, freely and voluntarily, whatever their means of communicating it and with the means of support required.“

Although the assessment report of the first phase of the 2014–2020 Action Plan of the Spanish Disability Strategy states that 96% of the actions were completed, the majority refer to action plans and the promotion of activities or measures integrated into other strategies, however, it does not define the measures to be developed. Although actions that include the commitment of the media stand out, such as the Capacitados Program (TV2) and the studies on the Media and use of language, of the 96 measures only 3 include DI:

35. Promote measures to promote access to employment for people with limited intellectual capacity *(accomplished)*

76. Ensure that all Spanish facilities abroad are fully accessible for people with physical, sensory, and intellectual disabilities *(in progress)*

92. Reduce the gap in the availability of accessible ICTs for people with intellectual disabilities *(in progress)*

Of the 1,216 parliamentary initiatives on disability, 20 were developed from the legislative function, 946 from the control function, and 250 from the policy orientation function. However, ID only appears in 23 initiatives, of which 22 belong to the control function, 1 to the policy orientation function, and none to the legislative function. In terms of ID, the questions by parliamentary groups to the Government with written responses from it reached a figure of 66.7%, compared to appearances by public of interest invited by parliamentary groups (29.2%) and non-legislative proposals (4.2%).

Regarding these issues, Fig. 1 shows that 41.4% of political attention was focused on initiatives for full inclusion and reducing the number of people below the poverty line, followed by 13.8% on employment (the need to increase job opportunities for people with ID) and education with 10.3%. Considering that Covid-related initiatives reached 10.2% in 2020, the rest is dispersed between initiatives on the rights of people with ID, violence against women, children and young people, and care in specific social centres. The political behaviour of the Government regarding these initiatives resides in the attitude with the presentation of plans, reports, or intentions in 45.8% and behaviour, with a scant 29% of actions and plans developed. Faced with these figures, it is worth noting that 25% correspond to expired or withdrawn initiatives.

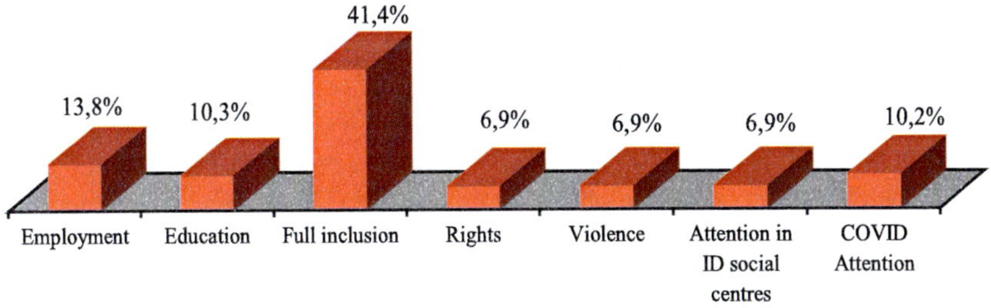

Fig. 1. Political interest issues (Source: own elaboration)

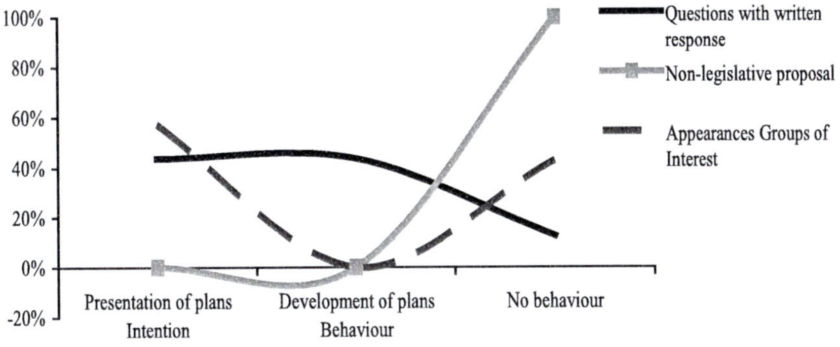

Fig. 2. Relationship between initiatives and level of behaviour (Source: own elaboration)

From the initiative-behaviour level (Fig. 2) bivariate analysis, the results show that questions with written answers are concentrated with the same weight between the presentation of plans (attitude) and the implementation of plans for their development (behaviour). Regarding the appearances of interest groups, the initiatives in the attitude phase are worth nothing (57.14%) compared to the absence of behaviour with 42.86% of the initiatives expired. The non-legislative proposal is a withdrawn initiative. Some interesting results were achieved for the type of issues, type of initiatives, and behaviour level. Sixty-six point seven per cent of full inclusion issues were addressed in interest groups' appearances and responded to a behaviour of attitude and intention, exposing reports or situations in the context of a particular problem of people with an ID. In the absence of behaviour, either because the initiative had expired, had been cancelled or had been withdrawn, 50% corresponded to appearances of interest groups and 16.7% to questions with written responses.

5.2 The Media Agenda

The media amassed a total of 742 news stories about "disabilities". Of these, only 123 or 16.6% addressed "intellectual disabilities". Although 82.1% of the news on ID used inclusive language, referring to a person/people with a disability, 17.9% continued to use the word disabled. The newspaper *El País* accounted for 57.7% and the newspaper *El Mundo* accounted for 42.3%. The presence of ID in the media increased progressively from 2016 to 2019 (13%, 18.7%; 31.7%, 32.5%). However, in 2020 it suffered a significant decrease (4.1%) until it disappeared from the press in 2021. The news source (Fig. 3) reflects the origin of the concern about ID and allows us to contrast the agent's behaviour with other variables. Relation of source and year, and given that interest groups had more presence in 2018, and the media in 2019, the data demonstrate a significant association between both variables (Pearson's Chi-squared test, $p = 0.004$).

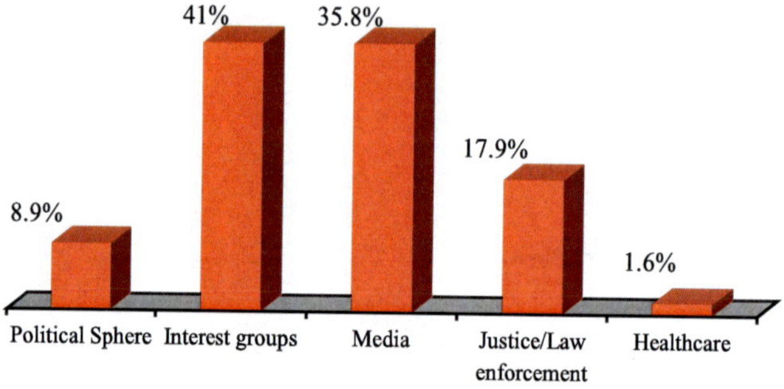

Fig. 3. Source of the object of the news (Source: own elaboration)

Table 3. Treatment of the media according to the news source

Agent/Source	Media treatment	
	Person with ID	Disabled
Political sphere	81.8%	18.2%
Public of interest	93.2%	6.8%
Media	86.4%	13.6%
Justice/Law Enforcement	59%	41%
Healthcare	–	100.0%

Affirmative actions for the ID collective were the most present issue in the newspapers (35.8%); issues on news, case, or testimony of stories and vital experiences of people with ID reached 29.3%; 16.3% referred to news about violence, sexist abuse, or school violence against people with ID, and universal suffrage accounted for 10.6% of the news stories. Although the language "person with a disability" was used in 82.1% of the means compared to the term "disabled" which persisted in 17.9%, the dependency relationship between the source and treatment variables was high (Pearson's Chi-square, $p = 0001$), therefore the source determined the language and emphasised the best use in the public agenda (Table 3).

Concerning responsibility, the media made ID issues visible to generate public opinion (LR1, dissemination, and visibility) in all the news stories, yet only 15.4% showed commitment and played an active role in the ID collective's issues (LR2). Even though almost 52% of the news did not refer to any of the principles of the 2014–2020 Action Plan of the Spanish Disability Strategy (Table 4), the full inclusion and participation of people with ID in society were present in 24.6% of the news stories, followed by civil dialogue between the agents to develop affirmative actions for the ID collective (21.3%).

Table 4. Principles of the 2014–2020 Action Plan of the Spanish Disability Strategy in the media agenda

Principles	Frequency
Civil dialogue	21.3%
Active inclusion and participation	24.6%
Universal design	5.7%
Universal accessibility	4.9%
Normalisation	16.4%
Equal opportunities	10.7%
Respect for difference	4.1%
Non-discrimination	7.4%
Independent living	13.1%
Dignity, autonomy, decision-making, independence	13.9%
None	51.6%

The principle-source bivariate analysis shows that the news in which the Plan reached the greatest presence was on the public agenda (interest groups) and in which all the principles appeared. However, the 5 main principles, in order, are: 1. Civil dialogue; 2. Full and effective participation and inclusion in society; 3. Respect for dignity, autonomy, decisions, independence; 4. Normalisation, equal opportunities and independent living; 5. Universal accessibility. The following principles are highlighted in the news whose source was the political sphere: 1. Full and effective participation and inclusion in society; 2. Civil dialogue; 3. Normalisation and non-discrimination. And the media as a source included full and effective participation and inclusion in society, and normalisation as more profuse principles. As for the behaviour of the agents of the news source and their active involvement with the Plan's principles, the media obtained a LR1 for 35.8% of the news originating in the public agenda as well as the media agenda, compared to 8.9% in the political agenda. The highest LR2 level is concentrated in the news that came from the media (52.6%) and interest groups (36.8%).

6 Discussion and Conclusions

In relation to the first objective, "to determine the presence and treatment of ID in the media and political agenda", we observed that both the news in the press and the parliamentary initiatives on ID occupied minimal space in their respective agendas in the overall context of disability. Interest groups, as involved and committed groups that seek to project their issues in the media agenda, bring the most abundant source of issues to the public agenda.

Although "disabled person" predominated in terms of treatment, in some news stories the term "disabled" was also found, therefore we still consider it necessary to gain knowledge and modify languages to improve the media's treatment of the ID collective. In relation to the media's active role,[5] the programme "Capacitados Issues/Disabilities" (Able) on channel TV2 to achieve the objective of promoting programmes related to disability in the media, where positive and normalising situations and behaviours are proposed in response to the diversity in people with disabilities, is still underway. And the measure "Studies on the Media and the Use of Language. Complaints submitted to the Ombudsman/Collective Agreement for Media Professionals" to fulfil the objective of promoting actions that guarantee the proper use of language on disability in social media is defined as dispersed. Although there are increasing initiatives on ID, the qualitative analysis showed more of a statement of intent than the actions taken. The correlation between the source and year of the news may have come from the modification of Organic Law 5/1985, of 19 June, of the General Electoral Regime to guarantee universal suffrage for people with disabilities. However, legislative advances, being important achievements that agree with the principle of full and effective participation and inclusion in society, is a specific action that would generically coincide with operational objective 3 of the Plan to Promote the Participation of People with Disabilities, under the conditions of equality in political, economic, and social life, although it does not respond to any of its measures because perhaps its design does not delve into the social issues of the ID derived from its variability. Likewise, measure 35 of the Plan is related to the principle of the labour market. Measure 76 would be included in the principle of universal accessibility and measure 92 would fit into the principle of universal design for all people. In view of the undefined and ongoing ID measures, there is still a long way to go before we see ID issues reflected on the political agenda. The issues on the political agenda, – the most abundant being that of full participation and inclusion in society – come from parliamentary groups and, exceptionally, lead to civil dialogue (the most reflected principle in the public agenda). The Government's responses to parliamentary questions refer to forecasts and to promoting positive actions, albeit, far from describing what the measures are and whether they are being implemented. Given the time frame of the Plan and this first evaluation, talking about future forecasts and actions is indicative of its stagnation. The political agenda shows a behaviour far from its attitude and the parliamentary groups raise the issues with the public of interest during the appearances. In summary, parliamentary initiatives respond to the control function and, in a very residual way, to the policy orientation function, but none of them responds to the legislative function.

The second objective, "know the level of responsibility in the relationship between the media, the political sphere, and the ID group", with the predominant LR1 of the media (especially with testimonies and life experiences), shows the media's low social

[5] The first phase of the report of the results by the State Disability Observatory describes the following actions aimed toward achieving the principles and objectives listed below.

involvement and the public servants scant intervention with the ID collective. Therefore, ID issues in the public agenda fail to be set in both the media agenda and the political agenda.

As for the third objective, "determine compliance with the Principles of the 2014–2020 Action Plan of the Spanish Disability Strategy in terms of ID" [19], the public agenda, with the presence of interest groups in the media and their appearances in commissions, and the media agenda with the presentation of ID issues are the agendas that most reflect the principles, while in the political agenda they are diluted with little significance in terms of full and effective participation and inclusion in society and social dialogue.

However, the direct or indirect exposure of the principles in both agendas does not mean their implementation or their manifest behaviour because 1) The answer refers to generic contexts and what is going to be done, but it is not very concise; 2) At the halfway point of the 2014–2020 Action Plan of the Spanish Disability Strategy, data available in 2021, the measures on disability were in process, scattered or pending and it contemplated few and indefinite measures for ID; and 3) The political agenda does not reflect the principles of the Plan and is still far from the issues on the public agenda. In summary and in relation to the objectives of relations with minorities:

- Affirmative actions are on the public agenda because the public of interest shows issues inherent to their fundamental purpose and objectives.
- There is little proactive and overt ID behaviour on the political agenda. It is the parliamentary groups who demand accountability, occasionally with interest groups, although with little follow-up and no response to ID issues showing the scant coverage with the aim of building an inclusive society. There is a gap between the public agenda and the political agenda.
- Although the media gives a fairly good reflection of the principles, its social function is mainly confined to the presentation of issues, complying with its LR1; its involvement in contributing to ID issues is still limited. There is a gap between the public agenda and the media agenda. There should be a greater social dialogue with interest groups, who should have a greater influence on decision-making.

In consideration of the above, the treatment of ID in political and media agendas confirms that it is the society that does not ensure compliance with the rights of people with disabilities by not establishing their issues in the political domain. Moreover, the sparse space, lack of recognition and legitimation of ID issues and their inadequate treatment in the agendas do not contribute to constructing the reality to which the group is exposed, favouring its status as a minority as presented from the social model.

Research. This article is the result of the work of the research line on the visibility of ID of the consolidated research group "Public relations, social responsibility, and communication with minorities" of the University of Alicante (Spain).

References

1. Araujo, K., Guzmán, V., Mauro, A.: El surgimiento de la violencia doméstica como problema público y objeto de políticas. Rev. Cepal **70**, 133–145 (2000). https://www.cepal.org/es/publicaciones/12204-surgimiento-la-violencia-domestica-como-problema-publico-objeto-politicas
2. Blumer, H.: Social problems as collective behavior. Soc. Probl. **18**(3), 298–306 (1971). https://doi.org/10.2307/799797
3. Carretón-Ballester, M.C., Lorenzo-Solá, F.: Niveles de responsabilidad de los medios en sus relaciones con las minorías. Epilepsia y autismo. Rev. Int. Relaciones Públicas **8**(15), 215–236 (2018). https://doi.org/10.5783/RIRP10.5783/RIRP-15-2018-12-215-236
4. Casado, D.: Comunicación social en discapacidad. Cuestiones éticas y de estilo. Ministerio de Trabajo y Asuntos Sociales. Real Patronato sobre Discapacidad, Madrid (2001). http://riberdis.cedd.net/bitstream/handle/11181/2887/132812.pdf?sequence=1&rd=0031628937897740
5. Cortés-Fuentes, J.A., Correyero-Ruiz, B.: Radio y empoderamiento social. Usos y gratificaciones del taller de radio para las personas con discapacidad intelectual o del desarrollo. Prof. Inform. **26**(1), 55–65 (2017). https://doi.org/10.3145/epi.2017.ene.06
6. Fernández, M., Chipre, L., Vidal, P.: Tratamiento de la discapacidad en los medios de comunicación. Observatorio de la Discapacidad Física. Observatorio del Tercer Sector, Barcelona (2017). http://hdl.handle.net/11181/5444
7. Horton, P.B., Leslie, G.R.: The Sociology of Social Problems. Appiclon-Century-Cropts, New York (1955)
8. Inza-Bartolomé, A., Bergantinos-Franco, N., Rivera_Escribano, M.J.: Las personas con discapacidad intelectual como protagonistas del proceso inclusivo. Lan Harremanak. Rev. Relaciones Laborales **29**, 217–228 (2014)
9. Jasler, V.I.: Responsabilidad Social y Medios de Comunicación: El rol del periodismo. [Tesis Doctoral de la Universidad de Palermo] (2009). http://dspace.palermo.edu/dspace/bitstream/handle/10226/1156/Jasler?sequence=1
10. Kingdon, J.W.: Agendas, Alternatives, and Public Policies. Little Brown, Boston (1984)
11. Lesly, P.: Lesly's Public Relations Handbook. Prentice-Hall, USA (1978)
12. Ley Orgánica 2/2018, de 5 de diciembre, para la modificación de la Ley Orgánica 5/1985, de 19 de junio, del Régimen Electoral General para garantizar el derecho de sufragio de todas las personas con discapacidad. BOE, no. 294 de 6 de diciembre: 119785–119787 (2018). https://www.boe.es/eli/es/lo/2018/12/05/2
13. Lorenc-Valcarce, F.: La sociología de los problemas públicos. Una perspectiva crítica para el estudio de las relaciones entre la sociedad y la política. Nómadas Rev. Crít. Ciencias Soc. Jurídicas **12**(2), 141–150 (2005). https://www.redalyc.org/articulo.oa?id=18153295010
14. Macbride, S.: Un solo mundo, voces múltiples. Informe de la Comisión Internacional para el estudio de los problemas de la comunicación. Fondo de Cultura Económica, Méjico (1980)
15. Ministerio de Sanidad, Consumo y Bienestar Social. Base estatal de datos de personas con valoración del grado de discapacidad. Informe a 31/12/2016 (2018) https://ceapat.imserso.es/InterPresent2/groups/imserso/documents/binario/bdepcd_2016.pdf
16. MINUSVAL. Dossier «Personas con Inteligencia Límite», Aproximación sociológica a las personas con DINAI. Madrid (2004). http://sid.usal.es/idocs/F8/8.2.1.2-139/145/13_34_dossier.pdf
17. Montesinos-Condo, R.A.: Medios de comunicación y ciudadanía. Rev. Invest. Comun. Desarrollo **2**(1), 16–24 (2011). https://www.comunicacionunap.com/index.php/rev/article/view/11
18. Muller, P., Surel, Y.: L'analyse des politiques publiques. Montchrestien, Paris (1998)

19. OED. Informe sobre la aplicación de la primera fase del Plan (2014–2016). Plan de Acción de la Estrategia Española sobre Discapacidad 2014–2020 (2018). https://www.observatoriodeladiscapacidad.info/wp-content/uploads/2016/12/Informe-Eval-Fase1-PAEED-OED-web.pdf
20. OMS. Clasificación internacional del funcionamiento, de la discapacidad y de la salud (CIF). Madrid, Imserso, Ministerio de Asuntos Sociales (2001). http://www.imserso.es/InterPresent2/groups/imserso/documents/binario/435cif.pdf
21. OMS. Informe Mundial sobre la Discapacidad (2011). Organización Mundial de la Salud, Malta (2011). https://www.who.int/disabilities/world_report/2011/summary_es.pdf
22. ONU. Informe de la investigación relacionada con España bajo el artículo 6 del Protocolo Facultativo. Comité sobre los Derechos de las Personas con Discapacidad (2017). https://www.cermi.es/es/actualidad/novedades/informe-de-la-investigaci%C3%B3n-relacionada-con-espa%C3%B1a-bajo-el-art%C3%ADculo-6-del
23. Piñuel-Raigada, J.L., Gaitán-Moya, J.A.: Metodología general: conocimiento científico e investigación en la comunicación social. Síntesis, Madrid (1999)
24. Proposición de Ley Orgánica de modificación de la Ley Orgánica 5/1995, de 22 de mayo, del Tribunal del Jurado, para garantizar la participación de las personas con discapacidad sin exclusiones. BOCG, no. 159 de 16 de octubre: 4–6 (2017). http://www.senado.es/legis12/publicaciones/pdf/senado/bocg/BOCG_D_12_159_1313.PDF
25. Real Decreto Legislativo 1/2013, de 29 de noviembre, por el que se aprueba el Texto Refundido de la Ley General de derechos de las personas con discapacidad y de su inclusión social. BOE, no. 289 de 3 de diciembre: 1–44 (2013). https://www.boe.es/eli/es/rdlg/2013/11/29/1
26. Sampedro, V.: Agendas de poder. Marco analítico y modelos del control político e informativo de los problemas sociales. Rev. Int. Sociol. **15**, 7–36 (1996)
27. Sánchez-De-Amo, A.: Los medios de comunicación ante la discapacidad. Rev. Acciones Invest. Soc. **17**, 183–214 (2003)
28. Schalock, R.: La nueva definición de discapacidad intelectual, apoyos individuales y resultados personales. Rev. Española Sobre Discapacidad Intelectual **40**(1), 229: 22–39 (2009). http://sid.usal.es/idocs/F8/ART11724/Schalock.pdf
29. Sierra-Bravo, R.: Técnicas de investigación social: teoría y ejercicios. Thomson Paraninfo S.A., Madrid (2005)
30. Suriá-Martínez, R., Bueno-Bueno, A., Rosser-Limiñana, A.M.: Prejuicios entre los estudiantes hacia las personas con discapacidad: reflexiones a partir del caso de la Universidad de Alicante. Alternat. Cuadernos Trabajo Soc. **18**, 75–90 (2011). https://doi.org/10.14198/ALTERN2011.18.04

Check for updates

The Emotions of the Outbreak. Topics, Sentiments and Politics on Twitter During Chilean October

Jarnishs Beltrán[1], René Jara-Reyes[2](✉), and Antoine Faure[2]

[1] Universidad de Valparaíso, General Cruz 222, Valparaíso, Chile
[2] Universidad de Santiago de Chile, Avda. Ecuador 3650, Estación Central, Santiago, Chile
rene.jara@usach.cl

Abstract. This paper interrogates the coherence and evolution of emotions circulating on Twitter in a specific context: the social and political outburst of October 2019 in Chile. Starting from the important literature that addresses the relationship between social movements, emotions and social networks, the paper asks about the particularities that this phenomenon in a country where the penetration and use of social networks is intense. By means of a sentiment analysis technique, more than 1,444,344 tweets published during a seven-week period are processed, putting particular interest in the description of the topics and emotions dumped in these messages. In the discussion we estimate how the exercise dialogues with results found in other similar situations, while in the conclusions we ponder its relevance for the analysis of emotions in situations of social conflict.

Keywords: Emotions · Social movements · Twitter · Social outbreak · Chile

1 Introduction

This paper is interested in studying the relationship between emotions, social protest movements and social networks. This relationship is being increasingly studied, in particular because of the expansive character that certain causes reach in the context of their diffusion through these platforms. We assume that this phenomenon can become more acute in contexts of high social conflict and uncertainty, as was experienced in Chile during those weeks.

This research analyzes this phenomenon based on the Twitter activity that took place in Chile during these days of crisis. The evidence gathered here covers seven weeks, taking October 18, 2019 as the starting date. A corpus of 1,444,344 tweets was constituted, which were systematically downloaded. From these messages, two types of analysis techniques were applied, aiming first to determine the content posted on Twitter via a modeling of the topics addressed and subsequently, a sentiment analysis of these messages. With these manipulations, we ask ourselves about the coherence and evolution of emotions found on social networks during the period. We then seek to raise evidence that dialogues with the reports found in other case studies. In the conclusions we evaluate the strengths and limitations of the analysis exercise proposed here.

© The Author(s), under exclusive license to Springer Nature Singapore Pte Ltd. 2022
Á. Rocha et al. (Eds.): ICOMTA 2021, SIST 259, pp. 216–226, 2022.
https://doi.org/10.1007/978-981-16-5792-4_22

1.1 Social Context

October 18, 2019 is the milestone of one of the strongest political and social events since the return to democracy in Chile (1990), which can be said today to mark a before and after. Among the characteristics of these intense protests, the violence of the rupture of the moral economy of domination (in Thompson's sense [1]) as well as the creativity and innovation of action repertoires [2] or the politicization of time in disputes over the synchronization of social and political temporalities [3] stand out. The overflow of social movement organizations and their disconnection with traditional actors [4, 5] has also become evident, even though the most important demonstration in the history of the country has taken place (October 25, 2019). We can emphasize at the same time the organization of citizens' meetings, public policy projects referring to a Social Agenda on the part of the government and the Agreement on a constituent process, still in progress at the time of writing this text, an agreement through which political professionals and traditional parties tried to retake the political leadership of the country.

Among the explanations and understandings under debate to understand these mobilizations, the emotions expressed in the heat of the mobilizations have been little addressed. According to an essay written during the first weeks of the social revolt - whose title is precisely "Rabia"-, it highlights manifestations arising from an emotion endowed with political sense: "The erratic handling of the first outbreaks of discontent, added to the attitude that was rightly denounced as "putting out the fire with benzine", strongly contributed to increase three types of emotions: surprise, anger and sadness" [6]. Using the survey "Pulso Ciudadano" of October 24, 2019, the same text notes the negativity of the emotions expressed: "The demonstrations produce feelings of anger and insecurity in equal parts, and only 18% feel "hopeful"" [7]. While sadness and insecurity can be linked in large part to looting and direct action as well as the uncertainty of a way out of the crisis, the ghost of the civil-military Dictatorship (1973–1990) provoked by the deployment of the Armed Forces in the streets provokes above all fear.

Although they agree on a certain distrust and fear generated by the social and political event, other subsequent studies, whether with quantitative or qualitative methodologies, show the strength of rather positive emotions, such as the joy of this awakening or the hope generated by the mobilizations. What is interesting is that these emotions reveal a projection towards the future and a certain enthusiasm for the possibility of generating social and political change oriented towards dignity, more socioeconomic equality and political participation. In a national survey conducted by the University of Santiago, it is evident that hope is characteristic of the 18–29 age range, preferably men and the C2 socioeconomic segment [8]. On the contrary, the upper classes and respondents over 50 years of age express sadness. Finally, according to the same survey, the lower income sectors show indifference, which reveals a radical hopelessness and the conviction that "nothing can change".

In a survey based in focus groups with people sample by Santiago and Puerto Montt, a team of sociologists exposes the articulation of these same emotions with the social and political context [9]. Again, fear and insecurity are revealed to be very strong when considering their repetitiveness in conversations. While they are linked to violence, the authors also highlight their relationship with the instability that the revolt provoked in everyday life and, specifically, for the work situation (employment, income or clientele).

The perception of the event is articulated around the rage, and its articulation, of those mobilized and specifically of young people. This anger as well as the sociocultural transversalization of the mobilizations are explained by an "emotional liberation" [10], that is, the loss of fear - felt until that event - of expressing oneself and protesting, and the courage given by the support of the masses. Finally, the indifference traced in the quantitative surveys is formulated as resignation in the focus group conversations. Faced with the future, all these emotions lead to a tension between suspicion and confidence in the future and the possibility of reducing what is perceived as "injustices".

2 Review of Literature

2.1 Twitter, Emotions and Protest Mobilization

We know that emotions have been studied with some intensity in the last ten years, particularly in the area of sociology of social movements. It has been emphasized that they have a function of cohesion and accompaniment to collective action [11], as well as a strong identity component to the struggles for people's visibility [12]. Emotions have been emphasized in their expression in the context of mobilization [13].

It is in this framework that a group of works have started to be interested in the link between social networks and emotions in contexts of protest mobilization or, as it has been called, under the "logic of connective action" [14]. In this sense, social networks make it possible to represent emotions and, at the same time, to provoke emotions [15]. It is thanks to this capacity that social networks seem to have this potential to escalate and de-escalate conflicts [16], which allows in the long run to estimate the true effect of online social protest [17].

Among these studies, particular interest has been paid to the use of Twitter in social protests [18]. A first question to be answered is whether there is a relationship between emotions expressed online and offline [19]. A second and larger body of work interrogates the functions that Twitter fulfills, in terms of the toolbox [20]. Teocharis, Jan W. van Deth and García-Albacete [21] identify that its main use is for political discussion and communicative protest information and much less for call of participation. That is, Twitter would serve only some functions of collective action, according to the list of possible ones identified by Cammaerts [22].

Since 2011, Chile has known massive protest movements, which have been accompanied by a consistent activity in social networks. The so-called digital activism [23], seems to be a central element within these mobilizations, which show the changes in the dynamics of collective action in the country. Regarding the former, network activity has been investigated as a source of participation and/or predictor of participation in protests [24, 25] and as an indicator of political engagement [26], as well as studies comparing the experience of student mobilizations in Chile and other Latin American cases [27]. Recently, the use of Twitter has also been used in environmental movements, identifying a relevant function of this digital activism as a launcher of alerts in the face of environmental catastrophes [28]. These studies suggest that certain behavioral patterns could have been repeated in the case of the so-called social explosion, which in turn represents a movement that brought together a large part of the demands raised in previous years.

3 Methodology

The work performs a double analysis on a common corpus of data extracted from the Twitter platform. For this purpose, hashtags that were trending topics and messages published during the period of interest were used. First, it performs a topic modeling (TP) and then a sentimental analysis (SA). The aim of the work was to understand the coherence and evolution of the emotions expressed on twitter with respect to the social outburst.

3.1 Techniques of Analyses

The first step was to have a list of the hashtags that marked trending topic week by week, for this we used the trendinalia website (http://www.trendinalia.com/). Then R software was used to download the tweets, process and visualize the results. R was connected through the twitter API using the R library "twitteR" [29], downloading some hashtags that were trending topic in the study period.

A data preprocessing was performed, which eliminated parts of the texts that do not contribute anything for the subsequent analysis, such as: URL, numbers, stopwords, punctuation marks, line breaks, emoticons, abbreviations, etc.

Then, two Natural Language Processing techniques were used: sentiment analysis and topic modeling. The first one consists in detecting through computational techniques the sentiments present in a text. The second consists of counting words and seeing which ones concur with which ones in the text, then the researcher decides which topics are encompassed by these words, which are usually nouns or adjectives. The mathematical process behind topic modeling is quite complex, but its connection with linguistics is well studied.

As for sentiment analysis, the present work is based on dictionaries. It contains a set of words with a predetermined emotional category: joy, fear, sadness, anger, disgust, surprise, anticipation and confidence, which are based on Plutchik's wheel of emotions [30] which identifies eight basic emotions in humans. The Syuzhet [31] package was used and from it the NCR dictionary that allows to perform analysis in Spanish, identifying the eight aforementioned feelings, in addition to having a classification of the words in polarities: positive and negative. The algorithm used by this package performed an association of the preprocessed tweets with the sentiment dictionary. If a word from the preprocessed tweets is contained in the dictionary, it is rated with "1" in the emotion to which it belongs and the polarity to which it corresponds. As an illustration of the tweet: "recuperemos la dignidad del pueblo" ("let's recover the dignity of the people"), you get:

Table 1. Example of sentiment analysis results for Tweets in R

Angar	Anticipation	Disgust	Fear	Joy	Sadness	Surprise	Trust	Negative	Positive
0	0	0	0	0	0	0	1	0	1

Regarding topic modeling, in this work we used the "topicmo-dels" package [32], which contains a machine learning algorithm known as Latent Dirichlet Allocation. In general, topic modelling consists of identifying themes (topics) in a text. This is achieved by detecting patterns within a collection of documents and grouping words in the document into topics by studying the probability of their concurrence in the text. Specifically, LDA assumes that each word in a document is generated from a topic that is taken from a distribution of topics for each document. The actual distribution of topics for each document is generated from a Dirichlet distribution which means that LDA allows a document to be part of several topics each with a different weight [33].

3.2 Sample, Textual Corpus

The analysis corpus has been constructed from downloading data from Twitter during a bounded period of time. This period starts on October 18, 2019 and the download started on October 21, 2019 and was extended until December 8, 2019. The data downloads were made week by week, during the last download day, since the Twitter App allows highlighting up to 7 days back. Details of the dates and number of messages downloaded are given in Table 2.

Table 2. Corpus of analysis

Week	Dates	Number of messages
Week 1	21-10-19/27-10-19	231.766
Week 2	28-10-19/03-11-19	322.222
Week 3	04-11-19/10-11-19	63.138
Week 4	11-11-19/17-11-19	314.791
Week 5	18-11-19/24-11-19	141.865
Week 6	25-11-19/01-12-19	220.074
Week 7	02-12-19/08-12-19	150.488
Total		1.444.344

4 Results

First, the "topicmodels" observed on Twitter during the seven weeks of the study in the context of the social revolt in Chile are presented, before addressing the sentiment analysis. Finally, a rather theoretical discussion of these results will be made.

4.1 Topic Modeling Analysis

The results of the topical analysis are presented in Table 1. They are ordered by week in the first column. The second column shows the three most significant topics out of a pool of six total topics computed. The four most significant terms of the topic were selected from a total of ten. The third column provides information on the type of orientation expressed by the topic in relation to the social movement (For, Against and Neutral) (Table 3).

The general reading of the table is that of an evolution of emotions and support for the movement. Out of a total of 21 topics studied, 13 topics expressed clear support, 6 topics against and 2 did not show a majority either for or against the movement.

In summary, there was a majority in favor of the movement, especially during the first six weeks. However, in the third and fifth weeks, topics showing dissatisfaction with the movement began to appear clearly, while in the seventh week this attitude became the majority.

Continuity between topics (1) and a certain recursiveness are also observed. For example, in reaction to the statements of the President of the Chilean Republic, Sebastián Piñera, who on the night of Saturday, October 19, 2019 spoke of a war against an internal enemy, it is noted that the topic "we are not at war" counts within the four most significant terms in the first week and "Chile is not at war" comes in second place the second week. A similar phenomenon happens with the topic "Chile Despertó", which became one of the slogans that identifies the event, and stood out during the first two weeks on Twitter. During weeks 3 and 4, this continuity shifted towards the condemnation of a dictatorial situation ("Piñera Dictator", "Chile in Dictatorship"). Finally, references to the Constituent Assembly appear, first as a claim in weeks 2 and 5, and then as opposition in week 3. In these ups and downs, they clearly reflect the polemic judgment about the future of the country and the ways out of the crisis. The support for a "new constitution for Chile" emerges precisely as a theme during the week of the Agreement on Peace and the New Constitution (November 15, 2019).

The interpretation of the topics supports the idea of an evolution of the attitude on Twitter towards the movement. The majority support at the beginning gave way to discourses that deepened the fear in front of the demonstrations in its multiple facets. Images from the past are appealed to, which become clear threats in the seventh week. These speeches are coherent with the story that has been constructed of this episode, where there were rumors of a coup d'état and a regression towards an authoritarian regime.

4.2 Sentiment Analysis

Before the analysis we must emphasize that the appearance of a feeling is given by the presence of a word that evokes such a feeling. For example, the word "happy" evokes the feeling joy.

During the period studied, two very differentiated groups of feelings are statistically observed. The first contains joy, anticipation, rejection and surprise, which are always under 12%. In the second group we find the feelings of confidence, anger, fear and sadness, which generally appear in more than 12% (Fig. 1).

The sentiment with the highest presence in tweets during the first four weeks was "fear". However, during the first week, the feeling of confidence is equivalent to "fear". During week 5, the predominant feeling was "confidence" and during week 6 "sadness", returning in week 7 to "fear".

Table 3. Topics Supporting/Against Chile's social outbreak movement.

Week	Topics/Concepts	Supporting/Against/Neutral topics
Week 1	(1) Luchamos/desobedienciacivil/prendió/chileprotesta (2) Chiledesperto/toquedequeda/noestamosenguerra/Estopasaenchile (3) chileviolatehumanrights/sitio/pineraviolalosddhh/vota	Supporting Supporting Supporting
Week 2	(1) chilenoestáenguerra/emoción/dispararon/preocupado (2) nomasmarchas/chiledesperto/pazparachile/loquelatelenomuestra (3) decente/chilesinmiedo/asambleaconstiyente/democrático	Supporting Neutral Supporting
Week 3	(1) Carabineras/Pinochet/chileencrisis/terrorista (2) Noalaasambleaconstituyente/fueracomunistas/constitución/quieren (3) ffaa/tontos/aprobación/piñeradictador	Against Against Supporting
Week 4	(1) matapacos/maldito/facultades/infraestructura (2) chileendictadura/nomastag/chalecosamarillos/prensaprostituta (3) fraude/ddhh/principios/violentas	Supporting Supporting Supporting
Week 5	(1) lamarchamasgrandedechile/libres/soñé/independientes (2) catrillanca/nuevaconstitucionparachile/Picoenelojo/laluchasigue (3) policiales/evidencias/pazparachile/suficiente	Supporting Supporting Against
Week 6	(1) incapaz/mayoría/violador/noparamosavanzamos (2) marchasincapucha/marchadenoviembre/yoparoelnsinmiedo/ paronacional (3) pacíficos/respeto/concentración/provocar	Supporting Supporting Neutral
Week 7	(1) militaresalacalle/pronunciamentomilitarya/ffaaporchile/pinochetazo (2) rngobiernoderotos/manofirmepresidente/notenemospresidente/ pronunciamientomilitaryapronunciamientomilitaryapronunciamientomilitaryacondiciones (3) pazparachile/vagos/instituciones/lumpen	Against Against Against

Source: By authors based on Twitter data

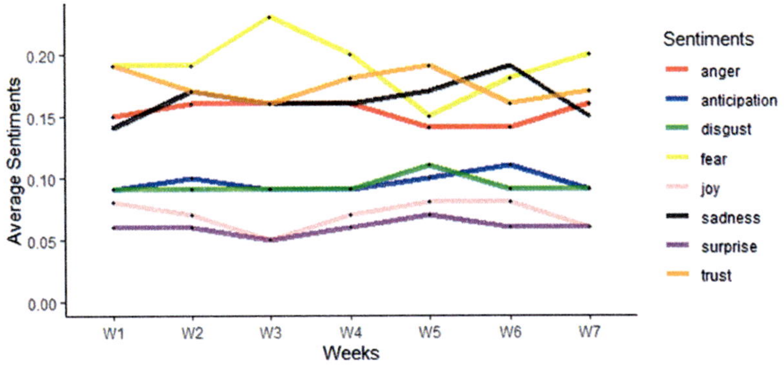

Fig. 1. Variation of sentiments in Twitter during Chile's social outbreak week to week. Source: By authors based on Twitter data.

During the first week a 50 - 50 ratio is observed in terms (words) implying positive and negative polarity. In the following weeks the curves separate, with the appearance of terms implying more negative polarity (Fig. 2).

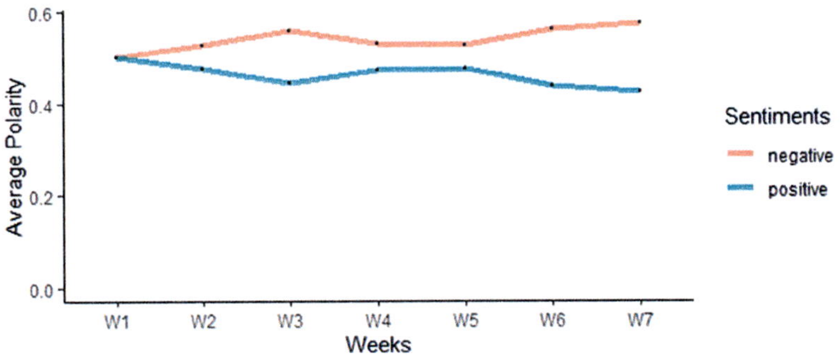

Fig. 2. Variation of polarity in Twitter during Chile's social outbreak. Source: By authors based on Twitter data.

The negative polarity of emotions coincides with the existence of tweets with a more negative connotation. This does not mean that the negativity is necessarily related to the mobilizations, as it only highlights the existence of messages with a more negative charge in their writing, either reflecting opposition to the government and the commodification of social rights or against the protesters. What is interesting is that this figure shows how, as a result of the social outburst, a certain form of polarization has become more acute on Twitter, which translates both in the topics and in the emotions that these entail.

4.3 Discussion

The evidence presented here endorses at least two types of issues that are collected in the specialized literature on emotions and social mobilization. In a context of great uncertainty about the destiny of a society, emotions at least have the possibility of expressing themselves in tune with these desires. In this way, they act in accordance with the offline reality, as discussed and presented in articles dealing with similar case studies. Uncertainty plays a central role in this case, given the weight that the presence of a recent past linked to the authoritarian legacy has for the Chilean case. The threat of a return to this situation contributed to accentuate fear, which as we have seen is one of the emotions most present in the messages analyzed. In this sense, topics and emotions indicate that the projection of change and collective action still seem to be framed, in Chile, by the risk of the past (the coup d'état and the civil-military dictatorship).

It is also possible to observe with relative clarity the presence of positive emotions and optimism. Taking this fact into consideration, which seems not to be sufficiently emphasized in the literature, helps to qualify the feelings of anger, instability, uncertainty and indifference with which the emotion of the protests is characterized. This fact seems to be an element that differentiates the expression of emotions in Chilean October and should make us think about the joyful and festive dimensions present in collective action. The opening of a future made of changes seems to be expressed in this positive emotionality. However, it is important to qualify this observation given that it is declared in the temporal regime of the immediacy of Twitter and the RRSS, without necessarily articulating a future project or contributing to temporal resynchronizations but rather to the "tyranny of presentist urgency", as historian Francois Hartog would say.

Ultimately, the evidence presented here reinforces the assumption that the emotions expressed on Twitter contribute to escalate and de-escalate social conflicts. Given the massive number of users that the platform reaches and its strong repercussion in terms of public opinion, it is possible to observe how the evolution of emotionality is synchronous with the events that take place during the mobilization period. In this sense, it is a coordination of online and offline activity, which reinforces and qualifies the unanimous character that the movement achieves during the successive weeks of the conflict studied.

5 Conclusions

The article set out to study the emotions expressed on Twitter during the social and political outburst in Chile. In this way, it was possible to verify a coherent itinerary of emotions expressed with varying intensity during the seven weeks covered by the study.

We must emphasize that the evidence gathered in this study endorses the results and conclusions reached by several specialized works on the subject. Perhaps the only particularity observed from the evidence gathered is the significant presence of positive emotions and optimism in the messages analyzed, most of the time related to the possibility of a constituent assembly and a festive celebration of the progress of the movement itself.

Within the limitations, we believe that a central issue to discern is the precise coding of the topics. In this regard, we should point out that the three categories used were not always adapted to the information collected. Establishing the link between the published message and its emotionality towards the movement may have underestimated other significant intentions (for example, rejection and/or support for the movement). However, distinguishing between these intentionalities and the attitude of support/rejection of the movement represents a difficult task, which probably requires another type of more sophisticated interpretation and coding.

Finally, the article concludes that the question of emotions constitutes a very fertile field of study to connect public opinion and activists. The evidence collected here shows a very fine connection between what is posted on Twitter and the ways in which this movement evolves. In this way, it will be possible to extend this type of exercise to other case studies, platforms (Instagram) and other types of publications (images), to understand more fully how much emotions collaborate in the public communication of protest.

References

1. Thompson, E.P.: The moral economy of the English crowd in the eighteenth century. Past Present **5**, 76–136 (1971). https://doi.org/10.1093/past/50.1.76
2. Faure, A., Maillet, A. : Chile Despertó. Mobilisations sociales et politisation au Chili. Revue IdeAs 15 (2020) https://journals.openedition.org/ideas/8364.
3. Faure, A.: ¿Se politizó el tiempo? Ensayo sobre las batallas cronopolíticas del octubre chileno. Universum **35**(1), 46–73 (2020). https://scielo.conicyt.cl/pdf/universum/v35n1/0718-2376-universum-35-01-46.pdf
4. Sehnbruch, K., Donoso, S.: Social protests in Chile: inequalities and other inconvenient truths about Latin America's poster child. Glob. Labour J. **11**(1), 52–58 (2020). https://doi.org/10.15173/glj.v11i1.4217
5. Somma, N., Bargsted, M., Disi, R., Medel, R.: No water in the oasis: the Chilean spring of 2019–2020. Soc. Move. Stud. (2020). https://doi.org/10.1080/14742837.2020.1727737
6. Stange, H., et al.: Miedos, abusos y desórdenes en el oasis chileno. Santiago de Chile, p. 68 (2019). www.icei.uchile.cl/dam/jcr:eeff3ee3-d6b4-4258-87fd-b03d6b968a14/RABIA.pdf
7. Activa Research, Pulso Ciudadano: Crisis en Chile, 24 de octubre de 2019. In: Stange, H., et al. (eds.) Miedos, abusos y desórdenes en el oasis chileno. Santiago de Chile, p. 126 (2019). www.icei.uchile.cl/dam/jcr:eeff3ee3-d6b4-4258-87fd-b03d6b968a14/RABIA.pdf
8. USACH, ACCH: Legitimidad, Miedo y Esperanza en el Chile post estallido. Encuesta Nacional 2019 (2019)
9. Mac-Clure, O., Barrozet, E., Conejeros, J., Jordana, C.: Escuchando a los chilenos en medio del estallido: liberación emocional, reflexividad y el regreso de la palabra "pueblo". CIPER Chile (2020). https://www.ciperchile.cl/2020/03/02/escuchando-a-los-chilenos-en-medio-del-estallido-liberacion-emocional-reflexividad-y-el-regreso-de-la-palabra-pueblo/
10. Jasper, J.M.: Emotions and social movements: twenty years of theory and research. Ann. Rev. Sociol. **37**, 285–303 (2011)
11. Milan, S.: From social movements to cloud protesting: the evolution of collective identity. Inf. Commun. Soc. **18**(8), 887–900 (2015)
12. Woods, M., Anderson, J., Guilbert, S., Watkin, S.: 'The country (side) is angry': emotion and explanation in protest mobilization. Soc. Cult. Geogr. **13**(6), 567–585 (2012)
13. Bennett, W.L., Segerberg, A.: The logic of connective action: digital media and the personalization of contentious politics. Inf. Commun. Soc. **15**(5), 739–768 (2012)
14. Duncombe, C.: The politics of Twitter: emotions and the power of social media. Int. Polit. Sociol. **13**(4), 409–429 (2019)
15. LeFebvre, R.K., Armstrong, C.: Grievance-based social movement mobilization in the #Ferguson Twitter storm. New Media Soc. **20**(1), 8–28 (2018)
16. Freelon, D., McIlwain, C.D., Clark, M.D.: Beyond the hashtags. Center For Media & Social Impact, Washington, D.C. (2016)

17. Gerbaudo, P.: Tweets and the Streets: Social Media and Contemporary Activism. Pluto Press (2012)
18. Youmans, W.L., York, J.C.: Social media and the activist toolkit: user agreements, corporate interests, and the information infrastructure of modern social movements. J. Commun. **62**(2), 315–329 (2012)
19. Theocharis, Y., Lowe, J.W., Van Deth, W., García-Albacete, G.: Using Twitter to mobilize protest action: online mobilization patterns and action repertoires in the occupy Wall Street Indignados, and Aganaktismenoi movements. Inform. Commun. Soc. **18**(2), 202–220 (2015). https://doi.org/10.1080/1369118X.2014.948035
20. Cammaerts, B.: Social media and activism. In: Mansell, R., Hwa, P. (eds.) The International Encyclopedia of Digital Communication and Society, pp. 1027–1034. Wiley-Blackwell, Oxford (2015)
21. González-Bustamante, B.: Evaluando Twitter como indicador de opinión pública: una mirada al arribo de Bachelet a la presidencial chilena 2013. Rev. SAAP. Publ. Ciencia Polít. Soc. Argentina Análisis Polít. **9**(1), 119–141 (2015)
22. Millaleo, S., Velasco, P.: Activismo digital en Chile. Repertorios de contención e iniciativas ciudadanas. Fundación democracia y desarrollo, Santiago de Chile (2013)
23. Valenzuela, S., Arriagada, A., Scherman, A.: The social media basis of youth protest behavior: the case of Chile. J. Commun. **2**(62), 299–314 (2012). https://doi.org/10.1111/j.1460-2466.2012.01635.x
24. Valenzuela, S., Correa, T., de Zuniga, H.G.: Ties, likes, and tweets: using strong and weak ties to explain differences in protest participation across Facebook and Twitter use. Polit. Commun. **35**(1), 117–134 (2018)
25. Valenzuela, S., Arriagada, A., Scherman, A.: Facebook, Twitter, and youth engagement: a quasi-experimental study of social media use and protest behavior using propensity score matching. Int. J. Commun. **8**(25) (2014). https://ijoc.org/index.php/ijoc/article/view/2022
26. Sola-Morales, S.: Las redes sociales y los nuevos movimientos estudiantiles latinoamericanos. La "Primavera Chilena" y el "Yosoy132". IC Rev. Científica Inform. Comun. (13), 153–193 (2016)
27. Mascareño, A., Henríquez, P.A., Billi, M., Ruz, G.A.: A Twitter-lived red tide crisis on Chiloé Island, Chile: what can be obtained for social-ecological research through social media analysis? Sustainability **12**(20), 8506 (2020)
28. Broitman, C., Jara, R.: Surviving the legacy media system: the place of local digital activism in the Chiloé Red tide crisis. In: Díaz-Pont, J., Maeseele, P., Egan Sjolander, A., Mishra, M., Foxwell-Norton, K. (eds.) The Local and the Digital in Environmental Communication. Palgrave-MacMillan, Londres, Reino Unido (2020)
29. Gentry, J., Gentry, M.J., RSQLite, S., Artistic, R.L.: Package 'twitteR'. Cran. r-project (2016)
30. Jockers, M.L., Thalken, R.: Text Analysis with R. Springer, Heidelberg (2020). https://doi.org/10.1007/978-3-030-39643-5
31. Da Silva, N.F.F., Hruschka, E.R., Hruschka, E.R.: Tweet sentiment analysis with classifier ensembles. Decis. Support Syst. **66**, 170–179 (2014)
32. Wöllmer, M., et al.: Youtube movie reviews: sentiment analysis in an audio-visual context. IEEE Intell. Syst. **28**(3), 46–53 (2013)
33. Liu, B.: Sentiment analysis and opinion mining. Synthesis Lect. Hum. Lang. Technol. **5**(1), 1–167 (2012)

Use of Technological Means and Personal Data in Electoral Activities: Persuasive Voters

Rosa María Ricoy-Casas(✉)

Faculty of Communication and Social Sciences, University of Vigo, Vigo, Spain
rricoy@uvigo.es

Abstract. Citizens today are the perfect target for an unscrupulous, post-truth and fake-news-infected political campaign which can help win an election. Likewise, voter profiling based on the illicit processing of personal data is a key and unavoidable issue at the moment of technological development in which we find ourselves, which can undermine crucial aspects of a democracy. This article aims to analyze the use of personal data in electoral activities in the world, making multiple references to specific cases at the global and European level, and reflect on the current technological means that help to modify, force or divert the will of the voters without them being aware of it, with a severe impact on the fundamental rights of citizens.

Keywords: Communication · Personal data · Political parties · Electoral activities · Political opinions · Ideology · Fundamental rights

1 Introduction

Some of the characteristics of the scientific name that Linnaeus assigned us in 1758 as Homo sapiens (wise man; rational animal; with capacity for abstract reasoning, introspection and speculation), are in decline. Each day we think less, all decisions are influenced (by our cultural and economic level, our aspirations, our environment, our gender, our age, and so on) and we have become "piratable animals". If in past decades the Ku Klux Klan, Nazism or apartheid were able to succeed en masse, now technology (neuromarketing, microtargeting, algorithms) is used to discover our tastes, desires, things that we reject, and then persuade, convince, bend our behavior to the letter. The very creator of the WWW has confirmed how the internet has drifted towards becoming a gigantic and powerful mechanism to spy on and monitor everything we do [1].

This is done with such precision that it is possible that the ancient Greek aphorism "know yourself" is in their power, moving from traditional marketing to digital "marketing 4.0" [2]. Companies begin to predict what the consumer wants before they ask for it, and that is why they conduct online and offline research. If big data involves the collection and use of large amounts of data, smart data focuses on the intelligent use of the data necessary for a purpose, this is what Smart TVs do, which can make proposals to our liking based on our previous viewings (automated processing and profiling). In 1932, Aldous Huxley wrote Brave New World, a dystopia about a society subjected

© The Author(s), under exclusive license to Springer Nature Singapore Pte Ltd. 2022
Á. Rocha et al. (Eds.): ICOMTA 2021, SIST 259, pp. 227–237, 2022.
https://doi.org/10.1007/978-981-16-5792-4_23

by science to full satisfaction, written precisely at a time when totalitarian states were struggling to dominate a part of the world [3]. Therefore, we have "hackable brains that vote" when they manage to hack us, they can not only predict our decisions, but also manipulate our feelings. (…) An algorithm can tell if someone is already predisposed against immigrants, and if their neighbor already detests Trump, in such a way that the first sees one headline and the second, on the other hand, another completely different one (…) the best method is pushing the buttons of fear, hatred or greed that we carry within. And that method has now begun to be used to sell us politics and ideologies [4].

2 Use of Technological Means and Personal Data in Electoral Activities: Persuadable Voters

We have become the perfect target for an unscrupulous political campaign. They could sell us anything, a product, a politician or a way of thinking. Lies and intoxication are as old as politics itself [5, 6], but what has changed is the scope, how it is distributed and how it has expanded. For example, by using hoax websites, millions of automated social media profiles, and a legion of bots, they are able to turn a lie into a shared trend millions of times. Social media bots became the source of 20% of messages about Hillary Clinton and Donald Trump in the 2016 US election campaign [7]. The traditional media have lost their monopoly on the history of reality, and those citizens who lack a minimum critical spirit now swallow, without questioning, everything that enters through social networks and cultural exposure.

And the propagation and dissemination of this type of information is aided and abetted, among others, by the so-called confirmation bias (tendency to favor, search, interpret, and remember, the information that confirms one's beliefs or hypotheses). Likewise, by those called by Eli Pariser [8, 9] as echo chambers (we spend time with our peers and the information, ideas or beliefs in this environment are amplified by transmission and repetition in a "closed" system, where different visions are represented in a minority, and even censored), and "bubble filters" (they are the result of a personalized search in which the algorithm of a web page selects, through predictions, the information that the user would like to see, based on information about himself –Based on elements such as your location, your search history, the elements you "clicked" on in the past, the "likes" or "I like" you have expressed, etc.). One fine day you wake up to find that everyone thinks like you. In the words of Gordon Allport and Leo Postman [10], "every rumor has its audience" (people often hear what they expect to see or hear, based on past experience). Eduard Punset [11], has stated that even when the brain perceives an explanation different from what it believes, it not only questions it, it cuts off the communication circuits so that it does not penetrate. What is termed cognitive dissonance is why we do not usually change our vote. That is, our brain blocks rational information that could make us change our mind, since we prefer emotional or moral convictions to rational or epistemological confirmations. It is worth reflecting as Sunstein does [12]; we only see what we want to see, we hear what we want to hear, and we read what we want to read. Is that good for democracy?

A team of researchers conducted a math test on more than 1,100 adults, noting that participants whose political beliefs aligned with a correct interpretation of the data were much more likely to solve the problem well, yet even the best mathematicians were 49% more likely to be wrong on the second question when the correct answer challenged their political beliefs. The problem was partisanship, political identity (identity that can also be associated with issues such as religion, nationalism, democracy, etc.). And this, to the point of justifying certain negative behaviors to defend them, which has been called "cognitive dissonance". People are often more interested in maintaining a positive relationship with their group than in perceiving the world accurately. Especially dangerous is behavior in politics. Researchers have observed that this polarization has grown in recent years, probably due to the effect of bubbles in social networks that act as echo chambers [13].

The business model of social networks particularly benefits from content that generates more interaction between users [14]. The problem is also found in the relationship between the dissemination of news and advertising, especially in those companies that do not make efforts towards brand safety, or those whose benefit for advertising attached to viral news (knowing wide dissemination will reach more recipients), without fact-checking, due to its great economic return, which compensates for the money lost to sanctions or brand damage, especially those web pages that centralize a target of interest to the company [15, 16], explain the appearance of some of these threats to their reputation in the transition from the traditional model through the one-way communication of organizations with their stakeholders, to the possibility that it has provided to stakeholders through digital social media.

In certain cases, the company contracting advertising loses control, since the provider places its advertisements in order to reach the agreed targets (regardless of the channel), and when buying by audience, rotation by sites or channels becomes more frequent, rather than by fixed locations which would be more easily controllable (programmed purchase). These are dangers that various institutions in the sector have already warned about [17–19]. All aimed at profit, even at the expense of reputation. The so-called fake news is not only fake, but also ways of presenting content (misleading information; inaccurate information; plagiarism taken from its original context; manipulated controversial content, etc.). In the words of Kostolany [20], fake news is dangerous, but false news exposure is even more dangerous. Likewise, the influence of audiovisual logic in contemporary political communication is undeniable, in which the phenomenon of the "emotivization of politics" is perfectly appreciated [21]. And so it has been since the first televised debate between Nixon and Kennedy, that political candidates also take into account their image, even reaching an agreement on essential elements of it, which greatly distort their objective [22]. Platforms such as Instagram, Twitter or YouTube have contributed to the development of a more human and close-up profile of the candidates as part of their electoral campaign. For this, marketing strategies (neuromarketing) are used, after analyzing the voter's brain (neuropolitics) [23–26]. With this knowledge, political parties offer what the citizen really wants, what catches his or her attention, what is capable of arousing emotion, with good results.

The Story-telling itself (a resource that seeks to capture attention through the telling of a story, tale, case, anecdote in an attempt to appeal to feelings; connect with audiences through emotions) is used in politics [27, 28]. Hopeful proposals that seem plausible, although not necessarily feasible (Lula da Silva –Brazil- "zero hunger"); build a unique identity ("Chavism", "Kirchnerism"); use easy-to-remember phrases and expressions that are repeated in the mind as an advertising slogan in the style of "I have a dream" (Yes we can, America first) - key messages for prime time, as the time that is worth gold on television is called; stories to tell or explain a political message (such as how Rajoy spoke of Pedro Sánchez's girl Valeria), photographs, videos strategically exhibited showing personal activities or their partners (Obama's family, Macron); presenting himself as a hero, leader, with strength (Putin, Macron); or advertising himself as an outsider –in the midst of the crisis of the democracy of the political parties-, a person who has nothing to do with politics, who is anti-establishment and/or "who does not need or does not want politics to get rich" (Trump, Mújica, Macri).

All over the world, political candidates participate in light-hearted shows, humor, gossip magazines, etc., probably also copied from the American style (Oprah, The Late Show with David Letterman, The Daily Show, The Arsenio Hall Show, Larry King Live!, or even in Russia the "Direct line with Putin", etc.). It is what Christian Salmon [27]. called the "Sheherazade strategy", after the princess of the tales of "the One Thousand and One Nights", who seeks to entertain the king with a story each night to stall him having her killed. This dramatization of politics, similar to what some authors have called infotainment [29, 30], politainment [31], or more recently "pop politics" [32], which, in turn, is the result of two phenomena: transnationality that has reduced the decision-making power of the nation-state to a minimum and the hyper-mediatization of society that assumes that political leaders no longer hold a monopoly on story and symbols [33]. Thus, according to Salmon, statecraft becomes "stagecraft" [34]. A rereading of "Foucaltian biopower": from Putins naked torso to Sarkozy's heeled shoes [33].

We are therefore facing an audience that sometimes seeks entertainment over pure information, also in politics. On many occasions, political advertising is even replaced with parodies, with the aim of questioning the original ideas -counter-advertising- (subvertising). Citizens even become authentic "media prosumers" in political communication [35]; they consume information, and produce content through wikis, blogs, social networks such as Facebook, Twitter, Flickr or YouTube [36–38], they become speakers. Any activity in the offline world can have transcendence in the online world, forming a "space of autonomy" [39] through "mass self-communication" [40], to mix "old information" with "new information", in the process referred to by some authors as "transmediation" [41]. It is the so-called "theatercracy" or the so-called "audience democracy" of Manin [42]. Perhaps all this has something to do with the loss of cognitive patience due to the acceleration of digital culture [43]. We process a lot of information in a short time, but partially and without reflection. Also with the so-called "infoxication" (more information than humanly possible to process), generating anxiety and other symptoms that characterize the information fatigue syndrome. As Ray Bradbury well put it in 1953 in Fahrenheit 451: Cram them full of noncombustible data, chock them so damned full of 'facts' they feel stuffed, but absolutely 'brilliant' with information. Then they'll feel they're thinking, they'll get a sense of motion without moving. And they'll be happy, because facts of that sort don't change. Don't give them any slippery stuff like philosophy or sociology to tie things up with. That way lies melancholy [44]. One more effect of the hyperconnected world.

We are "piratable animals" susceptible to piracy, we are "the product" to which are applied neuromarketing, microtargeting, algorithms, used in all the information we produce, for example through mobile phones (with the location, the places we frequent), the computer (the pages we consult), the television (what we see, from which it is possible to easily deduce ideology, cultural level), what we consume with the supermarket card (tastes, habits can be inferred), the credit card (economic level), the smartwatch (health status) and a long etcetera. Let's not forget that almost all of our "life" is concentrated in these 6 devices, soon some more such as home automation or connected appliances. We live in glass houses. What's more, according to a study by researchers from the Psychometrics Center from the University of Cambridge (United Kingdom) and the Department of Computer Science at Stanford University (United States), the behavior of Facebook allows a computer to make a more precise psychological profile of its users than their friends and even close family. If it had 300 likes at its disposal, the computer would have no rival. Even with this reliability, certain behaviors such as drug use, tendency toward depression, or political orientation could be predicted [45, 46]. The extractive and predictive capacity of these digital devices, social networks, and other technological colossi is such that even the acronym FANG, which is how the stock market refers to Facebook, Amazon, Netflix and Google, is premonitory. Let us remember, for example, that on December 4, 2009, Google extended the personalization of its search results to all users, something that until then only applied to queries made from a profile connected to a Gmail account.

A social network can also infer sexual orientation, and not only of its users, but also of friends who are not connected to the network [47]. And to give another example, among the many ways that these large platforms are obtaining data, contacts on Twitter can predict one's location [48]. That is why privacy is no longer an individual decision. If we believe that by not expressing our political or sexual orientation, or by not participating in social networks, we preserve our privacy, we are wrong. They are called shadow profiles (or ghost profiles). This is not by magic, although we could call it an illusion worthy of magicians, thanks to the fact that humans tend to connect with those who are similar to themselves (like attracts like) and, therefore, the predilection of users in the networks to connect with you want to share some characteristic (assortativity). Thus, they can know us even by the friends we have; "Tell me who your friends are and I'll tell you who you are". It should be added that computers have a couple of advantages over humans when it comes to analyzing a person's personality: machines can maintain and retrieve large amounts of information. And furthermore, all this data can be analysed with algorithms. This makes them less vulnerable to failure, forgetfulness, and the often irrational thinking of the human mind.

Some authors also speak of "electoral segmentation". There is reliable data on the lifestyle and consumption habits of Democrats and Republicans that allow campaign teams to influence or place advertising on certain products or media, as well as to go and find their voters where they are. One example was in 2008, when Obama's commercials appeared frequently in "Two and a Half Men", a series that Democrats like in polls. Thanks to these polls, campaign teams can also know that 46% of Republicans have a dog, compared to only 30% of Democrats; or that Democrats prefer to watch MTV or play video games while Republicans watch shows and series like 'Dancing with the stars',

'The Office' and 'The Mentalist'; or that most Republicans prefer American football or NASCAR while Democrats prefer to watch the NBA [49]. The "spin doctors", the advisers to political leaders, use this information to deliver their message with surgical precision.

They also use facial recognition programs for candidates in the electoral campaign (also already used in the human resources section of many companies), and applications such as Political Audience (from EmotionResearchLab.com), which allows for discovery of the emotional impact caused by videos or electoral posters, as well as any audiovisual content generated on social networks in a given population sample, in order to predict the success of a given campaign. Even the Neuropsychology software used in focus groups, to jointly analyze the statistics that result from the answer to the traditional questionnaire by the sample. With this, a comparative analysis is achieved between these data and the psychological records that allow the campaign to be directed towards the issues that generate the most positive emotions in the electorate, avoid those most problematic issues, and even select the most appropriate words, attitudes or behaviors to target so that the candidacy is convincing.

Obviously this is very easy when data provided freely by citizens through social networks is analyzed, more effective than the mainstream media, and even through geofencing (this allows data to be collected on smartphone users when they enter a certain geographical location) allowing campaigns to identify political leanings based on online and offline preferences (where you live, work, shop, play, etc.); and to segment ads based on inferred psychographic traits. A pro-Trump rally, for example, could be used to obtain information on hundreds of potential voters at the same time. Information from users enabled with this technology could be sent about events from nearby campaigns. Likewise, a smartphone-user visiting a rally, or a gun club, for example, is a good candidate for a political ad aimed at getting them to vote for Trump during the 2020 elections. Some authors have investigated psychological orientation such as an effective approach to mass digital persuasion [50]. This illustrates the feasibility and effectiveness of mass persuasion techniques implemented by companies like London-based Cambridge Analytica (CA), and exposes the risks inherent in this behavioral targeting, the main source of revenue for many tech giants.

In 2012, Facebook patented a technology for psychological profiling, which was later used by CA [51] (this is based on 5 pillars of personality and nicknamed the OCEAN model). Some authors responded with studies that showed the accuracy of such predictions, reflecting on their implications on the privacy of citizens [45], with repercussions in various press outlets such as The Financial Times [52, 53], which initially appeared to trigger a tightening of privacy policies on Facebook and other online platforms [54]. Thus, with all our digital fingerprint (the information we provide in various formats), and psychological profiling, they can publish dozens of advertisements aimed at certain specific personality types, adapted to people's fears, needs, tastes, emotions, etc., all in order to win an election. Obviously, we cannot analyze in retrospect (even in elections where we know that this methodology has been used), who voted, in what way, due to which announcements, since there are multiple variables. Another problem is if the virtual identity or psychological profile created is not correct (as we cannot know what data exists about us, the profile could be wildly inaccurate). Perhaps many details of the system remain to be discovered, but it is clear that its use will not go backwards even as it is further refined, despite the apparent efforts, and new regulations such as those approved in the EU.

Perhaps some governments may be involved, just remember the statements of Julian Assange (WikiLeaks), or some of the most devastating revelations Snowden's, such as the existence of the surveillance method known as PRISM, which he describes as a tool used "to collect data routinely from Microsoft, Yahoo!, Google, Facebook, Paltalk, YouTube, Skype, AOL, and Apple, including email, photos, video and audio chats, Internet browsing content, search engine queries, and all other data stored in their clouds. The scandals raised by Assange and Snowden are the premonition of totalitarian dystopias in which digital technologies have become instruments of control and not tools of emancipation [55]. In March 2018, the British television network Channel 4, released a series of videos showing the executive director of Cambridge Analytica, Alexander Nix, along with other company executives talking about the dirty tricks used in electoral campaigns. In these conversations, the executives say they have worked in approximately 200 elections around the world, including those in Nigeria, Kenya, the Czech Republic, India and Argentina [56]. Today it is also known that this has happened in many other places in relation to electoral processes or referendums such as Mexico in favor of the PRI - against the current President López Obrador [57], in the United States in favor of Donald Trump in 2016 [58], in the UK in favor of Brexit in 2016 [59], and in Kenya, to achieve the victory of the incumbent president, Uhuru Kenyatta, of the Jubilee party, in the national elections held in early 2017. His victory was later annulled by the Supreme Court [60–63]. That is why technologies that can even manipulate video in real time (audio can be manipulated more easily), without the need for high-end computers are disturbing; it is enough to have a YouTube news clip and a standard webcam on a laptop [64]. As this technology develops and proliferates at such low cost, almost anyone could make a compelling enough fake video, for example for political or partisan reasons.

Now exposed remains the great challenge of distinguishing legitimately expressed opinions from fake news (some of them generated by trolls, robots, applications), and some examples of political polarization. Certain programs such as PolitEcho.org (a Google Chrome extension), examine which pages, news, queries, your friends liked. With this information, the program allows us to know the political inclination or interests of our Facebook friends in a graph, and even give us a vision contrary to ours if we ask, which could also position us ideologically. The program allows profiling of third parties without their consent, even though we do not know the reliability and depth of this system, a mechanism that was used in the campaign between Hilary and Trump for the presidency of the United States. The candidates already know these technological means, and we can see it in that, for example, Trump has more than 3,000 websites (domain names or digital addresses) that he acquired before and after becoming President. The way Trump bought domains also shows how he methodically planned his political rise [65, 66].

As we have pointed out through some examples, the design of electoral campaigns with technological means and smart data are the present-day reality of political communication. With this and other information in the same vein from multiple world economic and technological powers, we are moving towards a de-globalizing political panorama, which focuses on national sovereignty, or regional in the case of the European Union, and which carries the great risk of destroying trust in the technology supply chain and a global internet system [67]. 2020 will mark the 75th anniversary of the enforcement of the United Nations Charter, signed in San Francisco in 1945. An anniversary that, however, coincides with a key moment in developments such as AI, 5G, that will undoubtedly create new spheres of influence and geostrategy, questioning current multilateralism.

3 Other Conclusions

The "appropriation" of citizens' data (even the most sensitive) has been increasing, also in the European Union. It is worrying how easy it is now to collect and process it on a large scale, with a single click, and the use of procedures aimed at modifying, forcing or diverting the will of the voters without them being aware of it. The public powers must promote the conditions so that freedom and equality are real and effective, and fundamental rights are protected, but precisely they are both the judge and the interested party, with scant discussions on the subject in the debates of national parliaments. Democracy is being hacked, even with the blessing of major research centers and Universities located in the Mecca (Silicon Valley) of technology.

Beyond the cases in which this digital dependence has been used to spread fake news or violate critical infrastructure, the advent or creation of uncertainty that generates fear, serves to make excuses for emergency limitations and interference with rights. Scenarios like the Patriot Act, which was reflected in countries of the European Union such as the United Kingdom and Germany, shake our democracies more and more frequently. The dystopia has become a reality. With limitations imposed overnight by COVID-19, unthinkable 15 days before, regarding the measurement of emotions, everything is possible, everything is imaginable.

We are likely to have more biases than we think, and hence it is more necessary than ever to find new information, a deliberate effort to question our initial intuition and evaluate analytically, verifying the sources of information and the information itself. We must reconsider the power of conversation, especially with those with diametrically opposed ideas and interests. Difficult work, since we have lost sociability, captured by our electronic devices in a hyperconnection that abstracts us from reality and that has disconnected us from ourselves. And the pandemic confirms what we all knew; that technology has a crucial place even in confinement, that there is still a digital divide (for example, a division by age and in accessibility to e-learning itself), and that the world is beyond our control. Awareness now is essential, because we cannot even imagine or know right now just how vulnerable we are to all the information out there "in the cloud".

References

1. Berners-Lee, T.: I invented the web. Here are three things we need to change to save it, The Guardian, 12 March 2017. https://www.theguardian.com/technology/2017/mar/11/tim-berners-lee-web-inventor-save-internet
2. Kotler, P., Kartajaya, H., Setiawan, I.: Marketing 4.0: Moving from Traditional to Digital. Wiley, New Jersey (2016)

3. Huxley, A.: Dust jacket of Brave New World. Chatto & Windus, London (1932)
4. Harari, Y.N.: Los cerebros "hackeados" votan, Suplemento Ideas de El País, 06 March 2019. https://elpais.com/internacional/2019/01/04/actualidad/1546602935_606381.html
5. Chomsky, N., Ramonet, I.: Cómo nos venden la moto. Icaria Editorial, Barcelona (1995)
6. Durandin, G.: La información, la desinformación, la realidad. Paidós, Barcelona (1995)
7. Gutiérrez-Rubí, A.: Bots para la comunicación Política (2016). https://www.gutierrez-rubi.es/2016/11/02/bots-en-comunicacion-politica
8. Pariser, E.: Cuidado con las burbujas de filtro. TED (2011). http://www.ted.com/talks/eli_pariser_beware_online_filter_bubbles?language=es
9. Pariser, E.: El filtro burbuja. Taurus, Barcelona (2017)
10. Allport, G.W., Postman, L.: The Psychology of Rumor. Henry Holt, New York (1947)
11. Punset, E.: Por qué somos como somos. Aguilar, Madrid (2008)
12. Sunstein, C.: República.com: Internet, democracia y libertad (Estado y Sociedad). Colección: Estado y Sociedad, Ediciones Paidós, Madrid (2003)
13. Van, Y.: Do politics make us irrational? TED: Ideas worth spreading (2020). https://ed.ted.com/lessons/do-politics-make-us-irrational-jay-van-bavel
14. Zuckerberg, M.: A Blueprint for Content Governance and Enforcement. Facebook, Menlo Park, 15 November 2018. https://www.facebook.com/notes/mark-zuckerberg/ablueprint-for-content-governance-and-enforcement/10156443129621634/
15. Floreddu, P.B., Cabiddu, F., Evaristo, R.: Inside your social media ring: how to optimize online corporate reputation. Bus. Horizons **57**(6) (2014). http://dx.doi.org/10.1016/j.bushor.2014.07.007
16. Maestro, L., Cordón, D., Abuín, N.: La comunicación publicitaria en entornos digitales: herramientas para garantizar la reputación corporativa. Prisma Soc.: Rev. Invest. Soc. **22** (2018). http://orcid.org/0000-0001-5603-0792
17. Comisión de Industria Publicitaria (CIP): Guía de Buenas Prácticas: Transparency, Ad Fraud & Brand Safety (2019). https://www.aimc.es/a1mc-c0nt3nt/uploads/2019/03/Guia_Transparency_Ad_Fraud_y_Brand_Safety_2019.pdf
18. DoubleVerify: Global Insights Reports (2019). http://dvtemp.doubleverify.com/wp-content/uploads/2019/06/DoubleVerify-2019-Global-Insights-Report-1.pdf
19. World Federation Advertiser (WFA): WFA's planning and strategic priorities for 2019. https://wfanet.org/knowledge/item/2019/06/18/WFA-launches-The-State-of-Advertising-report
20. Kostolany, A.: El fabuloso mundo del dinero y la bolsa, Wordpress (1985). https://homealldestination.files.wordpress.com/2018/04/el-fabuloso-mundo-del-dinero-y-la-bolsa-andrc3a9-kostolany.pdf
21. Sartori, G.: Homo Videns. La sociedad teledirigida. Taurus, Madrid (2012)
22. Soengas, X.: Los límites de la información en los debates pactados. Rev. Latina Com Soc. **64** (2009): http://www.revistalatinacs.org/09/art/875_Santiago/RLCS_art875.pdf
23. Cortina, A.: Neuroética y neuropolítica. Tecnos, Madrid (2011)
24. Marcus, G.E.: The sentimental citizen. Emotion in Democratic Politics. The Pennsylvania State University, Pennsylvania (2002)
25. Lakoff, G.: The Political Mind: A Cognitive Scientist's Guide to Your Brain and Its Politics. Penguin Books, London (2009)
26. Iacoboni, M.: This is your brain on politics. The New York Times (2007). https://www.nytimes.com/2007/11/11/opinion/11freedman.html
27. Salmon, C. Storytelling, la máquina de fabricar historias y formatear las mentes. Colección Atalaya, ediciones Península, Barcelona (2008)
28. Vázquez, P.: Storytelling personal en política a través de Youtube, Comunicac. y Hombre 12 (2016). https://comunicacionyhombre.com/article/storytelling-personal-politica-traves-youtube/

29. Brants, K., Neijens, P.: The infotainment of politics. Polit. Commun. **15**, 149–164 (1998). http://dx.doi.org/10.1080/1058460-9809342363
30. Moy, P., Xenos, M.A., Hess, V.K.: Communication and citizenship: Mapping the political effects of infotainment, Mass Communication & Society (2005). https://www.tandfonline.com/doi/abs/10.1207/s15327825mcs0802_3
31. Berrocal, G.S. (ed.): Politainment: la política espectáculo en los medios de comunicación. Tirant lo Blanch, Valencia (2017)
32. Mazzoleni, G., Sfardini, A.: Política pop. Bologna: Il Mulino (2009)
33. Castelo, S.: Reseña: La ceremonia caníbal (de perfomers y políticos). Beers&Politics (2015):https://beersandpolitics.com/resena-la-ceremonia-canibal-de-perfomers-y-politicos.
34. Salmon, C.: La ceremonia caníbal. Sobre la performance política. colección Atalaya, ediciones Península, Barcelona (2013)
35. Berrocal, S., Campos-Domínguez, E., Redondo, M.: Prosumidores mediáticos en la comunicación política: El "politainment" en YouTube. Comunicar **43**(XXII) (2014). http://dx.doi.org/10.3916/C43-2014-06
36. Toffler, A.: The Third Wave. Bantam Books, Nueva York (USA) (1980)
37. Chia, A.: Welcome to Me-Mart. Am. Behav. Sci. **56**(4) (2012). http://dx.doi.org/10.1177/0002-764211429359
38. Shaw, A., Benkler, Y.: A tale of two blogospheres. Am. Behav. Sci. **56**(4) (2012). http://dx.doi.org/10.1177/00027-64211433793
39. Castells, M.: Redes de esperanza y de indignación. Los movimientos sociales en la era de Internet. Alianza, Madrid (2012)
40. Castells, M.: Comunicación y poder, Alianza, Madrid (2010)
41. Cheong, P., Lundry, C.: Prosumption, Transmediation, and Resistance: Terrorism and Manhunting in Southeast Asia. Am. Behav. Sci. **56**(4), (2012). https://doi.org/10.1177/0002764211429365
42. Vallespín, F.: Teatrocracia. Los chismes de los partidos cotizan más, El País, 19 February 2015. https://elpais.com/politica/2015/02/19/actualidad/1424378170_930658.html
43. Wolf, M.: Lector, vuelve a casa. Deusto, Barcelona (2020)
44. Bradbury, R.: Fahrenheit 451, Planeta, Barcelona (1985)
45. Kosinski, M., Stillwell, D.J., Graepel, T.: Private traits and attributes are predictable from digital records of human behaviour. Proc. Natl. Acad. Sci. U.S.A. (PNAS) **110**(15) (2013). https://doi.org/10.1073/pnas.1218772110
46. Youyou, W., Kosinski, M., Stillwell, D.J: Computer-based personality judgements are more accurate than those made by humans. Proc. Natl. Acad. Sci. U.S.A. (PNAS) **112**(4) (2015). https://doi.org/10.1073/pnas.1418680112
47. García, D.: Leaking privacy and shadow profiles in online social networks. Sci. Adv. **3**(8), 8 (20170. http://dx.doi.org/10.1126/sciadv.1701172
48. Hutson, M.: People can predict your tweets—even if you aren't on Twitter. Science **21** (2019). https://doi.org/10.1126/science.aaw7254
49. Peytibi, X.: La segmentación electoral. Más poder local **13** (2012): http://www.maspoderlocal.es/files/articulos/110-F508305df1101350763999-articulo-1.pdf
50. Matz, S.C., Kosinski, M., Nave, G., Stillwell, D.J.: Psychological targeting as an effective approach to digital mass persuasion. Proc. Natl. Acad. Sci. U.S.A. (PNAS) **114**(48) (2017). https://doi.org/10.1073/pnas.1710966114
51. Nowak & Eckel: US Patent no. US20160283485A1. US Patent and Trademark Office, Washington, DC (2012)
52. Kosinski, M.: With big data comes big responsibility. Financial Times, 14 March 2013. https://www.ft.com/content/1c3e27ee-8b2f-11e2-8fcf-00144feabdc0

53. The Guardian: Ted Cruz using firm that harvested data on millions of unwitting Facebook users, 11 December 2015. https://www.theguardian.com/us-news/2015/dec/11/senator-ted-cruz-president-campaign-facebook-user-data
54. Varsity: University leaks show internal turmoil triggered by academic's Cambridge Analytica work, 21 March 2018. https://www.varsity.co.uk/news/15218
55. El País: Cuestión de derechos, 23 December 2019. https://elpais.com/elpais/2019/12/23/opinion/1577125258_935046.html
56. Channel 4: Revealed: Trump's election consultants filmed saying they use bribes and sex workers to entrap politicians, 19 March 2018. https://www.channel4.com/news/cambridge-analytica-revealed-trumps-election-consultants-filmed-saying-they-use-bribes-and-sex-workers-to-entrap-politicians-investigation
57. Forbes. Cambridge Analytica trabajó con el PRI: Channel 4 News, 30 March 2018. https://www.forbes.com.mx/cambridge-analytica-mexico-pri-enero-2018-channel-4-news/
58. CNN. Zuckerberg y Facebook, bajo fuego por filtración a compañía vinculada a campaña de Trump, 19 March 2018. https://cnnespanol.cnn.com/2018/03/19/mark-zuckerberg-y-facebook-enfrentan-criticas-por-filtracion-a-compania-vinculada-con-trump/
59. House of Commons RU: House of Commons Digital, Culture, Media and Sport Committee: Disinformation and 'fake news': Interim Report, 29 July 2018. https://publications.parliament.uk/pa/cm201719/cmselect/cmcumeds/363/363.pdf
60. Global Voices: Data and Democracy: What Role Did Cambridge Analytica Play in Kenya's Elections? 03 November 2017. https://globalvoices.org/2017/11/03/data-and-democracy-what-role-did-cambridge-analytica-play-in-kenyas-elections/
61. Privacy International: Voter profiling in the 2017 Kenyan election (2017): https://medium.com/@privacyint/voter-profiling-in-the-2017-kenyan-election-8d9ac1e52877
62. Comisión Europea: A multi-dimensional approach to disinformation Report of the independent High level Group on fake news and online disinformation. Publications Office of the European Union, Luxembourg (2018)
63. The Guardian: Thirty countries use 'armies of opinion shapers' to manipulate democracy Report, 14 November 2017. https://www.theguardian.com/technology/2017/nov/14/social-media-influence-election-countries-armies-of-opinion-shapers-manipulate-democracy-fake-news
64. CNN. When seeing is no longer believing Inside the Pentagon's race against deepfake videos. https://edition.cnn.com/interactive/2019/01/business/pentagons-race-against-deepfakes/
65. Pagliery, J., Yellin, T.: Por qué Trump tiene más de 3.000 sitios web. CNN, 20 February 2017. https://cnnespanol.cnn.com/2017/02/20/por-que-trump-tiene-mas-de-3-000-sitios-web/
66. Agencia EFE: La campaña de Trump compra un dominio web de iniciativa latina de Biden y se burla, 24 October 2019. https://www.efe.com/efe/america/portada/la-campana-de-trump-compra-un-dominio-web-iniciativa-latina-biden-y-se-burla/20000064-4095073
67. Steck, C.: La fragmentación del mundo tecnológico. Polít. exterior **34**(193), 70–75 (2020). https://www.politicaexterior.com/articulos/politica-exterior/la-fragmentacion-del-mundo-tecnologico/

Political Communication in Europe. The Role of the Lobby and Its Communication Strategies

Ana Almansa-Martínez(✉), Andrea Moreno-Cabanillas, and Antonio Castillo-Esparcia

University of Málaga, Málaga, Spain
{anaalmansa,amorenoc,acastilloe}@uma.es

Abstract. In the field of political communication, the various actors involved generate numerous communication strategies and actions. There are three main contexts that influence the public policy process: how and in what way people participate in the European institutions, the organizational structure of the interests in each country and the communication strategy planned, developed and implemented by the lobbies. In this sense, it is not enough for the European institutions to have mechanisms for citizen participation in community processes without the organizations knowing how to participate and on which institution to carry out their communication activities. Having an adequate and prepared organizational structure allows the best-organized lobbies to have a better chance of success, since access is essential. But it is also essential to know who to talk to, what messages to convey and how to get the information across.

Keywords: Lobby · Political communication · European union · Strategies of communication

1 Lobby and Political Communication

This text delves into the lobbying landscape in an international context, analyzing the role played by these organizations in the European Union [4, 5, 13, 21]. Lobbying must accommodate the organizational structure of the European Union, which is characterized by a regulatory system of lobbying action (Transparency Register), a weak media structure with a European perspective and a small, but complex, bureaucratic and civil service structure [23, 24, 27]. In this regard, the special configuration of the European Union must be kept in mind:

– There are institutions with a double power of co-decision, moving away from the traditional distribution of the States in Executive, Legislative and Judicial power, since there are bodies such as the European Council, the European Commission, the European Parliament that perform shared activities. This publication is going to focus on the analysis of lobbying relations in the European Commission (and its College of Commissioners) and in the European Parliament [30, 32, 36, 37].

© The Author(s), under exclusive license to Springer Nature Singapore Pte Ltd. 2022
Á. Rocha et al. (Eds.): ICOMTA 2021, SIST 259, pp. 238–248, 2022.
https://doi.org/10.1007/978-981-16-5792-4_24

- There is a regulation on the access of interest groups to European institutions, since, in political dynamics, the role of interest representation is a basic element in the formation of public policies [17, 25, 26]. In that registry, there are more than 12,000 interest groups that play an active role in the community decision-making process.
- There is no European media or European public opinion, so the grass-roots activity carried out by lobbies takes place in a different way. One of the objectives of the project is to find out how it is produced and what techniques it uses [3, 7, 14, 21].
- The volume of structures and civil servant staff is smaller than that in the states. Knowing this structure is essential, as the culture of shared effort in public policy making integrates the role played by lobbies [15, 17, 20, 38].

This situation is in line with a perspective, deeply rooted in the European Union, in which civil society participates in public policy planning processes. In this sense, numerous studies have pointed out that the increased role of the state leads to an increase in social initiatives towards institutions, with the aim of participating in institutional decisions [12, 17]. In the case of European regulations, there is an articulated system, in which the regulations are invoked and applied by the states, so that citizens, companies and associations transfer their demands and requests to the community institutions.

For interest groups it is basic to participate in public policy processes, although not all have the same capacity to access and act due to various factors [22, 26]. If we attend to this imbalance of forces of lobbies, a series of values that strengthen these capacities of political influence can be shown, such as:

- The capacity to mobilize lobby sympathizers or members as a sign of social support [8, 10, 31, 33].
- The lobby's financial capacity allows it to carry out a set of activities that cannot be carried out by lobbies with scarce economic resources. Hence, business or employer lobbies have greater resources than those that generate resources through the volume of their membership, such as NGOs, consumer associations, professional associations or trade unions [9, 18, 19, 35].
- Access to public authorities is essential to be able to engage in a dialogic process with decision-makers, since it is difficult to gain support for a proposal just by handing over documentation or through grass-roots campaigns. This capacity integrates the concept of revolving doors [20].
- Advocacy helps when there is a fit with social values, since it is easier for those in power to make decisions with social demands that are in line with what is acceptable to the population as a whole [1, 6, 33].
- Having a good social image facilitates the lobby's work, since its proposals seem to have a higher level of legitimacy [11, 27–29, 32].
- Occupying a strategic space in society or the economy also confers greater weight in the dialogue processes.

In essence, lobbying is linked to the political culture of each society and reflects, to a certain extent, its capacity to structure and manage social demands towards the political system. Social cleavages differ from country to country. Thus, within the European

Union, diverse societies with different problems are confronted with each other, which implies a difficulty in the decision-making process.

2 Strategies of Lobbies in European Union

Each society mobilizes through different communication techniques, based on its political culture, as shown in Table 1. This table, in turn, shows how various grass-roots actions are carried out differently from country to country.

The citizens of the different countries feel that the European institutions are distant entities and consider that they hinder citizen mobilization actions. In this context, lobbies develop more qualitative elements in the way they act.

Participation in administrative bodies of the commission, either with the College of Commissioners or with the general directorates into which this institution is structured. A very relevant aspect is that the number of civil servants assigned to the commission is scarce, so it is usual to set up expert commissions on multiple topics. In these expert commissions, the lobbies can participate and propose experts.

Contacts with the Commissioners through lobbying associations, to raise problems and situations of economic sectors, such as the automotive employers' association, which includes the Spanish ANFAC. These meetings held at the highest level focus on strategic postulates of the sectors involved.

To liaise with officials in the process of drafting specific regulations, providing the sector's perspective, generating supporting documentation or proposing prepared texts that can be considered by officials. In this action, the lobby's capacity for objectivity is essential to legitimize itself as a reliable entity, providing truthful information and becoming a valid interlocutor.

Actions on parliamentarians, to hold discussions on their proposals, to submit information from the sector, to establish personal relationships and, in short, to participate in discussions and in the drafting of legislation. All these actions of lobbies can only be carried out if they are registered in the Transparency Register. The Transparency Register was created precisely to regulate the participation of stakeholders in 2011, both the European Parliament and the European Commission. In order to manage this Transparency Register created their own structure: the Common Secretariat of the Transparency Register [2, 34].

Creating the register, it is possible to know what type of organizations want to participate, what interests they intend to defend or legitimize, which organizations participate in the defense of those interests and the economic and personal resources they have to carry out this representation activity (Fig. 1).

The evolution of the Transparency Register shows an upward curve, which is an example of the interest of lobbies in participating in the policies of the European Union.

Inclusion in the register implies a series of prerogatives for interest groups. In the European Parliament the advantages are access to the premises, the intervention as speakers in the public hearings of its committees, receiving notifications on the activities of the committees, co-organization of events with the parties of the Parliament, among others. In the case of the Commission, it is possible to hold meetings with Commissioners, members of Cabinets and Directors General; public consultations (they receive automatic

Table 1. Have you done any of the following activities in the last 12 months? Percentage answering yes. Base: total number of cases

	Total EU countries (10)	Sweden	Denmark	Netherlands	France	Spain	Italy	United Kingdom	Germany	Czech Republic	Poland
Signing a petition in a signature campaign	24,0	49,0	31,9	33,8	35,2	26,4	23,4	25,8	14,8	24,9	10,3
Buying certain products for political, ethical or environmental reasons	15,8	53,6	46,3	23,9	28,8	8,4	13,6	11,9	13,8	8,6	5,1
Boycott or stop using certain products for political, ethical or environmental reasons	15,1	43,3	30,1	21,3	28,3	8,9	12,6	10,8	15,6	4,9	3,8
Getting in touch with a politician or an authority or civil servant to draw attention to a problem	10,3	17,9	16,5	21,5	15,5	5,5	9,8	13,1	7,3	6,9	4,8

(continued)

Table 1. *(continued)*

	Total EU countries (10)	Sweden	Denmark	Netherlands	France	Spain	Italy	United Kingdom	Germany	Czech Republic	Poland
Taking part in demonstrations	10,3	7,7	5,3	2,8	14,0	23,2	14,3	4,0	7,3	9,3	3,6
Collaborate with a civic association or non-governmental organisation (NGO) to support social causes	9,6	13,2	18,4	15,7	17,5	14,9	8,7	5,0	5,9	5,1	5,0
Taking part in a strike	7,6	1,0	1,3	1,6	7,7	20,6	13,5	3,4	3,6	2,7	3,0
Participate in a self-organised protest movement via SMS, email, etc.	7,2	14,8	7,7	11,9	11,6	8,7	7,0	4,6	5,2	5,1	4,4
Giving money to a political party or organization	4,8	4,3	14,0	10,3	4,3	2,6	4,9	3,7	5,5	9,0	4,1
Contributing to the campaigns or activities of a political party	4,0	4,8	5,6	4,4	4,9	3,2	5,9	1,8	4,2	3,3	3,5

Source: Informe BBVA sobre participación ciudadana en la política/BBVA 2015 (Traslated: Report on citizen participation in politics)

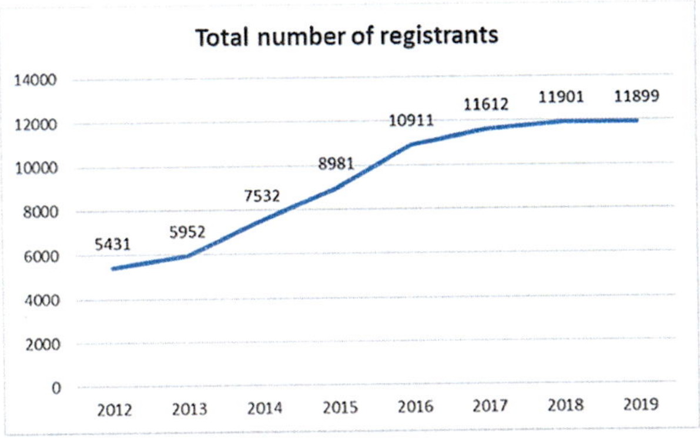

Fig. 1. Evolution of the number of registrants. Source: annual report on the operation of the Transparency Register (2019)

notification of consultations and roadmaps in the areas they have indicated); expert groups (registration in the Register is required for the appointment of certain types of members of expert groups); contacts with officials, for a meeting or an event.

As an example of the transparency policy of the European Union and the importance it has for citizens and its own institutions, is the fact that the Registry Secretariat offers informative courses on how the registry works and the most relevant aspects of interest groups. There have been numerous attempts to bring clarity to the actions of lobbies and recurring initiatives by the European institutions themselves or by independent bodies. This is the case of Transparency International, which has carried out studies on the role of lobbies, or that of its 2015 report, entitled Lobbying in Europe: Hidden Influence, Privileged, international, in which they demand a series of initiatives: require public institutions and representatives to proactively record and publish information on their interactions with lobbyists, including summaries of meetings, calendars, agendas and documentation received; ensure that a "legislative footprint" is created for each proposal, in order to ensure full transparency of decision-making processes; ensure that records apply to both direct and indirect lobbying efforts, targeting all institutions and individuals who play a role in public decisions; introduce a legal obligation for public authorities to strive for a balanced composition of advisory and expert bodies, representing a diversity of interests and viewpoints; make open calls to constitute the advisory/expert groups and ensure that common selection criteria are used to balance different interests; publish legislative footprints to track, in a uniform manner, contacts and input received on draft policies, legislation and amendments; ensure greater transparency regarding the composition and activities of expert groups by publishing information on the selection process of members, as well as the publication of detailed minutes of meetings.

The European institutions have produced initiatives to improve transparency in the work carried out by lobbies, which are based on two main postulates. The legislative footprint, as a mechanism that focuses on the traceability of the committee's regulations in Parliament, and which consists of a mechanism in which it is possible to observe how a regulation has been modified throughout the process and who has made these contributions. The publication of public agendas makes it possible to know with whom official meetings are held by the members of the commission, an element that is already in place today. The Commission has established that its members must make public the information on the meetings they hold, both themselves and the members of their cabinets with lobbyists, informing about the date of the meeting, the place where it is held, the name of the Commission member and/or cabinet member, the name of the organization or freelancer and the purpose of the meeting.

For a lobby, the communication strategy could focus on two different perspectives. On the one hand, the proactive strategy, in which the lobby takes the initiative in the definition, elaboration and approval of public policies, allowing it to raise situations and anticipate issues that may affect the interest group. Having the ability to be able to raise issues that may affect the interests of the lobby facilitates the structuring of the thematic, delimits the conceptual boundaries of the discussion and influences the approach to the solution to the problem [9, 16, 35]. On the other hand, the reactive strategy, which is delimited by a passive action of the lobby, which is only put into action when a decision affecting the lobby's interests is being considered, discussed or approved. This action does not allow the lobby to propose solutions, but starts from a defensive activity, which greatly reduces the field of action [13, 33].

3 Communication in the Commission and Parliament

Direct lobbying, understood as direct communication with politicians and public officials (either inside or outside the institutional premises) can take the form of: advice or presentations to officials, either on an ad hoc or periodic basis; delivering draft reports to public officials in which specific details of the policy itself are written; seeking informal contacts with individual politicians or branches of public officials, including having simple telephone conversations with such personnel; formal or invited consultation through institutionalized channels; participation in hearings, such as parliamentary committees; participation in a delegation or conference; and requested, or unsolicited, submission of information or documents to politicians and officials.

Indirect lobbying or grass-roots lobbying is one of the current trends in public affairs, in which a set of communication actions are produced on the political leader or officials, through the presence in the media, by direct requests from citizens or by generating spaces in social networks. In its most benign form, this type of citizen participation can be enriching for citizens. However, this technique can also involve something more reprehensible when it becomes astroturfing, the controversial practice of lobbyists hiding behind front organizations to give the appearance of popular support for a cause that is, in reality, funded by private interests. The activities associated with these off and online campaigns are: direct online citizen petitions; letters to the government or parliamentarians; public debates; leaflets and posters; demonstrations, among other activities, in order to pressure politicians to listen to them; use of related organizations such as advocacy associations; use of other entities such as think tanks; creation of blogs; cyber activists writing on social networks (Fig. 2).

Within the European Union, having a lobby that has the possibility of carrying out a proactive strategy opens up various possibilities for action, since it is a dynamic process in which there are divergent or convergent approaches among the actors participating in

List of meetings **Banco Santander, S.A.** has held with Commissioners, Members of their Cabinet or Director-Generals since 01/12/2014 under its current ID number in the Transparency Register: 799142914971-03.

Nr	Commission representative	Portfolio	Date	Location	Subject(s)
1	John Berrigan, Director-General	Financial Stability, Financial Services and Capital Markets Union (FISMA)	23/10/2020	Virtual meeting	Courtesy meeting
2	Andrea Beltramello, Cabinet member of Valdis Dombrovskis	An Economy that Works for People	30/09/2020	video conference	Digital finance, payments
3	Elisa Ferreira, Commissioner	Cohesion and Reforms	11/09/2020	Brussels	Introductory meeting with the new Managing Director – European Corporate Affairs of Banco Santander
4	Daniel Calleja Crespo, Director-General	Environment (ENV)	19/06/2020	Brussels	Green recovery, sustainable finance
5	Mirzha De Manuel, Cabinet member of Valdis Dombrovskis	An Economy that Works for People	12/05/2020	video-conferencing	Exchange of views on macro environment and COVID economic response.
6	Paolo Gentiloni, Commissioner	Economy	26/03/2020	Conference-call	Economic impact of COVID-19
7	Margrethe Vestager, Executive Vice-President	Europe Fit for Digital Age	26/03/2020	Brussels	To discuss digitalisation and competition
8	Jérôme Deslandes, Cabinet member of Valdis Dombrovskis	An Economy that Works for People	03/03/2020	Brussels	Basel III implementation with particular focus on operational risk;Resolution strategy for "multiple point of entry" model
9	Valeria Miceli, Cabinet member of Ursula von der Leyen	President	18/02/2020	Brussels, Belgium	The future of banking between digitalization and regulation

Fig. 2. Banco Santander report on meetings held (Source: Transparency Register, 2020).

the community institutions. This proactive strategy is approached from the creation of a series of indicators, such as:

- Those stakeholders whose presence in the Transparency Register has been in place for some time and who have registered in the early stages of the register (Permanence Indicator).
- The capacity for permanent and constant communication, with strategic communication planning, instrumented in a communication plan with objectives, timetable and personnel (Indicator strategic communication planning)
- The development of symmetrical dialogic communicative actions, which implies active participation in the committees, frequent meetings and the systematic preparation of documents (biological indicator).
- The purpose of the lobby, beyond the communicative activity, tends to fulfill an educational function on the objectives and functions of the lobby and a sensitizing function on the issues defended (Educational and sensitizing indicator).

- A large budget and staff available for lobbying activities, understood as exceeding the average budget in its category in the registry (Resources indicator).
- Constant, recurrent and planned participation in expert groups, both of the Commission and of the European Parliament (Participation indicator).
- Participation in meetings of experts and parliamentary committees in areas related to their field of action (Complementary indicator).
- The development of and participation in alliances with other interest groups with which they may share common interests (Coalition indicator).
- A follow-up with staff and budget of the regulations that have been approved and that may undergo modifications in the future, in order to accept the demands or requests of the lobby (Follow-up indicator).
- Evaluation of the communication campaigns carried out and analysis of the achievements obtained by applying measurement criteria, according to the Barcelona Principles of AMEC.

In short, lobbies' communication strategies should focus more on dialogic relationship elements, in which meetings, presence in committees and interviews are the central axis; and less on indirect lobbying actions.

4 Conclusion

In contemporary societies, it is necessary to highlight the role of lobbies as organizations that participate in the process of discussion, elaboration and implementation of public policies in the process of participatory democracies. To this end, lobbies develop direct and indirect communication strategies that seek to co-participate with political institutions. The capacity to generate communicative spaces through grass-roots lobbying implies that it is necessary to act on two essential mechanisms of political communication, such as thematization and framing. Hence, lobbying strategies are aimed at proposing topics for public discussion of those issues that affect them and to participate in the deliberative process, proposing the conceptual boundaries, terms and content of the discussion.

References

1. Almansa-Martínez, A., Fernández-Souto, A.-B.: Professional public relations (PR) trends and challenges. Prof. Inform. **29**(3) (2020). https://doi.org/10.3145/epi.2020.may.03
2. Almansa-Martínez, A., Castillero-Ostio, E.: Spanish lobbies listed in the European transparency register. Comunicação soc. Special Issue 109–126 (2020). https://doi.org/10.17231/comsoc.0(2020).2743
3. Arceneaux, K., Johnson, M., Lindstädt, R., Vander Wielen, R.J.: The influence of news media on political elites: investigating strategic responsiveness in congress. Am. J. Polit. Sci. **60**(1), 5–29 (2016)
4. Bernhagen, P., Dür, A., Marshall, D.: Information or context: what accounts for positional proximity between the European Commission and lobbyists? J. Eur. Public Policy **22**(4) (2015). https://doi.org/10.1080/13501763.2015.1008556

5. Beyers, J., Dür, A., Wonka, A.: The political salience of EU policies. J. Eur. Public Policy **25**(11), 1726–1737 (2018). https://doi.org/10.1080/13501763.2017.1337213
6. Biliouri, D.: Environmental Ngos in Brussels: how powerful are their lobbying activities? Environ. Polit. **8**(2), 173–182 (1999)
7. Binderkrantz, A.S., Rasmussen, A.: Comparing the domestic and the EU lobbying con-text: perceived agenda-setting influence in the multilevel system of the European union. J. Eur. Public Policy **22**(4) (2015). https://doi.org/10.1080/13501763.2015.1008553
8. Branton, R., Martínez-Ebers, V., Carey, T.E., Jr., Matsubayashi, T.: Social protest and policy attitudes: the case of the 2006 immigrant rallies. Am. J. Polit. Sci. **59**(2), 390–402 (2015). https://doi.org/10.1111/ajps.12159
9. Carty, V.: New information communication technologies and grassroots mobilization. Inform. Commun. Soc. **13**(2), 155–173 (2010). https://doi.org/10.1080/13691180902915658
10. Castillo-Esparcia, A., Carretón-Ballester, C., Pineda-Martínez, P.: Investigación en relaciones públicas en España. Prof. Inform. **29**(3) (2020). https://doi.org/10.3145/epi.2020.may.30
11. Castillo-Esparcia, A., Guerra-Heredia, S., Almansa-Martínez, A.: Political communication and think tanks in Spain. Strategies with the media. Prof. Inform. **26**(4), 706–713 (2017). https://doi.org/10.3145/epi.2017.jul.14
12. Chalmers, A.W., Macedo, F.S.: Does it pay to lobby? Examining the link between firm lobbying and firm profitability in the European union. J. Eur. Public Policy (2020). https://doi.org/10.1080/13501763.2020.1824012
13. Chari, R., Hillebrand O'Donovan, D.: Lobbying the European commission: open or secret? Social. Democr. **25**(2), 104–124 (2011). https://doi.org/10.1080/08854300.2011.579475
14. Cotton, C.: Competing for attention: lobbying time-constrained politicians. J. Public Econ. Theory **18**(4), 642–665 (2016). https://doi.org/10.1111/jpet.12202
15. Crepaz, M., Hanegraaff, M.: The funding of interest groups in the EU: are the rich get-ting richer? J. Eur. Publ. Policy **27**(1), 102–121 (2020). https://doi.org/10.1080/13501763.2019.1567572
16. De Bruycker, I.: Blessing or curse for advocacy? How news media attention helps advocacy groups to achieve their policy goals. Polit. Commun. **36**(1), 103–126 (2019). https://doi.org/10.1080/10584609.2018.1493007
17. De Bruycker, I., Beyers, J.: Lobbying strategies and success: inside and outside lobbying in European Union legislative politics. Eur. Polit. Sci. Rev. **11**(1), 57–74 (2016). https://doi.org/10.1017/S1755773918000218
18. Dempsey, S.E.: NGOs, communicative labor, and the work of grassroots representation. Commun. Crit./Cult. Stud. **6**(4), 328–345 (2009). https://doi.org/10.1080/14791420903348625
19. Dür, A.: Measuring interest group influence in the EU: a note on methodology. Eur. Union Polit. **9**(4), 559–576 (2008). https://doi.org/10.1177/1465116508095151
20. Dür, A., Bernhagen, P., Marshall, D.: Interest group success in the European union: when (and why) does business lose? Comparat. Polit. Stud. **48**(8), 951–983 (2015). https://doi.org/10.1177/2F0010414014565890
21. Flöthe, L.: The costs of interest representation – a resource perspective on informational lobbying. Eur. Polit. Sci. Rev. **11**(2), 161–178 (2019). https://doi.org/10.1017/S1755773919000055
22. Gallagher Cunningham, K., Dahl, M., Frugé, A.: Strategies of resistance: diversification and diffusion. Am. J. Polit. Sci. **61**(3), 591–605 (2017). https://doi.org/10.1111/ajps.12304
23. Holdo, M., Öberg, P., Magnusson, S.: Do citizens use storytelling or rational argumentation to lobby politicians? Policy Polit. **47**(4), 543–559 (2019). https://doi.org/10.1332/030557319X15613700896551
24. Junk, W.M.: Co-operation as currency: How active coalitions affect lobbying success. J. Eur. Publ. Policy **27**(6), 873–892 (2020). https://doi.org/10.1080/13501763.2019.1631377

25. Klüver, H.: Informational lobbying in the European union: the effect of organisational characteristics. West Eur. Polit. **35**(3), 491–510 (2012). https://doi.org/10.1080/01402382.2012.665737
26. Klüver, H.: Lobbying in the European Union: Interest Groups, Lobbying Coalitions and Policy Change. Oxford University Press, Oxford (2013). https://doi.org/10.1093/acprof:oso/9780199657445.001.0001
27. Klüver, H., Braun, C., Beyers, J.: Legislative lobbying in context: towards a conceptual framework of interest group lobbying in the European union. J. Eur. Publ. Policy **22**(4), 447–461 (2015). https://doi.org/10.1080/13501763.2015.1008792
28. Lowery, D.: Lobbying influence: meaning, measurement and missing. Interest Groups Advocacy **2**(1), 1–26 (2013). https://doi.org/10.1057/iga.2012.20
29. Marshall, D.: Explaining interest group interactions with party group members in the european parliament: dominant party groups and coalition formation. JCMS: J. Common Mark. Stud. **53**(2), 311–329 (2015). https://doi.org/10.1111/jcms.12163
30. Mayrhofer, E.M.: Lobbying the EU: the example of regional lobbies. Stud. Eur. **59**(1), 153–166 (2014)
31. Mergeai, S.; Gilain, H.: Analyse comparative des stratégies employées par le lobby pharmaceutique, gazier et automobile visant à influencer les réglementations de l'UE. Uni-versité Catholique de Louvain. Louvain School of Management, Louvain (2020)
32. Rasmussen, A.: Participation in written government consultations in Denmark and the UK: system and actor-level effects. Gov. Oppos. **50**(2), 271–299 (2015)
33. Rasmussen, A., Mader, L.K., Reher, S.: With a little help from the people? The role of public opinion in advocacy success. Comparat. Polit. Stud. **51**(2), 139–164 (2018). https://doi.org/10.1177/2F0010414017695334
34. Rasmussen, M.K.: The battle for influence: the politics of business lobbying in the European parliament. JCMS: J. Common Mark. Stud. **53**(2), 365–382 (2015). https://doi.org/10.1111/jcms.12156
35. Schnakenberg, K.E.: Informational lobbying and legislative voting. Am. J. Polit. Sci. **61**(1), 129–145 (2017). https://doi.org/10.1111/ajps.12249
36. Stevens, F., De Bruycker, I.: Influence, affluence and media salience: economic resources and lobbying influence in the European union. Eur. Union Polit. **21**(4), 728–750 (2020). https://doi.org/10.1177/2F1465116520944572
37. Woll, C.: Lobbying in the European union: from sui generis to a comparative perspective. J. Eur. Publ. Policy **13**(3), 456–469 (2006). https://doi.org/10.1080/13501760600560623
38. Wratil, C.: Territorial representation and the opinion–policy linkage: evidence from the European union. Am. J. Polit. Sci. **63**(1), 197–211 (2019). https://doi.org/10.1111/ajps.12403

Institutional Advertising in the Face of COVID-19 Hoaxes: Strategies, Messages and Narratives in the Spanish Case

Jesús Pérez-Seoane and Juan-Manuel Corbacho-Valencia(✉)

University of Vigo, Vigo, Spain
{pseoane,jmcorbacho}@uvigo.es

Abstract. The present work addresses the importance of institutional advertising to counter hoaxes during the first ten months since the outbreak of COVID-19. Institutional advertising campaigns run by Spanish central and regional governments have been studied from a quantitative point of view to establish their length, periodicity, views and interactions, and from a qualitative point of view in terms of strategy, intentionality, discourse and narrative and filming techniques. The main results suggest that institutional advertising campaigns are clearly focused on social networks and have not been the main tool to fight COVID-19 hoaxes, but rather to inform citizens. Their main characters are anonymous people, followed by affected individuals and health care workers, and these campaigns showed greater intensity during the first months of the pandemic and picked up again in December, due to fear of the consequences of a third wave. It can also be said that the different public administrations have fulfilled their duty to inform public opinion.

Keywords: Institutional advertising · Fake news · COVID-19

1 Institutional Advertising in Spain: Definition and Context

Being more than "a banal commercial activity" [1], public administration campaigns respond to the educational-social variation of institutional advertising, which is directly related to the educational and socializing role of the State apparatus. This type of campaign is aimed at bringing about changes in how citizens understand the world, introducing new values and arguments regarding life in society; thus, it must seek, above all, to benefit the citizens [2]. In this regard, [3] defines institutional advertising as a communication of public-social utility, while [4] considers it as an "essential means in the construction of a public image for public institutions and citizens, and the relationship

This work is part of the project "Digital narratives against misinformation. A study of social networks, themes and formats of Ibero-American fact-checkers", funded by the *Agencia Estatal de Investigación* [State Research Agency] of the Government of Spain, within the State Program of Research, Development and Innovation Oriented to the Challenges of Society (PID2019-108035RB-I00/AEI/10.13039/501100011033).

© The Author(s), under exclusive license to Springer Nature Singapore Pte Ltd. 2022
Á. Rocha et al. (Eds.): ICOMTA 2021, SIST 259, pp. 249–258, 2022.
https://doi.org/10.1007/978-981-16-5792-4_25

between them", in a sort of parent-child relationship. At times of growing tensions and uncertainties, such as that of COVID-19, public administrations must become a unique source of information, given the essence of the data to be transmitted, the principles of utility, efficiency, transparency, austerity, free competition and equality by which public information should be governed, and because "the State must inform citizens even without their request" [5].

Being a multifaceted field of study with multiple applications, it has resulted in different approaches to institutional advertising, particularly since the adoption of Law 29/2005, which relate with the discursive, rhetorical and cognitive sphere, but also with the legal sphere of institutional advertising in Spain [1–3, 6]. This aforementioned Law on Advertising and Institutional Advertising sheds light on the concept by defining institutional campaigns as "any activity aimed at spreading a message or common goal to a plurality of recipients, using a paid-for or transferred advertising platform", and being promoted and contracted by the General State Administration and other public sector entities. Institutional communication campaigns use "means of communication other than strictly advertising […] in order to disseminate a message or common goal to a plurality of recipients" by the same aforementioned subjects. Therefore, it generically refers to the messages that the Government and the different administrations send to citizens in the exercise of their executive function. The preamble to the Law states that "the duality between political and executive nature of Government action must be kept in separate communication spheres", with public utility, professionalization, transparency, and institutional loyalty being the objectives of institutional advertising and communication campaigns. In short, nowadays, and probably more than ever, institutional advertising understood as a public space, as a place for communication between individuals, groups and institutions [7], is not only a reflection of society, but must become a reliable information source.

2 Hoaxes, Fake News and Misinformation Regarding COVID-19

The Internet has democratized the creation and dissemination of all kinds of content. Although the "fake news" concept experienced a boom coinciding with Brexit and with Donald Trump's first presidential campaign, the use of false information dates back to much earlier times. While in the 20th century only a few entities had the capacity to misinform the public opinion (mainly governments and the media), for some time now it can be argued that such capacity is almost universal, at least in terms of creation and dissemination. Changes in media and information consumption patterns have been instrumental in this regard, as well as social networks, which have become a powerful platform for disseminating hoaxes, up to the point of influencing historical events worldwide. Between 2014 and 2016 there was a sharp increase in the number of fact-checking organizations [8]. The coronavirus pandemic is not an exception to the rule, but rather confirms it; since the outbreak of COVID-19 in March 2020, World Health Organization (WHO) had to warn about the spread of false information, which is considered by [9] as the first global infodemic caused by social networks.

In addition to this, fake news spreads faster than real news due to two factors [10]. On the one hand, fake news warns about a danger by spreading fear. From a cognitive point of view, pandemics create scenarios with unresolved fears that put public opinion on the alert. Disease prevention systems lead to both implicit and explicit safety measures, such as social isolation and less tolerance towards strangers. On the other hand, there is an intrinsic need for information. The lack of scientific information during the early stages of the pandemic fostered the search of explanations that did not exist, thus providing the perfect breeding ground for hoaxes and misinformation.

It is only natural that, in parallel with the boom of fake news and the tools to counteract them, the number of publications from the communication perspective has also increased, especially since the emergence of COVID-19. [11] state that there are many studies seeking to link misinformation about COVID-19 to social networks, as well as that users increasingly search for online health information that they do not only consume, but also share. Another phenomenon identified by the authors is that users assume that there is more information about COVID-19 than that provided by public administrations, and they claim different reasons for sharing health information: altruism, entertainment, socialization, leisure, information exchange and search for information. [12] argues that the current information ecosystem results from the proliferation of channels and platforms, the growing number of information providers an increased media competition, which makes it extremely difficult to stay well-informed. One of the consequences is information overload, which makes it harder for citizens to distinguish between true and false information, thus limiting the cognitive capacity of the recipient, who ends up creating his/her own mosaic of data and arguments [13]. As pointed out by [14], it is precisely through social networks that traditional news circulation has been disrupted and a new content distribution model is generated, combining the media's traditional vertical dynamics with those more horizontal which give prominence to users regarding data dissemination and even viral spreading. Therefore, a distinction must be drawn between the creation of hoaxes and their dissemination, as the latter is not necessarily ill-intentioned and can be aimed at informing others. Therein lies the complexity of countering the phenomenon. In addition to fact-checking, institutions must take on the responsibility of informing citizens under the pressure of having to provide answers in increasingly shorter periods of time in the race against fake news.

3 Methodology and Objectives

This study aims to analyze and establish the communication practices implemented by the different regional and central governments during the first three waves of COVID-19, particularly in the case of institutional advertising. Therefore, the main objective of this research is to determine how advertising campaigns were used by the various administrations during the first ten months of the pandemic.

Along with this, two specific objectives are proposed:

1. To identify what has been the role of advertising and communication campaigns in the management of the pandemic.
2. To know what channels have been used to fight hoaxes on COVID-19.

The present study covers ten months: from March 11, when WHO declared COVID-19 a pandemic, until December 31, 2020, when vaccination began. That new phase has been left out of this analysis because it has suffered several interruptions and has not made it possible to adopt a uniform strategy.

Within the context of a descriptive research, an analysis has been conducted of the audiovisual materials that were published by administrations in order to deal with COVID-19 pandemic during the reporting period and posted on their official communication channels, such as websites and YouTube. Out of a total of 335 videos, this study includes 97 videos that could be considered, strictly speaking, as institutional advertising resources (accounting for 28.96% of the identified institutional communication campaigns, with Andalusia, Asturias, Canary Islands, Balearic Islands and Madrid as the most active regions), as well as 238 videos from institutional campaigns.

The applied methodology encompasses several levels of analysis. From a purely quantitative perspective, this study collects the communicational activity by periods based on the three pandemic waves, as well as data on length, views and interactions. A content analysis of each video is conducted in terms of strategy, intentionality, discourse and narrative and filming techniques in order to understand the different ways to address the population's need for information since the outbreak of the pandemic. In addition, it will allow to establish potential patterns for a more effective crisis communication in pandemic scenarios.

4 Results

4.1 Analyzed Videos, Duration and Interactions

There are some descriptive aspects that allow us to know the audiovisual advertising production carried out by administrations during the first months of the pandemic. In that period, 335 videos were collected, 238 (71.04%) of which fall within institutional communication campaigns and 97 (28.96%) correspond to institutional advertising campaigns, designed to convey a message through paid-for or transferred means (Table 1).

When dealing with institutional communication about the pandemic through advertising campaigns, administrations tend to choose short messages, that is, commercial formats suited to television lengths (20 or 30 s) or to social networks (which usually last less than a minute).

That is the case in 71.3% of the analyzed ads, which are less than 60 s long (either from 0 to 30 s, or from 30 to 60 s). This percentage is in stark contrast to that of non-advertising audiovisual materials developed by administrations, almost half of which (45.80%) do not correspond to commercial messages (that is, more than 60 s long) (Table 2).

Turning our attention to the impact of the institutional advertising campaigns conducted during the first ten months of the pandemic, we see that almost 40% of the ads have more than 5,000 views, that is, a level of interaction higher than that obtained through other institutional communication campaigns, where 52.47% of the messages have less than 1,000 views (Table 3).

Therefore, it should be noted that, when it came to deliver messages to the population about the pandemic, administrations have mainly resorted to institutional communication campaigns, with advertising actions being the ones that had greater impact on citizens.

Table 1. Share of videos published by Spanish administrations during the first ten months of the pandemic that are part of institutional advertising campaigns.

	Institutional advertising	Institutional campaigns	% Advertising
Spain	6	33	15.4%
Basque Country	5	11	31.3%
Catalonia	8	30	21.1%
Galicia	8	8	50.0%
Andalusia	3	52	5.5%
Asturias	5	10	33.3%
Cantabria	0	3	0.0%
La Rioja	5	7	41.7%
Murcia	0	2	0.0%
Valencian Community	4	9	30.8%
Aragon	7	9	43.8%
Castile-La Mancha	2	15	11.8%
Canary Islands	12	9	57.1%
Navarre	7	3	70.0%
Extremadura	0	0	
Balearic Islands	3	29	9.4%
Madrid	17	7	70.8%
Castile and Leon	2	1	66.7%
Ceuta	3	0	100.0%
Melilla	0	0	
	97	**238**	

Table 2. Length of institutional advertising campaigns, compared to messages from other communication campaigns.

Advertising campaigns			Communication campaigns		
Length	Videos	Share	Length	Videos	Share
From 0 to 30″	34	35.05%	From 0 to 30″	53	22.3%
From 30 to 60″	35	36.08%	From 30 to 60″	76	31.9%
From 60 to 90″	15	15.46%	From 60 to 90″	64	26.9%
More than 90″	13	13.40%	More than 90″	45	18.9%
	97			238	

Table 3. Views obtained by institutional advertising campaigns and communication campaigns.

Advertising campaigns			Communication campaigns		
Views	Videos	Share	Views	Videos	Share
Less than 100	6	6.19%	Less than 100	31	13.90%
From 100 to 500	21	21.65%	From 100 to 500	55	24.66%
From 500 to 1,000	12	12.37%	From 500 to 1,000	31	13.90%
More than 1,000	19	19.59%	More than 1,000	45	20.18%
More than 5,000	7	7.22%	More than 5,000	9	4.04%
More than 10,000	32	32.99%	More than 10,000	52	23.32%
	97			223	

4.2 Strategy, Intentionality, and Discourse of Institutional Advertising Campaigns

From the point of view of dissemination, there are two different trends: that of institutional communication campaigns (where most of the videos (65%) are concentrated in the first four months of the pandemic) and that of advertising campaigns, which are much more seasonal.

Forty percent of the ads were made between March and June, aimed at making the population aware of the scale of the problem and the need for confinement and delivering information about de-escalation phases. The remaining percentage is divided into specific actions, such as the summer period, the return to school or, more particularly, Christmas time, all of which are periods where specific prevention messages were delivered (Fig. 1).

Regardless of the time of year in which messages are delivered, it is relevant to know what the intentionality and treatment of the different campaigns are. In this manner, it is possible to detect informational purposes (such as campaigns teaching how to put on the face mask), advertising purposes (continuing with the same example, those encouraging people to wear face masks) or propaganda purposes (those that tell us that a particular area is where people know best how to put on the face mask).

It is hardly surprising that the persuasive approach prevails within the context of institutional advertising campaigns; however, it is not accurate to say that all public announcements on COVID-19 are strictly intended for advertising purposes. It is noteworthy, to say the least, that 24.74% of the ads have an informational purpose (Table 4).

A similar trend can be seen in the construction of messages, which commonly have a strong rhetorical component (through figures of speech such as similes or other more conceptual resources), while a large number of messages are meant to meet informational needs.

It is worth mentioning that 21.65% of the analyzed ads base their argument on launching an appeal (whether individual or collective). This is a rare circumstance in conventional advertising (more focused on praising a product or service than on calling

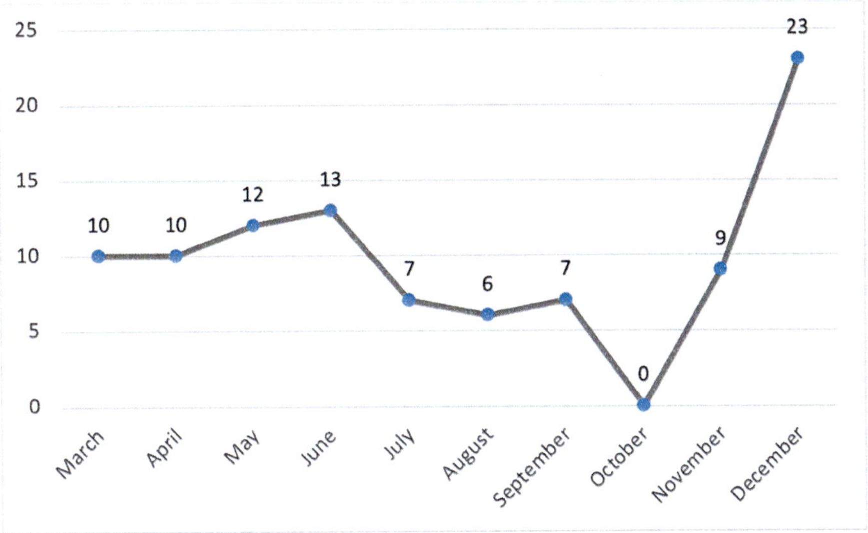

Fig. 1. The advertising activity of administrations in the face of the pandemic is less concentrated than in the case of institutional communication campaigns.

Table 4. Intentionality and argument in communication campaigns.

Intentionality	Videos	Share	Argument	Videos	Share
Informational	24	24.74%	Informational	25	25.77%
Propaganda	8	8.25%	Appellative	21	21.65%
Advertising	65	67.01%	Rhetorical	51	52.58%
	97			97	

for citizen mobilization), but it seems appropriate in a pandemic scenario, where many ads sought to boost people's morale and to ask them to keep complying with the necessary protection measures.

4.3 Institutional Advertising in the Face of COVID-19 Hoaxes

There are regions such as Canary Islands, Galicia or Castile-La Mancha that ended their ads with lines like "stay informed through official sources", but no specific advertising campaigns were identified; this is a striking fact given the importance of this matter during the first year of the pandemic, in which society has faced an unprecedented situation with many uncertainties and contradictory information.

In the remaining analyzed videos, only eleven (3.28% of the total and 4.62% of institutional communication campaigns) specifically addressed the issue of fake news and hoaxes, whether referring to COVID-19 symptoms, to certain groups (teenagers) or to the media through which the communication is delivered.

4.4 Narrative and Filming Techniques

The specificity of advertising, which implies condensing a message into an audiovisual piece of short duration, has led administrations to make specific productions for their ads. Such practice is different from that of other institutional communication campaigns, where it is much more common to create videos from stock footage or using animation techniques (Table 5).

Table 5. Type of production of advertising and communication campaigns.

Advertising campaigns			Communication campaigns		
Length	Videos	Share	Length	Videos	Share
Animation	16	16.49%	Animation	83	34.87%
Stock footage	6	6.19%	Stock footage	60	25.21%
Specific production	75	77.32%	Specific production	95	39.92%
	97			238	

When it comes to narration, most ads have an omniscient narrator. Seventy out of ninety-seven ads (77.31%) have a defined protagonist. In those cases in which the human figure is visible, the most common thing is to recreate the lives of anonymous people, but the creation of ads describing a real case through its protagonist or through experts (mostly health care workers), in order to add veracity to the messages delivered, is also significant in this regard (Fig. 2).

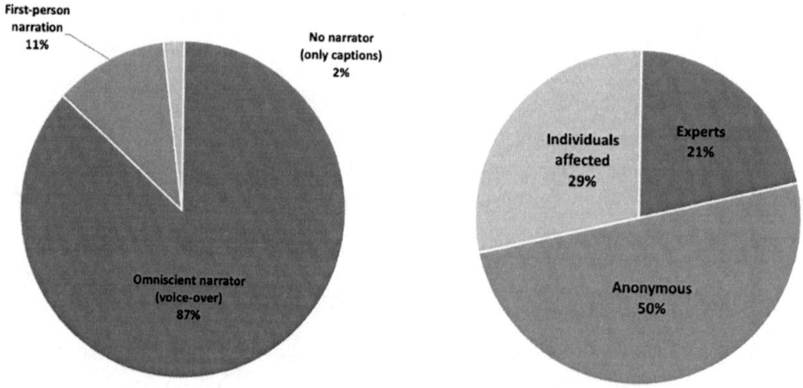

Fig. 2. Narration and human presence in advertisements.

5 Conclusions

Having analyzed institutional advertising campaigns during the first ten months, it seems evident that they were intended mainly for social networks, as reflected by the average length of most of the videos. Since advertising pieces are fewer in relation to other types of institutional communication videos, they tend to get more engagement, probably owing to their dissemination via mass media and social networks. Their publication/broadcast follows a seasonal pattern, with the highest incidence in the first months of the pandemic, in line with citizens' increased need for information, and it picks up again in December amid fears of a resurgence of cases that ended up happening in January 2021. As far as intentionality is concerned, a stronger persuasive component could have been expected, but one in four videos serves mainly informational purposes, with a higher ratio of individual appeals than what is usual in commercial communication.

In turn, institutional communication (non-advertising) campaigns emphasize the informational component, although they alternate between purely dissemination intentions and purposes of propaganda or of explaining the successes in the management of pandemic. These types of videos, of longer duration and with a more modest audiovisual production than advertising, prevailed at the beginning of the campaign and were the resource used to fight hoaxes and misinformation.

The fact that institutional advertising techniques have not been used to counter hoaxes is probably due to two reasons: firstly, because filming techniques are more sophisticated than in other institutional communication videos, and secondly, as a result of this, because they require investing more time, which makes it impossible to react immediately to potential fake news.

The predominance of voice-over as a resource, as well as the figure of influencers, seem consistent with this kind of crisis. In any case, it is striking that, in the videos featuring main characters, there is a predominance of anonymous figures, affected individuals and health care workers, in that order, compared to the leading role of experts that could be expected.

As stated above, the reporting period does not cover the beginning of vaccination, nor the impact of social networks on the dissemination of information. At the same time, such limitations open new lines of research such as studying how messages, contents and narratives evolve as the crisis progresses, until herd immunity is achieved. Another interesting topic would be to examine the demonization of certain groups singled out as guilty or the incidence of harsher or more explicit messages in terms of effectiveness.

Institutional advertising expresses ways of being a citizen [7] and the present study has revealed that public administrations have shown a proactive informational attitude, from the point of view of both advertising and institutional communication.

References

1. García Llorente, J.: El Gobierno de España como anunciante publicitario: La publicidad institucional y comercial de la Administración General del Estado (2006–2013). Razón Palabra **19**(1_89), 389–411 (2015)
2. Cortés González, A.: La publicidad institucional en España. Una década de perspectiva. Razón Palabra **75**, 1–23 (2011)
3. Martínez Pastor, E.: Publicidad institucional de las administraciones públicas: marco jurídico y controversias. Comun. Hombre **8**, 51–63 (2012)
4. Ruiz-Collantes, F.X., et al.: La construcción de la imagen pública de los organismos del Estado y la ciudadanía a través de las narraciones de la publicidad institucional televisiva. Questiones Publicitarias (Monográfico Publicidad Institucional), pp. 137–206 (2009)

5. Ibáñez Peiró, A.: La crisis del virus del Ébola en España y la gestión de la Información Pública en situaciones extraordinarias relacionadas con la salud. Cuadernos Artesanos de Comunicación, La Laguna (2017)
6. Magallón-Rosa, R.M.: La publicidad institucional en España. Evolución legislativa, tecnológica y social. Área Abierta **20**(3), 385–400 (2020)
7. García-López, M.: Publicidad institucional. Una necesaria reflexión a contracorriente. Redes **4**, 291–306 (2007)
8. Vázquez-Herrero, J., Vizoso, Á., López-García, X.: Innovación tecnológica y comunicativa para combatir la desinformación: 135 experiencias para un cambio de rumbo. Prof. Inform. **28**(3), 1–12 (2019)
9. Hao, K., Basu, T.: The coronavirus is the first true social-media "infodemic" (2020). https://www.technologyreview.com/2020/02/12/844851/the-coronavirus-is-the-first-true-social-media-infodemic/
10. Salvi, C., et al.: Going viral: how fear, socio-cognitive polarization and problem-solving influence fake news detection and proliferation during COVID-19 pandemic. Front. Commun. **5**, 1–16 (2021)
11. Apuke, O.D., Omar, B.: Fake news and COVID-19: modelling the predictors of fake news sharing among social media users. Telematics Inform. **56**, 101475 (2021)
12. Casero-Ripollés, A.: Impact of Covid-19 on the media system. Communicative and democratic consequences of news consumption during the outbreak. Prof. Inform. **29**(2), e290223 (2020)
13. Mora-Rodríguez, A., Melero-López, I.: News consumption and risk perception of Covid-19 in Spain. Comunicar **29**(66), 71–81 (2021)
14. Dafonte-Gómez, A.: Consumo y distribución de contenidos en la era digital: el papel de la audiencia en la propagación de noticias falsas. In: Renó, D., Gosciola, V., Renó, L. (eds.) Transformaçoes do Jornalismo na Nova Ecología dos Meios, Ria Editora, pp. 54–63 (2019)

Emotions and Pro-independentist Vote in Catalonia in the Elections of 2017

José Manuel Rivera Otero, Gonzalo Rodríguez Martínez(✉), and Álvaro González Gómez

Universidade de Santiago de Compostela (USC), Santiago de Compostela, Spain
josemanuel.rivera@usc.es, {gonzalo.rodriguez.martinez, alvaro.gonzalez.gomez}@rai.usc.es

Abstract. The Catalan "procés" represents an opportunity to analyze the influence of emotions on electoral behavior. The current Catalan political context, in which emotions have played such an important role, both in the construction of the independence narrative and in the discursive resources of the political and social actors, represents a unique case that allows us to measure the real impact of emotions on the construction of the independence vote decision. Assuming that, emotions directly and indirectly influence voting, we will show hox such influence is constructed through three dimensions: enthusiasm, anxiety and aversion. For this we will work with our own post-electoral survey, and we will use structural equation models as an analysis technique. Our analysis allows us to conclude that there is more enthusiasm and anxiety than aversion in the decision to vote of the Catalans on the pro-independence parties, confirming the importance of the emotional component in voting behavior.

Keywords: Emotions · Vote · Independentism · Electoral behavior · Catalonia · Procés

1 Introduction

The events that have taken place over the last years in Catalonia – largely associated to the "procés", the level of intensity reached in the demand for independence on part of the population, the massive participation of citizens in public demonstrations, the internationalisation of the conflict, or the imprisonment of some pro-independence leaders – has made the Catalonian electoral case a unique case for study.

Although the Catalan 'identity factor' has been historically present, the fact that is in as few as 10 years, the pro-independence movement in Catalonia, has gone from being a minority issue to become the main problem the Spanish democratic system must face nowadays.

In this study we address the explanation of the behavior of voters in the latest Catalan elections, trying to measure the impact of the emotional components in the decision to vote nationalist/pro-independence parties – JxCat and ERC. Our starting hypotheses, on the basis of both, the scientific literature and our previous work [1], are the following: 1) The effect of emotions on the voting decision is a dispersed effect, which is

© The Author(s), under exclusive license to Springer Nature Singapore Pte Ltd. 2022
Á. Rocha et al. (Eds.): ICOMTA 2021, SIST 259, pp. 259–269, 2022.
https://doi.org/10.1007/978-981-16-5792-4_26

directly or indirectly focalized through other political variables and especially on partisan identification; 2) In contexts of crisis, emotions associated to anxiety have a greater presence than the rest; 3) The intense confrontation associated to extreme polarization suggests that aversion emotions should play an important role in the decision-making of nationalist Catalan voters.

For our research, we will use our own post-electoral survey, which was conducted by the *Political Research Team* of USC in 2018[1]. Methodologically, we used Structural Equation Modelling (SEM), which has proved in previous own studies [1,2] and of other authors [3, 4] particularly effective in explaining the numerous relations between variables.

2 The Political Context: The Catalan "Procés"

The year 2017 was especially turbulent in the Spanish domestic political area and in the relations of the Central Government with the government of the Generalitat. Following a failed vote of no confidence against the Popular Party (PP) by Unidos Podemos with the support of other parties in June 2017, on the 1st of October of that year the self-determination referendum called by the Generalitat was held. The consequences of this referendum include the unilateral declaration of Independence by the government of Puigdemont and the ensuing destitution of the Government of the Generalitat by the central government and the calling of new elections that were held on 21st of December of that year. The December 2017 Catalan elections were a success for Ciudadanos after decades in which Convergència i Unió dominated the Catalan electoral landscape and held the government of the Generalitat. Even after its split from Unión Democrática de Cataluña (UDC), Convergencia Democrática de Cataluña (CDC) managed to win the 2015 elections in a coalition (JxSí) with, among others, Esquerra Republicana de Cataluña (ERC), this being the first victory of a purely pro-independentist candidacy. Despite this, the intensity reached by the "procés" and the pro-independentist demands by a part of the population – as well as the imprisonment of some of the politicians involved in the unilateral declaration of Independence and the flight abroad of several others – resulted in Catalan citizens losing trust in parties supporting the pro-independency "procés", which would have repercussions on electoral results.

If we analyze the support to Catalan nationalism, we may speak of a sustained growth of the exclusively Catalan sentiment (Fig. 1) since 2006, which reached its peak in 2017 (28.6%), precisely the year when the latest election was held.

[1] The *Estudio Emociones en Cataluña (EEC)* [Emotions Study in Catalonia] is a comprehensive study to analyse the political situation in Catalonia. Its sample size is 1,400 interviews with proportional allocation for age and sex and a provincial distribution, in a complex structure with a total of 18 thematic blocks and 82 questions and administered over the phone using the Computer Assisted Telephone Interviewing (CATI) system. Its universe is the population aged 18 or over residing in Catalonia.

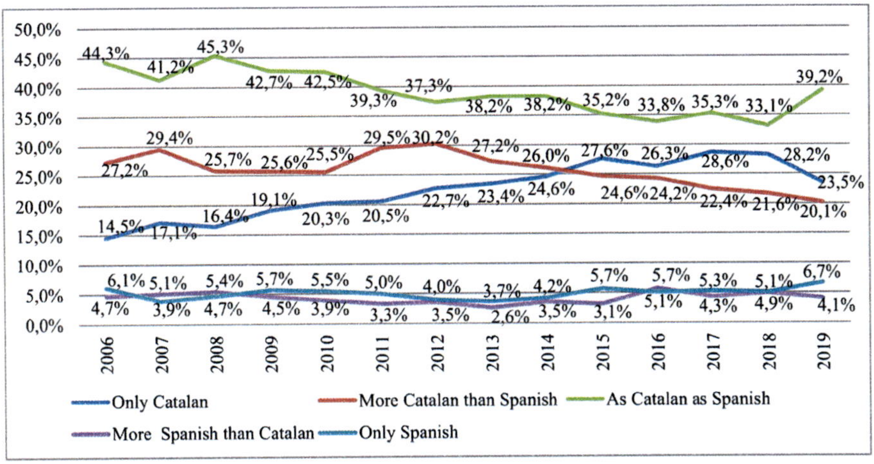

Fig. 1. Evolution of identity sentiment in Catalonia 2006–2019 (Source: Own preparation based on opinion barometers of *the Centre d'Estudis d'Opinió*)

Something similar occurs with the explicit support to independency, which, according to the data of the Centre d´Estudis d´Opinió, began to grow in 2010, reached its peak in 2013 (48.5%), and remained over 40% until 2017. However, the percentage of Catalan people who believe that Catalonia should be an independent State has progressively decreased down to 36.7% (Fig. 2).

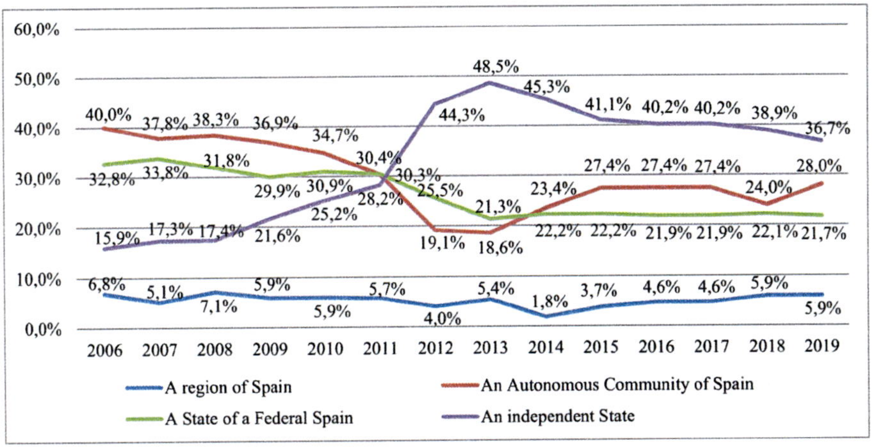

Fig. 2. Evolution of the support to the independency of Catalonia 2006–2019 (Source: Own preparation based on opinion barometers of *the Centre d´Estudis d´Opinió*)

As the data show, this increase in nationalist and pro-independence positions in Catalonia is true for an important section of the Catalan society and is reflected in an increase in the electoral support to pro-sovereignty parties. In other words, the "procés" becomes the master frame of Catalan politics and the key focal point of political competition, which is able to redirect identity and ideological positions around a single 'issue' [4]. An explanation of the electoral behaviour of Catalans in the 2017 elections will be strongly influenced by the political events of the time. If we considered the 2015 elections as a 'plebiscite' on the "procés" [2], the 2017 elections unequivocally gauged the support to independency on the part of Catalan people.

Within this special and effervescent political context in Catalonia, we consider that emotions are – more than ever – a factor when citizens make their voting decisions. But, in what way do emotions influence electoral behaviour? Which emotions have a greater influence, the positive or the negative? Is this a direct or an indirect influence? We will try to respond to these and other questions in the following pages, specifically regarding pro-independence parties or coalitions JxCat and ERC.

3 The Importance of Emotions in Explaining Political Behaviour

There is no novelty in saying that the most common approaches to explaining political behaviour rely on the hyperrationalism [5] that has dominated modern political science. Indeed, in the case of some of the most consolidated authors and approaches, when they have addressed the difference between rationality and emotion, they have done so to accept the former as the main driver of human decision making, while emotions were subsumed into the dark space of the irrational.

However, as we will see in the case of Catalonia, the traditional segregation of emotions and rationality is excessively narrow to understand the political events, obviates the existence of a conflict and encourages the displacement of politics for moral, law, economics or public management [5].

Some studies dealing with the reason/emotion dichotomy – and, in turn, the dependency between affective and cognitive signals as explanatory elements of electoral behaviour – have concluded that emotional elements have an important influence on voting decision [6–8].

The works of Campbell et al. [9] already mentioned a combination of beliefs, sentiments and behavioural intentions to refer to attitudes towards objects and there is no doubt that the explanatory paradigm of electoral behaviour based on partisan identification hides emotional components. However, the rational explanation of political behaviour has prevailed in most works explaining electoral behaviour. This is paradoxical as emotions have always been present in the centrality of the history of political thinking [10], which has led to believe that the problem lies, rather, in the difficulty of its analytic/scientific treatment [11].

The Theory of Affective Intelligence of Marcus and his colleagues [11] pointed to the primacy of emotions over cognitive aspects so that emotions are a prerequisite for the exercise of reason. In contrast to this, other approaches argue for the primacy of cognitive elements over the affective ones [12]. Our proposal, however, is based on the premise that reason and emotion are not two antagonistic dimensions, but they are complementary; they are not a dichotomy, but they go together so that reason in politics does not exist independently of emotions and vice versa [5, 13] and this enables their interpretation as socially constructed [14, 15].

Throughout this research we will show how emotions work by affecting voting behaviour, partisan identification or how variables that precede other classical variables act as mediating variables, thus showing through modelling the breaking of the reason/emotion dichotomy.

4 The Study of the Political Behaviour in Catalonia

The contributions to the analysis of electoral behaviour abound. None of them considers the impact of emotions, though. The fact is that there are few studies that address the effect of emotions on electoral behaviour [1], while research on the factors conditioning the vote of the Catalans are, however, numerous, some of them have focused on the so-called "voto dual", which means that voters' behavior changes on the basis of the type of elections [16–20]; on the retrospective analysis of voting [21]; on its spatial dimension [22, 23]; or even on an explanation underpinned by the national issue [16, 24, 25].

In our research, we have used our own post electoral survey, as there were no studies that included emotional variables in Spain, and specifically in Catalonia. The validity of surveys as a method to address emotions in political behaviour has been demonstrated in some earlier studies [1, 3]. Following the analysis of the existing literature and given some methodological problems regarding the measurement of the emotions observed in previous works, we designed our survey based on the proposal by Marcus [7], Marcus et al. [26, 27] on how to measure emotions in politics, differently from the approaches used in social psychology and applied his model first to the whole of the Spanish domain in previous works and subsequently to the case of Catalonia and the local domains.

Table 1. Emotions included in the research, dimension, and subsystem they belong to. (Source: own preparation from Marcus et al. [26])

Dimensions	Emotions	System
Enthusiasm	Tranquility, Enthusiasm, Hope and Pride	Dispositional system (Known political stimuli)
Anxiety	Disgust, Fear, Worry, Anger and Anxiety	Surveillance system (Unexpected political stimuli)
Aversion	Hatred, Contempt, Resent and Bitterness	Dispositional system (Known political stimuli)

There is no agreement in the domain of psychology – let alone in Political Science – on which emotions should be measured in order to explain political behaviour. The proposals within both fields of knowledge are numberless [11, 28–32]. In our research we opted for the model proposed by Marcus, which has already been tested several times in the domain of political behaviour [26][2]. The emotions they are asked about are thirteen,

[2] This proposal means introducing in the questionnaire a nominal filter question, which provides information on whether the respondent has ever felt a particular emotion towards a leader or a political party. If the answer is affirmative, they are asked about the degree of intensity with which they have experienced it and whether they still feel that emotion.

twelve of them correspond to the full set orthogonal proposed in the Pilot Study ANES 1995 [7]: proud, hope, enthusiastic, anxious, afraid, worried, hatred, contempt, bitter, angry, resentful, and disgusted; to which a further one was added, calm. These emotions are, in turn, grouped for their statistical processing in three dimensions: enthusiasm, anxiety and aversion (see Table 1), in accordance with the existing models, although as we will see in our analysis some data-conditioned adjustments are required. These three emotional dimensions were developed by Marcus from the work of Damasio [33, 34] and Gray [35, 36]. In his Theory of Affective Intelligence, Marcus notes the existence of two pre-conscious, emotional value systems which interfere with the behaviour of individuals. A first system, i.e., the disposition system, refers to the evaluation of the behaviours learnt on the go and corresponds to the emotional dimensions of enthusiasm and aversion as emotional responses to familiar political stimuli, whether they are positive in the first case or negative in the second case. On the other hand, the second system – the surveillance system – corresponds to the emotional response of anxiety, which occurs in new situations that require prudency. The hypothesis of these authors is that when individuals encounter known political stimuli, which confirm our positions, we can respond with emotions belonging to the domains of enthusiasm or aversion whereas when stimuli are unknown or unexpected and they pose a challenge, the response will be one of anxiety. In other words, anxiety only emerges in new or unknown situations. In our analysis we will test whether this distinction is confirmed for the case of Catalonia.

Two Structural Equations Models are introduced below to explain the vote to the two pro-independency parties which had the greatest percentage of vote in the latest elections to the Parliament of Catalonia: the coalition Junts per Catalunya (made up by the PDeCat and Convergencia Democrática de Cataluña (CDC)) and Esquerra Republicana de Catalunya (ERC). In all cases moderate levels of explanation and good adjustment indexes in the models (see Table 2) were obtained.

Table 2. Global levels of explanation and model adjustment measurements. (Source: own preparation from EEC)

	Pseudo R^2	NFI	CFI
JxCat voting model	0.52	0.973	0.977
ERC voting model	0.49	0.965	0.970

The analysis initially introduced a great number of variables in the two models, although finally only some of them are significant for explaining vote in the context of Catalonia (see models). Along with the variables already mentioned for the measurement of emotional responses towards political parties, the variables of the classical models for accounting for electoral behaviour are particularly noteworthy: sociodemographic, contextual variables, including the traditional ones and those specific to the current Catalan situation, the ideological and nationalist cleavages, the assessment of leadership and management, and variables to measure partisan identification.

Figures 3 and 4 graphically represent the result of SEM analyses for JxCat and ERC respectively.

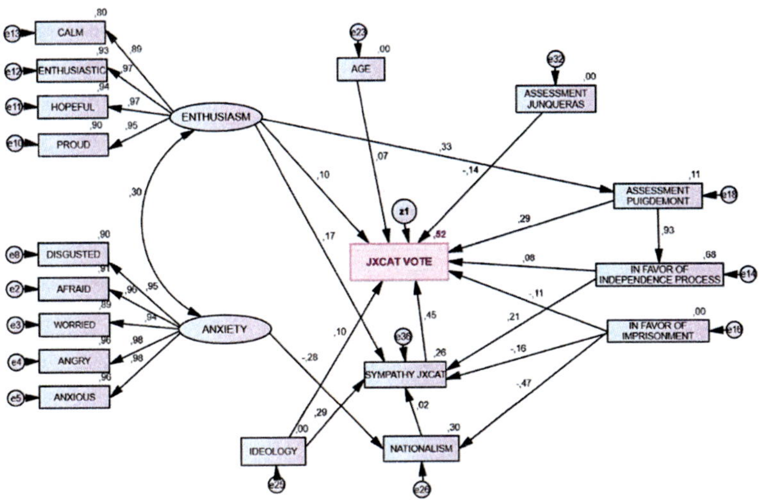

Fig. 3. SEM model of JxCat vote (Source: Own preparation form EEC)

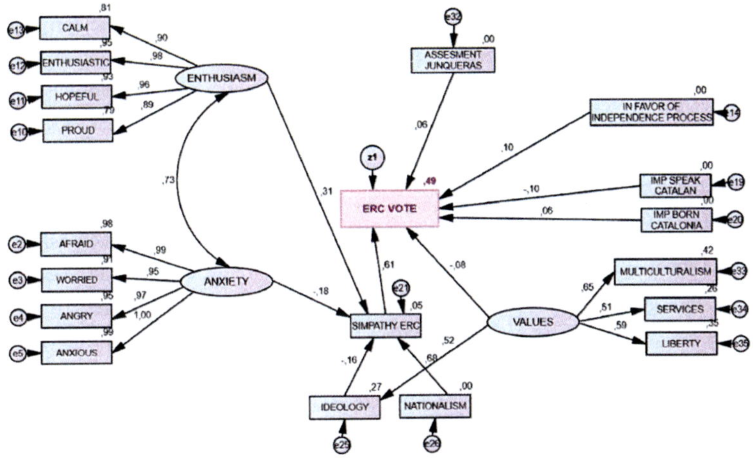

Fig. 4. SEM model of ERC vote (Source: Own preparation form EEC)

In the case of the JxCat model, like in that of ERC, the variable with the greatest predictive power is sympathy towards the party (partisan identification), followed, in the first of the models, by the assessment of the leader and former President of the Generalitat, Carles Puigdemont, who had fled the country. Also important is the explanatory power of ideology and the positioning in favor of the pro-independency process and against the incarceration of Catalan politicians. Again, the finding made in previous studies is confirmed: in the case of JxCat voters, the very process of independency is more important that the nationalist positioning itself [2], a position whose effect is indirect and with little relevance in respect of the rest of the explanatory variables. Age is also a conditioning factor in voting to this coalition so that the older the voters the more likely is their support.

As to the emotional space, we see how positive emotions of enthusiasm have a considerable influence on the vote to JxCat, both directly and indirectly, through sympathy to the party. However, the anxiety caused by JxCat among some citizens is negatively reflected in its nationalist position, which in turn has an indirect influence, albeit in a very limited extent, on the probability that they vote to this party.

Since presences are often as important as absences, it should count as a finding that aversion, contrary to what we might believe, is missing from the equation as the number of individuals who acknowledge they feel some of the emotions that make up such dimension is so small that is negligible. This is a fundamental element in our analysis which allows us to see a Catalan society galvanized in terms of enthusiasm and anxiety, but not in terms of aversion, something that sometimes does not seem to tally with the political or media narrative, which is much more heated and semantically fraught with discursive referents associated to aversion.

The model for ERC has many similarities with the one discussed above, and partisan identification is again the variable that best explains the vote to this party. Leadership, however, does not provide such an important explanatory contribution, which shows the explanatory weakness of the fact that Oriol Junqueras was already in prison; to which we should add the fact that the positioning before the imprisonments does not prove significant in this case, whereas the positioning in favor of independence is indeed significant, like in the case JxCat. Also noteworthy is the influence of two variables that have to do with a traditional nationalist reading. The first is the fact that attributing importance to having been born in Catalonia has a positive influence in voting to ERC, whereas the second, attributing importance to speaking Catalan, has a negative influence that speaks to us about the fact that the diacritic elements of primary identity – language, ethnicity, culture, history – have been now called into question in the constructivist nationalism of ERC voters, as suggested by previous studies [4].

This model of explanation of ERC vote has also the particularity that it includes three variables, which in the above model for JxCat were not significant and that make up a latent dimension we have called 'values', which refers to the positioning of voters in relation to postmaterialist values such as multiculturalism, the improvement of public services and social benefits and the security-freedom dichotomy. As it was only to be expected from a party that places itself in the left side of the ideological spectrum, positioning itself against migrants and the improvement of public services, and in favour of security reduces the probability of voting ERC.

Finally, the emotional dimensions of enthusiasm and anxiety are again present, this time exclusively in an indirect fashion, through partisan identification, in the composition of the vote to a party, while aversion is not significant either and is removed from the model.

The analysis of voting components, including the emotional ones, of the two pro-independent parties which had the greater support in the latest Catalan elections has provided us with interesting results, which in some cases confirm the results of previous research while, in other cases, have led to new hypotheses and lines of research.

5 Conclusions

Our research has contributed to highlight the importance of including emotional variables in the analysis of political behavior, particularly when explaining the electoral behavior and the decision making.

Firstly, the two models in our analysis confirm the persistence of the explanatory value of the variables associated to partisan identification, in the case of Spain, sympathy towards the party, variables which have been traditionally attributed to psychological components, although no attempt has been made to provide an in-depth explanation of the same. As our first hypothesis pointed out and as shown in other mentioned previous works, this analysis confirms that the impact of emotions in the voting decision is scattered and is expressed mainly through partisan identification. And this allows us to sustain the idea that the identification of voters with parties not only has emotional components, but it is expressed through clusters of specific emotions, associated to enthusiasm and anxiety.

Similarly, our analysis shows that such traditional cleavages as ideology or national identity, which had lost its weight in the direct explanation of voting, preserve this weight as antecedent variables of partisan identification, sharing this nature with emotions themselves.

Besides, the little presence and reduced effect of the sociodemographic variables on voting decision suggest that the fundamentally sociological explanation of electoral behavior that is characteristic of the earlier schools has lost relevance.

As to the behavior of the emotional variables, the composition of the factors is similar in both models. This shows that it is necessary to further develop into the perfecting of the methodology to measure the emotions.

Complementarily to Marcus' notion of the pre-eminence of the anxiety dimension in contexts of crisis, our work suggests that enthusiasm is also present in these contexts when such context opens the Structure of the Political Opportunity for some of the actors that are party to the conflict, as it is the case in Catalonia. The dimensions relating to enthusiasm and anxiety compose the latent variables with significant effects in both models while the scarce response obtained for items relating to the aversion dimension means that this third hypothesis is not significant in any of the models.

The absence of aversion, and in this regard, the negation of our third hypothesis, completes the emotional reading of the decision to vote nationalist parties. These results, as we have pointed out, broaden Marcus' reading whereby anxiety before political stimuli occurs at new or unexpected times. The drift of the Catalan process has resulted in extraordinary political events, leading to an exceptional situation that, in view of the data, seems compatible with stimuli able to cause anxiety in voters, but in this case, these stimuli also cause enthusiasm in certain sectors of the population which have both a direct and indirect effect on the voting decision.

Conversely, in contrast with the conflict situation that can be perceived in the Catalan society and politics – and exacerbated by the media – the resentment, hatred and bitterness that allegedly fuel the Catalan narrative seems to be absent from the emotional construction of citizens in the way we are told it is happening, or at least, these emotions do not play any role in the decision to vote to pro-independency parties.

Our analysis confirms what earlier studies on the pro-independence process of Catalonia suggested, the importance of the procés in the current Catalan political situation and the need to address this fact from a constructivist reading in order to be able to detach it from both the nationalist phenomenon and the pro-independence phenomenon.

To conclude that in the decision to vote Catalan pro-independency parties there is more enthusiasm and anxiety than aversion is tantamount to saying that the narrative exaggerates the emotions of citizens, and from this point of view, it is to be expected that the narrative ends up accommodating to the emotions rather than emotions to the narrative.

References

1. Jaráiz, E., Lagares, N., Pereira, M.: Emociones y decisión de voto. Los componentes de voto en las elecciones generales de 2016 en España. Rev. Española Invest. Sociol. (REIS) **170**, 115–136 (2020). https://doi.org/10.5477/cis/reis.170.115
2. Rivera, J., Jaráiz, E.: Modelos de explicación y componentes del voto en las elecciones autonómicas catalanas de 2015. Rev. Española Ciencia Polít. **42**, 13–43 (2016). http://dx.doi.org/10.21308/recp.42.01
3. Ciuk, D., Troy, A., Jones, M.: Measuring emotion: self-reports vs. physiological indicators. In: The 2015 Annual Meeting of Midwest Political Science Association (2015)
4. Cazorla, A., Rivera, J.: De la nación primordial a la nación en proceso: la nueva identidad nacional catalana. In: Rivera, J., Montabes, J., Lagares, N. (eds.) Cataluña en Proceso. Las elecciones autonómicas de 2015, pp. 261–288. Tirant Lo Blanch, Valencia (2017)
5. Máiz, R.L.: hazaña de la razón: la exclusión fundacional de las emociones en la teoría política moderna. Rev. Estudios Polít. (nueva época) **149**, 11–45 (2010)
6. Marcus, G.: The structure of emotional response: 1984 presidential candidates. Am. Polit. Sci. Rev. **82**, 735–761 (1988). https://doi.org/10.2307/1962488
7. Marcus, G.: Emotions in politics. In: Polsby, N. (ed.) Annual Review of Political Science, vol. 3, pp. 221–250. Annual Reviews, Palo Alto (2000)
8. Ragsdale, L.: Strong feelings: emotional responses to presidents. Polit. Behav. **13**, 33–65 (1991)
9. Campbell, A., Converse, P.E., Miller, W.E., Stokes, D.: The American Voter. Willey, New York (1960)
10. Neuman, W., Marcus, G., Grigler, A., Mackuen, M.: The Affect Effect. University of Chicago Press, Chicago (2007)
11. Marcus, G., Neuman, W., MacKuen, M.: Affective Intelligence and Political Judgment. University of Chicago Press, Chicago (2000)
12. Lazarus, R.: Emotion and Adaptation. Oxford University Press, New York (1991)
13. Bodei, R.: Geometria delle passioni. Feltrinelli, Milano (1991)
14. Turner, J., Stets, J.: The Sociology of Emotions. Cambridge University Press, Cambridge (2005)
15. Clarke, S., Hoggett, P., Thompson, S.: Emotion, Politics and Society. Palgrave Macmillan, Basignstone (2006)
16. Montero, J., Font, J.: El voto dual en Cataluña: dimensiones, sujetos y factores. Mimeo, Barcelona (1989)
17. Pallarés, F., Font, J.: Las elecciones autonómicas en Cataluña 1980–1992. In: Del Castillo, P. (ed.) Comportamiento político y electoral, pp. 221–273. CIS, Madrid (1994)

18. Riba, C.: Voto dual y abstención diferencial. Un estudio sobre el comportamiento electoral en Cataluña. Rev. Española Invest. Sociol. **91**, 59–88 (2000). http://dx.doi.org/10.2307/40184275
19. Riera, P.: L'Evolució del vot dual a Catalunya. In: Working Papers 278/09. Institut de Ciències Polítiques i Socials, Barcelona (2009)
20. Mo-Groba, D., Pereira, M.: Los componentes del voto en las elecciones autonómicas de 2015–2016 en Andalucía, Cataluña, Galicia y País Vasco. RIPS: Rev. Invest. Polít. Sociol. **17**(1) (2018). https://doi.org/10.15304/rips.17.1.4973
21. Pérez-Nievas, S., Fraile, M.: Is the nationalist vote really nationalist? Dual voting in Catalonia 1980–1999. In: Estudios/Working Papers 147, CEACS, Madrid (2000)
22. Padró-Solanet, A., Colomer, J.: Espacio político-ideológico y temas de campaña (El ejemplo de las elecciones autonómicas de Cataluña de 1992). Rev. Estud. Polít. **78**, 131–159 (1992)
23. Bacells i Ventura, L.: ¿Es el voto nacionalista un voto de proximidad o un voto de compensación?: una nueva aproximación "espacial" al voto en dos dimensiones. Rev. Española Ciencia Polít. **16**, 61–88 (2007)
24. Pallarés, F., Virós, M., Canals, R.: Els eixos de competència electoral, Estudis Electorals 10, Fundació Bofill, Barcelona (1991)
25. Argelaguet, J.: Subjective national identities in Catalonia. Natl. Ethnic Polit. **12**, 431–454 (2006). http://dx.doi.org/10.1080/13537110600882643
26. Marcus, G., MacKuen, M., Wolak, J., Keele, L.: The measure and mismeasure of emotion. In: Redlawsk, D. (ed.) Feeling Politics: Emotion in Political Information Pocessing, pp. 31–45. Palgrave Macmillan, New York (2006)
27. Marcus, G., Neuman, W., MacKuen, M.: Measuring emotional response: comparing alternative approaches to measurement. J. Polit. Sci. Res. Methods **5**(4), 733–754 (2017). https://doi.org/10.1017/psrm.2015.65
28. Watson, P.: Civil society and the politics of difference in Eastern Europe. Transit. Environ. Transl.: Feminisms Int. Polit. 21–29 (1997)
29. Watson, D., Tellegen, A.: Issues in dimensional structure of affect—effects of descriptors, measurement error, and response formats: comment on Russell and Carroll (1999)
30. Plutchik, R, Conte, H.: Circumplex models of personality and emotions. American Psychological Association (1997)
31. Russell, J.: A circumplex model of affect. J. Pers. Soc. Psychol. **39**(6), 1161 (1980)
32. Abelson, R., Kinder, D., Peters, M., Fiske, S.: Affective and semantic components in political person perception. J. Pers. Soc. Psychol. **42**(4), 619–630 (1982). https://doi.org/10.1037/0022-3514.42.4.619
33. Damasio, A.: Descartes' Error: Emotion, Reason and the Human Brain. G. P. Putnam's Sons, New York (1994)
34. Damasio, A.: The somatic marker hypothesis and the possible functions of the prefrontal cortex. Philos. Trans. R. Soc. London Ser. B-Biol. Sci. **351**, 1413–1420 (1996). https://doi.org/10.1098/rstb.1996.0125
35. Gray, J.: Causal theories of personality and how to test them. In: Joyce, J. (ed.) Multivariate Analysis and Psychological Theory. Academic Press, New York (1973)
36. Gray, J.: Brain systems that mediate both emotion and cognition. Cogn. Emot. **4**(3), 269–288 (1990). https://doi.org/10.1080/02699939008410799

Media, Applied Technologies and Communication

Media Interactivity in China. Hierarchical Cluster Analysis of China's English-Language Media

Daniel Barredo Ibáñez[1,2](✉), Linsen Su[3], and Narcisa Jessenia Medranda[4]

[1] School of Human Sciences, Universidad del Rosario, Bogota, Colombia
daniel.barredo@urosario.edu.co
[2] Fudan Development Institute, Fudan University, Shanghai, China
[3] Department of Communications, Beijing Jiatong University, Beijing, China
[4] Carrera de Comunicación Social, Universidad Politécnica Salesiana, 170517 Quito, Ecuador

Abstract. The Chinese cybersphere is one of the world's most active online spaces. On one hand, there are traditional mainstream media outlets, which are part of the State or either subject to commercial market needs. On the other hand, social media platforms have arisen: there, users are empowered, and they even allow journalism without the need for journalistic organizations. Using content analysis, we examined the interactive features of 20 English-language media located in mainland China. We found that the media incorporated more options related to usability or promotion through social media than user-generated content. Through hierarchical cluster analysis, we identified a new typology for understanding the roles adopted by the selected media: we observed a distinctive category of online information organizations—source-oriented media. Such media do not attempt to establish user communities: their target is consultation and shared social media platforms.

Keywords: China · Social media · Online media · Online journalism · Interactivity

1 Introduction

The rise of social media has been crucial to developing a more active public opinion in China. It is a country whose media outlets are under a government surveillance [10–12, 23, 25, 31] and where official media coexist with commercial media organizations [30]. But it seems that methods of communication are being transformed. According to a report of China Internet Watch [9], at the end of December 2018, there were 1.131 billon active mobile Internet users in China; they spent on average 5.7 h a day using those devices. Thus, a type of citizen has emerged who uses technological skills and features to boost online participation: the netizen. Some authors have found that the Internet constitutes an important tool for sharing opinions and mobilizing the Chinese people [13, 17, 27]. For example, through microblogging, it is possible to spread fragmented breaking news [7]. At the same time, as netizens are more exposed to international news

© The Author(s), under exclusive license to Springer Nature Singapore Pte Ltd. 2022
Á. Rocha et al. (Eds.): ICOMTA 2021, SIST 259, pp. 273–284, 2022.
https://doi.org/10.1007/978-981-16-5792-4_27

[11], they quickly learn how to avoid the moderation systems triggered by social media. Many websites demand active user participation; thus, to engage users, moderators have to be very flexible with their constraints [29]. The digital arena is apparently infinite; so, if a website has tight restrictions, quoted authors point out that users can leave that place and join a different website. According to King, Pan and Roberts [19], the Chinese government's aim with Internet surveillance is not reducing criticism but controlling social mobilization. This means that technology is often used to express discontent under certain circumstances; however, mobilization is stymied because it can cause chaos and disorder in the world's most populous country.

The Chinese Internet includes also interactive features promoted by local governments to encourage citizen participation [8, 15, 28], and official state media accounts on Sina Weibo (Chinese Twitter) which share official viewpoints [27]. Moreover, the Chinese government is making efforts to enhance the cybersphere towards promoting the state's ideals. President Xi Jinping has demanded faster "media integration" [35] towards developing more credible, influential and sustainable online media; that move is evidently the result of both the social impact and economic transformation produced by the cybersphere. According to Wang and Sparks [33], there is a shift in advertising from legacy media to new online outlets. Thus, social participation is stimulated by both online and offline media [33]. In that sense, interactivity is one of the most distinctive features in the relationship among netizens and social media. To determine trends of online informative design, we have analyzed the interactive features of some of the most important English-language online media based in mainland China.

2 Research Questions

This study focuses on the interactivity design of China's most important English-language media. Those outlets have two kinds of potential audience. First, they are information platforms directed at foreigner residents in mainland China. Second, those media are also used by Chinese who want to improve their English, as observed by Gil and Adamson [14]. Those authors found that such media play an essential role as they are a "link between speakers of different languages" (p. 30): they are a window for finding news about China and its agendas and also a common platform for sharing ideas and opinions with other users. Thus, we propose the following research questions:

- **RQ1:** What are the information design trends in implementing interactivity in the most important English-language online media in mainland China?
- **RQ2:** To what extent do such media incorporate UGC features?
- **RQ3:** To what extent do these English-language media sites stimulate the development of online communities?

3 Materials and Methods

The present study adopts a descriptive, correlational, non-experimental, cross-sectional design. It has a quantitative scope: we chose content analysis to address the above research questions; this technique allows investigation of a phenomenon using a systematic, objective, replicable approach [3]. The instrument used was proposed by Rodríguez, Codina and Pedraza [26]. It consists of a set of 36 variables divided into 8 factors related to media interactivity. The instrument was used in a previous study [4]. In line with that investigation, we standardized all the variables using a dichotomous scale of 1 or 0. Thus, if a medium had the interactivity feature observed, it received a score of 1; its absence was accorded 0. Content analysis considered only the manifest aspects [3]—not latent aspects—in each evaluated medium. Our aim was to make the media selection as exhaustive as possible. We chose both English-language versions of Chinese-language online media and other English-language media according to the following three criteria. First, the media chosen had to be information websites. Second, all the media newsrooms analysed had to be located in mainland China. Third, all the media chosen had to have updated front pages. If there were signs of abandoned or ghost media, we did not include them in our sample. As proposed in a previous study, the unit of analysis was the entire media website [22]. Thus, we did not use a sampling method: one coder analysed all the websites from 1 to 19 June 2019. The sample included the websites of the following 20 media outlets: Beijing Review; Caixin Global; China Central Television; China Daily; China Economic Net; China Global Television Network; China Military; China Plus; China Tibet Online; China Youth International; Chongqing Evening Paper; Eastday; Global Times; Guangming Daily; People's Daily; Shanghai Daily; Shenzhen Daily; Six Tone; The Economic Observer and Xinhua News Agency. Cronbach's alpha analysis for internal consistency produced a high value ($\alpha = 0.761$). That value may be considered stable and reliable: according to Huh, DeLorme and Reid [18], the indicator should be regarded as consistent when equal to or greater than 0.6. For our interpretation, we first used descriptive statistics. And, in second place, we employed a hierarchical cluster analysis, which is recommended with small samples [32]. To avoid outliers, we fixed a threshold of $+1$; thus, if a variable lacked at least two answers, it was excluded. The hierarchical cluster analysis considered 26 variables for the sample. We conducted the analysis using SPSS software, version 25. The clusters presented below emerged post hoc; they were designed according to Ward's method, with the distance calculated with a size difference for binary variables.

4 Results

Our RQ1 examined information design trends related to interactivity within our sample. As evident in Fig. 1, the analysed media tended to apply most interactive features for easier user navigation and to promote published content through Web 2.0 platforms; in the analysed media, only one of two proposed Web 2.0 tools was implemented. This finding is consistent that of previous studies: Repnikova and Fang [25] recorded that some Chinese media have a very active online profile in their platforms; they even lead in the popularity rankings of Sina Weibo. Thus, the selected media showed deeper implementation of features linked to selective interaction, i.e. better adaptation for user experience or navigation. This result is in line with our RQ2: the least adopted features were user-generated content and implementing the users' registration process. However, if we compare our findings with those in other countries, we observed more UGC than was reported for national media in Mexico and Ecuador, though less than in Colombia [4].

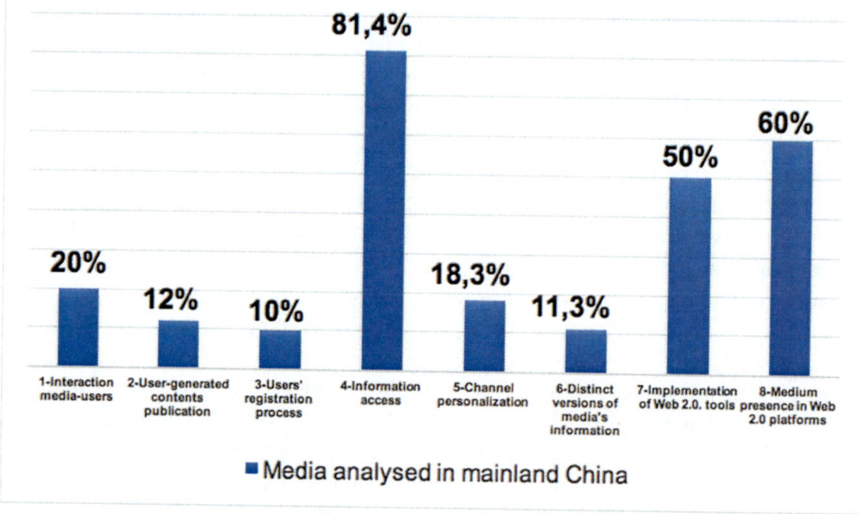

Fig. 1. Interactive features in China's English-language media (2019)

With respect to the most frequent interactive features, our analysed media often incorporated features related to usability—one of the most demanded aspects for an online information platform [5]—and the presence on social media platforms; that was because they offer many benefits for media organizations. For example, by linking their websites to such platforms, online media can be assisted by their users to enhance their news spread [17] (Table 1).

There were some features that related to facilitating the contact between users and the editor or newsroom. However, we found that the least frequent features were in line with those predicted by previous studies. Huang and Lu [17] observed that a well-known Chinese broadcasting organization, such as CCTV, considers its online users part of its "audience" (p. 782), i.e. passive consumers rather than active producers [6] (Table 2).

Table 1. Frequent interactive features in China's English-language media (2019)

Variable	%
4.1. Access to information through front page	100
4.3. Information access through related news	100
4.3. Information access through related news	95
4.4. Internal finder of news	95
7.1. Users can share news with other users	95
8.5. Medium is present in friendship social media platforms (e.g. Facebook)	95
8.6. Medium is present in microblogging social media platforms (e.g. Twitter)	95
8.7. Medium access through external social media platforms	95
1.2. Users can contact editor or newsroom	80
4.7. Medium access through external social media platforms	80

Table 2. Infrequent interactive features in China's English-language media (2019)

Variable	%
1.4. Users can vote on published news	0
1.6. Users can modify or correct informative content	0
2.4. Users can send their videos for publication	0
6.2. Users can compare global or national information treatments	0
8.3. Medium has developed its own social media	0
2.1. Users can create blogs in the medium	5
3.2. Users can contact other registered users	5
5.1. Users can adapt the interface according to their interests	5
6.3. Constant updated version of offline medium	5
7.2. Blogs published by the medium outlet	5

No analysed media allowed users to modify or correct published content; likewise, they could not adapt the interface according to their own interests. Thus, the investigated media were still deciding their agenda as gatekeepers. In RQ3, we asked to what extent the media stimulate the development of online communities. The general pattern we found was that the selected media did not frequently incorporate features related to registration processes: those could actively intervene to create a sense of community around online media. Only in one case among the media examined was it possible for users to contact other registered users.

5 Hierarchical Cluster Analysis

As noted in the Methodology section, to obtain a deeper response to RQ1, we conducted a hierarchical cluster analysis to determine the interaction of variables from a post hoc perspective. Three clusters emerged using Ward's method and distance based on size difference. The first cluster related to 10 variables that tended to appear frequently together (Fig. 2). That cluster identified media that incorporated features related to their presence in Web 2.0 platforms, implementation of Web 2.0 tools and options for information access. Such online outlets also let users contact the editor or newsroom. Those media did not attempt to enhance an active assembly of users or producers. Among such media, there was in fact a lack of characteristics related to community building, such as UGC publication, channel personalization and user registration processes.

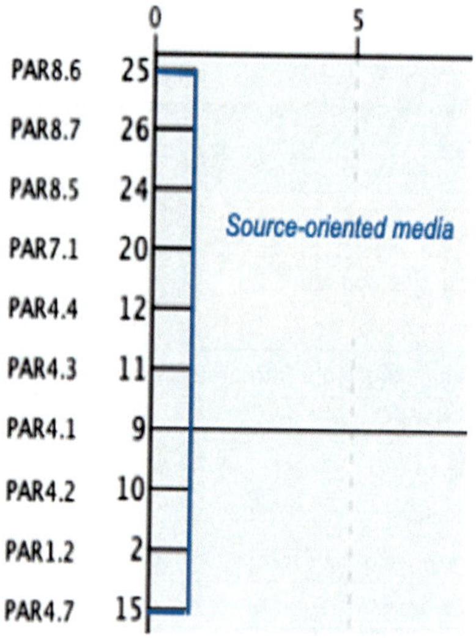

Variables	Factor
8.6. Medium is present in microblogging social media platforms (e.g. Twitter)	8-Medium presence in Web 2.0 platforms
8.7. Medium access through external social media platforms	8-Medium presence in Web 2.0 platforms
8.5. Medium is present in friendship social media platforms (e.g. Facebook)	8-Medium presence in Web 2.0 platforms
7.1. Users can share news with another users	7-Implementation of Web 2.0 tools
4.4. Internal finder of news	4-Information access
4.3. Access information through related news	4-Information access
4.1. Access to the information through the front- page	4-Information access
4.2. Access to the information through sections	4-Information access
1.2. Users can contact with the Editor or newsroom	1-Interaction media-users
4.7. Medium access through external social media platforms	4-Information access

Fig. 2. First cluster: source-oriented media interactive features in China's English-language media (2019)

Thus, the first cluster could be defined as source-oriented media: they attempted to establish a role as sources for other information platforms or be spread through social media. These source-oriented media are designed such that they do not necessarily engage with users. They function simply as information sources that can be consulted and shared. Some authors, such as Alvaro [1], have stated that some of China's English-language media function as a kind of "spokesperson" (p. 297) to spread the government's message. Accordingly, source-oriented media can be distinguished in terms of two core values: responsibility and information impact. This means that they are consulted by local and regional media, which may replicate or share the information since it is regarded as official. Among the media characterized by this trend, encouraging user participation is not regarded as important. Their aim is basically to influence the reading audience through other platforms (Fig. 3).

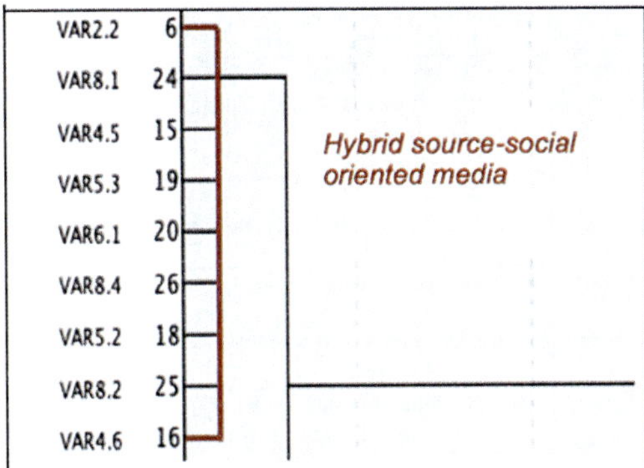

Variable	Factor
4.5. Sitemap available	4. Information access
8.2. Medium is present in photographic social media platforms (e.g. Flickr)	8. Medium presence in Web 2.0 platforms
4.6. News access through user recommendations	4. Information access
8.4. Medium is present in professional social media platforms (e.g. LinkedIn)	8. Medium presence in Web 2.0 platforms
8.1. Medium is present in audio-visual social media platforms (e.g. YouTube)	8. Medium presence in Web 2.0 platforms

Fig. 3. Second cluster: hybrid source-social oriented media interactive features in China's English-language media (2019)

This second cluster suggests that media organizations are mainly adapted from offline versions: they have not clearly defined their online presence through a deeper social concept. They seem to in the first steps of the convergence process—before they delineate a distinctive online version. Certain factors can intervene with this second cluster: they slow down user integration owing to such factors as technical costs or lack of diagnosis or quality control.

Finally, the detected third cluster (Fig. 4) suggests more dynamic social construction. These social-oriented media constitute a trend related building user community: they aim to establish a complex interaction that enhances and stimulates most of the features possible with Web 2.0. They do of course offer information since they are primarily information outlets; however, they basically want to develop deeper social participation. Accordingly, the reading audience should be considered active users or produsers [6]—even though some of the media analysed established a boundary or clear separation between information and UGC. These socially oriented media include more advanced features of participation; for example, users can send their photos or videos, and there

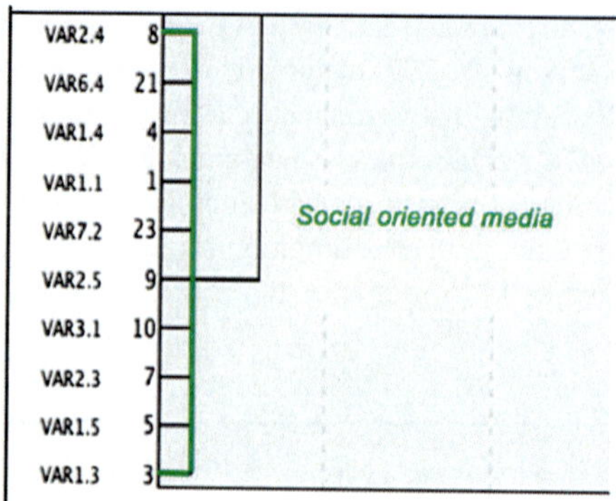

Variable	Factor
2.2. Users can send their texts for publication by the medium	2. User-generated content publication
6.1. Offline version available	6. Different versions of media information
5.3. Subscription for alerts or newsletters	5. Channel personalization
1.5. Users can comment on posts of hosted blogs	1. Interactive media users
2.3. Users can send their photos for publication by the medium	2. User-generated content publication
2.5. There is an exclusive section available for UGC	2. User-generated content publication
5.2. Syndication availability	5. Channel personalization
3.1. Users can be registered	3. User registration process
6.4. Offline version available adapted to Web 2.0	6. Different versions of media information
1.3. Users can comment on news	1. Interactive media users
1.1. Users can communicate with news authors	1. Interactive media users

Fig. 4. Third cluster: social-oriented media interactive features in China's English-language media (2019)

are one or more sections specifically for publishing UGC. At the same time, users can register, and there is an evident increase in features related to a deeper relationship between media and users. Thus, these media aim to present a social focus: along with the information, the aim is to promote user communities via the website.

6 Discussion

English-language media in mainland China are important platforms owing to social, international and economic reasons. First, they provide a meeting point for foreigners living in China and also for Chinese speakers wanting to learn English. Second, such media can be considered an opportunity for spreading Chinese culture overseas. Third, as Gil and Adamson [14] state, some Chinese economic sectors depend on English, such as tourism and leisure, business and management. Thus, improving the quality of online English-language media can be regarded as a way to engage users, provide a window to encourage better understanding of China, and promote international corporations, services or products in that regard.

Our results suggest possible innovations in the studied media. First, the Internet has to be considered a way for complementing available information sources [30]. The public space undergoing development in the digital arena establishes a multidirectional means of communication; that is in contrast to offline media, which are characterized by unidirectionality [29]. In that sense, interactivity is the key to expanding the communication possibilities of media outlets. Thus, interactivity has to be seen primarily as a "source of revenue" (p. 193) [28]: according to those authors, it functions in response to social media companies. However, with most of the media examined in some countries (México, Colombia or Ecuador) [4], there was a clear separation between user contributions and information.

Second, interactivity helps focus a user community around a media outlet. Thus, interactivity can be identified as a major factor for engaging users [8]. This point is more relevant for young users, who are more influenced by technological platforms than by legacy media [11]. However, interactivity should also be regarded as a factor that can promote broader participation with media outlets. Contrary to what might be supposed, Chinese governments (both national and local) offer many citizen interaction opportunities. Some interesting interactive initiatives encouraged by China's government have emerged in recent years, such as the mayor's mailbox on local websites [15]: those are direct channels of communication between local authorities and citizens. A direct, friendly style is evident with some Sina Weibo accounts on state media [27]. There has even been the online adoption of information websites [16], which has led to the launching of online versions in Chinese, English and other languages. So, a transformation has taken place through the efforts of public authorities, activation of Chinese netizens [27] and convergence of offline media towards promoting an online presence [16]. Accordingly, we found some indications pointing to partial adaptation of online procedures. We observed communicative interaction to be less frequent than selective interaction; thus, the media were more equipped for consultation and dissemination rather than user integration and community building. We support this inference with reference to a typological explanation regarding the online editorial trends of Chinese online media in English: we found that some media apparently do not place emphasis on intensifying the user experience; they are prominent organizations whose news is going to influence a great number of secondary sources (e.g. local media).

We did, however, observe a curious paradox: interactive communication spaces (e.g. posting a comment) could be seen as possible sources of disharmony or social mobilization; however, their omission on online media encouraged users to move away and interact through social media platforms. Such collaborative spaces cannot be easily moderated or supervised [7, 28]: users quickly learn how to avoid observation—just as journalists adopt tactics to evade the censorship apparatus [31]. Thus, social media induces uncertainty in China, where national identity is associated with generalized use of technology.

Contemporary journalism derives from both media organizations and from social media [20, 24]. This means that every citizen is potentially a journalist if they open an account in, for example, Sina Weibo or Tencent Weibo. In fact, "collective action" (p. 326) [19], which is apparently the main focus of Internet surveillance, is more likely to occur with social media than with online media. That conclusion can be explained by Appelgren [2]: the delusive practices orchestrated by online media outlets organize social participation through a filtered process, which does not apparently exist on social media. At the same time, restrictions imposed on online media relocate users to social media platforms: the exclusion of interactive proposals of Web 2.0 results in isolation [24].

There are legal, technical and professional problems that affect UGC implementation; therefore, content moderation is the solution that has been developed by media organizations that present an inclusive response. Indeed, content moderation is the main reason for the greater likelihood of social mobilization through social media than in interactive communication spaces managed by online media. Professional journalists can define the limits of Chinese public opinion, but that can lead to confusion among netizens. That is why in China, it is necessary to develop a creative transformation: netizens and journalists should work together—as their predecessors did during the Cultural Revolution [25] by combining art and propaganda.

This article has demonstrated that Chinese online media outlets based in mainland China conform to a distinctive typology. President Xi Jinping asserts that online Chinese media have be transformed through more "media integration" [35]; thus, it is necessary to implement deeper communication interaction with features related to UGC publication to get users more involved with "interactive participatory persuasion" (p. 777) [25]—and also to attract advertisers, which are moving away to new online outlets [34]. Thus, in line with the indicated typology, source-oriented media should progressively change to socially oriented media platforms, where users can actively discuss topics related to their interest communities. In that regard, China Daily is a very good example of a socially oriented medium that is run by the state but manages to sustain a complex, dynamic online community of English-language users.

In future studies, it would be interesting to examine and compare the present results with those of online media in Chinese. It would also be interesting to investigate user perceptions of such media. From our analysis, we propose a deeper implementation of interactive features; however, such features would not automatically result in a more collaborative culture. It is imperative to educate new journalists in what Mackay and Tong [21] describe as "more pro-active" (p. 69) moderation. This means that contemporary communication professionals who specialize in online media need to be able to promote a more dynamic conversation with users [13]: that would result in the identification of errors or transgressions; it would also help promote a more positive dialogue, which would enrich media outlets and citizen participation in general. That suggests another interesting line of research in continuing the findings of the present study: how to create a dialogue between journalists and users through media platforms in a complex online scenario, such as in China.

Acknowledgements. This article was funded through the Fudan Development Institute (FDDI) as a result of a visit by Daniel Barredo to Fudan University (Shanghai, China) from 25 May 2019 to 30 June 2019. The authors acknowledge and recognize all the support provided by the FDDI, Universidad del Rosario and Fudan University. We thank the Edanz Group (www.edanzediting.com/ac) for editing a draft of this manuscript.

References

1. Alvaro, J.J.: Discursive representations of a dissident: the case of Liu Xiaobo in China's English press. Discour. Soc. **24**(3), 289–314 (2013)
2. Appelgren, E.: An illusion of interactivity. Journal. Pract. **12**(3), 308–325 (2018)
3. Bardin, L.: Content Analysis, 3rd edn. Akal, Madrid (2002)
4. Barredo, D., Díaz-Cerveró, E.: Interactivity in Latin American digital journalism. An analysis of the main cybermedia of Colombia, Mexico and Ecuador (2016). Rev. Lat. Comun. Soc. **72**, 273–294 (2017)
5. Barredo Ibáñez, D., De la Garza, D., Freundt-Thurne, Ú., Pinto, K.T., Días, D.L.: Questioning the existence of the prosumer in Ibero-America. A study on university students from Colombia, Peru Chile, and Spain. LETRAL **20**, 183–205 (2018)
6. Bruns, A.: Gatekeeping, gatewatching, real-time feedback: new challenges for journalism. Braz. Journal. Res. **7**(2), 117–136 (2011)
7. Chan, Y.: Chinese journalists circumvent government's tight testrictions. Nieman Rep. **65**(1), 53–57 (2011)
8. Chen, Q., Xu, X., Cao, B., Zhang, W.: Social media policies as responses for social media affordances: the case of China. Gov. Inf. Q. **33**, 313–324 (2016)
9. China Internet Watch. China saw 1.1 billion active mobile devices in 2018, 2 September 2019. https://www.chinainternetwatch.com/28796/mobile-device-trend-2019/
10. Cui, D., Lin, T.T.: Professional intervention and organizational incorporation: examining journalistic use of microblogs in two Chinese newsrooms. Asian J. Commun. **25**(4), 351–370 (2014)
11. Di, C., Fang, W.: New channels, new ways of becoming informed? Examining the acquisition of public affairs knowledge by young people in China. Inf. Dev. **20**(10), 1–15 (2018)
12. Fu, J.S., Lee, A.Y.L.: Chinese journalists' discursive Weibo practices in an extended journalistic sphere. Journal. Stud. **17**(1), 80–99 (2016)
13. Gao, F., Martin, R.: New scheme of communication: an exploratory study of interactivity and multimedia use in Chinese j-blogs and the implications. Asian J. Commun. **21**(1), 69–83 (2011)
14. Gil, J., Adamson, B.: The English language in mainland China: a sociolinguistic profile. In: Feng, A. (ed.) English Language Education across Greater China, pp. 23–45. Multilingual Matters, New York (2011)
15. Hartford, K.: Dear mayor: Online communications with local governments in Hangzhou and Nanjing. China Inform. **19**(2), 217–260 (2005)
16. Hassid, J., Repnikova, M.: Why Chinese print journalists embrace the Internet. Journalism **17**(7), 882–898 (2016)
17. Huang, L., Lu, W.: Functions and roles of social media in media transformation in China: a case study of "@CCTV NEWS". Telemat. Inform. **34**, 774–785 (2017)
18. Huh, J., DeLorme, D.E., Reid, L.N.: Perceived third-person effects and consumer attitudes on preventing and banning DTC advertising. J. Consum. Aff. **40**(1), 90–116 (2006)
19. King, G., Pan, J., Roberts, M.: How censorship in China allows government criticism but silences collective expression. Am. Polit. Sci. Rev. **107**(2), 326–343 (2013)
20. López Parra, R.: Revolutionize the way of doing journalism in China. Revista Mexicana de Comunicación 43–48 (2013)
21. Mackay, H., Tong, J.: Interactivity, the global conversation and world service research: digital China. Participations J. Audience Recept. Stud. **8**(1), 48–74 (2011)
22. Massey, B.L., Levy, M.R.: Interactivity, online journalism, and English-language web newspapers in Asia. Journal. Mass Commun. Q. **76**(1), 138–151 (1999)

23. Peidong, Y., Lijun, T.: "Positive energy": hegemonic intervention and online media discourse in China's Xi Jinping ra. China Int. J. **16**(1), 1–22 (2018)
24. Peters, C., Witschge, T.: From grand narratives of democracy to small expectations of participation. Journal. Pract. **9**(1), 19–34 (2015)
25. Repnikova, M., Fang, K.: Authoritarian participatory persuasion 2.0: netizens as thought work collaborators in China. J. Contemp. China **27**(113), 763–779 (2018)
26. Rodríguez, R., Codina, L., Pedraza, R.: Indicators to evaluate the quality of online journalism web sites: an analysis of Web 2.0 interaction and adoption. Rev. Española Doc. Científica **35**(1), 61–93 (2012)
27. Song, Y., Chang, T.K.: Managing impressions online: microblogs and the state media's adaptation of online logics in China. Journalism **18**(8), 1064–1081 (2017)
28. Stockmann, D., Luo, T.: Which social media facilitate online public opinion in China? Probl. Post-Commun. **64**(3–4), 189–202 (2017)
29. Tang, L., Sampson, H.: The interaction between mass media and the internet in non-democratic states: the case of China. Media Cult. Soc. **34**(4), 457–471 (2012)
30. Xie, W., Zhao, Y.: Is seeing believing? Comparing media credibility of traditional and online media in China. China Media Res. **10**(3), 64–73 (2014)
31. Xu, D.: Online censorship and journalists' tactics. Journal. Pract. **9**(5), 704–720 (2014)
32. Vilà, R., Rubio, M.J., Berlanga, V., Torrado, M.: How to perform and interpret an exploratory factor analysis using SPSS Statistics. REIRE **7**(1), 113–127 (2014)
33. Wang, Q.: Participatory journalism in the Chinese context: understanding journalism as process in China's participatory culture. Journalism **18**(4), 501–517 (2017)
34. Wang, H., Sparks, C.: Chinese newspaper groups in the digital era: the resurgence of the party press. J. Commun. **69**, 94–119 (2019)
35. Wei, X., Desheng, C.: Xi urges greater use of new media, 26 January 2019. http://www.chinadaily.com.cn/a/201901/26/WS5c4b4cbea3106c65c34e69af.html

Community Radio in Ecuador: Cayambe Radio Message Case

César Andrade-Martínez[1](✉), Luis Álvarez-Rodas[1](✉), Ángel Hernando[2](✉), and Abel Suing[3](✉)

[1] Salesian Polytechnic University, Cuenca, Ecuador
{candrade,lalvarez}@ups.edu.ec
[2] University of Huelva, Huelva, Spain
angel.hernando@dpsi.uhu.es
[3] Private Technical University of Loja, Loja, Ecuador
arsuing@utpl.edu.ec

Abstract. Community radio is the media with the greatest penetration and significance in the world, providing cognitive and methodological contribution to the production of knowledge and the processes of democratization of culture. In Ecuador, community radio is part of the history of indigenous villages and nationalities linked to social claims especially vulnerable sectors, such as spaces for the recomposition of the social groups, intercultural education, and the construction of ancestral identities. Community Radio "Message" of Cayambe, from its beginnings, was the alternative that exploited and unprotected communities have used in the defense of nature, land and human rights; but also for the production and survival of the peoples. The research is qualitative with an exploratory, descriptive and interpretive approach and scope with an ethnographic design. For this purpose, several people linked directly and indirectly to the station were interviewed to obtain data regarding the sociocultural contribution that Radio Message has had since its creation. The results of the investigation show a high index of reliability regarding the social work of Radio Message. Currently the community radio station continues to be the voice of the indigenous and peasant communities of Cayambe and Pedro Moncayo, which for a long time were subordinate to the information broadcast by traditional media.

Keywords: Community radio · Indigenous nationalities · Ancient languages · Alternative radius · Freedom of expression

1 Introduction

Community radio in Ecuador, a multicultural and plurinational country, is the non-profit media. Its main objective is to inform, educate, entertain and amuse the audience through productions in different genres, styles, types of programs according to the communicative needs of collective societies with identity, values and cultures, producing "social senses provoking processes related to Aboriginal identities and with intercultural dialogue" (p. 104) [12].

© The Author(s), under exclusive license to Springer Nature Singapore Pte Ltd. 2022
Á. Rocha et al. (Eds.): ICOMTA 2021, SIST 259, pp. 285–294, 2022.
https://doi.org/10.1007/978-981-16-5792-4_28

It is the place where listeners can identify, recognize and communicate with each other, facilitating and encouraging their participation in processes that affect the community and that, together, achieve responses to social problems. "Building community can then be an attempt to strengthen the local versus the national or global. It implies building the local public sphere, the space for meeting and democratic debate at that level" (p. 14) [13].

Currently, the Ecuadorian community radio is strengthened and resurfaces thanks to the Organic Law of Communication LOC, the same one that in Art. 106 distributes with 34% of the radioelectric spectrum in its favor, which allows to cover new spaces for the benefit of the various Ancestral communities and peoples of Ecuador [14].

Applying social responsibility is imposed on the economic aspect to promote the direct participation and defense of citizen interests, informing in a timely, truthful and transparent manner. Respecting the opinion of all members of society, promoting cultural diversity, listening to the participation and voice of women, without any discrimination or censorship, "these types of stations belong to groups, individuals or entities that organically represent the indigenous movement or local peasant" (p. 76) [2].

Having the advantage of easy reach and immediacy within society as a means of mass communication, community radio allows all members of the community to freely express themselves, express their ideas and opinions on facts and events of which they are direct and indirect actors. In the search for the truth, achieving possible solutions to problems and concerns that arise in common in educational, political, cultural, social issues, among others.

Rights that, established in the law, are not complied with, evidencing that the ancestral peoples in Ecuador "have been passive subjects in relation to the use of the media, not of their own free will, nor because they lack the ability to use technology, but because of the continuation of the inequalities established since long ago" (p. 60) [19]. However, community radio promotes the unity and participation of community members, achieving the imaginary of the circumstances and conditions in which the population develops, forming a world of color, voices, sounds, music, acoustic images, soundscapes, innovation and environmental creativity, and other radio elements.

Under these technical and humanistic conditions, on the functions of the radio, the investigation exposes the importance of the community radio stations in Ecuador; specifically to Community Message Radio (RMC) located in the Cayambe canton of the province of Pichincha. Station that during the last four decades maintained a regular miscellaneous and musical programming, as a result of the lack and economic self-support. Eight years ago the radio replaced its grill with an active, monothematic and inclusive programming; a situation that generated a change in the productive life of the members of the indigenous and peasant communities of the Cayambe and Pedro Moncayo cantons who live in the sector in precarious situations.

2 Research Methodology

The research is qualitative, which allowed "the collection and analysis of data to refine the research questions or reveal new questions in the interpretation process" (p. 7) [10]. As research tools, the method of unstructured interviews was used focused as "a specific form of social interaction that aims to collect data for an inquiry" (Behar [5], p.55); activity that was carried out during the period from November to December 2020 to several people directly and indirectly linked to the station in order to obtain objective data regarding the sociocultural contribution that RMC has had since its inception. The characters who were interviewed are: Javier Herrán Gómez, director Cayambe's Salesian house; José Juncosa Blasco, anthropologist and researcher at the UPS Salesian Polytechnic University; Armando Grijalva Brito, UPS researcher professor; Carlos Cisneros, former director of RMC; Sofía Cuascoto, indigenous leader of the Cayambe community; Pablo Tera, current director of RMC; Gina Tafur, coordinator of the station; and Wilson Fabián Alba, member of the Cayambe community.

To develop the interviews, the actors in question were selected, as a voluntary sample or intentional sampling, in accordance with the criteria of representativeness, relevance and adequacy. The invited participants, predisposed, contributed more and better information to the research. The interviews were developed with questions of unrestricted or open characteristics.

The scope of the research was exploratory and descriptive because there are no previous works related to RMC, the interpretive paradigm was applied because it focused on the experiences and opinions that social actors have regarding the formation of RMC. A bibliographic and hemerographic review of the literature was also carried out in Wos, Scopus and Google Scholar.

3 Research Results

3.1 Community Radio in Latin America and Its Use in Education

The appearance of radio that arises at the service of all humanity and without distinction of economic condition, were also identified as popular stations, but they did not distance themselves from community stations as alternative media, since they imposed themselves against multiple needs of society, and to counterpoint the dictatorial speeches of the power elites of the time. "In Ecuador, community radio stations were the first media that were created and had an educommunication purpose" (p. 129) [17]. In addition, these stations were the basis of a true educational process to combat illiteracy in depressed and marginalized communities and peoples.

In Ecuador, community radio had its beginnings thanks to social development work inspired by the Catholic Church, which created the Popular Radio Schools of Ecuador ERPE. The process was initiated by Monsignor Leónidas Proaño, who dedicated his life to the vindication of indigenous and peasant peoples, whom he made literate through radio as the most effective means of communication for this purpose, "decided to found the Popular Radio Schools from Ecuador and in March 1962 it began emissions" (p. 28) [18].

And it is precisely through the ERPE that it was taken during the indigenous and peasant uprising, by the Confederation of Indigenous Nationalities of Ecuador CONAIE in May 1990. From there messages were issued in Quichua about the paralysis of activities throughout the country, demanding from the government of President Rodrigo Borja Cevallos, the fulfillment of the mandate for the ethnic, educational, social and legalization rights of their ancestral lands.

For the 90s' The Coordinator of Popular Educational Radio of Ecuador CORAPE, with 30 years of experience in the construction and strengthening of alternative, popular, citizen and community media, manages to manage the acceptance of community radios before the Ecuadorian State in the Constitution of the country, the same that is maintained to this day [8].

The community radios have their objective of focused attention on their towns, who tune in to the station while they carry out their agricultural and productive work tasks from the early hours of the morning, allowing the active participation of their listeners. Its mission is to democratize communication, ensuring the participation and inclusion of all. Assessing and identifying all kinds of opinions that are raised as possible solutions to the problems that arise in the community in a supportive and timely manner.

It has served as an educommunicative tool in the rescue of ancestral mother tongues of the different peoples and nationalities of Ecuador. Generating an active and effective intercultural communication not only to inform, but also to educate according to their natural environments of life with the Paccha Mama [17] consider that "locating talking radios in spaces where there is little access to the media, enables social actors to acquire tools and thus empower themselves by exercising their right to free expression of their reflections and needs" (p .129).

Article 14 of the LOC goes hand in hand with Article 36, which, on the right to intercultural and plurinational communication, assumes "indigenous, Afro-Ecuadorian and Montubian peoples and nationalities have the right to produce and disseminate in their own language, content that expresses and reflect their worldview, culture, traditions, knowledge and knowledge" (p. 8) [14].

The same Constitution of Ecuador in Section III, Article No. 16 that refers to Communication and Information, grants people, individually or collectively, the right to "free, intercultural, inclusive, diverse and participatory communication, in all areas of social interaction, by any means and form, in their own language and with their own symbols" (p. 30) [3].

The rights enshrined in the laws and constitutional regulations are rights that are the product of the constant social struggle of the communities throughout a process of equality and democratization of communication, which has resulted in the distribution of radio frequencies for various communities in Ecuador, as seen in the following table (Table 1):

Radio is a strategic and privileged space for nationalities and peoples of Ecuador to exercise their right to communication, as it is a medium based on orality, in the word, as well as low cost and high impact (p. 203) [4].

For Geovanna Gasparello, the management of community radio stations is to spread the reality of indigenous peoples, according to their experiences, their vision and their language. Radio is an invaluable instrument for the strengthening of languages in the face of the decrease in speakers, as claimed by the announcers of Ñomndaa Radio, of the Autonomous Municipality of Suljaa (Xochistlahuaca) of the State of Guerrero in Mexico. The only station in the indigenous Amuzga language. "All the radios of the nationalities, now the ancestral and intercultural languages are channels of communication with the communities and a way of transmitting their knowledge, ways of life and needs from their own actors and local voices" (p. 99) [16].

Table 1. Community Radios of the Peoples and Nationalities of Ecuador as of 2016

Radios	Nationality	Languages	Province
La Voz de Nae 89.7 FM	Achuar del Ecuador	Achuar Chicham	Morona Santiago
Tarimiat 93.5 FM	Shiwiar del Ecuador	Shiwiar	Pastaza
La Voz de la Frontera 95.9 FM	Andwa del Ecuador	Kichwa	Pastaza
Nase 92.7 FM	Nación Sapara del Ecuador	Sapara	Pastaza
Wao Apeninka 91.1 FM	Waorani del Ecuador	Huao Tiriro Kichwa	Pastaza
Tasanda Jenfa 90.0 FM	A¨I Kofán del Ecuador	Ai'Ingae	Sucumbíos
La Voz de Tuna 94.7 FM	Federación de Nacionalidad Shuar de Pastaza	Shuar Chicham	Pastaza
Jatari Kciwa 92.3 FM	Asociación de Comunidades Indígenas de Araujo-Kichwas	Kichwa	Pastaza
Ñucanchi Muskuy 92.3 FM	Organización de comunidades Kicwa de Loreto-Orellana	Kichwa	Orellana
Stereo Espera Siapidaarade 90.7 FM	Éperara Siapidaara del Ecuador	Sia Pedee	Esmeraldas
Chachi 89.5 FM	Federación de Centros Chachi de Esmeraldas	Cha Palaa	Esmeraldas
Somba Pamin 102.5 FM	Tsáchila	Tsá Fiqui	Santo Domingo
Ampara Su 90.7 FM	Federación de Centros Awa del Ecuador	Awapit	Imbabura-Ibarra
Radio Siona 89.7 FM	Organización de Nacionalidades Siona el Ecuador	Paicoca	Sucumbíos-

In January 2017, the Agency for the Regulation and Control of Telecommunications ARCOTEL of Ecuador, reported the list of assignments of the public tender of frequencies for radio and television with open signal, where 61 frequencies were assigned to community media of which 49 are radios, 26 of them affiliated with CORAPE as indicated in Table 2 [1]. But, only two years later, in January 2019, ARCOTEL reports that "there is a total of 1,064 radios, of which 64 correspond to community radios, which represent 6% of the total frequencies" [7]. In December 2020, the National Government of President Lenin Moreno resolved to assign 3,096 FM radio frequencies, of which 168 would be destined for community stations [9].

Table 2. 26 Ecuadorian Community Radios affiliated with CORAPE

Radios Comunitarias	Provincias
Antena Libre	Esmeraldas
Católica de Cuenca	Azuay
Católica de Manabí	Guayas, Manabí
Chaguarurco	El Oro, Loja
El Buen Pastor	Azuay, Loja, Morona Santiago
ERPE	Bolívar, Chimborazo, Tungurahua
Frontera	Carchi
Guamote	Chimborazo
HCM1	Pichincha
Ideal Tena	Napo, Orellana, Pastaza
Ilumán	Imbabura
Irfeyal	Imbabura, Pichincha
La Voz de Ingapirca	Azuay, Cañar, Morona Santiago
Latacunga	Bolívar, Cotopaxi, Guayas, Los Ríos, Manabí
Luz y Vida	Loja
Matovelle HCM3	Azuay, El Oro, Loja, Zamora Chinchipe
Mensaje	Pichincha
Ondas de Paltas	Loja
Puyo	Morona Santiago, Napo, Pastaza
Runacunapac	Bolívar
San Francisco	Nacional
Santa Cruz	Galápagos
Sonoonda	Azuay, Chimborazo, Loja
Sucumbíos	Carchi, Napo, Orellana, Sucumbíos
Voz del Santuario de Baños	Pastaza, Tungurahua
Voz del Upano	Azuay, Cañar, Zamora Chinchipe

3.2 Cayambe Radio Message: Alternative Means of Training and Community Development

The indigenous populations of the Cayambe and Pedro Moncayo cantons located 70 km away from Quito in the northeastern area of the province of Pichincha, have been victims, since the time of the colony, of constant labor exploitation and expropriation of their lands, submerging them in a world of total poverty.

It is until the 1950s with the appearance of the Salesian Society that a transformation begins in favor of the inhabitants of the sector. José Ignacio López Vigil [15] cited by Chimbo et al., States that "Inti Pacha in Cangahua, Cayambe canton, was the first indigenous radio station, which led to the emergence of others in Imbabura, Chimborazo and Bolívar that, little by little, consolidated a concept of community indigenous radio stations" (p. 144) [6].

With the aim of promoting evangelization and social promotion; and by management of Monsignor Isaías Barriga Naranjo, Radio Message a Seed of Hope was founded on November 23, 1967 in Tabacundo, where socio-cultural work began to educate an indigenous and peasant population through the radio where 50% did not he could read or write. This is pointed out by José Juncosa, an anthropologist and researcher at the Salesian Polytechnic University of Quito, who narrates that, thanks to the initiatives and experiences on the radio teaching system, carried out by Monsignor Leónidas Proaño in the city of Riobamba, province of Chimborazo; The educommunication method that had already been used by Sutatenza radio in Colombia was applied. (Juncosa J. Personal interview, December 16, 2020).

The literacy process began using short wave radio-receivers so that the population of the rural sectors of Cayambe and Pedro Moncayo can receive the information. However, the problems appeared immediately; for example, there was demotivation in the population, since the reality or the context of the situation was not reported; on the other hand, the station signal became intermittent, which caused lags in the teaching process (Juncosa J. Personal interview, December 16, 2020).

In the 1980s, the Salesians created the Peasant House of Cayambe Foundation and set their sights on the critical situation of poverty and marginality of the indigenous people of the sector, giving way to the construction of various educational works. Starting in 1990, with the encouragement of Father Javier Herrán Gómez, Director of the peasant house of Cayambe, the station became a work of the community. In August of that year the radio transmission from Cayambe was restarted on the dial 1590 AM https://bit.ly/2QHI01L Since then and motivated by the Salesian charism, under the figure and thought of Saint John Bosco, radio programs of joy, motivation, information, education and entertainment [11].

In May 2012, with the canonical visit of Father Marcelo Farfán, Inspector of the Salesians, it was decided to make the proposal to the Social Communication career of the Salesian Polytechnic University in Quito (UPS) so that the radio could become a laboratory of practices for students and as a link in the proposals of connection with the community. Thus, on November 30 of the same year, with the presence of Father Javier Herrán, rector of the UPS; the master Viviana Montalvo, Vice-rector of the Quito headquarters; the master's degree María del Carmen Ramírez; Director of the Social Communication Career; authorities, teachers and students, the RMC relaunch program is carried out (Grijalva A. Personal interview, November 14, 2020).

The experiences, anecdotes multiplied among the community, once it was coordinated so that the same indigenous and peasants of the sector; besides learning to read, write, add, multiply and divide; They can carry out community work in mingas and campaigns for planting and harvesting vegetables, reforestation, agricultural production and consumption of quality milk were coordinated, says the former director of the station Carlos Cisneros. These activities gave way to the formalization of several grassroots organizations, where their respective leaders formed the Association of savings and credits through a community system.

Currently, RMC has modern and digital equipment, where both Communication students, as well as the different instances of the UPS, works of the Salesian Community and local organizations, develop direct communication spaces with the communities of the city and the country, doing living experience with the rural and urban population of the Cayambe and Pedro Moncayo cantons to the north of Pichincha, as well as in the southern part of the Imbabura province, points out Pablo Terán Puente, current director of RMC. "One of the main activities to highlight is the participation of Communication students in Bonding projects, training radio producers, benefiting around 100 participants, who emerge as their own managers of live radio programming" (Terán P. Personal interview, November 14, 2020).

Interculturality is the main ingredient in RMC programming. Local and international events are promoted and reported thanks to the satellite system. RMC, today, is the official voice of the Salesian Work in Cayambe. It has an integrated mobile communication system that allows live broadcasts to the air and direct from neighborhoods and communities [11].

Gina Tafur, coordinator of RMC explains that "the radio is frequently requested for interviews by public institutions, covering municipal events in both Cayambe and Pedro Moncayo, as well as interviews with officials from the Secretary of Public Procurement SERCOP, Ministries of Health MSP, and of Economic and Social Inclusion MIES, etc." (Tafur G. Personal interview, November 14, 2020).

Sonia Cuascoto, leader of the Cayambe canton and coordinator of the Luciérnaga Comunitaria radio program, explains that RMC has helped the community mainly as a means in which we talk about our products, at the beginning when we did the program listening to my colleagues, I am sincere the first times we spoke with the microphone we were shaking, they stutter to speak, now they function well. I have listened to the programs and they are quite informative, it is a pure reality, because it comes from the mouths of the members themselves, who may not be the right words, but they speak as they say "lo cholo", their truth is their reality. (Cuascoto S. Personal interview, December 16, 2020).

Wilson Fabián Alba, resident of the Cayambe community assures that RMC has allowed him to be involved in a participatory way with caring for the environment and agricultural production in the sector, seeking that the community create habits about garbage collection and tree planting to protect nature (Alba W. Personal interview, December 16, 2020).

4 Discussions and Conclusions

The community radios of Ecuador that arose from the need to express the rejection of the inhumane exploitation of which, since colonial times, the peoples and nationalities of the country have been victims, constantly fight to remain active and inclusive in interculturality with their own language and customs, during the current society of media convergence. And despite the fact that the Organized Communication Law (LOC) benefits the country's communities and social organizations in a percentage, it is not complied with; since, to obtain a radio frequency, the legal process is complex and cumbersome, so you can see the imperious and urgent need to continue in the struggle to fulfill, until now, a utopia of marginalized peoples.

From the inquiries made based on interviews with social actors, it was found that with 54 years of operation the RMC station is an alternative that has allowed the indigenous and peasant communities of Cayambe and Pedro Moncayo to be given a voice, who for a long time had to be subordinate to the information transmitted by the commercial media. It is about the community radio space, which grows stronger every time and with the passing of time, and of which the inhabitants of Cayambe have a good acceptance, trust and credibility on the part of the rural and urban sector; with favorite programs in the audience, where interviews, reports, communiqués, community announcements, musical greetings, etc., messages, ideas, opinions, needs and desires that connect the broadcasters with the receivers as part of a coordinated radio grid hand in hand of the community.

From what has been investigated, several ways to follow are suggested. Questions are raised and future lines of research are exposed; even though this work limited the inquiry to the audience levels in the different parishes and communities to measure the incidence of radio in the periphery of the Cayambe canton.

Unlike other community radio stations, which in most cases are copies of models of traditional radio stations, RMC has become a means of communication with visible potential for survival that has championed community development in the educational, religious and cultural spheres. Productive of the marginalized and excluded indigenous communities of the dominant system in Ecuador, contributing to the sociocultural construction and the identity of the indigenous communities of the sector.

RMC represents a space for communication, interaction, promotion and collective participation of ancestral knowledge and knowledges; and opportunities for the benefit of the entire sector community; and role model in other vulnerable communities where media literacy and community empowerment and development are required.

References

1. Arcotel: Agencia de Regulación y Control de las Telcomunicaciones (2017). https://bit.ly/2WUYDqc. Obtenido de
2. Arroyo, C.: Las radios comunitarias y su relación con el desarrollo local. Revista Punto Cero, **9**(8), 75–78 (2014). https://bit.ly/3u0YDTT. Obtenido de
3. Asamblea-Nacional: Constitución de la República del Ecuador. Quito: Asamblea Nacional (2008). Obtenido de. https://bit.ly/3rzIy7I
4. Barragán, V., Garzón, B.: La interculturalidad en las radios comunitarias del Ecuador, las radios de las nacionalidades. Redes.com: revista de estudios para el desarrollo social de la Comunicación, pp. 194–215 (2016). https://bit.ly/34LBbQL. Obtenido de
5. Behar, D.: Introducción a la Metodología de la Investigación. Cuba: Shalom (2008). https://bit.ly/354fuvr. Obtenido de
6. Chimbo-Mayancela, M., Sarango-Macas, L.: Comunicación comunitaria y sostenibilidad económica de la radio Ilumán 96.7 FM, en Ecuador. Ciencia e Interculturalidad **23**(2), 241–257 (2018). https://doi.org/10.5377/rci.v23i2.6580

7. Coque, M., Guatemal, S., Medranda, N.: Participación ciudadana en la creación de la radio comunitaria. Radio Bocina de La Merced de Quito. In: Sánchez, R., Ramírez, M.D. (eds.) Derechos a la comunicación: Ética y competencias del comunicador, pp. 89–119. Quito: Editorial Universitaria Abya Yala (2020). Obtenido de. https://bit.ly/3hRK1nr
8. CORAPE: Coordinadora de Medios Comunitarios y Populares y Educativos del Ecuador (2021). Obtenido de. https://bit.ly/3ub5Alh
9. Gasparello, G.: Donde crece la flor de la palabra. Reflexiones sobre la radio comunitaria indígena en los Estados de Guerrero y Oaxaca, México. Nómadas. Crit. J. Soc. Jurid. Sci. **29**(1), 1578–6730 (2011). https://bit.ly/37U2f2d. Obtenido de
10. Hernández-Sampieri, R., Fernández, C., Baptista, M.: Metodología de la Investigación (6ta. ed.). México D.F.: McGraw-Hill/Interamericana Editores (2014). https://bit.ly/2KV2Tnk. Obtenido de
11. Herrán, J.: Salesianos Ecuador (2020). https://bit.ly/3mCiuVq. Obtenido de
12. Huergo, J., Morawicki, K., Ferreyra, L.: Una experiencia de radio comunitaria con aborígenes wichí. Revista científica de Comunicación y Educación Comunicar, **13**(26), 103–110 (2006). https://bit.ly/3fyjHvD. Obtenido de
13. Kaplún, G.: Las radios comunitarias uruguayas: entre la legalización y la legitimación social. In: Martínez, M., Mayugo, C., Tamarit, A. (eds.) Revista Enfoques de la Comunicación. Consejo de Regulación, Desarrollo y Promoción de la Información y Comunicación. Retos y desafios de los medios comunitarios, pp. 11–34. Quito: Creative Commons (2019). https://bit.ly/2WPEtOm. Obtenido de
14. LOC: Ley Organica de Comunicación. Obtenido de LexisFinder (febrero de 2019). https://bit.ly/3fxDcEK
15. López-Vigil, J.: Manual Urgente para Radialistas apasinados y apasionadas. Quito: Inti Barrientos (2005). https://bit.ly/3hjgbpo. Obtenido de
16. Moretti, M.: Idiomas ancestrales e interculturales en los medios comunitarios del Ecuador. In: Martínez, M., Mayugo, C., Tamarit, A. (eds.) Revista Enfoques de la Comunicación. Consejo de Regulación, Desarrollo y Promoción de la Información y Comunicación. Retos y desafíos de los medios comunitarios, pp. 93–108 (2019). https://bit.ly/2WPEtOm. Quito: Creative Commons. Obtenido de
17. Patiño, I., Medina, S., Ramírez, M.D.: Pluralidad y diversidad en la comunicación: la radio parlante Pamba Radio como herramienta de participación ciudadana para el cambio social. In: Montoya, R.S., Ramírez, M.D. (eds.) Derechos a la comunicación: Ética y competencias del councador, p. 121 (2020). https://bit.ly/3poPmTB. Quito: Abya Yala. Obtenido de
18. Pousa, X., Yaguana, H.: La Radio, un Medio en Evolución. Comunicación Social Ediciones y publicaciones, Salamanca-España (2013)
19. Vásquez, F.: Radio comunitaria, música y lengua en el pueblo Ayuujk. Academia Premium, pp. 6–118 (2013). https://bit.ly/3f50L8M. Obtenido de

Credibility in Local Journalism, a Look at the Fourth Estate

Paola Malo, Cesar Pineda, Esperanza Namicela, and Ana María Beltrán-Flandoli(✉)

Universidad Técnica Particular de Loja, San Cayetano Alto S/N, Loja, Ecuador
ambeltran@utpl.edu.ec

Abstract. Media credibility continues to be a relevant issue in the country. Various audiences make decisions and guide their actions from informing themselves through social networks on matters of local interest on an indicator. Thus, the work analyzes several concepts of credibility and journalistic ethics provided from the Organic Law Communication (LOC-2013) to make the positions in favor and contrary. In this sense, this study aims to demonstrate the credibility and integrity that journalism in Loja has (Ecuador), analyzing the professional practice of eight journalists who participate in the case study. The collected data based on an applied survey to twenty-four face-to-face students and twenty teachers of the Communication career of the UTPL. In addition, eight **interviews** were carried out with journalists from Loja to contrast both parts of the investigation and conclude with positive or negative aspects of the journalistic exercise. The results indicate that journalism in Loja still generates uncertainty and uneasiness about our citizens' credibility, compared to the credibility that our journalists practice.

Keywords: Credibility · Journalism · Information · Veracity

1 Introduction

As the object of interest of this study is the applied concept of journalistic credibility, it is worth defining it initially through some elementary theses. First, it is essential to refer to its multidimensional nature, analyzed from the perspective of social psychology, consumer practices, and communication sciences [1]. In the journalistic field, two nuances are distinguished: persuasion as a fundamental principle of personal interpretation in the first instance, and, on the other hand, the notion of audience affiliation with some specific media processing [2]. These characteristics are determined and are the ones that influence positions on the informative consumption of the neo-readers and the audience from their communicative capacity.

The trust approach in the news and media spun to the viewer's construction in terms of quality. It focuses as relevant in a precarious moment for journalistic credibility in the world [3, 4]. Disinformation campaigns, primarily through social media [5], journalistic manipulation, and the famed "fake news" often techno-fabricated [6] constitute some of the main challenges for journalists today. In the words of Alsina [7], in the post-truth era, journalism cannot renounce the ethics of responsibility because it can be a mortal wound to the value of its informative media discourse.

© The Author(s), under exclusive license to Springer Nature Singapore Pte Ltd. 2022
Á. Rocha et al. (Eds.): ICOMTA 2021, SIST 259, pp. 295–303, 2022.
https://doi.org/10.1007/978-981-16-5792-4_29

1.1 Media Representation of Reality

According to Osuna et al. [8], social media offer us a "representation" of the world, a mediated and biased version of it. As previously stated, journalistic composition involves taking some approaches and leaving others.

However, this does not imply and should be far from the distortion of information. Beyond that, viewers repeat this process, create their own experience, and judge a particular position on the media and its production.

Thus, Frau-Meigs [9], from the field of media education, clearly related to the deontological values of journalistic training and practice, presents a series of paradigms to conceptualize and highlight the problem of the veracity and credibility of the media from a critical sense that starts from the audience, among these: realism, presence, and absence, denouncing bias and stereotypes, commitment to data, creativity, and online freedom.

In the same sense, for Arguelles [10], in the news market, there are two conceptions of the way information is demanded: 1. the natural conception, where consumers or readers demand accurate and authentic information; and 2. the modern conception that understands readers as individuals who want to see their preferences fulfilled, for which they choose a bias of information, but does not disregard accuracy in its entirety. (p.7).

Though it determines the other construction pole, the journalist "naturally" biases the information according to his criteria. One factor that can define and differentiate the journalist's professionalism would be to create a prominent link to the viewers since the discursive narrative allows users to remain faithful to whom he gives the information. Likewise, corroborating that everything that comes out of his mouth is true, the journalist has done his part to keep others up to date.

As a tie point of this research, there is the insertion of the antecedent in the local context. The transgression of specific journalism quality indicators associated with critical credibility of the news from a changing paradigm from traditional to digital has favored a passionate discussion in the Ecuadorian case [11–13], also marked by the jurisprudence of the Organic Law of Communication of Ecuador LOC 2013 [14], whose Art. 22, states the "Right to receive truthful information of public relevance."

Precisely, Carro [15], in addition to the critical role in the informative perception of the viewer, insists that when the receiver asks questions, pursues issues, or momentarily places himself in the place of the journalist, an integrating perspective of the responsibilities from the profession obtained. It gives journalism its identity.

Thus, the present research work intends to obtain a perspective about credibility and affiliation to the veracity of journalistic production, through the vision of a collective involved in the academic formation of social communication, to propose in a first stage parameter of analysis that allows incurring in a priori reflections on this phenomenon.

2 Methodology

Given that the main objective of this research is to analyze positions regarding credibility in local journalism, taking into account the subsequent relationship both with the professional praxis of journalists in the context, as well as with the informative consumption of users; a non-experimental, descriptive and correlational methodological design was determined to observe the relationship between perceived credibility with respect to variables such as the contrast and coherence of facts and their verification by the audience.

The data collection framed in particular articles of the Organic Law of Communication of Ecuador (such as Art. 22) was carried out through mixed research techniques in a specific population group, adopting the studies case or closed sample [16]. Due to its direct connection with the subject of analysis, it understands the variables and the research conclusions that cannot be generalized yet but generates some first discussion parameters extensible to future research in this field.

From this slogan, a questionnaire of 13 questions had been applied to 20 professors of the Communication career of the UTPL, linked to journalistic writing subjects, social networks, and traditional and digital media, and an average of 6 students per academic cycle of the face-to-face modality of the same career, making a total of 24 students. Table 1 presents the structure and categorization of the reagents of the instrument based on the following parameters: general/contextual, informative consumption, perception of truthfulness/credibility, and deontology, which link to the purpose of this research work.

Table 1. Structuring parameters of the questionnaire

Nª of Question	Category	Rationale/Objective of implementation
1,2	General/contextual data	Arias & Aristizábal [17] Data, information, recognition
3,6,7,8	Information consumption	Romero & Aguaded [18] "unmoderated information consumption can have dysfunctional consequences on cognitive processes and decision making" (p.38)
4,5,9	Perceived veracity/credibility	Roses, Sergio; Gómez-Calderón, Bernardo (2015) [19] "Credibility is the result of a process in which the individual subjectively examines and evaluates the qualities of an issuer, content, source, or other informational instance" (p. 433)
10,11,12,13	Deontology	Vargas [20] "Ethics and deontology are nowadays essential for any profession and even more so for those who provide services and deal with disadvantaged people" (p.65)

Information provided by teachers and students based on a selection of questionnaire itself; structured interviews conducted with eight local journalists, chosen for their popularity, assessed through indicators and metrics of their social networks as well as the year's career experience, in order to deepen the views about their actions and the perception of their journalistic quality and credibility.

Some of the questions implemented were: What type of content do you broadcast (entertainment, entertainment, sports, informative), what authors or references (bibliographical or epistemological) you know and mention to speak of veracity and credibility in journalism and Social Communication? In your opinion, what is the role of journalism in today's world? What percentage of the published information is correct? Which article from the Organic Law of Communication do you consider fundamental? What type of sources do you consult to elaborate on informative pieces?

3 Results and Discussion

The results of the presented research follow a pattern of the core issues that have served as a direction: local information consumption, preferences, and perceptions about journalistic work and the relationship of this with the concept that handled its quality, from the knowledge, attachment, and practice of the notions of truthfulness and credibility. In addition, the findings questionnaires discussed theoretical background and journalists' answers from the interview based on the LOC Ecuador paradigm. Finally, a profile of the journalists consulted presents establish criteria for reflection and analysis of the state of the fourth journalistic power in local environments.

From the data obtained, women represent most responses in both surveys (see Table 1). The students' section represents 79%, while the teachers who responded makeup 60%. In the student's sample, the age range of 15 to 26 years (the majority) (Fig. 1) responded that they are not sure if this law applies in the news concerning the use of LOC in the news. It seems that age is a crucial factor in the knowledge of this section, which is not the case for teachers, with a negative response on this issue.

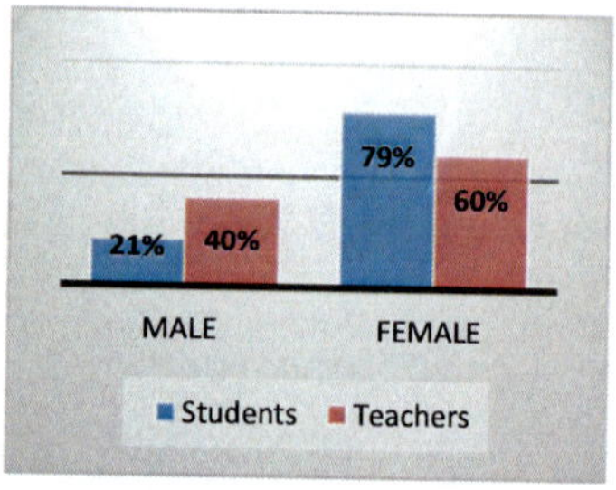

Fig. 1. Respondent demographic data

As shown in Fig. 2, the social networks most used for information by female students are in parity Facebook and Instagram, unlike female teachers who prefer Twitter. The trend is maintained in the male sex since students prefer Instagram, and teachers prefer Facebook, thus evidencing what Del Hoyo et al. [2] state. Each person maintains a different posture of information consumption.

In the questionnaire asked about the level of credibility of local media, according to the perception of teachers and students of communication, the results obtained indicate that 12 female students trust the digital media Primer Reporte, as do 11 female teachers

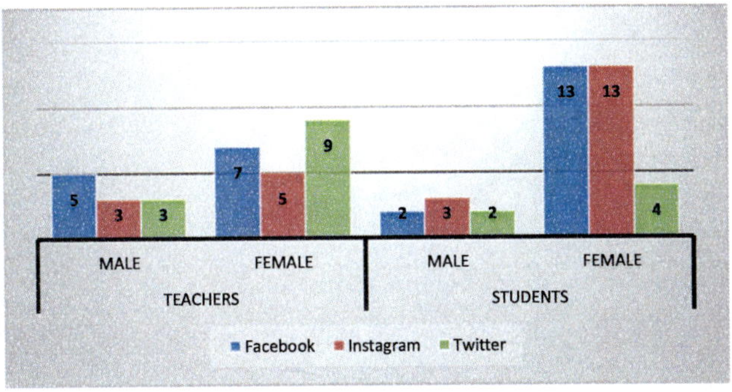

Fig. 2. Social network preference by gender

who choose the same media for the consumption of local information. On the other hand, teachers and students prefer different media in Loja regarding veracity and credibility. As shown in Fig. 3, in both surveys, women represented the majority of responses.

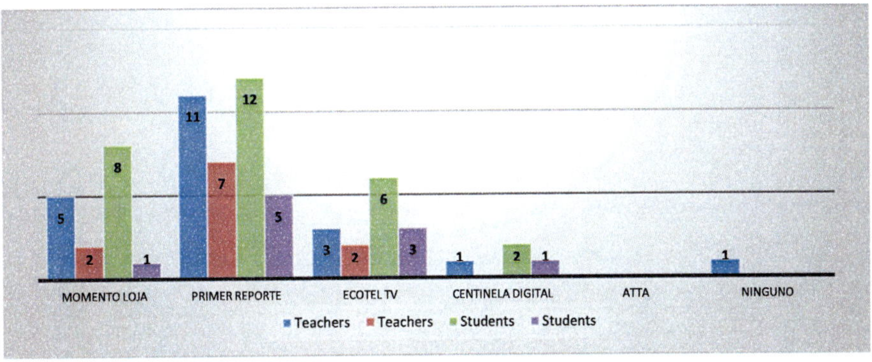

Fig. 3. Perceived credibility of local media by gender

According to Rodrigo-Alsina and Laerte [7], the social emergence networks, the communicative ecosystem, and the notions of information relevance and veracity varied enormously. It is also reflected in the questionnaire responses since most teachers and students consider that credibility is medium. In the same proportion, some are "not sure" of the veracity of the information.

In this sense, one of the most followed professionals is Boris Sarango (see Fig. 4), a journalist from Lojano who maintains a relevant number of followers on social networks such as Facebook and Instagram. In connection, the data received indicate that 80% of teachers follow Lojano journalists. At the same time, many students prefer to follow national journalists, and it follows that national credibility is more significant than local credibility.

Considering the two conceptions for news consumption of Arguelles (2020) [10]; the natural one, in which readers demand accurate and factual information, and the modern

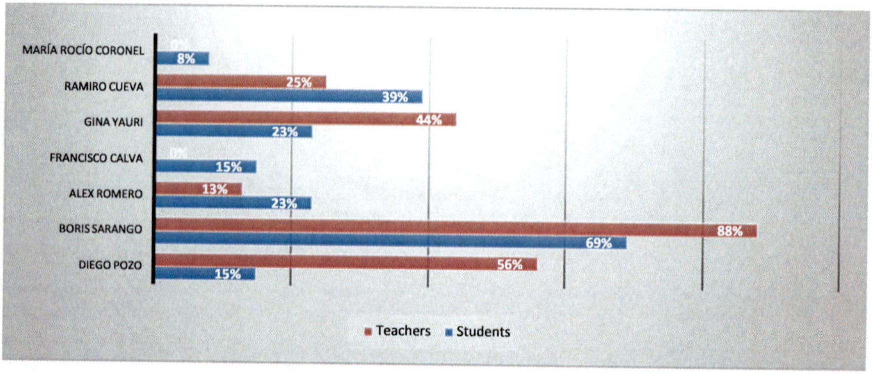

Fig. 4. Journalists followed in social networks

one, consumers want to see their references fulfilled. Teachers in 95% and students in 83% verify the information in other media. Regarding the mechanisms, as shown in Fig. 5, 39% of students and 26% of teachers decide to read the newspaper because it is an accurate way to get information and avoid falling into fake news.

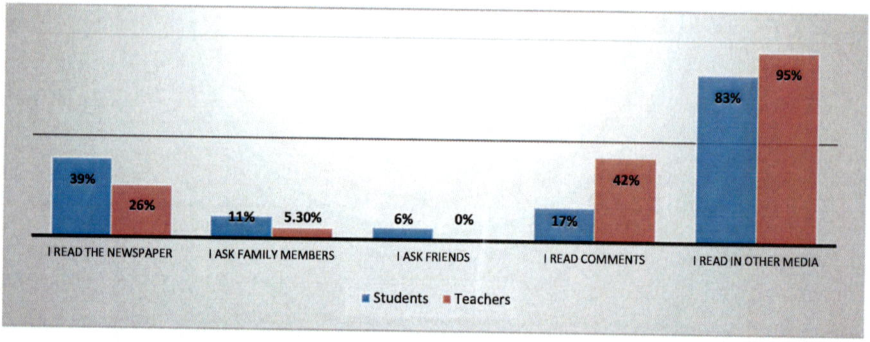

Fig. 5. Methods of verifying the users of information

The contrast of the answers from both academics and professionals' training communication, expressed in the interviews with the newsmakers, allowed the confirmation of Table 2, like an x-ray of construction credibility and consumption methods and techniques. It is discussed in subsequent lines.

The analysis of Table 2 shows several situations. Eight journalists interviewed work in four different thematic areas: sports, news, entertainment, and education. Only one of the professionals dedicates to the sports genre, and seven are inclined to the informative branch. In the case of entertainment, three professionals broadcast this content. The educational branch does not work in this city. Considering Osuna's postulates [8], and on the basis that most journalists appear as part of a media or group, it infers that their interventions represent an editorial line.

Table 2. Profile of Lojano journalists.

Journalist/Media	Content they produce	Sources	Technical resources	Validation of content (veracity)	Basis in the LOC	Deficiency in local journalism
Freddy Cabrera, Radio Satelital	*Sports*	Athletes, authorities, fans Deportistas, autoridades, aficionados	Voice recorder, Cellular phone, Notebook	85%	Does not socialize LOC	-
Stephany Patiño, Antena 7	*Informative, entertaining*	Web page, Digital press	Archives, Audiovisual products. Infographics, Arts	90%	Art. 17. Right to Freedom of Expression	Egoism
Anita Soto, Radio La Hechicera	*Commercial, entertainment*	Digital press, television, radio	Photographs, videos, podcast	95%	Art. 9, Art. 39, Art. 5, Art. 103	Lack of financial resources
Lindon Sanmartín, Portal Digital SR Radio	*Informativo, entretenimiento y farándula*	Municipality, Prefecture, Governor's Office	Photographs, videos, podcast	100%	Does not socialize the LOC	Lack of preparation, lack of knowledge
Freddy Aponte	*Political and environmental*	National and International Press, Twitter	Photographs, infographics, and videos	100%	No socializa la LOC	Lack of research
Daniela Gallardo, Radio Poder	*Informative*	Professionals, Analysts	Press archives, research	95%	Art. 100, national production. Art 101.independent national products	No innovative tools. No doors open to young journalism
Lourdes Quezada, Radio UTPL	*educational, and entertainment*	Official sources	Visual pieces, podcast	95%	Art. 25	Little research, low pay, ethics, lack of government support
Yina Yauri, Lo del Momento Loja	*News and research*	Other media	Cellular, recordings	100%	Art. 9	Confor-same

The elaboration of news is a resource used by Freddy Cabrera. He uses it as an example of institutions, organizations, and authorities, while Stephany Patiño, a young journalist, relies on websites and digital media; digital press, television, and radio, which are the platforms where she highlights her informative pieces, similar to Ana Játiva, a radio broadcaster.

On the other hand, Lindon Sanmartín, like the other local journalists, relies on public and private institutions, while Freddy Aponte uses national and international press and scientific reports. Daniela Gallardo's (28 years old) sources are public and private sector personalities. Finally, Lourdes Quezada and Gina Yauri rely on direct and official sources.

The technical resources most used by journalists are photographs, videos, and podcasts, leaving aside traditional narratives for data collection, such as notebooks and recordings.

Journalists in Loja had stated that their news is 85% to 100% credible. Before disseminating it, they contrast sources, investigate both sides to write, and carry out a process of argumentation according to their self-perception of the procedures of news construction.

According to the results obtained through the interviews, several of the journalists have a theoretical basis for their daily journalistic practice. They point out, for example, articles 9, 25, 100–101, 39, 5, 103, and 7 of the Organic Law of Communication (LOC 2013) [12]. However, journalists question if there are articles in which they do not agree, and most of them were able to emphasize that the law is not the problem but that the problem lies in the distorted forms of interpretation.

According to this criteria, journalism in Loja may suffer from a lack of veracity and credibility due to selfishness, attachment to morbidity, and speculation of reality. In addition, they point out that several media do not like to invest in hiring new journalists or in the technical updating of personnel; on the contrary, conformism and lack of innovation prevail. On the other hand, they state that institutionally, the laws and ordinances stipulated in the LOC are not respected, which means that the rights of communicators are not taken very seriously.

4 Conclusions

The research conducted in Loja with local journalists shows a particular uncertainty among citizens in general. Students and teachers linked to this profession agree that credibility plays an important role; however, depending on the journalistic exercise of the professionals, the notion of its implementation in the actual field is not reflected or defended.

It is evident in the analysis of surveys and interviews conducted in Loja, representing a certain degree of insecurity for the public. Teachers and students involved in these studies believe that the professional reputation of journalists plays an important role, depending on the media where they work.

All the journalists interviewed take into account Organic Law of Communication on which to base themselves. However, in the professional exercise, it does not apply in a primordial way. This action turns out to be essential to carry out the informative notes; thus, there is knowledge, but it is not exercised. In addition, in the applied surveys, the lack of usability of this law is reflected.

In this sense, the journalists in Loja do not positively influence the future journalism professionals of the Communication career of the UTPL; therefore, the lack of credibility and periodicity of the local journalist is questioned; the young person prefers national journalism.

Finally, Boris Sarango, journalist of Primer Report, is the professional with the highest degree of credibility in the city of Loja, being one of the most followed journalists in social networks, which reflects the acceptance and trust of the information disseminated.

References

1. Mayoral, J., Parratt, S., Morata, M.: Desinformación, manipulación y credibilidad periodísticas: una perspectiva histórica. en Historia y Comunicación Soc. **24**(2), 395–409 (2017)
2. del Hoyo Hurtado, M., García-Galera, M.D.C., Blanco-Alfonso, I.: Disinformation and the erosion of journalistic credibility in the context of fake news. a case study. Estudios Sobre El Mensaje Periodístico **26**(4), 1399–1409 (2020). https://doi.org/10.5209/ESMP.70238
3. Rodrigo-Mendizábal, I.: Credibilidad de medios y periodistas en Ecuador en el año 2015. Razón y Palabra **20**(95), 659–678 (2016)

4. Nelson, J.L., Kim, S.J.: Improve trust, increase loyalty? Analyzing the relationship between news credibility and consumption. Journal. Pract. **15**(3), 348–365 (2021). https://doi.org/10.1080/17512786.2020.1719874
5. Szostek, J.: Nothing is true? The credibility of news and conflicting narratives during "information war" in Ukraine. Int. J. Press/Politics **23**(1), 116–135 (2018). https://doi.org/10.1177/1940161217743258
6. Wagner, J., Sonmez, F.: About 80 Percent of the Media are 'The Enemy of the People,' Trump Says (2018)
7. Rodrigo-Alsina, M., Cerqueira, L.: Periodismo, ética y posverdad. Cuadernos.Info (44), 225–239 (2020). https://doi.org/10.7764/cdi.44.1418
8. Osuna, A.S., Fraug, M.D., Marta, L.C.: Educación mediática y Formación del Profesorado. Educomunicación más allá de la Alfabetización Digital, Revista Interuniversitaria de Formación del Profesorado **91**(32.1), 29–42 (2018)
9. Frau-Meigs, D.: Media and Information Literacy (MIL): Taking the digital social turn for online freedoms and education 3.0. The Routledge Companion to Media and Human Rights, London: Routledge (2017)
10. Arguelles Quezada, J.: Competencia entre compañías de noticias y su impacto en el sesgo de la información. Tesis de maestría. Centro de Investigación y Docencia Económicas. Obtenido de (2020). http://hdl.handle.net/11651/4278
11. Punín Larrea, M.I., Rencoret Quezada, N.A.: Cambios en el mapa mediático del Ecuador: los medios públicos que tenemos y los medios que queremos. Telos: Revista de Estudios Interdisciplinarios en Ciencias Sociales, **16**(3), 434–446 (2014). Recuperado a partir de. https://dialnet.unirioja.es/servlet/articulo?codigo=5655342
12. Reyes Aguinaga, H.: Activismo estatal y democratización social en Ecuador: tensiones contrahegemónicas frente al poder mediático (2007–2013). Nueva Sociedad **249**, 108–118 (2014)
13. Checa-Godoy, A.L.: Banca y la propiedad de los medios: el caso de Ecuador. Rev. Lat. Comun. Soc. **67**, 125–147 (2012). https://doi.org/10.4185/RLCS-067-950-125-147
14. Ley Orgánica de Comunicación de Ecuador - Google zoeken. (s. f.). Ley Orgánica De Comunicación de Ecuador. Recuperado 29 de mayo de 2021, de (2013). https://bit.ly/3wysepk
15. Carro, M.J.: Periodismo y sentido de la realidad. Teoría y análisis de la narrativa periodística. Madrid: Fragua (2005)
16. Piñeros-Piza, C., et al.: Credibilidad percibida del periodismo a través de la Internet: una visión desde la psicología del consumidor. Diversitas Perspectivas en Psicología, **7**(2), 225–238 (2011)
17. Arias, J., Aristizábal, C.: El dato, la información, el conocimiento y su productividad en empresas del sector público. Scielo **14**(28), 95–1109 (2011). http://www.scielo.org.co/pdf/seec/v14n28/v14n28a7.pdf. Obtenido de
18. Romero, L., Aguaded, I.: Consumo informativo y competencias digitales de estudiantes de periodismo de Colombia Perú y Venezuela. Scielo **23**(70), 1405–14035 (2016)
19. Roses, S., Gómez-Calderón, B.: Credibilidad de los medios en España: divergencias de percepción y caracterización de los escépticos. Profesional de la Información **24**(4), 432–440 (2015)
20. Vargas, L.P.: Deontología y código deontológico. redalyc, pp. 65–79 (2011). https://www.redalyc.org/pdf/3497/349733228009.pdf

Check for updates

Marketing and Digital Press: Information Consumption Patterns in Colombia During COVID19

Verónica Crespo-Pereira[1](✉), Ana Cecilia Vaca-Tapia[2,3], Roberto Xavier Manciati-Alarcón[3], and Sofía Isabel Cabrera-Espín[3]

[1] Universidade da Coruña, A Coruña, Spain
veronica.crespo@udc.es
[2] Universidade de Santiago de Compostela, Santiago de Compostela, Spain
[3] Universidad UTE, Quito, Ecuador
sofia.cabrera@ute.edu.ec

Abstract. COVID19 has had enormous consequences in the media. The pandemic has affected journalism by encouraging new informational newspaper consumption trends. This phenomenon has inevitably changed newspaper newsrooms since print versions started to decline in favor of digital ones. Since the beginning of the mentioned health crisis, information provided by media has become a highly citizenship demand. The study of the dynamics of information consumption is very relevant for understanding the potential journalism business transformation nowadays and in the years to come. Such a health crisis might open a scenario of opportunities and challenges to face by journalism worldwide. The objective of this research is to analyze the influence of COVID19 on newspaper digital edition consumption patterns. We have conducted an exploratory investigation based on the secondary data from Similarweb. Data focus on providing a portrait of Colombian newspapers reading habits during the most critical moments of COVID 19, the outbreak, from March to May 2020 (confinement and first wave), and the following months, from September to November 2020 (second wave). The results confirm the high impact of Covid-19 on digital edition demand on 15 Colombian newspapers during the first wave. Citizens who have traditionally been far away from media might have now been connected with media. However, results also reveal a dramatic decrease in unique visitors in the second wave, thus the potential audience benefits for media and advertisers might have been considered a missing opportunity to retain and maintain Covid-19 outbreak readership habits.

Keywords: Marketing · Press · Colombia · COVID19 · Journalism · Consumption habits

1 Introduction

COVID19 has encouraged the debate on the role of the media in crisis situations. There is no doubt that information on the outbreak has become a valuable asset for citizenship. Media credibility and their public service nature are two central aspects considered

© The Author(s), under exclusive license to Springer Nature Singapore Pte Ltd. 2022
Á. Rocha et al. (Eds.): ICOMTA 2021, SIST 259, pp. 304–313, 2022.
https://doi.org/10.1007/978-981-16-5792-4_30

by academics regarding the need for society to support journalism. However, different aspects should be considered when assessing media social value.

1.1 Journalism and Citizen Journalism in Colombia

As mentioned, the public service nature of media has centered many debates around its role during the pandemic. Its educative function around preventive protocols to avoid the dissemination of the disease centered the academic research, among many other different approaches and topics [1]. Some other studies reflect about news production challenges such as information overload, sensationalism, ideological biases [2], fake news, or disinformation [3, 4], as well as censorship and political pressures. Much of the information provided by journalists come from official government sources and official institutions. Information practices have important repercussions in the citizenship reality configuration. Studies suggest that informational treatment of the Colombian press (Cali) did not facilitate citizen awareness of the disease [5]. Colombian media operated with data provided by the Ministry of Health and Social Protection through a regularly updated map [6] and other entities such as the Secretariats of Health and Safety or the Metropolitan Police. Studies indicate that political sources were responsible for the promulgation of disinformation, specifically considered "half truth" (manipulated information, partially false or misleading and out of context). Sources conditioned the framing under a perspective on which citizenship living conditions were not visible [5]. Manipulated information and information out of context was also provided by Latin American media [7]. Colombia is considered as one of the three Latin American countries along with Argentina and Mexico that presents a greater number of disinformation. Paradoxically, Colombia has also the largest number of news classified as "true" in Latin America. A large part of them come from reliable sources such as members of the government, other public officials, as well as the media [7].

Traditional media, and in particular press, are the most credible media compared to social networks [8]. During the pandemic, it was not social networks nor messaging platforms the most relevant sources of information for citizens but newspapers and television [2]. However, citizenship reluctance towards the media is evident. Newspaper editorial line and ideology that outline the agenda and the approaches is identifiable and recognizable by readers [2], and therefore, it contributes negatively to the trust placed in the media.

The lack of credibility and trust in media is a growing phenomenon worldwide [9]. Nordic countries, territories that traditionally have high levels of press freedom, also register a trust decrease in the last years. Although the pandemic could help improve the image of the media, the downward trend continues [2]. It should be noted that citizenship educational level influences the perception of credibility. People with a lower educational level have a more positive attitude towards the COVID 19 media coverage compared to those with a higher educational level [10]. The urgent need for health information might not have been positively capitalized by media to gain and improve credibility and trust. Citizen journalism coverage during the pandemic was key for its contribution to reporting about topics and perspectives not covered by the official sources and media. Citizen coverage has contributed to making visible the dimension of health problems in Latin American countries due to the lack of censorship filters. This is the case of Ecuador, a country whose citizen journalism viralized videos with corpses in the streets of Guayaquil attracted worldwide media attention. Although the access to news through social networks and private messaging is growing and contributes to overcoming censorship this might be a risky route. "Informational disorders" [10] such as the lack of quality health information [11] or hoaxes [7] always become an obstacle for this type of informational initiatives. WhatsApp was widely used as a means of information. However, it must be taken into account that the platform makes easy the proliferation of hoaxes and its messages have a high level of acceptance among its users [12]. Also, social networks were used to set the agenda with political [13], propaganda and commercial interests and purposes [14] during Covid-19.

1.2 Digital Journalism vs. Printing

The confinement reduced the newspapers print editions considerably or even totally.

The transition to the digital context has forced newspapers to rethink their business model and work dynamics. The pandemic made visible the great capacity of the digital platform to satisfy the social demand for information. Accordingly, paid newspapers increased their subscribers [2]. The need for information is greater and more continuous. Up to 78% of citizens stated that they inform themselves more frequently and the consumption habits changed to a slower reading [15]. COVID19 news coverage represented 63.7% in digital media [16]. The young population group is especially relevant. This group represents a very important consumption of health information through the Internet and official websites [17].

New technologies have contributed to accelerating new information consumption patterns. Smartphone time of use has increased. At the same time new technologies appear to encourage teleworking and supply social contact through apps [18]. Also, the need for constant, up-to-date and immediate information has benefited the appearance of new consumption patterns by traditional readers. At the same time, readers who traditionally would not consume media started to have contact with digital editions. This new consumption could solidify given the foreseeable fall of the printed newspaper and the incidence of the pandemic on the sector [19, 20]. This research carries out an analysis of the consumption patterns of digital newspapers in Colombia in order to detect and compare citizen digital press readership consumption along the first 9 months of the crisis.

2 Methodology

Research on the impact of COVID19 on the consumption of the media, and specifically on the press, is a phenomenon that, although it has been approached from several perspectives, not so profusely in Latin America. Various studies address media consumption during the pandemic in the United States and Spain [2, 10] the treatment of journalistic images (fake images) [4], press vignettes [21] or the presence of infographics in the daily press [22] in times of COVID19. The role of digital press in times of pandemic has been fundamental [16] and points to the hybridization between the traditional and digital systems [2].

In the Latin American scenario, different approaches have found, such as the treatment of COVID19 through humor in the Ecuadorian press [1], or the press informative agenda in Colombia and Ecuador [5]. Andean community countries have a minimal representation in media studies on Google Scholar and Scopus. Health, education and socioeconomic and political issues derived from COVID19 that are most abundant topics. The Scopus database has been searched using Boolean operators to identify the volume of research associated with the territory under study, such as "Colombia AND Covid19"; "Colombia AND Covid19 AND media", "Latin America AND Covid19 AND media"; "Latin America AND Covid19 AND press", without success. The study encourages a debate on the press consumption in a territory sensitive to natural and health disasters.

The health crisis in Colombia began on March 6, 2020. On March 19 the quarantine is ordered by the Alcaldía Distrital and on March 23 a national quarantine is ordered [23]. Although it is considered that Latin America has not finished the first wave [24], in Colombia a second peak begins in the month of August [25] that continues in October 2020 [26]. This research analyzes the consumption patterns of Colombian digital newspapers in the early stages of the crisis (March-May 2020), comparing these patterns with the second coronavirus wave (September-October-November 2020). The study analyzes, in a descriptive and exploratory way, the evolution of relevant indicators for digital business models that represent a turning point in daily newspaper consumption. The study of positioning, engagement, monthly visitors, internationalization, origin by channels, search traffic or social network traffic are some of the variables that have been collected through the Similarweb platform. Studies under platforms similar to the one mentioned have been used with relevant results [10, 16]. The aim is to reflect about the role citizenship confered to national press in times of international health crisis.

3 Results

Digitization fosters total freedom of media consumption if the right conditions exist, such as the access to technological devices and to the internet. Half the Colombian's population does not have access to the Internet despite the fact that national development plans seek to overcome this restriction, which affects more than 23 million people [27].

Data reveal an extremely high demand for news in digital newspaper editions (for almost the entire set of newspapers analyzed) in March 2020. The news interest generated by the outbreak of the health crisis declines progressively over the following months in a very different way for the newspapers (Table 1). In other words, this need for information decreases in the subsequent months (April, May) and in the last period analyzed (September to November) (Table 1). It is El Nuevo Liberal and the regional newspaper Magangue Hoy and El Tiempo the newspapers with the greater growth of visits.

Information consumption is clearly higher in the first wave of the pandemic (March-April-May). Unique visitors in March, reached more than 16 million in the newspaper El Tiempo. Many other newspapers have also increased the visitor percentage. This phenomenon is consistent with studies that consider information as a fundamental resource for citizens, especially in challenging situations such as the Covid-19 pandemic that increases the demand for high volumen of updated information [2]. On the other side,

Table 1. Percentage of visits per month

Journal	March	April	May	Sep	Oct	Nov
El Tiempo	70,19%	−8,17%	−13,68%	0,44%	1,80%	0,44%
El Espectador	54,14%	0,79%	−17,90%	−2,76%	−2,75%	10,37%
El Nuevo Siglo	25,96%	−5,50%	−9,28%	5,74%	−2,17%	−11,10%
Q'Hubo	−14,23%	−29,64%	−42,84%	−13,15%	7,69%	−23,76%
Extra	−2,21%	−26,77%	−44,01%	0,29%	12,99%	−20,18%
Publimetro	24,53%	−21,47%	−27,04%	−10,46%	−23,6%	1,84%
La República	71,47	32,74%	−16,47	1,89%	−3,74%	1,62%
Portafolio	50,77%	6,42%	−17,51%	0,62%	0,78%	0,27%
El Colombiano	60,79%	−11,99%	−16,61%	−7,97%	4,12%	−1,52%
El Mundo	26,78%	3,31%	−13,66%	−23,81%	4,71%	−15,22%
El Heraldo	26,46%	−11,60%	−249,00%	12,44%	−2,64%	14,30%
El Universal	35,78%	−13,07%	−20,09%	−6,90%	12,98%	13,98%
Magangue Hoy	180,16%	26,17%	−64,48%	−62,55%	−2,02%	−10,84%
La Patria	49,00%	31,00%	−27,69%	−10,32%	−2,75%	−2,75%
El Nuevo Liberal	191,72%	−2,24%	−22,74%	−11,99%	19,73%	−59,72%

Source: own elaboration

data also point out a dramatic decrease on the number of people interested in the news provided by digital newspapers in the following months, especially, during the second period of analysis (August-November). The informative need decreases considerably over time (Table 2).

Studies indicate a revitalization of mass media consumption among citizens around the world, especially in the digital press and television in the pandemic [2, 10]. The prominence of the media is indisputable. Interest in the pandemic has prompted new routines among casual and regular readers. Studies have even reveal a positive assessment of media coverage by an audience profile characterized by low information consumption [10]. The attention gained should motivate press to bet on innovation and the generation of added value to maintain and retain occasional readers and increase the satisfaction of those who are already regular consumers. Identifying and satisfying audience expectations through significant innovative marketing changes could lead to audience retention and a higher potential profitability [28]. Data point out that Colombian digital newspaper consumption might have not won new readers in the long term as seen on Table 2. On the other hand, the loss of visitors over the months might have had a positive impact on the time of consumption, since those readers who remain interested in news stayed for a long time in the digital edition (Table 3).

Covid-19 has affected the media and the way of accessing and evaluating information. The informal education promoted by the press during the pandemic has socially enhanced its relevance. Likewise, studies show a positive increase in the assessment

Table 2. Unique visitors per month

Medio	Marzo	Abril	Mayo	Sep	Oct	Nov
El Tiempo	16.73M	15.58M	14.68M	2.366M	2.383M	2.407M
El Espectador	7.909M	7.923M	7.580M	849,726	816,359	818,201
El Nuevo Siglo	226,053	191,941	201,725	–	–	59,701
Q'Hubo	113,769	85,071	81,879	–	–	–
Extra	630,034	481,22	462,695	–	–	–
Publimetro	4.923M	4.170M	2.989M	–	–	–
La República	1.837M	2.387M	2.099M	–	–	–
Portafolio	2.863M	2.951M	2.510M	–	–	–
El Colombiano	3.392M	2.963M	2.599M	–	–	–
El Mundo	270,208	279,484	259,429	–	–	–
El Heraldo	3.178M	3.041M	2.289M	–	–	–
El Universal	1.618M	1.599M	1.251M	–	202,906	202,906
Magangue Hoy	21,44	23,154	10,234	−5000	−5000	−5000
La Patria	566,082	838,87	570,814	102,876	99,103	99,103
El Nuevo Liberal	15,626	13,687	12,102	−5000	5090	−5000

Source: own elaboration

of media coverage and credibility according to Casero-Ripollés [10]. Local news coverage has provided information of interest not only to national but to foreign markets. Digital editions allow proximity issues coverage with a potential worldwide distribution. Although most of the readers come from Colombia (March 80.94% - November 72.54%), there is a considerable percentage of foreign countries that pay attention to Colombian coverage during the COVID19. Diasporas might play a key role here. United States is the territory that has the greatest impact on Colombia digital newspaper consumption (4.27% - 3.67%), followed by Mexico (2.53% -2.77%), Argentina (1.54 -1.08%) and Spain (1.06% -1.15%). Peru, the territory with the lowest percentage in March (0.49%), increases its weight exponentially in the second period of analysis, mainly October (1.44%) and November (1.42%) (Table 4).

Traffic to digital newspaper websites is generated from different sources (Table 5). Organic search, carried out using search engines like Google, is the most common way to achieve visitors (60.21%). Traffic generated from social networks in the first month of the crisis reaches 9.23% in March and decreases in April (6,3%).

Mobile phones are the main tool to access the digital editions. 71% visitors used these devices to read news meanwhile computer reading reaches 28% in March. The rise of instant messaging networks and platforms has generated profound changes in the traditional media-audience relationship. As stated by Casero-Ripollés [10], social networks have spread false news and contributed to the chaos in the public sphere; in addition to fragmentation or excessive supply of information. On the other hand,

Table 3. Digital edition consumption in minutes

Newspaper	March	April	May	Sep	Oct	Nov
El Tiempo	0:02:54	0:02:50	0:05:36	0:03:56	0:04:13	0:03:30
El Espectador	0:02:00	0:01:58	0:02:13	0:03:14	0:03:33	0:03:42
El Nuevo Siglo	0:01:40	0:02:00	0:01:54	0:02:07	0:03:09	0:02:39
Q'Hubo	0:05:30	0:05:56	0:05:40	0:08:56	0:11:44	0:06:19
Extra	0:01:23	0:01:19	0:01:52	0:02:39	0:02:10	0:01:47
Publimetro	0:03:01	0:03:01	0:40:38	0:21:37	0:24:58	0:17:43
La República	0:01:34	0:01:34	0:02:22	0:02:36	0:02:01	0:02:12
Portafolio	0:01:28	0:01:22	0:09:20	0:02:21	0:02:21	0:02:22
El Colombiano	0:02:46	0:02:48	0:03:43	0:04:08	0:04:09	0:04.14
El Mundo	0:01:03	0:01:00	0:01:45	0:01:03	0:01:33	0:01:14
El Heraldo	0:02:16	0:02:04	0:03:18	0:03:31	0:03:23	0:03:14
El Universal	0:02:48	0:02:35	0:03:10	0:04:32	0:04:55	0:04:55
Magangue Hoy	0:01:11	0:01:17	0:09:15	0:03:24	–	0:02:24
La Patria	0:02:39	0:02:33	0:03:03	0:03:47	0:04:08	0:04:08
El Nuevo Liberal	0:00:40	0:01:07	0:01:57	0:04:10	0:00:47	0:04:58

Source: own elaboration

Table 4. Readers by countries

Country	March	April	May	Sep	Oct	Nov
Colombia	80,94%	80,28%	81,33%	78,21%	80,75%	72,54%
United States	4,27%	3,33%	3,96%	4,56%	3,97%	3,67%
Mexico	2,53%	1,82%	2,64%	3,25%	3,05%	2,77%
Argentina	1,54%	1,53%	1,09%	2,26%	1,20%	1,08%
Spain	1,06%	1,20%	1,10%	1,59%	1,02%	1,15%
Peru	0,49%	0,61%	0,90%	0,75%	1,44%	1,42%

Source: own elaboration

social networks have also constituted a powerful window to make visible and give access to information from digital newspapers. Traffic generated by social networks to the Colombian digital editions websites is distributed mainly between two platforms, Facebook (77.60% - March; 65,79% Nov.) and Twitter (15.14% - March; 20,69%-Nov.). If the first platform stands out for the great coverage it reaches, the second does so because it is a markedly informative social network. YouTube reaches a 3,15% in March and Whatsapp Web a 0,0203% in the same month.

Table 5. Source type

Source type	March	April	May	Sep	Oct	Nov
Direct	33,01%	37,44%	35,62%	30,63%	30,33%	29,98%
Email	1,28%	1,98%	3,23%	1,50%	1,39%	1,36%
Referrals	0,76%	1,36%	0,57%	0,58%	0,51%	0,63%
Social	9,23%	6,30%	7,75%	7,05%	8,03%	8,81%
Organic Research	55,69%	52,30%	52,74%	60,21%	59,70%	59,14%
Paid Research	0,00%	0,00%	0,00%	0,01%	0,00%	0,02%

Source: own elaboration

4 Conclusions

Covid-19 health crisis has the potential to accelerate changes in print and digital editions. Although media stand as fundamental pillar for the dissemination of information among citizens in time of crisis, the presence of citizen journalism and the loss of media trust worldwide, affect the current and future media consumption. The appearance of new informative habits among the occasional audiences that are more alien to the news could have generated a positive precedent regarding the stimulation and democratization of news access by the public opinion.

The research carried out yields comparative data on the Colombian digital press edition consumption behavior in two specific periods, the beginning of the Covid-19 pandemic and the second wave. Data show that information consumption intensifies in periods of crisis regardless of its nature. This trend is also observed, not only in Colombia but also in other countries. The role of television and newspapers during this period of analysis might contribute to the enhancement of their social value in a panorama dominated by a profound loss of media trust and credibility.

Colombian's digital newspapers register a considerable increase in audience in the first months of the outbreak of the pandemic, but the demand for information gradually decreased over the following months. Despite the fact that the period of analysis does not allow great conclusions about the use of social networks as a traffic generator, it is considered of interest to open new lines of research about its strategic value to motivate visits and revalue the work of journalism. Not need to mention that local news coverage has provided information of interest not only to national but to foreign markets and diasporas. However, the demand for Covid19 information has a limit. New possibilities in the digital panorama must be taken into account for the survival of the press since worldwide distribution is a reality. Although technology is key, contents become the pillar to attract and, what it is more important, maintain people's interest.

References

1. Bravo-Mancero, J., Larrea Naranjo, C., Ruales Parreño, R.: Tratamiento del Covid 19, Ecuador mediante el humor periodístico. Braz. J. Health Rev. **3**(2), 3523–3541 (2020)

2. Masip, P., Aran-Ramspott, S., Ruiz-Caballero, C., Suau, J., Almenar, E., Puertas-Graell, D.: Consumo informativo y cobertura mediática durante el confinamiento por el Covid-19: sobreinformación, sesgo ideológico y sensacionalismo. Prof. Inform. **29**(3) (2020)
3. Toledo-Ibarra, G.A., et al.: The COVID-19 pandemic from the multidisciplinary visión of 28 University Professors of Nayarit, México. Rev. Bio Ciencias **7**, e976 (2020)
4. Andreu-Sánchez, C., Martín-Pascual, M.-Á.: Fake images of the SARS-CoV-2 coronavirus in the communication of information at the beginning of the first Covid-19 pandemic. Prof. Inform. **29**(3), e290309 (2020)
5. Manrique-Grisales, J.: La prensa en modo pandemia: una aproximación a las agendas informativas de Expreso y El País sobre COVID19. Rev. Española Comun. Salud Suplemento S142–S157 (2020)
6. Cobarsí-Morales, J.: Datos cuantitativos de muertes de la pandemia Covid-19 en España: notas para una discusión técnica. Blog Informática++, Estudios de Informática, Multimedia y Telecomunicación de la Universitat Oberta de Catalunya (2020)
7. López-Pujalte, C., Nuño-Moral, M.V.: La "infodemia" en la crisis del coronavirus: Análisis de desinformaciones en España y Latinoamérica. Rev. Española Doc. Científica **43**(3), e274 (2020)
8. Austin, L., Lui, B.-F., Jin, Y.: How audiences seek out crisis information: exploring the social-mediated crisis communication model. J. Appl. Commun. Res. **40**(2), 188–207 (2016)
9. Newman, N., Fletcher, R., Kalogeropoulos, A., Nielsen, R.K. Reuters institute digital news report 2019. Reuters Institute for the Study of Journalism, Oxford (2020)
10. Casero-Ripollés, A.: Impact of Covid-19 on the media system. Communicative and democratic consequences of news consumption during the outbreak. Prof. Inform. **29**(2), e290223 (2020)
11. Jiménez-Sotomayor, M.R., Gomez-Moreno, C., Soto-Perez-de-Celis, E.: Coronavirus, Ageism, and Twitter: an evaluation of tweets about older adults and COVID-19. Am. Geriatr. Soc. 1–5 (2020)
12. Moreno, A., Fuentes-Lara, C., Navarro, C.: Covid-19 communication management in Spain: exploring the effect of information-seeking behavior and message reception in public's evaluation. Prof. Inform. **29**(4), e290402 (2020)
13. Pérez-Dasilva, J.-Á., Meso-Ayerdi, K., Mendiguren-Galdospín, T.: Fake news y coronavirus: detección de los principales actores y tendencias a través del análisis de las conversaciones en Twitter. Prof. Inform. **29**(3), e290308 (2020)
14. Al-Rawi, A., Shukla, V.: Bots as active news promoters: a digital analysis of COVID-19 tweets. Information **11**, 461 (2020)
15. Asociación de prensa de Madrid. Aparecen algunos síntomas de saturación informativa en el consumo de medios durante el confinamiento. https://www.apmadrid.es/aparecen-algunos-sintomas-de-saturacion-informativa-en-el-consumo-de-medios-durante-el-confinamiento/. Accessed 19 Jan 2021
16. Lázaro-Rodríguez, P., Herrera-Viedma, E.: Noticias sobre Covid-19 y 2019-nCoV en medios de comunicación de España: el papel de los medios digitales en tiempos de confinamiento. Prof. Inform. **29**(3), e290302 (2020)
17. Igartua, J.-J., Ortega-Mohedano, F., Arcila-Calderón, C.: Communication use in the times of the coronavirus. A cross-cultural study. Prof. Inform. **29**(3), e290318 (2020)
18. Gil-Torres, A., Martín-Quevedo, J., Gómez-García, S., San José-De la Rosa, C.: El coronavirus en el ecosistema de los dispositivos móviles: creadores, discursos y recepción. Rev. Latina Comun. Soc. **78**, 329–358 (2020)
19. Meyer, P.: The Vanishing Newspaper. Saving Journalism in the Information Age. University of Missouri Press, Missouri (2004). ISBN 978 0 8262 1877 3
20. Martínez-Fernández, V.-A., Castellanos-García, P., Juanatey-Boga, O.: Del papel a los metamedios: la prensa ante el fin del ciclo impreso. Prof. Inform. **25**(3) (2016)

21. Cairo, H.: Geopolítica popular del coronavirus: el poder de las viñetas editoriales de la prensa diaria. Geopolítica(s). Rev. Estud. Sobre Espacio Poder **11**(Especial), 303–317 (2020)
22. Salvat-Martinrey, G., Aranda-Martínez, S.: Análisis de contenido de la prensa diaria Española sobre el uso de informar de la crisis sanitaria de la COVID19. Rev. Comun. Salud **10**(2), 185–210 (2020)
23. Roselli, D.: Covid-19 en Colombia: los primeros 90 días. Acta Neurológica Colombiana (2020)
24. BBC News Mundo, Qué lecciones está dejando la segunda ola de covid-19 en Europa (y cómo pueden prepararse los países que apenas se están recuperando de la primera). https://www.bbc.com/mundo/noticias-55016466. Accessed 12 Feb 2021
25. Llaneras, K.: La segunda ola europea superará pronto las muertes de la primera. El País. https://elpais.com/politica/2020/11/27/actualidad/1606486774_748425.html. Accessed 14 Feb 2021
26. Infobae Este es el panorama de la segunda ola del Covid-19 en Colombia. https://www.infobae.com/america/colombia/2020/12/09/este-es-el-panorama-de-la-segunda-ola-del-covid-19-en-colombia/. Accessed 14 Feb 2021
27. Mintic, La mitad de Colombia no tiene Internet. MinTIC. https://www.mintic.gov.co/portal/inicio/Sala-de-Prensa/MinTIC-en-los-Medios/100837:La-mitad-de-Colombia-no-tiene-internet. Accessed 15 Feb 2021
28. Rivas-de-Roca, R., García-Gordillo, M., Caro-González, F.J.: La construcción del periodismo "localizado" en medios digitales europeos. Estudios de casos. Rev. Latina Comun. Soc. **75**, 1–26 (2020)

National Survey on Educommunication in Spanish Universities During the COVID-19 Pandemic: Methodology and Results

Ingrid Gil(✉)

Universidad Jaume I-Universidad Pontificia Comillas, Madrid, Spain
ingrid.gil@comillas.edu

Abstract. Since the end of 2019, the world is experiencing the COVID-19 pandemic. Many countries have been forced to take exceptional measures, such as closing many economic activities and educational institutions. In this context, many universities have seen their work routine altered. This investigation aimed at studying how students have adapted to this new circumstance and how they have changed their traditional face-to-face methodology to a distance methodology in a few days. The lack of time to prepare the new materials, together with a lack of knowledge of the technical means to carry out this task, has caused an unprecedented situation. The objective of this research is to survey the perceptions of Spanish university students on the application of this teaching methodology and to analyze the difficulties encountered. To achieve this, we relied on a quantitative methodology, based on the administration of a questionnaire, which allowed us to obtain answers that can help establish the necessary future guidelines. Although they have understood that the exceptional circumstances required online teaching, the results show that students tend to prefer face-to-face education.

Keywords: Media competence · Digitalization · COVID-19 · Online education · Questionnaire · Educommunication

1 Introduction

We are immersed in a true digital revolution. We have moved from an atom-based to a bit-based culture [1]. The implications are huge, especially since digital technology removes the need to be in the same place at the same time to meet for whatever purposes. Space-time coordinates were, until recently, the frame of reference for any human activity [2].

In the era of digitalization in the classroom, it is assumed that institutions, teachers, or students —at any level— are ready to face the challenge of online or blended education from a computer [3]. It is sufficient to enter the words "classroom", "digital", or "online education" in the computer's search engine to find multiple options, specialization courses and, ultimately, a flood of information for all ages. Nevertheless, are we really prepared?

The general assumption is that Information and Communications Technologies (ICTs) favor teaching and learning processes [4], which implies that teaching institutions:

© The Author(s), under exclusive license to Springer Nature Singapore Pte Ltd. 2022
Á. Rocha et al. (Eds.): ICOMTA 2021, SIST 259, pp. 314–324, 2022.
https://doi.org/10.1007/978-981-16-5792-4_31

> [...] must adapt to be competitive in what they offer and guarantee their students the best means and resources. But it is not only necessary to modernize the existing technologies in educational centres, but an update of the entire community and educational organization is required. (Author's translation) [4]).

In this sense [5]:

> [...] If we say that society is capable of permanent learning and that ICT allows us to design and develop spaces for the generation and transmission of knowledge in an efficient way, we must reorganize our universities to make them as dynamic as the very context in which they are immersed. (Author's translation) (p. 83) [5].

The current COVID-19 crisis has forced us to ascertain if we are in fact prepared to handle ICTs and generate online training resources for higher education. The fact that it has affected all levels of education and that both teachers and students have had to adapt to this situation virtually overnight, has generated the appropriate context to find out how this situation has been managed, what actions have been implemented, and what learning and updating requirements exist in this field.

This investigation was conducted in the context of the national lockdown that was declared in Spain on March 14, 2020, due to the COVID-19 pandemic. This measure forced Spanish universities to lockdown and move from face-to-face to online teaching from March to June 2020.

The first section will review the literature on the concept of educommunication, which provides the theoretical context of this research. The second will describe the research design, the research question, and the methodology. The third and the fourth sections will present the data and the results of the research. The fifth section will discuss the results, while the sixth will deal with the limitations of the study and provide some lines for future research.

2 Literature Review

This research is based on the theoretical approach of educommunication, which postulate the incorporation of technology and digital resources into the educational process. On the importance of dialogical education, understood as an interactive process based on the exchange of knowledge [6–9]. On the other hand, has been argued [10] that for literacy to become an instrument of liberation, students must become autonomous subjects, capable of working in a collaborative environment, based on reflection and dialogue. Along similar lines it has been observed that knowledge is effective when students can relate technology with their personal learning process [11].

ICTs can become transformative instruments of the educational environment [12]. ICTs can be particularly useful to manage a volume of information that is constantly growing because they offer instruments to convert this information into knowledge, thanks to their formalism and connectivity. Formalism operates in a specific way by following a series of specific commands and actions that must be mastered. Here, the metacognitive skills that the user needs to apply come into play to understand the operation of the processes and the uses of ICT. Connectivity allows us to create online communities and establish information networks, which is important for the generation of collaborative learning environments.

Vygotsky's conceptualization of learning processes [13] is very much in line with what ICTs allow us today in terms of social interaction. Vygotsky developed the theory that every formative function appears first at the social (interpersonal) level and then at the personal (intrapersonal) level. Cognitive processes are generated from common social processes. However, the central aspect is interactivity, which facilitates constant learning. Along these lines, the user must interact with the technological medium, which will provide a series of stimuli to which the user will respond with some feedback that will allow them to redirect their actions. This behavior requires users to play a leading role. This way, they will feel that they have control over their knowledge, which will act as a catalyst for motivation and promote student understanding and learning.

Technical advances and the information society have led to the integration of technological and digital tools in the classroom, thus becoming part of an emerging educational process. However, despite its potential advantages, this process still raises doubts about its correct implementation. First, it would be necessary to determine the level of literacy and media competence of teachers and students, and then design and generate digital contents that focus on clear objectives and specific curricular competencies.

Likewise, to move with ease in the labor market and society at large, it is increasingly necessary to acquire digital and technological competences, together with the necessary media competence. These skills must be acquired in the educational environment either in schools, through vocational training, or in universities. Students need to be trained to work with the technological environment surrounding us. New educational scenarios and actions need to be designed [14]. We must propose a specific educational policy for the digital environment and apply new technologies to education, devising educational scenarios where students can learn to move and in the new telematic space.

ICTs have opened possibilities for a new communicative environment that can be applied in the classroom, thus giving rise to the emergence of a new communicative space, that is virtual education [15]. Virtual education is usually conceived as an educational opportunity for those who are forced to break from the spatio-temporal paradigms of classical training due to lack of time or the need to reconcile work life and studies. At the same time, scholars are analyzing the possible difficulties of ICTs and the challenges to be overcome [16, 17].

In a context in which ICTs are increasingly imposed in the educational system, both teachers and students face a series of challenges [18, 19]. The relative novelty of ICTs requires that more studies be conducted to understand how to implement them effectively and how they impact in the perception of students and teachers.

To contribute to this literature and to further understand the advantages and disadvantages of the use of ICTs in education, this study explores the perceptions of Spanish students during the first months of the COVID-19 pandemic in Spain. From March to June 2020, due to the lockdown, Spanish universities were forced to move their teaching from the physical to the online space. What were the perceptions of students about the online teaching that took place during this exceptional moment? As such, this study presents a series of specific characteristics. First, the adaptation to the online methodology was carried out in a forced and unnatural way, with limited time. Moreover, the change was abrupt. This means that students and teachers could not be previously trained in the use of the technology necessary to implement the online teaching. To this must be added an extraordinary social situation, characterized by the concerns with the social and health consequences of the pandemic and with home isolation. All this has caused online teaching to not be as accurate as it should. This offers a good opportunity to explore this process in motion and to highlight current needs in terms of online and face-to-face educommunication.

3 Design and Method

Research question and objectives:
Based on the literature review, the main research question that guides this investigation is:

What are the students' perceptions about the implementation of online teaching during this situation?

Based on the research question, this study aims to explore:

- The online teaching from March to June 2020.
- Their own media competence and the media competence of their teachers.
- The process of adaptation of teachers and universities to the online teaching.
- The possible future implementation of online teaching.

Method: the survey
To answer these questions, this study was based on the collection of empirical data using a questionnaire disseminated online from May to June 2020.

This tool offers several advantages, such as its low cost, the possibility of being disseminated online, and the possibility of obtaining rapid results. Moreover, we can standardize data, which allows its computerized treatment and statistical analysis.

As for the items, each question had to respond to a specific need for knowledge and had to be adapted accordingly. From the data obtained, general trends were extracted. These were related with the following variables: university, educational level, sex, and media competence.

The questionnaire had 20 questions and was composed of closed-scale questions (nominal and Likert).

The items were organized into 8 thematic blocks for the survey questions to be logically ordered, and to facilitate the subsequent extraction of data and trends:

- Items 1–4: Initial students' data (university, degree, type of training, and sex).
- Items 5–7: Self-perception of the students in the personal realm (if the personal situation has affected the academic life of the students; if they have suffered stress; personal problems).
- Items 8–11: Relationship with the university and perception of its actions (emotional attention by the university and the teaching staff; convenience of the price of the fees)
- Items 12–13: Media competence (before and after the COVID-19 lockdown).

- Items 14–17: Difficulties of the online method (adaptation to the new method; communicative sensations in the online class; academic problems; level of demand of the online method).
- Item 18: Digital tools used.
- Items 19–25: Perception of the teaching staff and subject (difficulties of the teachers; feedback received; adaptation of the evaluation criteria; assessment of the management of the students by the teacher; management of students with special needs).
- Items 26–28: Prospects and general assessment.

The potential problem with these types of surveys is that often there is no exact option on the list that matches the answer that the subject wishes to provide; therefore, we have added the option "others" whenever necessary.

Some multiple-choice questions (for example, question 16), in which the subjects are provided with many answer options, may lead them to select those that are best known and used by the sample without reading all the options. It can also happen that, even after reading them, they lean towards the first (error of primacy) or the last (error of recency), even if they are not the answers that they would have marked if they were in another order. For this reason, the options rotate randomly in the online version of the questionnaire. In scale questions, by convention, low numerical values usually correspond to the absence or the lowest level of the trait that we are measuring; therefore, the answer options are listed starting with those values.

Regarding the means of capturing the sample, we used the CAWI system (Computer-Assisted Web Interview). The questionnaire was sent by email, using a chain of contacts, and requesting that it be forwarded.

The survey was launched on May 18, 2020, after two months of forced online education. A total of 206 responses were obtained. Before analyzing the results, the surveys were reviewed to verify that they had indeed been answered correctly, filling in the necessary fields, and that the subjects met the required profile. Regarding the sample, it includes university students who participated voluntarily.

4 Results

To interpret the data, we extracted the most significant trends, considering the division of the questionnaire into blocks of questions.

4.1 Baseline Data of the Subjects

The students belong to 13 Spanish universities (public and private). Most study a double degree, or one degree. They study different branches of knowledge, although they are more numerous in the area of Human Sciences. Regarding sex, the majority are women (78.2%). Nevertheless, the results did not show any correlation between the participants' answers and sex.

The variable university was cross-referenced with the following variables, yielding the following trends:

- University and media competence (before March 2020): there is no correlation between the two.
- University and future predisposition to study at a distance: there is no correlation between these two variables since the lack of predisposition to study online is uniform and common in all universities.
- University and tools used: there is no correlation between both variables, but the same tools have been used uniformly in all universities (Moodle, e-mail, and Blackboard Collaborate), except on a few occasions.
- The variable sex was cross-referenced with the following variables, showing the following trends:
- Sex and stress: there are no clear trends, since both men and women have reported having suffered stress; however, men have suffered these episodes less frequently than women.
- Sex and communication in the online classroom: both agree that the most frequent sensation is that of feeling less participative and motivated.
- Sex and educational method: Both agree to opt for the face-to-face method, with no clear differences in this regard.
- Sex and assessment of online teaching: equally, both men and women, agree in their preferences and they are clear that what they value the most when organizing the subject is that the teacher is empathetic and that the schedules are clear.
- Sex and general assessment of the experience: there are no trends or significant relationships between these two aspects.

4.2 Students' Perception About Their Personal Feelings

The trends in terms of the emotional state experienced by students in this specific period of online teaching are quite clear. More than 85% state that their personal situation has affected their academic situation and more than 80% have suffered stress. The personal problems that have affected them the most are the workloads (46.1%) caused by the performance of domestic tasks, problems of coexistence with relatives (34.5%), and health problems of their own or of relatives (33%). 8.7% indicated problems of access to computer media.

4.3 Students' Perception About the University and Their Actions in the Online Teaching Period

40.8% indicate that universities have occasionally taken these personal and emotional problems into account, while 25.7% say they have not. 33.5% affirm that this was always the case. Most of them positively or very positively evaluated both universities and teachers (47.6%); 19.5% negatively or very negatively; and 33% gave an average evaluation. Regarding the payment of fees, 48.3% do not agree to pay the same prices in face-to-face and non-face-to-face classes, although 20% agree, and 31.7% are not very clear about it. This is an issue that universities should address in the future and make clear to families and students.

When cross-referencing the variable university with those of initial media competence and degree of subsequent preparation, there are no clear trends related to the university of origin.

The university variable was triangulated with the variable media competence, and with the assessment of teachers and universities, yielding the following trends:

- There is no relationship between university and initial media competence or the student's perception of learning (see below in "media competence").
- There is a relationship between assessment of the university and learning: the lower the first, the lower the second.

4.4 Media Competence

Most of the students report basic competence in mastering online teaching tools (75.3%). While they indicate that they feel sufficiently prepared, in almost no case do they report a high level of knowledge (Table 1). These data show that, even though students see themselves as digital natives, they do not master the tools related to online teaching, research, or study, and need training in this regard. If we relate the perception of their initial competence with the perception of their current preparation, the data show that they have improved their learning (Table 1). In this sense, there is an improvement in preparation. Those who initially felt unprepared or ill-prepared are fewer and the number of students who feel more prepared to face online teaching increases.

Table 1. Comparison of initial competence and current preparation

Initial competence		Current preparation	
None	21.4%	None	2.9%
Little	40.8%	Little	20.9%
Sufficient	23.3%	Sufficient	42.7%
Moderate	11.2%	Moderate	28.6%
Strong	2.4%	Strong	4.9%

Source: created by author

We have cross-referenced the media competence variable with the following data, reflecting the following trends:

- Initial media competence and university: no correlation.
- Initial media competence, university and university assessment: the better the university has been valued, the higher learning students have reported, and vice versa, indicating that when the university and the teaching staff are involved, students are more motivated and feel that they learn more.

- Media competence and current student preparation: there is no correlation, since students feel that there has been an increase in their preparation, although this does not depend on the university.
- Media competence and motivation to receive online teaching in the future: the lack of desire that students indicate to study remotely is not related to the initial media competence or their current perception of preparation. Although this preparation has increased according to the survey data, this increase in the students' competences does not lead to an increased desire for the online method, and there is no relationship between the two variables.
- Initial media competence and adaptation to the online method: it shows that those who had indicated less initial knowledge have adapted worse, and vice versa.
- Media competence and academic problems and difficulties: there are no clear trends. The same types of problems (loss of time, demotivation) are reported regardless of the initial competence of the students.

4.5 Difficulties of the Online Method

Almost 75% of students consider that they have done it regularly or well enough with the online method, although they indicate that it was costing them less work after they developed technical skills and time organization. This shows the need to train students in media competence oriented toward online methodology.

As for the negative feelings that the online method produces, these are: the feeling of wasting time (55.3%); the lack of motivation (40.8%) and little desire to participate (49.5%); loneliness and isolation (39.6%); and the perception of lack of preparation on the part of the teaching staff (30.1%). The academic problems that the students have experienced throughout this experience are: that the online method is more demanding and that they have to work more and more independently (64.1%) and that, on many occasions, the teachers have not adequately prepared the online classes (53.9%). These ideas will need to be explored through a series of in-depth interviews in successive phases of the investigation.

Digital tools used: The tools that students have used the most are Moodle (86.9%), e-mail (68.4%), and Blackboard Collaborate (71.4%).

4.6 Perception About the Teaching Staff

Students were also asked questions about their teachers, in terms of digital competence and preparation.

The negative aspects that students report are: poorly managed workload (64.1%); ignorance of digital tools (68.1%); difficulties in controlling the class from a distance (63.7) and in teaching with distant and unmotivated students (58.3%); and the perception that the teacher might face a work overload (43.1%). Regarding the feedback and evaluation criteria, 53.9% affirm that it was not useful and not very useful, while only 16.2% think it was useful and very useful. 29.9% affirm that it was averagely useful.

The positive aspects that the students indicate are the teachers' capacity to understand their difficulties (73.5%); that the schedules are clear (50%); the visual support through video classes (49%); and the continued student-teacher contact (40.7%).

Regarding the possibility of adaptation of students with special needs, most of the students consider that it will be more difficult to monitor them effectively in the online teaching (57.1%).

The activities that students believe that are lost, that cannot be developed in the same way, or that are negatively affected by the online method include the lack of access to libraries (64.8%), the lack of collaborative work in face-to-face groups (54.6%), or the impossibility to attend their internships programs (62.2%).

4.7 Prospects and General Valuation

Regarding the method preferred by students, or with which they claim to feel more comfortable, more than 75% opt for the face-to-face method, while almost 20% think that the online and face-to-face method could be alternated. This trend is consistent with what was indicated previously, in the media competence section. It is curious how, even though students report an improvement regarding the management of online education, they do not show much interest in this method. Students still prefer direct contact and face-to-face communication, although they think that the experience was not necessarily negative. 35.9% evaluate the experience as negative and very negative. 40.3% averagely evaluate it. 23.8% affirm that it was positive and very positively. Despite this relatively positive assessment, more than 65% do not feel like studying remotely in the future. Remarkably, only 1% declare to prefer the online education. In future studies, it will be necessary to explore more the reasons for this skepticism regarding online teaching.

5 Conclusions

After analyzing the data, we can extract some trends:

- More than 60% of students admitted little, very little, or no prior preparation to cope with online learning.
- Students have little prior knowledge about non-face-to-face education and about how to adapt to it (62.2%).
- Students, generally, are not motivated (53.9%) and do not know how to organize their time when the teacher is not present (46.1%). Their responses show a difficulty to organize their work in an autonomous way.
- Students value more the emotional proximity of the teacher (73.5%) and the organization of schedules and subjects (50%) than the originality of the sessions or digital artifacts (15.7%).
- Student's associate personal problems with academic problems and academic problems caused them more stress (89%)
- What students like the least about online teaching is the feeling of loss of time (55.3%), the low participation that this model allows (49.5%), and the disconnection and demotivation that can imply (40.8%).
- Students believe that teachers do not have sufficient media competence (68.1%) and that online teaching augments the teachers' workload (43.1%).
- The most used tools have been Moodle (86.9%), Blackboard Collaborate (71.4%), and e-mail (68.4%).

- Students work with less than 5 tools and do not know what benefits or disadvantages each one of them can bring.
- Students are not particularly attracted to a remote method and tend to prefer the traditional method (75% prefer face-to-face method).
- Students consider that the remote method is, generally, more difficult to be used (64.1%).
- Students have positively valued their work during the lockdown but are aware that much better can be done and that they have a long way to go in terms of media competence (64.1%).
- Students perceive that universities have reacted as well as they could to adapt classroom courses to online in record time, train teachers, and support students (80.6%).
- Nevertheless, this adaptation is mostly perceived as an emergency remedy that has been implemented quickly, but also partially improvised.

According to this study, students exposed to online teaching report feeling isolated, unmotivated, and uninvolved, claiming that the interaction and the provision of feedback are insufficient. In fact, both are crucial to foster constant learning and make students feel part of the process (Vigotsky, in Daniels, 2003). The impression is that we are not teaching students' how to interact with technology, without falling into the trap of banking education (Freire, 2005). Technology is not simply a vehicle for the transmission of knowledge. At the same time, information cannot be confused with knowledge, or access to information with learning. For this reason, educational institutions need to devote adequate resources to learning how to generate content and activities, and how to communicate with and motivate students.

References

1. Negroponte, N.: Being Digital. Aldred A. Knopf, New York (1995)
2. Pérez, M.A.: La paradoja de la comunicación sin fronteras: la «fractura digital». Portularia: Rev. Trabajo Soc. **3**(Ejemplar dedicado a: Nuevas realidades familiares), 299–310 (2003)
3. Mosquera, Í.: Las cifras no mienten: la digitalización en las aulas es una realidad a nivel mundial. Rev. UNIR. La Univ. Internet (2019). https://www.unir.net/educacion/revista/noticias/las-cifras-no-mienten-la-digitalizacion-en-las-aulas-es-una-realidad-a-nivel-mundial/549203639125/. Accessed 1 Dec 2020
4. Domínguez, R., Hernández, A., Chica, E.: Construcción y validación de un cuestionario para la evaluación del uso de las TIC en los centros educativos de secundaria. Digit. Educ. Rev. **34**, 1–26 (2018)
5. Gisbert, M.: La digitalización de las universidades. Tecnol. Marcha **17**(3), 81–89 (2004). https://dialnet.unirioja.es/ejemplar/377463
6. Aparici, R. (ed.): La revolución de los medios audiovisuales: educación y nuevas tecnologías. Madrid: Ediciones de la Torre (1996)
7. Aparici, R. (ed.): Comunicación educativa en la sociedad de la información. UNED, Madrid (2003)
8. Aparici, R. (ed.): Educomunicación: más allá del 2.0. Gedisa, Barcelona (2010)
9. Aparici, R. (ed.): Conectados en el ciberespacio. UNED, Madrid (2010)
10. Freire, P.: Pedagogía del oprimido. Siglo XXI, México (2005)

11. Gutiérrez, A.: Alfabetización digital. Algo más que ratones y teclas. Gedisa, Barcelona (2003)
12. Coll, C., Martí, E.: La educación escolar ante las nuevas tecnologías de la información y la comunicación. In: Coll, C., Palacios, J., Marchesi, Á. (eds.) Desarrollo psicológico y educación: Psicología de la educación escolar, vol. II, pp. 623–651. Alianza, Madrid (2001)
13. Daniels, H.: Vygotsky y la pedagogía. Editorial Paidós, Madrid (2003)
14. Echeverría, J.: Educación y Tecnologías telemáticas. Rev. Iberoamericana Educ. **24**, 12–23 (2000). https://rieoei.org/historico/documentos/rie24a01.htm
15. Rama, C.: University virtualisation in Latin America. RUSC. Univ. Knowl. Soc. J. **11**(3), 32–41 (2014)
16. Zabalza, M.: El estudio de las buenas prácticas docentes en la enseñanza universitaria. Rev. Docencia Univ. **10**(1), 17–42 (2012)
17. Durán, R., Estay-Niculcar, C., Álvarez, H.: Adopción de buenas prácticas en la educación virtual en la educación superior. Aula Abierta **43**(2), 77–86 (2005). https://doi.org/10.1016/j.aula.2015.01.001
18. Adell, J., Castañeda, L.: Tecnologías emergentes, ¿pedagogías emergentes? In: Hernández Ortega, J., Pennesi, M., Sobrino López, D., Vázquez Gutiérrez, A. (eds.) Tendencias emergentes en educación con TIC, pp. 13–32. Asociación Espiral, Educación y Tecnología, Barcelona (2012)
19. Castañeda, L.: Debates regarding technology and education: contemporary pathways and pending conversations. RIED. Rev. Iberoamericana Educ. Dist. **22**(1), 29–39 (2019). https://doi.org/10.5944/ried.22.1.23020

Digital Interaction and the Transition in the Information Consumption of the New Generations

Daniel Javier de la Garza Montemayor(✉)

Universidad de Monterrey, 66238 San Pedro, NL, México
daniel.delagarza@udem.edu

Abstract. There are many studies focused on analyzing, the level of disinformation generated by social networks, whether there is a deeper discussion on public issues that, in general terms, impacts the participation in contemporary societies. In order to add value to this ongoing debate, it was proposed to carry out a qualitative study on the perceptions of this phenomenon by key actors who have observed this transition from the classroom: university professors. To do this, interviews are conducted with teachers from two emblematic Ibero-American nations: Mexico and Spain. Both countries have different systems but have been at the forefront of digital interaction by digital media. The results found that, despite the differences between the two countries, the perceptions of the Mexican and Spanish teachers have more coincidences than differences.

Keywords: Social networks · Internet · Youth · Teachers and Digital interaction

1 Introduction

Studies on social and virtual media interactions show how different they can be between cultures, generations, and political climates. Far from being a fleeting trend, social networks in public affairs can be confirmed at different moments in history, all around the world [1].

One example is the 2008 elections 2008, when the now former President of the United States of America Barack Obama became elected. The internet became a platform for the political campaign to influence the voters in their decision in a way that was equally effective as any other traditional platform. Thus, creating a new trend for influencing the public [2].

In the Ibero-American context, Spain, Mexico and Chile experience their own social movements that emerged from the internet as a platform for change [3]. However, there were some reservations on the true impact that a social network can have in the public, and their effectiveness to promote (or discourage) a political ideology.

Only time will tell, if this new platform will begin to replace the more traditional sources of information, especially among the younger generations, particularly university students. However, since 2015, the electoral processes in many countries have shown

© The Author(s), under exclusive license to Springer Nature Singapore Pte Ltd. 2022
Á. Rocha et al. (Eds.): ICOMTA 2021, SIST 259, pp. 325–332, 2022.
https://doi.org/10.1007/978-981-16-5792-4_32

signs that social media has become a medium with equal, if not more, influence that any other form of communication [4].

Analysts have concluded that social media is more than a way to influence people, it is also a tool for citizens to express their discontent against political oppression or traditional ideologies. This is possible by creating networks that allows for a more open and free conversation [5].

It is a fact that in the recent years, there is an increase of consumption of information on politics. Key actors have been identified to be the ones to recognize the transition of digital narratives, which are none other than university professors, because millennials are rarely aware of this process. For this reason, this key witness has been chosen to provide testimonies on events that have marked the political climate in Mexico and Spain in the last five years but also provide a panoramic view of these changes and the responses of the citizens when they were informed.

2 Digital Consumption of the New Generations

2.1 New Paradigm

The Internet and social networks have allowed for younger people to create their own universe in which new patterns of consumption, creation and spreading of audiovisual content have been established [6]. Traditional media have been overtaken in this process by multiple devices with internet connection by virtue of their availability to adapt and learn from users [7]. At present, these consumer demands of young people are being adequately served by automated platforms, which show greater competition, to the extent that they have strategies that are closer to the way they interact and their way to express themselves. It is possible to argue that the transition to digital is not just a step to a new form of content distribution. The input and output of information is changing like never before in history. As a result of this process, it is expected that there will be an alteration that will possibly change the rules of engagement and how people, not just new generations, actively seek information [8].

It is important to establish that there is evidence that digital content has a more ephemeral effect than content received through the mass media. The excess of information received through digital platforms can end up being exhausted relatively quickly [9]. But is also possible to argue that it can have an important effect on the perception that is generated about important events [10].

In the midst of the Covid-19 pandemic, it was proven that the way it was reported through social networks had serious implications on its perception and social evaluation, especially in the case of new generations. The Coronavirus crisis accelerated the integration of social media in our lives in an alarming rate as information technology and telecommunication sources [11].

2.2 Risk of Misinformation

The distortion of information during the digital age has also raised a serious discussion about the absence of ethical limits for digital media. It is, however, possible that some sensitive issues can sensitize some people and decision makers, but if they are handled in an irresponsible way, they can have harmful effects on social life [12].

Notwithstanding the above, it is possible to argue that one of the main counterweights to misinformation that have characterized these mass media comes from society itself. But it is also important to establish that combating misinformation is not easy, since it requires the verification of the authenticity of a certain source be carried out by reliable sources. In other words, the credibility of mediators is fundamental so they can contribute to counter-act the misinformation [13].

Through an experimental study, they confirmed that users tend to trust more news that is close to their convictions, even when confronted with solid evidence that denies its authenticity. This generation perception affects the social coexistence, and it is what some authors called the post-truth era [14, 15].

On several occasions, diverse actors called to challenge on the streets social distancing measures and health protocols in different countries around the world, because they considered that the guidelines were part of a conspiracy. Situation like these, which confirmed the misinformation originated from digital media, could lead to situations that endanger the health of the citizens [16].

3 Methodology

3.1 Research Design

As explained in the previous paragraphs, for some years, there has been a migration in consumption from conventional to non-conventional media, specifically linked to social networks. This change has led to the search for the reasons why social networks are so attractive to their users, as well as to verify whether this consumption and the activity that takes place in them has an impact on the social field. These digital platforms have become a media where users inform themselves, exchange ideas and positions about what happens in daily life. The interest in this phenomenon arises from the changes that have been manifested in the consumption of the media, migrating from a traditional block, to the digital media.

Given this argument, the following questions arise: What are the factors that influence social networks to make media attractive to users? Does social media contribute to building trust in a determined environment? We have also set ourselves the general objective of analyzing the impact that social networks have on contemporary democracies through interviews with university professors from Mexico and Spain, that can provide testimony about the changing consumption of information of a generation. The professors that were selected, had at least 5 years of interaction with students. Also, they all belonged to social science departments. Ten university teachers from each country were selected, with a total of twenty interviews.

Additionally, as specific objectives, we propose, first of all, to know the factors that influence the consumption of social networks, as well as to analyze the impact that interaction in social networks have on the development of the quality of social coexistence. Secondly, we seek to know if the participation that takes place in social networks has an impact on the political effectiveness and the formation of social capital.

The previous objectives and questions are relevant because they promote the relationship between the consumption factors of non-conventional media, which can influence the development of social coexistence. Various studies over the past decade have shown that there is a close relationship between the information circulating in the media and the impact of this information on the interaction of individuals [17–19].

The innovation of this study lies in the approach on the impact that social networks now have in the public sphere, replacing traditional media, such as print, radio and television. The testimony of the teachers has been chosen, because they have witnessed, from the classroom, a change in the way students are informed.

It is possible that the narrative of this transition may be clearer from an external actor perspective because social networks have become a means of youth socialization and may not be seen with the same objectivity. For this reason, we consider that information on this phenomenon that has been studied can be provided by complementing the research that has been done in this area.

Due to the nature of this phenomenon, the scope of this study is divided into two parts, an in-depth interview to the test subjects, and the collection and analysis of data. To make the research more objective and broader, two different contexts were compared: Mexico and Spain.

Phenomenological: The phenomenon studied is influenced by several elements: the generational change in media consumption, the perception on the impact that the political participation has inside and outside the line in the public sphere, the use of social media, as well as the trust they have in these spaces as a way to strengthen democracy.

In-depth interviews: 20 interviews were conducted with university professors from Mexico and Spain, specialized in the social sciences of public universities. In the case of Mexico, the professors interviewed were from public universities in Mexico City, Puebla and Sonora. In Spain, teachers from the cities of Granada and Seville were interviewed.

Hermeneutics: As a study that aims to know the changes that are presented in the communicative processes of a generation and the impact of these on participation in public affairs, hermeneutics is relevant because teachers interpret these processes of change in their student's media consumption.

Comparative Method: When analyzing various movements that have been strengthened by social media, it was considered advisable to draw a comparison between two countries to know if this phenomenon had significant similarities or differences that could be contrasted. These techniques were carried out in three stages: the first was the analysis of documents, followed by interviews with Mexican professors, culminating in interviews with Spanish professors. The fieldwork was carried out from February to July 2019. All data obtained through the application of the described method and techniques were analyzed with NViVo software version 11.

3.2 Results. Most Used Social Networks and Consumer Preferences: Mexico and Spain

In the case of Mexico there is a clear differentiation in consumption, depending on age. Young students between the age of 18 and 25 use social media without checking the information they share and read. In contrast, people 35 and older also use social media, but mainly to communicate with their nearest environment, share ideas, images, among other functions. In general, users over the age of 35 do not perceive a use of social media as a channel to inform themselves about issues of public interest.

There are elements of coincidence in the consumption of Spanish and Mexican users, because they prefer Facebook, Instagram and Twitter. The main characteristic is that there is no difference in consumption based on the age range, by-which the majority (young and older adults) are mainly informed by social networks or by digital media. Like Mexican and Spanish professors, they agree that the immediacy of information is important for the users of social networks.

3.3 Fake News: México and Spain

There is a coincidence among all social media users - young people and adults- in Mexico and Spain, because both groups create and share information about public affairs that in some cases is false, especially during the election season. In many cases, the purpose of influencing the electorate is achieved by ensuring the circulating such news. Due to the high circulation of fake news on social networks it is important to analyze the impact that this type of news has on social network users. This type of news also affects the perception of users on how they visualize candidates, how they influence electoral preferences, and gives us an idea of the final effect they have on the democratic process.

3.4 Main Attraction on Social Media: Mexico and Spain

The main attraction that teachers from both countries find in social networks, is the possibility of consulting a high content of images, allowing them to have social relations with individuals who, for reasons of time, place of residence or exposure, would have been difficult in any other historical context. In both countries it is noted that in social networks, users share facts that they consider relevant in their lives, such as travel, family photos, professional achievements, which in some way causes them to feel like public figures and even, feel like they have some kind of influence with their nearest surroundings. In the traditional media this feeling could only be experienced by artists, politicians or socially recognized people, therefore social networks allow this type of exposure to any individual. The basis of social networks is the image, this being the main attraction they have, so consumption is related to the exposure or management of images, beyond the management of reliable information.

Given that there are few spaces for discussion and enough characters to present ideas, Mexican interviewees believe that the impact that social networks have on democracy is rather negative. Some even consider that the discussion on the essential issues of a democracy is trivialized by social media's own characteristics. Another factor to consider is that social networks determine the topics or advertising they present to their users. By consumption preferences, generating a bias in the information that could be presented on the user's devices. In other words, the algorithm causes advertising to be targeted to the user based on their search history.

3.5 Information They Share on Social Media that Impacts the Public Sphere

The results of the study have helped identify the main elements that are shared in social media related to the public sphere:

1. They approach public reality through humor with "memes".
2. They pursue ideals of community life through the "hashtag".
3. Signed petitions through Change.org.
4. They manifest for some cause through virtual media.

The results show that Spaniards and Mexicans interact in a similar way by addressing issues of public interest on social media, sharing basically the same things. Digital media, in both contexts, have a greater impact on the call for demonstrations for specific causes.

3.6 The Importance that Politicians Confer with Leaders on Citizen's Manifestation on Social Media

In both studies there is the same agreement on this paragraph. The leaders (politicians, communicators, entrepreneurs) know the importance of social networks today, as it has migrated, as we have seen, from conventional to unconventional media, that's why politicians pay attention to the expressions that individuals have on social media. In addition, the different elected positions use social networks to position themselves, articulate demands that are trending topics, and present arguments, among other actions. In the case of public life issues, the interviewees agreed that, although politicians tend to attach great importance to these spaces, that there is no real evidence that any demand made on social media has been translated into a measurable and evaluable public policy, so the effectiveness of social networks in the implementation of public actions is still in doubt.

3.7 Contribution of the Social Media to Social Coexistence

There are two positions on the contribution that social media make to democracy. Some interviewees report that social networks have trivialized discussions on relevant public issues, while others mention that they have strengthened democracy. Through the analysis of the data obtained from this research we can conclude that the impact on democracy is presented as follows:

1. Social networks do not allow for an in-depth discussion on issues of public interest.
2. Due to the amount of information that is generated and the immediacy of it, it is difficult to verify its validity and make a distinction between the data that are true and those that are not.
3. Since the emergence of social networks, new forms of political participation have not really manifested themselves. In general, what has happened is that the calls to participate in the spaces of conventional politics such as the exercise of the vote, manifestations, public opinion, among others, are given in an easier way, with the potential that they can reach more people. Some of these movements (which have taken place both in Mexico and in Spain) have become multitudinous, attributing strength to information and communication technologies.
4. The political and social actors of both countries attach great importance to social networks, in order to present positions and disseminate their public image. In matters of social problems, if any request or social movements "go viral", they can pronounce

on them, but there are not many precedents around which of these expressions end up strengthening the creation of new public policies.
5. Social networks usually generate trust between users, so both contexts, fake news tends to emerge strongly.
6. Fake news affects the development of public opinion, being a negative factor for the development of democracy.
7. In both countries, the sense of empowerment among young people has crystallized; this underscores the conviction that their individual actions can contribute to greater social change.

4 Conclusions

It is important to underline that, even when there may be differences in the social life of both countries, the perception of university professors had more similarities than differences. This could mean that the change in the consumption of information on politics of a generation has to do more with a historical process than with a different historical and political juncture. In general terms, it is noteworthy that the university professors agreed on some of the promises of the social partners, even though in some cases they expressed reservations. There is recognition that reality has changed and that social networks have become a fundamental aspect of the way in which societies are shaped, organized and even reclaimed from their subjects.

It is also relevant to note that in both contexts there are doubts about the quality of the information shared on social media. As an accountability mechanism, despite the potential that these tools initially had, it is not clear how much social media has contributed to improving governance. This leads us to reflect on the real contribution of information and communication technologies to the democratic process in both countries. In both nations, it was considered that social media can be a catalyst for social interactions, but that actions can be ephemeral.

The study has clear limitations: these are perceptions of what a key player has witnessed throughout the last five years. But the purpose of this is to insist on the need to deepen the analysis from different perspectives on the effects of social networks in recent historical moments. As mentioned at the beginning of this text, there is a consensus that social media is now part of the way that the public inform each other, and therefore act. However, assessing the quality of this process, which involves, inter alia, assessing the contribution of technology to the quality of public debate, remains a pending task for further research.

References

1. Zeynep, T.: Twitter and Tear Gas: The Power and Fragility of Networked. Protest. Yale University Press, New Haven (2018)
2. Soní-Soto, A.: Mitos y símbolos en la campaña de Barack Obama. Palabra Clave **14**, 67–82 (2011)
3. De la Garza, D., Peña-Ramos, J., Recuero, F.: Online political participation of young people in Mexico, Spain and Chile. Comunicar **27**(61), 83–92 (2019)

4. De la Garza, D., Barredo, D.: Democracia digital en México: un estudio sobre la participación de los jóvenes usuarios mexicanos durante las elecciones legislativas federales de 2015. Index Comunicación **7**(1), 95–114 (2017)
5. Leon, E., McLeod, J.: Engaging with change: information and communication technology professionals' perspectives on change in the context of the 'Brexit' vote. PLos One **12**(11) 1–26 (2017)
6. Fernández, A., Lazkano, I., Eguskiza, L.: Nativos digitales: consumo, creación y difusión de contenidos audiovisuales online. Comunicar **26**(57), 61–69 (2018)
7. Tana, J., Eirola, E., Nylund, M.: When is prime-time in streaming media platforms and video-on-demands services? New media consumption patterns and real-time economy. Eur. J. Commun. **35**(2), 108–125 (2020)
8. Raustiala, K., Sprigman, C.J.L.: Segunda disrupción digital: el streaming y el amanecer de la creatividad impulsada por datos. N. Y. Univ. Law Rev. **94**, 1556–1620 (2019)
9. Billard, T.J.: Evidencia experimental de diferencias en los efectos prosociales de los programas de televisión vistos por atracones versus programas de televisión vistos por citas. Journal. Commun. Q. **96**(4), 1025–1051 (2019)
10. Ballesteros, C.: The digital spread of the coronavirus: measuring engagement of entertainment on the emerging social network TikTok. Revista Española De Comunicación en Salud **1**, 171–185 (2020)
11. Arana, E., Mimenza, L., Narbaiza, B.: Pandemia, Consumo Audiovisual y Tendencias de Futuro en Comunicación. Revista de Comunicación y Salud, **10**(2), 149–183 (2020)
12. Roberts, T., Marchais, G.: Assessing the role of social media and digital technology in violence reporting. Contemp. Read. Law Soc. Justice **10**(2), 9–42 (2018)
13. Ardèvol-Abreu, A., Delponti, P., Rodríguez-Wangüemert, C.: Intentional or inadvertent fake news sharing? Fact-checking warnings and users' interaction with social media content. Profesional de la Información, **29**(5), e290507 (2020)
14. Kim, A., Dennis, A.: Says who? The effects of presentation format and source rating on fake news in social media. MIS Q. **43**(3), 1025–1039 (2019)
15. Muhammad, W., Nauman A.: Role of social media in diagnosis and management of COVID-19; an experience of a Pulmonologist. Ann. King Edward Med. Univ. **26**, 233–234 (2020)
16. Mcintyre, L.: Post-Truth. MIT Press, Cambridge (2019)
17. Gil de Zúñiga, H. Veenstra, A., Vraga, E., Shah, D.: Digital democracy: reimagining pathways to political participation. J. Inf. Technol. Politics **7**(1), 36–51 (2010)
18. Vesnic-Alujevic, L.: Political participation and web 2.0 in Europe: a case study of Facebook. Public Relat. Rev. **38**(3), 466–470 (2012)
19. Oser, J., Hooghe, M., Marien, S.: Is online participation distinct from offline participation? A latent class analysis of participation types and their stratification. Political Res. Q. **66**(1), 91–101 (2013)

Twenty-First Century Trends and International Cross-Cultural Perspective: The Post-dramatic TV Series Model in the United States vs. Spain's Neoclassical Hesitancy in Television Serial Fiction

Miguel A. Orosa(✉), Daqui Lema(✉), and Viviana Galarza-Ligña(✉)

Pontificia Universidad Católica del Ecuador, Ibarra, Ecuador
{maorosa1,cdlema,vngalarza}@pucesi.edu.ec

Abstract. At the beginning of a scientific chapter addressing the new artistic-dramatic trends of the twenty-first century, in particular the comparison of the television fiction phenomenon in the United States and Spain, we open the portico of this reflection with the analysis of an international situation of a cross-cultural nature, the hybridization of cultures, from a legal and constitutional perspective linked to the development of human rights in the world and especially between the American and Spanish tv serial post-drama. In the midst of this scenario we have just referred to, we examine the postulates and characteristics of the American model of television series, of a post-dramatic stamp, and we compare it with the fundamental patterns of the phenomenon of series fiction in Spain produced for television. While the United States is betting on an avant-garde inspired by popular anti-classical liberties and the narratives of libertarian improvisation so typical of Spanish dramatic culture, Spain takes refuge in a neoclassical dramatic model, fundamentally of Saxon origin, renouncing its own culture and tradition of the Golden Age for the sake of who knows what objectives and at the risk of missing the train of aesthetic contemporaneity. Comparisons of models and cultures, descriptions of (post-)dramatic patterns, analysis and information made available to science for further reflection and discussion.

Keywords: North American post-drama TV series · Twenty-first century TV series in Spain · (Post-)dramatic trends of the twenty-first century in TV fiction

1 Introduction

The movements and trends brought about by global communication and interdependence have been elaborating a continuous defragmentation, relocating the different cultural components that societies embody, whether in their daily practices and chores or in their global aspirations and ideas. The mutations resulting from these conceptual redesigns, also of a legal nature, feed new interconnections that lead to hybrid results, culturally speaking, so that an ever wider public makes a new language with unprecedented and enriching suggestions its own.

© The Author(s), under exclusive license to Springer Nature Singapore Pte Ltd. 2022
Á. Rocha et al. (Eds.): ICOMTA 2021, SIST 259, pp. 333–343, 2022.
https://doi.org/10.1007/978-981-16-5792-4_33

Along this path, interculturality understood as a horizontal process of recognition and reciprocal feedback of cultural diversities has been opening the way to interesting experiences through the use of public policies, including affirmative actions. This general principle interacts in an important way with the practice and respect for human rights, thus leaving a significant platform for social transformation that allows rhizomatic unions in a perspective open to interactions that also produce transcultural processes that can hardly be understood at their peak, but that definitely show us coming changes aimed at the construction of a common idea of humanity [1, 2].

2 Methodology

The present work, of mixed approach with predominance of the qualitative paradigm, has as its object of study the aesthetic organization of the North American serialized post-drama and the current fiction tv series in Spain. For this purpose, the analytical-synthetic method will be used: first, there is a decomposition of the works in several of their constituent parts and, subsequently, the common characteristics are synthesized in order to be able to draw relevant conclusions.

We are not talking about a simple description of facts or a theoretical exposition of the state of current narrative trends in the field of serialized fiction in the United States and Spain devoid of a methodology and results, although sometimes not all the steps we followed in the process are marked in bold. It is not necessary; the reader who spends a little time reviewing this study will see that an authentic scientific framework has been developed, made up of two empirical models that highlight the variables of our research in the fields of post-dramatic TV series in the United States and the more neoclassical ones in Spain (by the way, unpublished studies to date, as far as we have been able to verify). From here, it is possible to pose the main research questions of this paper, that is: what patterns and variables reveal the two serialized trends mentioned, what is their identity?, and, subsequently, from a panel of works cited and explicitly exposed, to see how the variables of the models mentioned are fulfilled, to check if the initial premise is satisfied: one, is there a fictional serialized post-drama in the United States? and two, are we witnessing a non post-dramatic phenomenon in Spain, essentially neoclassical in these manifestations?, which validates the models used in this article.

3 Theoretical Framework

The Spanish language culture of popular and festive character, as well as narrative, liturgical and celebratory (which always revolves around an event) stands out for its freedom, participation and ability to improvise [3]. In contrast to this attitude, classical dramatic cultures are more intellectual, not born of the people but are perfect, studied, rational, full of harmonious rules in search of balance and beauty. Fictional television series in the United States have discarded the classical models of Greek Elizabethan origin to welcome an avant-garde and a know-how inspired by the dramatic culture of Spanish tendency (obstinately present in the contemporary European post-theater). Meanwhile, fiction TV series in Spain, renouncing their own dramatic tradition of the Golden Age, surrender their own identity on the altar of a neoclassical culture under the pretext of who knows what objectives. Some of the Spanish series try to get out of such dramatic confinement, but they do not succeed in finding the proper techniques of our time, especially present in North American fiction television.

3.1 TV Series Fiction Post-drama in the United States of America

When describing the patterns that characterize the post-dramatic movement of series produced for television in the United States, we have studied and analyzed many works that are encompassed within this model from its origins to the present day. To list a few examples, tentatively rather than exhaustively, we could mention (without necessarily fulfilling all the notes of this post-dramatic paradigm) The Sopranos, Sex and the City, Six feet under, 24, The O.C., Prison Break, Lost, Mad Men, True Blood, In treatment, Game of Thrones, Boardwalk Empire, The Witcher, The Magicians, Watchmen, Black Mirror and many others of recognized prestige and international recognition [4, 5].

3.2 Spain's Neoclassical Hesitancy in Its Current Serialized TV Fiction

Next we are going to introduce in Table 2 and in alphabetical order a list of some of the most famous TV series in Spain, which does not mean that they are the best or the most prestigious, but that they enjoy a good diffusion and recognition and this is for exemplary but not limiting purposes.

As we have already mentioned, Spain is faithful to a neoclassical model in its TV fiction series typical of the dramatic cycle and, paradoxically, alien to its own performing culture that comes from the Middle Ages to the Golden Age. This neoclassical paradigm is fundamentally and basically based on the following patterns in Table 3 below.

We have already referred to this neoclassical model and its characteristics in several articles cited in references below. In fact, the Spanish model is quite simple and focuses on categories 2 and 3 of this Table 3, namely, a neoclassical dramatic organization and the intensive use of dramatic tension.

4 Discussion

4.1 TV Series Fiction Post-drama in the United States of America

Some of these categories and their components described in Table 1 have already been discussed in the works cited earlier in this article. We would like to make a special reference to some issues perhaps less covered in previous reflections such as the changes of roles in the characters so typical of this post-dramatic model of tv serial stamp, the second act and the spectacular speech or some considerations of relevance in their relationship with the dramatic tension.

With reference to role changes, the same character can play a role as protagonist within one of the themes of a play - independently of the functions that he/she fulfills within the scope of other themes of that same piece - and, in that same theme, we insist, and soon after, go on to perform other functions such as, for example, deuteragonist or, surprisingly, as antagonist and, suddenly, become a dramatic target, as we have just mentioned above.

Table 1. Patterns of North American post-dramatic TV series model

	Category	Component
1	Five to seven themes. Unveiling of the themes as the episode progresses Tendency to the thematic organizational labyrinth	Themes are always in motion, they are not static. Themes are subject to permanent change and, moreover, since there are so many of them and they are subject over and over again to fusions and mixtures between them, as well as to changes or mutations of all kinds, it is not easy to establish with clarity and security what these themes are, to identify them Doubts and intrigues about the constitution, essence and identity of the themes, creating a labyrinthine effect
2	Disclosure and change in the hierarchy of themes	We can go through the work with highly anti-hierarchical spaces in which the themes tend to take on a similar importance. The strategy and attitude regarding this issue goes through a concrete philosophy: to make the present moment the decisive and truly important thing
3	Dismemberment and fragmentation of themes	The basic forces of a dramatic nature (protagonists, antagonists…) are fragmented into each of their components and come to life independently and end up, many times, forming or constituting their own autonomous themes
4	Mutant themes. Obliqueness in the presentation of the themes. Discontinuous or non-parallel development of themes	The themes are mutating, changing in nature and substance over and over again. One enters the new topic in an indirect, oblique manner, linked to another issue from which one moves on to the new topic in question. The mutant theme can be developed in a way that is intertwined with other related issues that are entered into indirectly so that this theme becomes other ones. The development of the themes in time is not synchronous or, at least, does not run similar or adjusted to the rhythm of the different contexts

(*continued*)

Table 1. (*continued*)

	Category	Component
5	Change of roles of the characters in relation to the dramatic forces (agonist, antagonist and deuter forces). Fragmentation and deconstruction of characters	One and the same character can play a role as a protagonist within one of the themes of an episode and shortly afterwards go on to perform other functions as a deuteragonist or as an antagonist and suddenly become a dramatic target There is a permanent reinvention and multi-perspective of the characters throughout this new model
6	Conflict and other matters	Oppression would be one of those substances that is always present within the teleserial discourse. And this burden, this substance or component, would be an element formed, in turn, by two others: tension and agon, that is, doses or traces of confrontation
7	Permanent change. The destructuring of dramatic categories. The compositional breakdown. Communicative and artistic architecture: forces of dramatic tension	The decategorization or contamination of the dramatic concepts opens in the new model the doors towards the total freedom, towards a creation without barriers guided only by the impulse of the moment, the intuition, the creative formal eagerness The technical form yields its privileges and supremacy to the dramatic tension in order to give unity to so much centrifugal forces and compositional breakdown

Source: Orosa, M.Á. [6–9]

We can also witness processes of fragmentation and deconstruction of the characters in this model. When we speak of fragmentation we refer to that lost and broken piece of the mirror in which a character is reflected, in one of the aspects of his or her multiple, varied and complex personality (there are other scattered pieces…); and when we speak of deconstruction we mean the side or facet of a character's personality that arises, at a given moment, on the specific referential context on which he or she is situated, in precise circumstances. These two characteristics (fragmentation and deconstruction) are constants in this new post-dramatic model and we cannot but refer to them. There is a permanent reinvention and multiperspectivism regarding the characters in all these fiction series produced for television.

In the pilot episode of The Sopranos, if we take a close look at Dr. Melfi, we can observe how she plays different dramatic roles depending on the moment and development of the action. We see her in a deuteragonist role throughout the chapter trying to help Tony Soprano to discover the cause of his depression in order to treat it. But she also comes up as the dramatic target of a weak and dreamy love theme on the part of Tony Soprano, when he comments in therapy to his psychiatrist that his mother, Tony's mother,

Table 2. Panel of Spain's most popular TV series of recent years

	Title	TV production company/Year
1	Alguien tiene que morir	Netflix/2020
2	Alta mar	Bambú Producciones/2019
3	Días de navidad	Filmax y Netflix España/2019
4	Élite	Zeta Audiovisual, Netflix España/2018
5	Hache	Netflix España, Weekend Studio/2019
6	La catedral del mar	Atresmedia Televisión, Diagonal Televisión, Televisión de Galicia (TVG)/2018
7	La casa de papel	Vancouver Media, Atresmedia Televisión/2017
8	La valla	Atresmedia Televisión, Globomedia, Good Mood/2020
9	Las chicas del cable	Bambú Producciones, Netflix España/2017
10	Los favoritos de Midas	Nostromo Pictures, Netflix España/2020
11	Mar de plástico	Boomerang TV/2015
12	Nevenka	Newtral/2021
13	Perdida	Atresmedia Televisión, Big Bang Media/2020
14	Tiempos de guerra	Atresmedia Televisión, Bambú Producciones/2017
15	Toy Boy	Plano a Plano/2019
16	Valeria	Plano a Plano/2020
17	Vis a vis	Globomedia/2015
18	Vivir sin permiso	Telecinco, Alea Media, Ficción Produccnes, Mediaset España/2018

Source: Orosa, M.Á.

would have liked her, Melfi, to be his daughter-in-law. Not to mention the role that the psychiatrist plays as the main character in a meeting of friends with Dr. Cusamano or, in the same role, when she meets Tony in an important restaurant in the city and they greet each other as if they were friends or even, we dream it, as if they were going to be a sentimental couple in the development of the action. And what to say, to mention another of the moments of change of dramatic force in the doctor, of her role as antagonist, in the same chapter, opposing the darkest of Tony Soprano's character and making him reach, in spite of himself, into the depths of his soul and observe how lonely he is, to understand the importance of communication between human beings.

Tony Soprano is a very complex character who shows, in relation to the fragmentation and deconstruction of the characters, some admirable symptoms of rupture and breakdown in its constitution to the point that makes him a museum piece for the universal dramatic literature. Soprano is, without a doubt, a friend and a good friend, as befits a serial mobster. He is also a vulnerable and melancholic man, not without a certain romanticism. Very human and impressionable in the face of the passing of time or the change of values, sensitive to the lack of communication between colleagues to the point

Table 3. Neoclassical dramatic panel

	Category	Component
1	Plot	Plot: turning points. Emotional projections Selection of facts (story): not all the life or legends of the hero, but only the events necessary to tell the theme of the work
2	Dramatic organization	External: blocks or acts Middle: themes, movements (exposition, conflict, resolution) Unity of action (a protagonist who seeks an objective)
3	Dramatic tension	Conflict or confrontation (obstacles that separate the protagonist from his/her objective) Activation: style, spectacular speech, intellectual discourse, characters, music
4	Narrative organization within drama Type of narrative organization	Narrative organizations involved in the field of drama (arrangements/organization of the "novel" that appears within the drama)
5	Technical-formal organization	Situation, formal drawing, intensity, duration, colors and textures, tempo, story

Source: Orosa y López-López [10]

that this causes him a depression with severe panic attacks and loss of consciousness in public places. Affectionate with his children, protective; understanding to unsuspected limits with his wife, a tremendous cynic who does not understand him and wants to ignore what she herself is not interested in; schizophrenic in the defense at all costs of a family that he essentially betrays every time he feels like it. Faithful philosopher in his search for the truth about life and the human being and also about the cause that motivates his profound illness. He is a ruthless ruler and, at the same time, a person of dialogue. He likes to explore multiple perspectives when it comes to solving the problems of the Mafia and its business (which he has had to face in a historical moment that is not to his liking). In short, he is implacable with his enemies and, if necessary, an irredeemable murderer so as not to lose those values that tradition has placed in his hands and that he, as long as he lives, is obliged to safeguard.

In regard to conflict and the style of confrontation within the panorama of the new North American model, we must refer to one of its founding notes, the feeling of overwhelm. In our opinion, overwhelm would be one of those substances that is always or on many occasions is present within the serial TV discourse, conferring on it a certain aroma that is peculiar to it and that gives it a flavor quite tasty and generally desirable. And this burden, this substance or component, in our opinion, would be an element possibly made up of two other ingredients, namely: tension and the so well-known agon, that is, doses or traces of confrontation. This feeling of overwhelm, which we are dealing with, depends to a great extent on a very intense experience of what is happening on stage at "this moment", the full awareness of the present time we are living right now, the result of the masterful use of dramatic tension. In turn, the agon and the dramatic tension tinge somewhat with its aroma the use of what we call activation, that is: the plot and its components, the stylistic discourse, the spectacle and the constitution of the new characters, together with what the canonical tradition calls the intellectual discourse.

Another of the essential patterns of the serial TV model is the permanent change, the uninterrupted substitution of situations, characters, manners and forms, objectives, struggles, goals and, therefore, of dramatic categories so that the intrigue and the structural puzzle are the organizational and labyrinthine constant of creative tendency within this new (post-)drama. Hence the use of so many themes at the same time, which the spectator has to guess slowly; hence the use and change of ambiguous hierarchies that move in time as life does, ...hence a constant fragmentation and dismemberment of the themes from their forces of origin, the substantial mutation of themes or their oblique presentations, the constant changes of roles and functions of the characters, the creation of a new concept of the second act (essential to Western drama), the fusion of genres or, why not, of different worlds (real, fantastic) or so many other novelties that are nothing more than an invitation to do what we feel is most appropriate when the specific circumstance arises that can open the doors to the seduction of the everlasting spectator.

Of course, all this enormous freedom leads the drama to an architecture that would be chaotic, and possibly not artistic or not dramatic, if there were not some kind of unitive element of compositional character to give cohesion to so much labyrinth and disorganizing and centrifugal tendency. Everything turns out to be intrigues in its disorganization, ruptures, inadequacies and lack of unitive cements to go from here to there. The new writer, without ceasing to make use of the old technical-formal structures, has to get hold of a new instrument that gives some kind of union to so much "nonsense" and this will be no more and no less than one of a historical and traditional character: the dramatic tension, the illustrious and ancient dramatic organization in terms of attentive interest that Aristotle so wisely describes and develops in his first Poetics [11].

Perhaps this change of hierarchy (between formal techniques and dramatic tension) is showing that the (post-)drama more typical of our times (of serial and North American TV) is betting a little more on communication and seduction, on capturing the attention of a more intelligent and educated audience and perhaps a little less on the creation of artistic structures that, although beautiful, would die without being born in case of losing the favor of an audience that today is measured more one by one, in terms of subscribers to a cable station, than in numbers of viewers in the thousands and millions capable of capturing a good ad that is explosive (in multimillionaire financial figures) for an old generalist channel in an outdated concept of what was, but will no longer be, the new and current television.

A brief and last mention to the spectacular discourse that within this post-dramatic model for television takes place, not only in great scenes of spectacle, battles, explosions or huge events of this nature, in general terms, but in all the staging of everything that surrounds the script. It is enough to watch two of the HBO productions kicking off the year 2010 and 2011 (Game of Thrones and Boardwalk Empire) to realize that this spectacular discourse, many times, has to do with the magnificent and credible staging of the dramatic action to which the script is inviting.

4.2 Spain's Neoclassical Hesitancy in Its Current Serialized TV Fiction

There are basically two cases in which Spain's TV series try to break away from this dramatic model of neoclassical character to find freer, more contemporary paths; ways that run through rhizomatic juxtapositional elaborations and notions of a more post-dramatic character (which would link much better with the Spanish tradition). We refer to some infrequent moments of Money Heist (La casa de papel) and, above all, to Elite.

Elite is a TV series that employs a very slightly arched dramatic organization with a strong narrative component (typical of the Spanish tradition) that overlaps and sometimes replaces the dramatic one. It has a pathos, an emotional element of sensuality sometimes relevant, a very significant stylistic language of agonic tendency and a construction of the plot that constantly appeals to the conflict as a fundamental part of the organizations of dramatic tension, which it constantly seeks. To this last end, it does not fail to make use of the elements of activation cited in Table 3, category 3, namely: conflicting stylistic resources, a varied cast of characters, a spectacular and sentimental discourse very much in accordance with the canons of the dramatic tradition, constant appeals to in-depth themes that capture the viewer's attention and, of course, the recourse to both diegetic and extradiegetic music.

We are witnessing a permanent decomposition of the classical dramatic structure (Setup, Confrontation, Resolution) for the benefit of the second act in order to favor dramatic tension in the action, as we have mentioned. This may seem very contemporary, with mutant themes that are the result of the evolution of previous ones, an intense fragmentation of the action and the dramatic process, very flat architectures, the resignation of composition in favor of communication and attentive interest (although the second season tends to pursue form with more intention and tenacity, whether technical or narrative) or the use of collage effects and multi-plane and simultaneist techniques. We have already said that all this may seem somewhat post-dramatic, and it is a good attempt, but the truth is that it is no more than an attempt to search for contemporaneity because both the scripts and the audiovisual narrative are still quite classical and the excessive atomization and decomposition of the dramatic discourses does not generate, in our opinion, a sense/nonsense effect, a game of order and chaos that may result in contemporary rhizomes/forms of interest. When the creators of this TV series want to escape from this excessive atomization, they end up again in neoclassical forms: in short, the series does not work completely and totally well from an artistic point of view.

5 Conclusions

The path followed by the American post-drama in fictional serial television implies a partial relinquishment of its Elizabethan tradition and a bet for freedom, surprise, permanent dramatic change as a constant, the seduction of the spectator, the abandonment of dogmatic dramatic categories for the sake of a narrative feeling absolutely immersed in the mentality of our time. It has been an enormous transformation in the organization of the plays: the development and evolution of their themes, the way of presenting them, the constitution of the characters, the conception of the second act, the role to be played by the dramatic tension in the juxtapositional gear of these productions and the relegation of the composition techniques to a second tier for the sake of audiovisual communication as a fundamental component of these artistic manifestations.

This de-categorization of the classical scenic worldview has too much to do with the history and the phenomenon of dramatic culture in the Spanish language. It is not being claimed that American scriptwriters are directly familiar with the works of the great playwrights of the Spanish Golden Age, which could be the case. What can be clearly seen is that there is a parallel between the Spanish dramatic phenomenon and the North American tv serial post-drama. Perhaps this influence is direct, perhaps it is produced through the European post-drama [12–16] of our days (which has also undergone the same process of decategorization as a result of the Spanish dramatic culture, in our opinion) or, in any case, what we see on the American screen in our days is a process and a result of artistic freedom on the stage, that has always been a legacy of the Spanish stage culture.

In any case, the United States of America ensures the future of its television industry linked to post-dramatic series thanks to a cultural process that runs parallel to the dramatic culture of Spanish-speaking countries, a festive, popular, imaginative culture, very much given to narrative celebration and improvisation.

Meanwhile, fiction TV series in Spain, betraying its own dramatic tradition, approaches a neoclassicism of Saxon origin already outdated, that includes certain varnishes of renovation based on merely spectacular issues.

References

1. Kacowicz, A.: Globalización, regionalización y fragmentación. Nueva Sociedad 214, marzo - abril (2008). ISSN 0251-3552
2. Mato, D.: Des-fetichizar la "globalización": basta de reduccionismos, apologías y demonizaciones; mostrar la complejidad y las prácticas de los actores. In: Mato, D. (ed.) Cultura, política y sociedad. Perspectivas latinoamericanas. CLACSO, Buenos Aires (2005)
3. Orosa M.Á., Lema D., Galarza-Ligña V., Culqui A.: Ecuador: the popular liturgical and festive origins of the Latin American indigenous post-drama and its specific conflict. Comparisons with the Spanish and European post-drama. In: 15ª Iberian Conference on Information Systems and Technologies, pp 279–288. Springer, Heidelberg (2020)
4. Doidge, K.: 100 best TV shows of all time. https://thestacker.com/stories/980/100-best-tv-shows-all-time. Accessed 18 June 2020
5. Matus, D.: Las mejores series de HBO Now y HBO Go. https://es.digitaltrends.com/entretenimiento/mejores-series-hbo/. Accessed 21 June 2020
6. Orosa, M.A., Collado-Campaña, F., Galarza-Ligña, V.: The (post-)theatre of the twenty-first century in Spain and the North American post-drama TV series: a political, historic and comparative research. Playwrights, patterns and all-embracing point of view. In: Rocha, Á., Reis, J.L., Peter, M.K., Cayolla, R., Loureiro, S., Bogdanović, Z. (eds.) Marketing and Smart Technologies. SIST, vol. 205, pp. 573–584. Springer, Singapore (2021). https://doi.org/10.1007/978-981-33-4183-8_45
7. Orosa, M.Á.: El cambio dramático en el modelo teleserial norteamericano. Publicia, Saarbrücken (2012)

8. Orosa, M.Á., López-Golán, M., Márquez-Domínguez, C., Ramos-Gil, Y.: The American postdramatic television series: the art of poetry and the composition of chaos (How to understand the script of the best American television series). Rev. Latina Comun. Soc. **72**, 500–520 (2017). http://www.revistalatinacs.org/072paper/1176/26en.html. https://doi.org/10.4185/RLCS-2017-1176en
9. Orosa, M.A., López-Golán, M., Márquez-Domínguez, C., Ramos-Gil, Y.T.: El posdrama teleserial norteamerciano: poética y composición (Cómo entender el guion de las mejores series escritas para la televisión en los Estados Unidos). Rev. Latina Comun. Soc. **72**, 500–520 (2017). http://www.revistalatinacs.org/072paper/1176/26es.html. https://doi.org/10.4185/RLCS-2017-1176
10. Orosa, M.A., López-López, P.C.: Postdrama culture in Ecuador and Spain: methodological framework and comparative study. Comunicar **57**(XXVI), 39–47 (2018)
11. Aristóteles: Poética, ed. trilingüe de Valentín García Yebra. Gredos, Madrid (1974)
12. López, J.G.: La escena del siglo XXI. Asociacion de Directores de Escena, Madrid (2016)
13. López, J.G.: Tendencias en el teatro europeo actual. Teatrología, pp. 184–201 (2010)
14. Sarrazac J.P.: El drama no será representado. Teatrología, pp. 92–103 (2010)
15. Carlson, M.: Postdramatic theatre and postdramatic performance. Rev. Bras. Estudos Presença **5**, 3 (2015)
16. Cornago, Ó.: Teatro postdramático: las resistencias de la representación. Artea. Investigación y creación escénica [en línea, sin paginación]. www.arte-a.org. Accessed 15 Nov 2014

Podcast as an Emerging Branded Content Tool: The Case of Luxury Fashion Brands

Isabel Garcia Hiljding[1] and Paula Gárgoles[2](✉)

[1] Innovación y Tecnología, ESNE Escuela Universitaria de Diseño, Madrid, Spain
isabel.garcia@esne.es
[2] University of Navarra, Pamplona, Spain
pgargoles@unav.es

Abstract. Luxury brands position themselves on creating offers through opening their world to their consumer, where exclusivity and prestige go hand in hand. This positioning is frequently supported by substantial brand heritage which is linked to history and the past. However, time changes and with time, evolution and technology have become new factors to take into account in order to establish the communication strategies for luxury brands. Communications moves fast, and the luxury brands have in the past had difficulties in embracing changes and adapting to new formats. Therefore, the purpose of this paper is to analyze the podcast as a branded content tool for luxury fashion brands.

The sample is the Chanel, Gucci, Hermes and Dior podcast during the 2019–2020. This paper seeks to meet three objectives: stress the importance of branded content for the luxury brands; highlight the podcast format as a tool for creating brand content for fashion brands and focus attention on how each brand builds branded content in the podcast format, where a visual industry creates a sound universe. Our discussion and conclusions highlight that the podcasts of these luxury brands are a channel for generating content that unites the brand's values with its cultural and social interests. Most of them offer inspirational content far from promoting their products.

Keywords: Branded content · Podcast · Luxury brands

1 Introduction

The luxury industry is idiosyncratic. Luxury is more than the material offering (even if the offering is a service). Luxury brings symbolic and experiential value in addition to its functionality [1, 2]. Luxury brands, unlike mass brands, do not communicate their advantages to their consumers, nor do they push them to buy, but rather the opposite. We can say that luxury brands are early adopters, while mass brands are their followers, in terms of innovation in the strategies they follow [3, 4].

When brands started to use digital communication, luxury brands were reluctant to change. Selling without consumers being able to touch the product and experience the customer journey they were used to, bewildered brands. The main reason for the skepticism of luxury brands in undertaking their digital strategies lies in the very attributes of

© The Author(s), under exclusive license to Springer Nature Singapore Pte Ltd. 2022
Á. Rocha et al. (Eds.): ICOMTA 2021, SIST 259, pp. 344–353, 2022.
https://doi.org/10.1007/978-981-16-5792-4_34

luxury and the Internet: while luxury is synonymous with rarity, inaccessibility and exclusivity [5, 6], the Internet is characterized by accessibility and democracy [7]. Kapferer and Bastien (2012) [5] coined the term "Internet dilemma" for luxury brands in this context.

Although they were "lazards" in ecommerce, luxury brands have been ahead in traditional communication strategies. In the case of podcasts, it is pertinent to note that mainstream brands are not using this digital tool to connect with their audience or to make branded content even in a general way. While other industry sectors, such as technology or entertainment, have already embraced podcasting, it seems that the fashion industry has not yet widely adopted podcasting as a media format.

For the audio format of the podcast, the fashion industry's reluctance seems reasonable, as fashion communication is very focused on visual aspects. But this is not the case for luxury brands. According to the article "Why fashion brands are launching podcasts" published by BoF in January 2019, "luxury companies have always been rich storytellers and content creators. The podcast is a rising format within that same tradition" [8]. Podcasts are one of the fastest growing media formats. According to a report by emarketer [9] on podcasts, between 2022 and 2023, Spotify will gain ground on Apple, reaching 37.5 million listeners worldwide. The same study predicts that by 2024, U.S. agencies will spend $1.83 billion on advertising within audio content.

This study's aim is to examine the branded content used by luxury firms through the creation and distribution through audio platforms such as Spotify, Apple Podcast, etc. of a corporate podcast of four selected luxury brands: Chanel, Hermés, Dior and Gucci. Additionally, this study also aims to identify the frames (source and creativity), the longevity, the duration, related media and the language used in order to understand how the podcasts are becoming a successful strategic communication tool for luxury brands.

2 Literature Review

2.1 Branded Content in the Luxury Industry

The communication departments of luxury brands have different means to reach potential customers. The evolution of advertising and brands began with product placement as an integration of brands in movies and television series [10] but the market developed by integrating products and brands in entertainment contexts to attract their public [11]. Thus, branded content was born as "a symbiosis between advertising and entertainment content, whose main objective is to attract the public to the values of a brand in an attractive and suggestive way" (p. 729) [12].

Through the development of branded content, the concept of storytelling has also grown, which "its use for the construction and dissemination of brand identity is a recent trend that has grown under the protection of branded content, as this has created the possibility of telling brand stories in a more subtle, more emotional way and more likely to generate true connection with the audience" (p. 319) [11].

2.2 Podcasting

The term podcast has its origin, on the one hand, in the device through which the podcast was mostly accessed at the beginning of its existence, the Ipod, which is the music player manufactured by Apple, and on the other hand, in the term broadcasting [13]. The term podcast was defined by Bonini (p. 21) [14] as "a technology used to distribute, receive and listen to on-demand audio content produced by traditional publishers such as radio stations, publishers, journalists and educational institutions, as well as content created by independent radio producers, artists and radio amateurs".

The main difference between podcasting and radio is their content. While the goal of a radio program is to provide interesting stories for a broad audience and address local issues in its service area, podcasts focus on special communities of listeners and are especially popular on niche topics [15]. Podcasts are emerging as a tool for the production and dissemination of audio content [16].

2.3 Podcasting as Branded Content Strategy for Luxury Brands

Digital media allows brands to connect with younger audiences, something that all fashion brands seek. In many ways, the luxury industry has been a "digital laggard" [13, p. 31] most likely due to the important visual aspect inherent in fashion [17]. In November 2017, businessoffashion.com published an article titled "Fashion Wakes up to Podcasts" which asks whether the fashion industry can successfully conquer this fast-growing form of media: the podcasts [17]. The article's discussion of the untapped use of podcasts within the fashion industry highlights the poor knowledge about the fashion industry and public relations.

There is currently scarce academic literature on the role of podcasts as a branded content strategy in the fashion industry. One of the few papers on podcast and fashion is by Bratchter [17] who claims that podcasts have the potential to be useful in building brands' stories and awareness. According to the author "podcasts serve as more long-forum platforms that allow detail and explanation by speakers. Brands' goals for podcasts do not seem to be centered on the sale of products – particularly in the form of quick and concise marketing messages we're used to seeing. Instead, podcasts are meant to inspire and elaborate on the already well-known products and morale of the brands" (p. 14) [18].

While social media communication is immediate and fast, the podcast allows for more relaxed, longer conversations. In this sense, the tempo of the podcast is better suited to the tempo of luxury brands that need more time to do their storytelling. Podcasting combines radio's intimacy with the personalization of digital media forms to create a new and interesting space for media and cultural interaction [19]. Despite their audio and non-visual nature and limited reach, podcasts are becoming a popular communications tool for fashion companies.

3 Methodology

The sample of podcasts analyzed was drawn from Interbrand's ranking of the top 100 brands of the year 2020 [20]. The luxury brands that appeared on the list were in order:

Louis Vuitton (17), Chanel (21), Hermes (28), Gucci (32), Cartier (73), Dior (83), Tiffany & Co (94), Burberry (97) and Prada (99). The requirements for analyzing the brands were that they were luxury and that they had a podcast from at least the year 2020. After an exploratory search on Apple Podcast and various podcasting platforms, these four brands were found: Chanel, Gucci, Hermés and Dior.

A quantitative study was conducted analyzing the number of episodes in 2019 and 2020, longevity [21]; How long are the episodes? [13]; Diffusion [21] and the language used. It has also been analyzed from a qualitative perspective: a content analysis has been carried out on the Creativity Category [30] and Source-based Frames [17]. Regarding the Creativity Category, the content frame was analyzed and the categorization of Bratcher, T. R. (2021) [30] was followed in which it is divided between: Inspiration Frame; Design-detail Frame and Signature or Icon Frame. With reference to the Source-based Frames, Bratcher, T. R. (2021) [17] distinguishes between expert and celebrity but after the analysis, we have also included the category of artist, since in many episodes, we have found a large number of artists because of the strong link that luxury brands have with culture.

4 Results

The authors of the paper have analyzed a total of 130 episodes with a total duration of 2634.5 min that are summarized in Table 1.

4.1 Chanel Podcast

The Chanel podcast is a pioneer among luxury and fashion brands and was created in November 2017. The podcast is titled Chanel Connections 3.55, in honor of the iconic 2.55 bag. Their podcast is according to the brand "a conversation with artists and friends of the brand, about their sources of inspiration and creation" [22]. It has a total of 46 episodes, between the years 2019–2020, although there are two series, La première fois and Chanel á la opera, which are repeated in English and French. We can highlight the division into series of the podcasts and that all episodes of the same series are published on the same day. The frequency of publishing is variable, and the average duration of each episode is 16,06 min. The predominant language of the podcasts is English, although there are also episodes in French, Spanish, Italian, Russian, Arabic and Asian languages.

The last series of the 2020, Métiers d'art show, was recorded in ten different languages. A brand ambassador from each country read an excerpt from a text written by Fanny Arama about the Château de Chenonceau, which was the inspiration and backdrop for the 2020/2021 Métiers d'art show "Le Château des Dames". The podcast of the firm has its own section on the website of Chanel where apart from being very intuitive, their followers and public can see the different series, a brief synopsis of each of them and there is an access to listen to the episodes directly from there. The website also contains images of videos of the recordings of the episodes, inviting the public to enter both visually and aurally in the universe of the Maison.

Despite the fact that this study analyzed the podcast between the years 2019 and 2020, we can observe an evolution in the content of the firm's podcasts. Chanel starts

Table 1. Episodes analyzed

	CHANEL	GUCCI	HERMES	DIOR
Longevity	Nov. 2017	May 2018	Feb. 2019	March 2020
Frequency	Variable (series)	Variable	Variable (series)	Variable (series)
How long are the episodes? Average	16,06 minutes	28,3 minutes	13 minutes	26.5 minutes
Language	French (16/46) English (20/46) Italian(1/46) Spanish (1/46) Asian languages(5/46) Russian (2/46) Arabic (1/46)	English (26/27) Spanish (1/27)	French (15/28)& English (13/28)	English 22/29 French 6/29 Italian 1/29
Diffusion	Chanel web	Podcast Platform	Hermes web	Own web
Number of Podcast (2019-20)	46	27	28	29
Predominant frame	Inspiration frame	Inspiration frame	Signature o icon frame	Inspiration frame
Source-based frames	Expert	Celebrity	Expert	Expert

Source: authors

in 2017 with podcasts focused on its products, such as the Handbag Stories series, in which influential women in the fashion industry are interviewed about Chanel's style and about its handbags. Over the years, the content has become increasingly inspirational, connecting the brand with culture and art, a very characteristic of luxury companies and of Chanel indeed.

4.2 Gucci Podcast

The Italian brand GUCCI, which has been part of the KERING group for more than two decades, launched its podcast in May 2018. GUCCI podcasts, consists of interviews between two or more people, whose common link is that the interviews are conducted with people who have a relationship with the brand and who collaborate with it. Podcast hosts can vary according to the subject matter covered in each episode. During the two years in which the analysis was carried out, the brand produced a total of 27 episodes. They are published monthly (although in some cases two episodes are published in the same month, or there is a month in which no podcast is published). The average duration is 28,3 min. GUCCI's podcasts are entirely in English, except for one episode that is repeated in English and Spanish, which is about the Gucci Osteria that has opened in Beverly Hills.

Gucci podcasts talk about social concern. The themes that are most present in the episodes are sustainability, integration of all people in society, racism and equality. One of the podcast series is about Chime for Change. GUCCI founded in 2013, the CHIME FOR CHANGE campaign, through which, the brand aims to inspire its audience to participate in a collective community, bringing together people from around the world and all generations in the fight for equality [23]. Gucci podcasts that are published on podcasts platforms, are mainly divided into series: #guccigig, chime for change and #gucciabsolutebeginners are some of them, and it is interesting to highlight one of the series, in which Gucci makes four episodes in collaboration with the American magazine Fast Company. The series was recorded during the European Innovation Festival and the main themes of the episodes deal with climate change and the technological revolution.

Therefore, we could conclude that in the case of Gucci, the framework for the vast majority of the firm's podcasts, a total of 85%, is an inspirational framework, where on very few occasions, the podcast is about a product, collection or something more directly related to the brand. Its branded content does not focus on its products directly, but the brand uses podcasts to give voice to topics that are of interest to it.

4.3 Hermès Podcast

Luxury brand Hermès started their podcast called Podcasts from Le Monde d'Hermès in February 2019. They have issued 28 podcasts in total in 2019–20. The frequency of publishing is variable through 3 different series and the average time is 13 min. The languages are French and English in which they duplicate episodes except for two podcasts which are in French only. For the brand, the podcast is a way to communicate the universe of Hermes through the people who work in the brand as its best ambassadors and its iconic products. That is why they give voice to the designers, store director, cultural director of the patrimony of Hermès or the Manager of external relations.

It is a podcast between reality and fiction because everything is focused on dreams, on the dreamlike. For example, the first series is called The Faubourg of Dreams. Faubourg is the street where the first store of the brand was opened in 1880 by the son of Thierry Hermès, the founder of the brand. The second series is called "Around a dream" in which they interview several personalities of the Maison and tell their most extravagant dreams. All of them offer a vision -utopian, fantasy or humanist- of their profession.

The last series is the most fiction-focused and is called "Penelope's Investigations" in which a detective named Penelope investigates whose cases are linked to iconic objects of the brand such as the silk carré. The podcasts are hosted on the corporate website and also on podcasting platforms such as Apple Podcast or Spotify. Therefore, we could say that during 2019–20, 26 podcasts have been interviews with internal experts: that is, people who work in the brand and the last 4 podcasts have invented a fictional character of a researcher in which her cases are related to Hermès objects. The frame of the podcast is the Signature or icon frame. Their way of elaborating branded content is very focused on the brand itself: the title is significant: the world of Hermès. The brand tells the story of the brand through its employees and its iconic objects.

4.4 Dior Podcast

Luxury brand Dior started its podcast called Dior Talks on March 8, 2020, International Women's Day. The date is part of the intention and message of the podcast. They have broadcasted 29 podcasts during 2020. The majority language is English (22/29), although there is one series that is in French (6/29) and one episode in Italian. The frequency of the episodes is variable and the average time is 26.5 min. Maria Grazia Chiuri is the brand's first female creative director and since 2017, she has positioned Dior in favor of feminism. A symbol was the T-shirt from the spring-summer 2017 collection printed with the message "We Should All Be Feminists". It was one of the most viral clothing garments during 2017. The podcasts are hosted on a specific website for the podcast [24] and also on podcasting platforms such as Apple Podcast or Spotify.

The format of the podcast is through conversation with artists, collaborators of the Maison in which they talk about their work and the challenges of tomorrow. The most recurring theme is the role of art, always from a feminist perspective. In fact, of the 29 chapters, only 4 are interviews with men. The frame of the podcast is the inspirational frame. The first series is called Feminist Art and consists of interviews with artists related to Maria Grazie Chiuri. The second season is about the women of Christian Dior and was recorded at the Victoria & Albert Museum in London. The third season of this podcast series explores how the work of female photographers and creative professionals collaborating with Dior offers a radically new and progressive image of women.

The fourth season is about the artistic director of the jewelry and costume jewelry collections of the house of Dior. It is the only series in French. The fifth season, which revolves around the 5th edition of Dior Lady Art, presents the ten contemporary artists and collectives who, in the coming weeks, will share their personal experience. Dior with its podcast shows a brand committed to feminism and connected to culture. They are always artists linked to the brand by some collaboration with a collection or friendship with the creative director. It is an inspirational content through art and social issues of today's world such as the role of women in fashion and art [25].

5 Discussion

As a summary of the most important aspects of each brand, we could highlight Chanel's relationship with culture, the look towards Asia: it is the only one that has Japanese, Korean and Chinese episodes. Gucci stands out for its corporate activism with themes such as gender, black lives matter, women and also for its use of hashtags in its campaigns. With the Hermès podcast: the entire internal universe of the brand is transmitted. You could say that it is the most "egocentric" since all the topics of the podcast revolve around the brand. From the history, the store, the employees, the products. Hermes is the only one to do fiction in its podcasts. The Hermès podcast can be said to have the perceptive function: it connects with emotions through its dream-focused subject matter. In the case of Dior, it is striking the feminist perspective they have given to each series of the podcasts and their connection with arts.

We have also found similarities between brands, for example: Chanel and Gucci have made collaborations with magazines: Monocle and Fast Company respectively, in which the informative function of the podcast is accentuated. Gucci and Dior have also used the podcast in order to create awareness regarding different social issues. They use the podcast as a tool for brand activism and unifying their voices with issues of social interest. Gucci, which is part of the Kering group whose focus is sustainability, addresses this issue in several of its podcasts, as well as gender and black lives matter. In the case of Dior, whose creative director has expressed her concern about feminist issues, the podcast contains this approach in all its episodes. Brand activism is a corporate practice in which companies voluntarily take a stance on what they believe is "good" or "right" for society; making public statements and occasionally, adapting their operations to support that stance. Sometimes the topics selected are not directly associated with the company's products or operations [26]. Nowadays, brands are increasingly betting on taking a stance on social issues as a way to connect in a coherent way and generate empathy. The podcast format allows luxury brands to tell their storytelling in a slower tempo, something that is impossible in social media or fashion films. The average length of Chanel's podcast is 16.06 min, Gucci's 28.3 min, Hermès' 13 min and Gucci's 26.5 min. This is another advantage that luxury brands can find when generating branded content in podcast format.

After the analysis, the predominant frame from which they create branded content is inspirational: interviews with artists, photographers in the case of Chanel, Gucci and Dior. Hermès has focused more on the brand itself and its frame is the Signature or icon frame. It has been interesting to analyze the languages of the episodes to understand the target audience and the diversity in fashion [27]. The predominant language is English with a percentage of 62.3% because they are global brands that operate globally. The next most important language is French (28.5%), which can be said to be the language of luxury. In fact, three of the four brands analyzed are French: Chanel, Hermès and Dior. The other languages account for 9.2%. Chanel is the oldest podcast in this format and is the only one to have episodes in Asian languages such as Chinese, Japanese and Korean, as well as Arabic and Russian. With this selection of languages, it is possible to make an X-ray of the origin of the luxury consumer. Chanel and Hermès have decided to host their podcasts on their own corporate websites, while Dior has created a specific website for its podcast and in the case of Gucci has chosen to host it on podcasting platforms such as Apple Podcast or Spotify.

6 Limits and Conclusion

One of the limitations of the study is that the sample is small. Only four brands have been analyzed and the timeline is also limited: it has not been analyzed the total number of podcasts published by each firm, but only the episodes broadcasted in 2019–20. It has also not been possible to investigate the number of listeners and downloads of the podcast, so we do not know if the podcasts have had an impact. Another way this study is limited is by its lack of exploration on how audiences are interacting and engaging with brands' podcasts. For the future lines we would research the evolution of the podcast in the luxury fashion brands and how the podcasts are embedded in the communication strategies in the luxury and no luxury brands.

In conclusion, after analyzing the four podcasts of the world's leading luxury brands, it can be said that they use podcasting as a tool to create branded content, provide value to their customers or potential customers and generate engagement with their audience. All of them have transmitted the DNA of the brand [28] in audio format. Most of them create valuable content by interviewing artists and, in the case of Hermes, its employees. It is a way to connect with their audience and transmit the brand's values without the need to sell their product. Audio allows to generate a close and intimate connection and luxury brands are using it to generate brand experience through interviews or tell stories related to the company. Luxury brands have managed to generate a sound universe in a visual industry in which the image had been the main tool until now. The luxury industry is a differentiated offer that provides symbolic value and is strongly connected to artistic and cultural language. They are the ones who have led a new format in which to generate branded content. Just as they were the ones who started with fashion films, in the case of Prada in 2012. Will non-luxury brands copy the podcasting format to generate branded content?

References

1. Berthon, P., Pitt, L., Parent, M., Berthon, J.P.: Aesthetics and ephemerality: observing and preserving the luxury brand. Calif. Manage. Rev. **52**(1), 45–66 (2009)
2. Chung, Y., Kim, A.J.: Effects of mergers and acquisitions on brand loyalty in luxury brands: the moderating roles of luxury tier difference and social media. J. Bus. Res. **120**, 434–442 (2020)
3. Grigorian, V., Petersen, F.E.: Designing luxury experience (No. 14-04). ESMT Working Paper (2014)
4. Bazi, S., Filieri, R., Gorton, M.: Customers' motivation to engage with luxury brands on social media. J. Bus. Res. **112**, 223–235 (2020)
5. Kapferer, J.N., Bastien, V.: The Luxury Strategy: Break the Rules of Marketing to Build Luxury Brands, 2nd edn. Kogan Page, London (2012)
6. Jacob, I., Khanna, M., Rai, K.A.: Attribution analysis of luxury brands: an investigation into consumer-brand congruence through conspicuous consumption. J. Bus. Res. **116**, 597–607 (2020)
7. Hennings, N., Wiedmann, K.P., Klarmann, C.: Luxury brands in the digital age – exclusivity versus ubiquity. Mark. Rev. St. Gallen **29**(1), 30–35 (2012)
8. Schiffer, J.: Why fashion brands are launching podcasts. Business of Fashion (2019). https://www.businessoffashion.com/articles/news-analysis/luxurys-surprising-embrace-of-the-podcast. Accessed 13 Apr 2021
9. Emarketer 2021 report. Insider Intelligence (2021)
10. Méndiz Noguero, A.: Diferencias conceptuales entre publicidad y propaganda: una aproximación etimológica (2007)
11. Méndiz Noguera, A., Regadera González, E., Pasillas Salas, G.: Valores y storytelling en los fashion films: el caso Tender Stories (2014–2017), de Tous. Rev. Comun. **17**(2), 316–335 (2018)
12. Ramos-Serrano, M., Pineda, A.E.: advertainment y las transformaciones de los formatos en el ámbito publicitario: el caso de los fashion films. Tripodos Extra **2009**(2), 729–737 (2009)
13. Dietrich, L.F., Bug, P.: Exploring the role of podcasts in the fashion industry (2019)
14. Bonini, T.: The "Second Age" of podcasting: Reframing podcasting as a new digital mass medium. Quaderns del CAC 41, 18 July, pp. 21–30 (2015)
15. Krugmann, D., Pallus, D.P.: Podcasting—Marketing für die Ohren. Gabler (2008)

16. Iskold, A.: Will podcasting survive? ReadWriteWeb (2007). http://readwrite.com/2007/08/28/will_podcasting_survive. Accessed 13 Apr 2021
17. Ahmed, O.: Fashion Wakes Up to Podcasts. Business of Fashion. https://www.businessoffashion.com/articles/news-analysis/popping-the-fashion-podcast-bubble (2017). Accessed 13 Apr 2021
18. Bratcher, T.R.: Purses, pencil skirts, and podcasts: a content analysis of fashion brand PR. Public Relat. J. **14**(1) (2021)
19. Wrather, K.: Making 'maximum fun' for fans: examining podcast listener participation online. Radio J.: Int. Stud. Broadc. Audio Media **14**(1), 43–63 (2016)
20. Interbrand. Best Global Brands 2020 (2020)
21. Antunes, M.J., Salaverría, R.: Examining independent podcasts in Portuguese iTunes. In: Stephanidis, C., Antona, M. (eds.) HCII 2020. CCIS, vol. 1226, pp. 149–153. Springer, Cham (2020). https://doi.org/10.1007/978-3-030-50732-9_20
22. Chanel.com (2021). https://www.chanel.com/gb/fashion/podcasts/3-55/. Accessed 13 Apr 2021
23. https://equilibrium.gucci.com/about-chime/. Accessed 13 Apr 2021
24. https://podcasts.dior.com/. Accessed 13 Apr 2021
25. Maryam, M., Khalid, A., Khunti, N., Mohan, M.: Media, fashion and beauty: influence on women empowerment (2021)
26. Craddock, J., Boichuk, J., Cian, L., Parmar, B.L.: Brand activism (2018)
27. Ma, J.: Reconnecting with customers through culture–revisiting the concept of cultural diversity in luxury fashion brands. J. Text. Sci. Fashion Technol. **5**(2) (2020)
28. del Hoyo, C.R., Molano, M.M.: El branded content como estrategia (no) publicitaria. Pensar la Publicidad. Rev. Int. Invest. Publ. **14**(1), 65–76 (2020)

Check for updates

Media, Fear of Crime, and Authority: Focus Groups in Lima (Perú)

Lilian Kanashiro[1](✉), Lucía Dammert[2], and Wilson Hernández[3]

[1] Universidad de Lima, Lima, Perú
lkanashi@ulima.edu.pe
[2] Universidad de Santiago de Chile, Santiago de Chile, Chile
lucia.dammert@gmail.com
[3] GRADE, Lima, Perú
whernandez@grade.org.pe

Abstract. Lima's news agenda focuses on the media's exposure and coverage of crime. This paper aims to analyze the relationship between news consumption, fear of crime, and trust in authority. To this end, twelve focus group discussions were conducted with residents of Lima. The findings revealed significant vicarious fear: respondents admitted to feeling greater fear for their children and other relatives as they remembered recent news reports. Additionally, the focus groups related news consumption to a paucity of trust in authority and evidenced a subjective consonance with their environment.

Keywords: News coverage · Insecurity · Vicarious fear · Legitimacy of authority

1 Introduction

Crime-related violence is the highlight of the information diet of Lima's citizens, and the media's spectacularization of such events serves to increase the citizenry's fear of crime [1]. The extant studies do not agree on the relationship between greater news consumption and increased fear of crime [2, 3]. The appropriate addressal of this complex association demands due consideration of the profound changes visible in the contemporary media [4]. The ways in which the media are perceived may be probed through their productive routines, regular coverage, the credibility of their content and enunciators, and modifications effected in their content formats and approaches.

The perception of insecurity stemming from the fear of crime includes both an emotional state of unease and the belief that one is a probable future victim of a criminal act [5, 6]. Additionally, the concept of vicarious fear is incorporated as a serious concern for family members (children, partners, parents) and is much more evident in women [7]. Quantitatively-oriented criminology studies have privileged variables such as victimization, vulnerability, social disorder and disorganization, and sex [8].

In Latin America, the social consequences of crime range from an increase in the perception of insecurity to the erosion of the legitimacy of institutions charged with law enforcement. Further, the contagion effect spreads the civic distrust of authority to other

© The Author(s), under exclusive license to Springer Nature Singapore Pte Ltd. 2022
Á. Rocha et al. (Eds.): ICOMTA 2021, SIST 259, pp. 354–364, 2022.
https://doi.org/10.1007/978-981-16-5792-4_35

institutions fulfilling totally dissimilar functions [9]. The spatial scale in the informative treatment becomes relevant in the public perception of the media. In Latin America, the fear of crime is higher at the national plane than at the regional level [4].

The perception of insecurity due to potential violent crime is significant in Perú: fear of crime was 85.5% from May to October 2019; it dropped to 81.8% in 2020 [10]. Despite the fear, a clear gap exists between actual victimization and imagined suffering in the future. Thus, it is pertinent to probe whether this fear is generated by the media coverage, the impact of witnesses [11], or the influence of natural interpersonal communication. A recent study based on the Peruvian situation established discrete effects resulting from the perception of insecurity triggered by levels of violence, noting that damage to physical or sexual integrity generated greater fear than the mere presence of firearms. That study further reported that the adopted protection practices exerted a scant impact on the reduction of fear [12].

Security practices manifest the perception of insecurity. A qualitative study of the lower-income sectors of Lima found that fear and anger predominated these communities. Conversely, the study also indicated that communal surveillance and neighborhood entrance barriers (bars) represented primary protection practices for these communities [11]. An ethnographic approach highlighted the coincidence between a more significant neighborhood-based commitment to community safety and intense crime news coverage [13]. The institutional legitimacy variable proposed by Hernández [9] should be reconsidered in the context of this relationship between news coverage of crime and public perceptions of insecurity. Thus, the following pages propose to examine the relationship between information habits, perceptions of insecurity, and the legitimacy of the law enforcement authority.

2 Agenda-Setting, Fear of Crime, and Legitimacy of the Authorities

The present study is tethered to three conceptual axes: news consumption, fear of crime, and legitimacy of authority. Agenda-setting vis-à-vis news updates was selected as the apt approach for the first aspect, and the extant literature on sociologically oriented criminology was referenced for the other two facets.

In principle, the agenda-setting theory contends that communication media produce public interest issues in a hierarchical manner, privileging some news items over others and controlling news exposure and consumption. In the current context, such agenda-setting actions by the media are not said to be performed to elicit fear; rather, they position the insecurity sensed by citizens on the public agenda [3, 14]. Thus, three conceptual levels emerge: the relationship between the media and public objectives; the ranking of attributes in terms of actors, narrative styles, and frameworks; and agenda melding [14].

First, the need to orient audiences through the relevance and subsequent uncertainly of the agenda is emphasized [15]. Second, certainties are established about the changes in the attributes and narratives relating to news items that increase the public sense of insecurity. For instance, the media may highlight anecdotal reports and exaggerate events to add to distorted representations and exacerbate imagined victimization [16]. Recent research has evidenced that insecurity and violence influence the autonomy of journalists as they produce information [17] and that the ability of news items to incite fear is a relevant predictor of their informational relevance [18].

Third, agenda melding refers to the configuration of each topic of an agenda network to satisfy individual orientation needs. Agenda melding encompasses the combination of traditional and alternative media agenda networks and personal preferences relating to news items [15]. The notion of subjective consonance is added to this view, denoting that people pay increased attention to news that is congruent with their immediate environment [4].

In terms of the perception of insecurity, the search for predictors such as sex, socioeconomic status, and age has been accomplished by quantitative criminology. In this context, the fear of crime is related to four widely studied concepts: victimization, vulnerability, disorder, and social disorganization. It is recurringly hypothesized that victimization increases the feeling of insecurity; however, conclusions are not definitive [19] [20]. Vulnerability describes the risk of victimization due to the severity of the consequences and the potential of controlling situations. It has been classified as personal or physical (sex, age, health), social (race and socioeconomic level), and situational (residence and neighborhood) [21]. Social disorder denotes dysfunctions of the social and physical environment: for instance, the presence of graffiti, vandalism, annoying noise, or prostitution, among other elements [22]. Finally, social disorganization signifies characteristics that make a community unable to achieve social control and tackle crime. Such communities consequently lack social capital and collective efficacy [23].

The variable of trust in the authorities assumes a certain degree of legitimacy and recognition of the role and effectiveness of administrative agencies. Notably, this study alludes to the authorities as national (National Police) and local (Serenazgo, non-armed district security) officials with direct influence to fight crime. Criminological studies regard the impact of trust in the authorities as a non-tangible or non-economic cost. In this sense, scant literature has managed to measure this effect. However, it should be noted that crime exerts a significant influence on interpersonal or institutional trust. In the latter instance, delegitimization extends to institutions that do not influence public security and thus do not affect the legitimacy of democracy [9].

3 Methodology

This study used empirical evidence obtained from testimonies and opinions articulated under group pressure to examine the fear of crime and evaluate and its association with the news media and trust in authority. To achieve this objective, the general research question was posed as, "What role do news media play in relation to the fear of crime and the legitimacy of authority?" The following specific questions were also asked:

(1) "What is the relationship between news consumption and fear of crime?" This question was included because it was deemed essential to ascertain the roles discharged by the different types of fear contemplated by previous studies in the context of intense shifts in information production routines, regardless of whether the media elicit fear in audiences [5–7].

(2) "What is the relationship between news consumption and trust in authorities?" This query was necessitated to measure the scope of the situation apropos chronically weak democracies [9].

(3) "What is the association between reported news items and personal opinions about the authorities?" The notion of subjective consonance was considered pertinent to determine whether the media confirmed an already weakened legitimacy or whether they actively generated the public distrust of the authorities.

This qualitative study adopted an empirical-analytical methodology, which involved deconstructing participant-generated data into three components, fear of crime, agenda-setting, and trust in the authorities. The categories of victimization, vulnerability, and social disorder were taken into account to assess the fear of crime. The distinctions made between the media, the public, and agenda melding were considered for agenda-setting. Finally, trust in the authorities was ascertained by distinguishing aspects related to public security from other representative state institutions. This approach allowed a broad panorama enabling the perception of insecurity in the communicative environment of the respondents.

The qualitative methodology is based on collecting perceptions and interpretations of everyday life. The selected technique for data collection involved focus groups because they allow the compilation of experiences and compel opinions to be articulated in the context of group pressure [24]. The present study was limited to adults aged between 25 and 50 years who were residents of Lima. The qualitative sampling criteria included sex and socioeconomic status identified through residence locations. In total, 12 focus groups were conducted, three for each indicated variable: AB women, AB men, DE women, and DE men.[1] Each focus group comprised an average of eight participants, and a total of 95 people participated in the study.

The focus groups were administered three instruments: (1) a pre-study sociodemographic questionnaire, (2) a focus group guide, and (3) informed consent. The sociodemographic questionnaire purposed to confirm the characteristics of the focus group participants and used a conventional model to collect data such as age, place of birth, current district of residence, and education level.

Table 1. Variables and indicators

Variables	Indicators
Social agenda	National, city, and neighborhood issues
Habits and consumption	Media and credibility
News agenda	News recall and feelings
Expectation toward authority	Feelings toward the police and Serenazgo

The indicators were taken into account by the focus group guide, which was validated in four sessions conducted with three participants, one for each sampling variable.

[1] Socioeconomic levels (SES) are categories formulated by the Peruvian Association of Market Intelligence Companies (APEIM), an entity that groups together market research and public opinion pollsters in Peru. Socioeconomic levels in Peru encompass five levels: A, B, C, D, E; SES A owns the most resources and the SES E has the least resources.

These sessions measured the duration and effects of group dynamics, phrasing, and comprehension of prompts. The validation was performed in January 2018. The instrument was modified according to observations attained during the validation process.

Participants were recruited by personnel charged with verifying characteristics marked by the sampling criteria (age, residence, sex, and education level). The focus groups were held between February 26 and March 3, 2018, at the University of Lima. All the focus group sessions were conducted by the same researcher, who was aided by an assistant in the discussion room to ensure that the group dynamics followed the same guidelines. The sessions were audio and video recorded and lasted around 90 min on average.

The transcripts of the focus group discussions were subsequently processed via NVivo and programmed in three stages: (1) encoding according to the structure of the instrument, (2) axial coding by sampling variables, and (3) coding by research question. Information demonstrating saturation in three areas was prioritized: by focus group, by sample variable, and by theoretical category. Constant comparison analysis was used, and dissent data were eventually released when they contributed new information to the study objective [25]. Finally, the focus groups were conducted within the framework of a mixed study of greater scope. The obtained results were expected to complement the comprehension of behavior. The technological support was meant to compensate for the limitations of other methods [26] in the context of the contributions offered by quantitative techniques [27].

4 Results

The findings of the study are presented in three sections according to the three conceptual cores of the study: habits, fear, and authority legitimacy. Each section outlines the relevant results, prioritizing those that achieved total saturation in every focus group, then stating outcomes that reached saturation by socioeconomic level, and finally revealing the findings by sex.

4.1 Media and News Consumption

News habits must be ascertained to recognize the impact of the media. The participants indicated that they resorted to more than one medium to inform themselves, and they indistinctly combined traditional media with social networks. No one medium was exclusively utilized.

Facebook and television achieved saturation point in all 12 focus groups. Participants agreed about doubts apropos the credibility of Facebook, warning of the presence of fake news. However, the access to media of their choice or the aggregation of content was asserted as an advantage of this platform.

With respect to print media, the participants differentiated between two types of newspapers: the serious and the *chicha* press (popular newspapers). The DE SES evinced a consensus in opining that serious newspapers were reliable even though they do not have the means to buy them. This viewpoint revealed that the dependability of such newspapers was a belief rather than a proven fact. In addition, participants affirmed the predominance of news related to insecurity and crime in popular newspapers:

> Blood, pure blood. For example, I have a colleague […] who sells newspapers. […] and he says, right? Well, today I am happy because I sold enough newspapers, but my newspapers must be dripping blood. If they don't drip blood, I won't sell, he says. […] Pure death. (Male, 30 years old, high school studies, DE SES)

Online newspapers manifested as a consumer trend for the AB SES. Participants designated in this group pointed out that the online versions were identical to the paper newspapers but more easily accessible. They also carried a variety of information, and the participants valued the freedom to select information of their interest.

The women highlighted the immediacy of online news sources over conventional media. While they acknowledged that Facebook was their major source of information, this social network platform was easily accessible and aggregated news items from varied sources, acting in interaction with other media in the information environment. Television did not escape criticism. The men agreed on the loading of sensational items and censored interests described as corrupt in the news coverage:

> In journalism one realizes how badly they work to ask such bad questions, […] they ask a father who is crying "Excuse me sir, and how do you feel about your daughter crying?" Tell me, is that journalism? (Male, 33 years old, university studies, AB SES)

The AB SES women criticized the news coverage, emphasizing the predominance of celebrity-related news reports. Most agreed that the crimes represented the primary news items on television. However, neither the SES nor the sex achieved saturation with respect to this perception.

Unlike the aforementioned media, radio was generally lauded for its credibility. The men from the DE SES underscored that the information provided on the radio was more professional because there were more specialists who dedicated more time to intensively discuss the offered information. The DE SES women also agreed on the news and permanence of the radio, highlighting the live coverage of events.

4.2 News Consumption and Fear of Crime

The responses obtained from the 12 focus group to the question about how media were related to the fear of crime revealed a semantic relationship between the term fear and words such as death, robbery, cell phone, and children. A pattern was consolidated that the news about the theft of money, wallets, or cell phones was the most frightening.

However, respondents used figures, not facts, to reflect the reasons for their fear. The news fed their vicarious fears by intensely projecting imagined scenarios relating to children or relatives. The twelve groups agreed that they felt the most intense fear when news of insecurity caught their attention was the fear that their children or relatives could suffer from a similar incident (vicarious fear). Stressful situations are created from this worry within families as adults attempt to exercise greater control over their children's activities.

> A: I put as an example, the news about the 16, 17-year-old boy who was killed for his cell phone. I very much identify with that because my son spends all day with

> a cell phone, so I always tell him if they rob you, hand it over. Several women: Sure. (Women, 41 years old, university studies, AB SES).

The comments regarding fear of death were more recurrent in the DE SES. The participants of DE SES and the majority of the BA thought that the news caused fear for two reasons: first, because they automatically positioned themselves in the situation narrated on the news as possible victims and/or because the news report resonated with personal circumstances of victimization they had previously experienced. Most AB SES groups highlighted the aggression of such events. The majority of the DE SES groups registered astonishment or indignation at the features of certain events. Besides the actual robbery or even sexual attack, it is the ferocity of the act that influences fear. People were perplexed about the rationales for armed robberies or about the fact that some robberies that resulted in death involved trivial objects like cell phones. The groups also discussed additional cruelties that accompanied cases of rape, such as the burning of the body or the death itself.

> A: [...] because now they not only rape you, now they kill you. Before they raped you, now they kill you and dismember you, a[...] B: They burn you and[...] A: They burn you. B: They burn you, rape you and dis[...] (Women, 47 years old, high school studies, DE SES)

Vicarious fear manifested more strongly in women. AB SES women's groups were more vocal in displaying their fears, associated experiences, and the likelihood of being victims.

The aspects mentioned above match attributes that make an incident more newsworthy in terms of journalism. The news agenda does not report all criminal events; it disseminates only those incidents that satisfy the characteristics of attracting the most attention from the audience.

4.3 News Consumption and Trust in the Authorities

The remarks made during the news recall included critiques on the authorities. In the instance of Perú, two types of agents are specifically linked to the fight against crime: the police (national) and the Serenazgo (local). The 12 focus groups negatively appraised the police authorities as corrupted, highlighting aspects such as bribe-taking and even asserting that the police were sometimes accomplices to crimes. The participants delved deeper into descriptions of real or imaginary occurrences once a criminal was caught, showcasing that the justice system was ineffective and favored criminal elements, while citizens acting in self-defense or police officers who fulfilled their duties suffered judicial processes.

> The system, right? The entire system is corrupt because many times the police capture them, take them to jail and before the Judiciary. The criminals already know how much, how much they ask, 10 thousand soles, right? [...] Eh, the judges demand, "Hey, they're offering 15 thousand soles," ok, so criminals sometimes have their little savings... (Male, 30 years old, master's degree, AB SES)

The 12 focus groups evinced the same stance for the Serenazgo (local authorities), who do not represent trained personnel. The focus groups alleged that they were former criminals hired to better confront criminality.

The AB SES participants were aligned in adversely evaluating the Serenazgo in comparison to the police. Broadly speaking, the participants indicated that the Serenazgo were more disadvantaged as a unit because their powers were limited, and they did not have adequate authority. Nevertheless, they also pointed out that not everything was negative and that much depended on the district. The Serenazgo were respectful and collaborated with security officers in districts that had more resources. The DE SES men highlighted experiences of abuse of authority by the Serenazgo, either because they were wont to treat people badly or because of their abuse of informal vendors. This perception was summarized as the statement that the Serenazg were abusive with street vendors and fearful of criminals. Although the criticism of the authorities was elicited from the news recall, opinions were linked more to the social experiences of participants than to the content projected in the news.

5 Discussion and Conclusion

The feelings associated with crime news coverage are mixed: they lie somewhere between fear and distrust. To answer the general research question about how the media are related to the fear of crime and the legitimacy of authority, the fear is associated with the future probability of a close family member becoming a victim of a crime, and the distrust of authority is based on experience.

This study also posed a specific research question the relationship between the media and fear of crime. A notable aspect of the obtained results concerns the role of vicarious fear as a particular type of fear of crime that relates to news coverage. The present study's results are congruent with Haynes and Rader's findings of the intensity with which this fear affects women [7]; however, the connection of this fear to journalism and news coverage is relevant. The outcomes of the present study indicate that family circumstances add an element that contributes to the increase of fear regarding crimes, especially in the age group represented by the sample.

Another significant facet involves the linking of news coverage to the public agenda. The findings of this study revealed that news reports generate feelings of uncertainty which are expressed as a part of the public agenda. This finding is aligned with the assertions of McCombs [14] and Rodríguez and Quinde [3]. However, the present study highlighted that participants criticized the media they consumed and censored the claims of plurality and depth in news coverage. The relationship of participants with the media and its agenda was not uncritical, and it did not indicate the satisfaction of the needs of the citizenry.

This study confirmed the transformation in editorial narratives: for example, the emphasis on the anecdotal and the exacerbation of imaginary victimization [17, 18]. The in-depth qualitative analysis revealed an alert that should motivate studies focused on media coverage of gender violence. If their news consumption causes women to believe that they can be sexually assaulted and moreover, suffer even more cruel forms of violence, the extent to which such coverage of cruelty contributes to the normalization, submission, and consent of women to less aggressive but more quotidian forms of violence is worth probing.

Studies conducted by Killias and Clerici [21] have examined the functioning of different types of vulnerability (personal or physical, social, and situational). The present study's findings reveal some of these vulnerabilities in relation to news coverage. The appearance of vicarious fear as imaginary victimization in recalling news items is intimately linked to the vulnerability of women.

The second specific research question inquired about the media and the legitimacy of authority. According to Kessler and Focás [4], national news reports elicit more fear than local items. The present study corroborated the significance of the geographical scale from the perspective of the legitimacy of the security-related authorities from responses received on their types, local or national. The findings suggest that distrust of authority is greater for local agents than for the National Police authority. This viewpoint was expressed in remarks unconnected to news content but relevant to the participants' experiences of their environment.

The abovementioned distrust is connected to the variable of social and situational vulnerability and indicates the erosion of the legitimacy of institutions as a non-tangible cost, the contagion effects of such feelings, and their impact on the credibility of democracy as indicated by Hernández [9]. From a qualitative standpoint, the findings point to the occasional mention of corruption by the participants in their narratives about insecurity. The results suggest that such narratives transcend citizen insecurity and are transformed into a systemic discourse of delegitimization. Thus, it is important to delve into perceptions of spatial scales.

This study must acknowledge certain limitations, which can serve as opportunities for future research initiatives. First, it must be admitted that the qualitative approach allows room for further study and is limited in its scope and generalizability. In the present instance, the drawback concerns the focal attention on experiences pertaining to the capital city. Although circumscribing the study to the capital offers the advantages of population concentration and is beneficial because Lima is home to the national media, regional experiences must not be underestimated. It is thus suggested that future research endeavors should center on the spatial scale concerning the legitimacy of authority and accord special emphasis on the local authorities and their associations with the citizenry's fear of crime.

A second limitation is found in the qualitative sampling variables, which prioritized SES and gender in the context of the city of Lima in this study; both variables were significant. However, studies incorporating the situational variable in their sampling are necessary for more intensive comparisons between the national versus regional capitals. Finally, the indirect effects of the spectacularization of cruelty or the showcasing of the grotesque may include the normalization of daily violence. This outcome was a non-contemplated element of the present study that points to specific topics of the news coverage and must be probed further by prospective researchers.

References

1. Martín-Barbero, J.: Pistas para entre-ver medios y mediaciones. Signo y pensamiento **21**(41), 13–20 (2002)
2. Sherman, A., Etchegaray, N.: Consumo de noticias y temor al delito en Chile. Estudios sobre el Mensaje Periodístico **19**(1), 563–575 (2012)
3. Rodríguez, J., Quinde, M.: Miedo al delito y medios de comunicación tradicionales: un estudio exploratorio con universitarios venezolanos. Espacio Abierto **25**(2), 145–165 (2016)
4. Kessler, G., Focás, B.: Responsables del temor? Medios y sentimiento de inseguridad en América Latina. Nueva Sociedad **249**, 137–148 (2014)
5. Ferraro, K.F., Grange, R.L.: The measurement of fear of crime. Sociol. Inq. **57**(1), 70–97 (1987). https://doi.org/10.1111/j.1475-682X.1987.tb01181.x
6. Narváez, M.: La identificación del miedo al delito: Un límite conceptual en el método de medición. Revista Crítica Penal y Poder **8**, 94–119 (2015)
7. Haynes, S., Rader, N.: Concerns about crime for self and others. an analysis of individual and contextual effects. Crim. Justice Rev. **40**(3), 303–321 (2015)
8. Kanashiro, L., Dammert, L., Hernández, W.: Percepción de inseguridad: Determinantes y narrativas. [pdf] Consorcio de investigación económica y social. bit.ly/38WE0Bf. Accessed 21 March 2021
9. Hernández, W.: Costos sociales de la victimización en América Latina: Percepción de inseguridad, capital social y percepción de la democracia. Lat. Am. Res. Rev. **54**(4), 835–853 (2019). https://doi.org/10.25222/larr.23
10. Instituto Nacional de Estadística e Información (INEI): Estadística de Seguridad Ciudadana, no. 6 [pdf]. Instituto Nacional de Estadística e Información. https://www.inei.gob.pe/media/MenuRecursivo/boletines/informe_seguridad_ciudadana.pdf. Accessed 21 March 2021
11. Kanashiro, L.: Entre el miedo y la ira. Prácticas de seguridad en los sectores de menores recursos en Lima, Perú. Revista Mexicana de Ciencias Políticas y Sociales **66**(241), 317–345 (2021). https://doi.org/10.22201/fcpys.2448492xe.2020.241.69997
12. Hernández, W., Dammert, L., Kanashiro, L.: Fear of crime examined through diversity of crime, social inequalities and social capital: an empirical evaluation in Peru. Aust. N. Z. J. Criminol. **53**(4), 515–535 (2020). https://doi.org/10.1177/0004865820954466
13. Tufró, M.: Mediatización(es) de las prácticas políticas. Los vecinos, la "inseguridad" y el ecosistema mediático. La Trama de la Comunicación **20**(2), 145–161 (2016)
14. McCombs, M.: A look at agenda-setting: past, present and future. Journal. Stud. **6**(4), 543–557 (2005)
15. McCombs, M., Shaw, D.L., Weaver, D.H.: New directions in agenda-setting theory and research. Mass Commun. Soc. **17**(6), 781–802 (2014)
16. Focás, B.: Inseguridad: En busca del rol de los medios de comunicación. La Trama de la Comunicación **17**, 163–174 (2013)
17. Garcés-Prettel, M., Arroyave-Cabrera, J., Blatar-Moreno, A.: Professional autonomy and structural influences: exploring how homicides, perceived insecurity, aggressions against journalists, and inequalities affect perceived journalistic autonomy in Colombia. Int. J. Commun. **14**, 3054–3075 (2020)
18. Wong, J., Harraway, V.: Media presentation of homicide: examining characteristics of sensationalism and fear of victimization and their relation to newspaper article prominence. Homicide Stud. **24**(4), 333–352 (2019). https://doi.org/10.1177/1088767919896391
19. Dammert, L., Lunecke, A.: Violencia y temor: análisis teórico-empírico en doce comunas del país. Centro de Estudios de Seguridad Ciudadana, Santiago (2002)
20. Triana Sánchez, J.: Percepción de inseguridad en polígonos geográficos prioritarios en Acapulco. Espiral Estudios sobre Estado y Sociedad **24**(70), 221–249 (2017)

21. Killias, M., Clerici, C.: Different measures of vulnerability in their relation to different dimensions of fear of crime. Br. J. Criminol. **40**(3), 437–450 (2000)
22. Sampson, R.J.: Analytic approaches to disorder. Br. J. Sociol. **60**(1), 83–93 (2009)
23. Sampson, R.J., Groves, W.B.: Community structure and crime: testing social-disorganization theory. Am. J. Sociol. **94**(4), 774–802 (1989)
24. Krueger, R., Casey, M.: Focus Groups: A Practical Guide for Applied Research. Sage, London (2015)
25. Onwuegbuzie, J., Dickinson, W., Leech, N., Zoran, A.: Un marco cualitativo para la recolección y análisis de datos en la investigación basada en grupos focales. Paradigmas **3**(1), 127–157 (2011)
26. Cyr, J.: The unique utility of focus groups for mixed-methods research. Polit. Sci. Polit. **54**(4), 1038–1042 (2017). https://doi.org/10.1017/S104909651700124X
27. Guerrero, L., Xicola, J.: New approaches to focus groups. In: Methods in Consumer Research, vol. 1, pp. 49–77. Woodhead Publishing (2018). https://doi.org/10.1016/B978-0-08-102089-0.00003-0

First Studies of the Migration of Television Content to Twitch in Spain

Natalia Quintas-Froufe(✉) and Ana González-Neira

Department of Sociology and Communication Sciences, Universi dade da Coruña, A Coruña, Spain
n.quintas.froufe@udc.es

Abstract. Within the framework of the complex current media ecosystem, traditional television must share space with video streaming platforms like Twitch, which has led new audiovisual consumption habits. This live-streaming video platform focusing on video games has recently spread outside this field and is now in general use, particularly among the younger generations who see it as a new means of accessing and viewing audiovisual content. The potential for interaction with young people that Twitch offers its streamers is one of the keys to its growth and success. Through the analysis of some examples of television content migration involving Ibai Llanos, one of the streamers with the highest number of followers, our aim is to make a first approach to the synergies between television and this platform. In this way, it can be seen that Twitch is no longer a platform linked to gaming, but an audiovisual entertainment channel for a more active and selective audience.

Keywords: Twitch · Television · Audiences · Streaming

1 Television in the Current Media Ecosystem

The current media ecosystem is extraordinarily complex and convergent due to the dynamics brought about by digitalization and the use of devices which have, to a greater or lesser extent, affected all and every type of mass media. Within this context, television is one of the media which has had to face up to most changes in the last few decades, as we can now watch TV contents on the multiple platforms and screens that have expanded the audiovisual experience assisted by the social networks. Through second screens, the TV channels attempt to complement this experience by making it more flexible and interactive for the user. In fact, according to the AIMC [1], 42.8% of surfers use the internet on a second device while watching television, a practice that is on the rise.

In addition, the high-level reach of the new OTT viewing platforms (Netflix, Amazon, etc.) has called into question the value of the linearity of television and even the strength of the media itself. Traditional television has to contend with formats created by internet, on demand consumption, pay-tv and audiovisual content distribution platforms [2]. This is a complex panorama which has intensified the process of hyper-fragmentation of the audiences [3] and means that many voices have been raised anew to proclaim the death of

© The Author(s), under exclusive license to Springer Nature Singapore Pte Ltd. 2022
Á. Rocha et al. (Eds.): ICOMTA 2021, SIST 259, pp. 365–373, 2022.
https://doi.org/10.1007/978-981-16-5792-4_36

television [4]. As some authors state, it appears that "the rise of new media has indicated that only sports and other great events will uphold the flow, linearity and liveness of traditional television" (p.606), [5]. However, at the present time it is still the media with the greatest penetration and audience in Spain [6].

The traditional supremacy of television increased during the Covid-19 pandemic. This extraordinary lockdown situation brought about a change in people's media consumption patterns at all levels. Digital and TV consumption were, undoubtedly, the big winners [7]. Referring to the medium of television, which is our concern, we can see that there was great growth of consumption during the months of lockdown. The television viewer numbers in Spain broke all records since ratings began, and even the youngest consumers, who normally use television less, were drawn to it [8, 9]. However, young people do not use the TV media solely to view contents but also for other uses (OTT viewing, videogames, etc.) as they wish to experience shared consumption [10], one of the keys to Twitch.

1.1 Transformation of Audiovisual Consumption Habits

In this new context of redefining television or of post-television [11], with different consumer conditions, other media practices have arisen in which the viewers decide what, when and where to view audiovisual contents, independently of the type of broadcaster and the time and place limits. For this reason, platforms such as Netflix, Amazon or Youtube, based on streaming consumption, attract a younger public that will not be controlled by the strict timetables of TV schedules and has replaced the concept of prime time with my time [12] and become their own programmers.

The migration of audiovisual contents to the online area means that live-streaming has become an extremely interesting context for participatory online media, spearheaded by services such as YouTube, that have put the traditional consumer into the role of content creator [13]. We may think, as pointed out by Sjöblom & Hamari [14], that streaming may be another type of entertainment like online videos, but "for many users it is a more manifold and holistic communication channel than mere video media content, particularly due to the high levels of interaction" (p.985) [14]. These authors also highlight an interesting difference between streaming as a technological solution, and the cultural phenomenon of live broadcasts of user-generated content, also commonly referred to as streaming. This latter approach is the basis for the success of Twitch.

We must also take into account that streaming "is a route to reach a market of over a hundred million with highly relevant products" (p.324) [15]. Many advertisers have already seen how to reach a broader audience which it would be difficult to impact through more traditional media.

From this setting emerged Twitch, which many insist on considering as a true rival to television as the audience numbers it achieves could compete with even the most successful traditional television channels[1] (Woodcock & Johnson, 2019). However, Twitch does not aim to compete with television but rather boosts one of the basic characteristics

[1] So far, the Twitch broadcast with the biggest audience (2.4 million viewers) was on the Spanish streamer channel TheGrefg on 11 January 2021.

of the media, as it "may be understood as representing a return to linear-TV with its emphasis on live streaming" (p.606) [5].

2 The Origins of the Platform

Twitch, a spin-off of Justin.TV, was introduced in 2011 as a video platform with live or recorded broadcasting which offered the possibility of interaction with the content creators (the twitchers/the streaming performers). The main difference from other similar platforms is that it was one of the first fully dedicated to videogames,[2] specifically to gamecasting and video game competition (also known as e-sport), because seeing how others play is crucial for gaming culture [16]. From 2015, when it was acquired by Amazon, it started to make extensions into non-gaming streaming, by introducing new categories such as 'music', 'creative' and 'IRL' ('in real life')" [16].

It is indispensable to understand that Twitch began as a platform mainly dedicated to video-gaming culture and e-sports and this is what differentiates it from other similar platforms such as YouTube. It has many similarities with YouTube, as stated by Pires & Simon [17], although YouTube is geared towards a much wider public. However, at present Twitch has a much broader sample of channels that broadcast in streaming than YouTube, as the latter platform was not created for this purpose. In addition, the fundamental difference between the two platforms is that the capacity to offer live television content on this scale is exclusive to Twitch [15].

As has been noted, the Twitch phenomenon is not original, but what is, is the growing momentum of its development in the last few years, particularly in the year 2020 due to the pandemic situation. According to the StreamElements report, the year-on-year growth of the platform in viewer hours was 83% [18]. Currently, Twitch has 30 million daily visitors from almost every country in the world, almost half of whom are between 18 and 34 years old, and 21% between 13 and 18 [19].

Although Twitch began as a video game platform, the introduction of new contents allows for the adoption of a new research angle which may compare it with other types of contents produced by other media such as television [19]. Some viewers, particularly younger ones, find contents more suited to their interests on Twitch than on the television, as "watching Twitch was not 'one thing', it was a compilation of multiple ways of viewing and interacting that took place along a continuum from small, densely-knit community channels to big, mass-audience channels resembling traditional mega-sized television productions" (p.611) [5].

In short, Twitch, as stated by Gutiérrez-Lozano & Cuartero [21], not only highlights a change in trends in young people's audiovisual consumption, but has brought about a broader transformation in the way in which this audience interacts with an audiovisual product, as we shall see in the next section.

2.1 Twitchers and Audiences

Twitchers fit in with the model for the creation of user-generated content in which any user may create content and broadcast it. Therefore, the potential to create and broadcast

[2] To compete with Twitch, in 2015 YouTube created the YouTube Gaming channel and Facebook launched Facebook Gaming in 2018.

content is no longer in the hands of large communication companies, as indicated by Pires & Simon [17], because any person can become a TV provider. Anyone with minimal technology and little audiovisual training can reach a large audience, and so there is a process of democratization of broadcasting. In addition, the platform encourages users to take this step and makes it really easy to go from being a Twitch-watcher to a Twitch-streamer [5].

Streamers may be considered as "social media influencers", a term that, as noted by Woodcock and Johnson [14], has become a widespread, if sometimes nebulous, way of describing a digital celebrity who is able to inform and encourage particular consumer choices. While it is true that only streamers with big audiences seem to stand out, there are streamers with less visibility who will interact with different sized audiences. At present Twitch has seven million streamers with monthly broadcast [19].

The interaction of the streamer with their audience is one of the keys to the platform's success. Twitch "offers real-time human interaction between the streamer and viewers, facilitating their ability to interact with each other" (p.58) [22]. It should be noted that, as believed by Spilker, Ask & Hansen [5], we conceptualize Twitch viewers primarily as audience, as opposed to, for example, gamers, in order to explore ways of theorizing new media practices. The viewers watch the content offered by the streamer, but may also interact directly with him/her. This facilitates a two-way connection where streamers directly acknowledge and respond to viewers, and viewers can actively participate in, and influence, live-stream broadcasts [14].

The platform has multiple interactive tools through which the streamer can connect with the audience. For example, it includes a chat in which the users may communicate with the streamer and participate directly and actively in the viewed content; in this way, there is an instant response from the streamer. Diverse elements are also introduced to improve the viewing experience in order to constantly increase the interaction and the number of channel subscribers. Streamers must carefully choose which tools are most suitable for their individual stream and streaming community [23]. Twitch provides two different forms of collaboration for their creators, the affiliate program (lower-level access to revenue and services) and the partnership program (higher-level access to revenue and services). The streamers must also pay special attention to the demands of their audience, and so personalise the viewer's experience by giving them a greater share through various actions or practices (calling them by name, giving personal thanks) using the tools which the platform provides.

Social recognition by other viewers or by the streamer himself makes engagement with this platform appealing. This is definitive because "motivations to engage in live-stream entertainment have a strong social and community emphasis compared to engagement in mass media such as television" (p.65) [22]. The streamers "gamify" the stream-viewing experience so as to keep the users longer on the platform and make them more active [22]. Depending on the type of streamer (big or small) and the number of followers they have on the channel, the relationship between them will be more fluid and will strengthen the sense of community which is key for the platform. This sense of community is one of the eight socio-motivations for live-stream engagement together with entertainment, information seeking, meeting new people, social interactions, social support, social anxiety and external support (p.59) [22].

It should be stressed that the viewing experience on Twitch is of an individual nature, but it is also social as it is shared with many other viewers. Therefore, Twitch may be considered as a "virtual third place, in which informal communities emerge, socialize, and participate" (p.1) [24].

3 Methodology

The objective of this article is to address the Twitch phenomenon from the perspective of media studies, and not from that of game studies, which has been common in academic literature. Twitch was chosen because, at present, it is the biggest live-streaming platform.

This is an exploratory study in the Spanish area. Spain was chosen as the country under study for two reasons: on the one hand, Spanish is one of the two main languages on the platform; and, on the other, the main streamers on the platform are Spaniards. The aim of this article is to show some of the synergies between Twitch and the medium of television by analysing of the case of the Spanish streamer Ibai Llanos. To do so, the migration of TV formats to the Twitch platform has been analysed, with particular emphasis on the audience data in order to quantitatively measure the phenomenon under study.

One of the problems to be taken into account in this research is the limited theorisation of the phenomenon, as stressed by Gandolfi [25] among others. The academic studies regarding the platform are quite recent and most focus on analysing its technical characteristics and its content. The Twitch platform has been studied principally from the perspective of game studies, so what has been researched is the main motivations and gratifications of the users [14, 20, 22, 26, 27]; the formation of communities [24]; e-sports [28]; or the determinants of live streamers' continuance broadcasting intentions [29]. Other works have attempted to understand the viewing practices of Twitch [5] or classify the content and types of streams on Twitch [30]. And yet other publications have appeared which address Twitch from the strategic communication [15]; education [31]; audiovisual communication [21], or gamification perspectives [23].

4 The Case of Ibai Llanos

Ibai Llanos is one of the "social media influencers" and the streamer (both on YouTube and Twitch) with the greatest impact on the e-sports community both in Spain and at an international level. He began his streamer career as a videogames commentator, later joining the Liga de Videojuegos Profesional and subsequently joining G2 Esports which he left in January 2020 in order to create his own digital entertainment project called "Ibailand". Currently, he creates contents mainly for Twitch and has won the accolade for the best streamer of the year (2020) in the Esports Awards.

The first example of audiovisual content migration to the Twitch platform was the Campanadas de Fin de Año (New Year's Chimes), one of the television events which have traditionally brought together a large part the Spanish audience since they were first broadcast on television in the 1960s, as they favour collective viewing [3]. On 31 December 2020, for the first time in the history of the platform, Ibai Llanos broadcast the New Year's Chimes, a four-and-a-half-hour event with 552,345 users at midnight. This figure includes the total of single devices connected to his broadcast. This fact is highly significant as its audience ratings were higher than a generalist channel like Cuatro (269,000 viewers) [8]. Moreover, on this occasion television consumption during the broadcast of the New Year's Chimes broke a historical record with 22.3 million viewers watching the television in the last minute of the year 2020 [9]. This outstanding fact must be placed in context within the framework of the pandemic and the restrictions on movement which obliged people to stay in their homes and thus form part of a potentially captive audience.

At present, the comparison between the audience numbers reached on Twitch by one channel and the number of viewers watching a television channel, for example, Cuatro, cannot be made on an equal footing as the Twitch audience is global while the audience for a channel like Cuatro is limited to Spanish viewers. Another point to be taken into account which impedes the comparison of both audiences is that the data offered by Twitch correspond to the number of connected users, without allowing for the fact that several people may be simultaneously connected to a single screen, which does not occur with the audience data offered by the ratings for the television channel.

The other case for analysis was the broadcast of an episode of First Dates on the streamer's channel. First Dates is a reality dating show by Spain's Cuatro which is broadcast from Monday to Friday on prime-time. On this occasion, the team led by Ibai Llanos went to the set of the program to organise their own live dating show and broadcast it on his Twitch channel. Carlos Sobera, the programme presenter, welcomed them to the set to make the handover. "Buscando el amor en IbaiLand", as they called the format, was broadcast on 16 February 2021[3] for two hours during which it brought together 210,548 viewers, reaching 269,632 at its peak moment. Apart from the participants in the competition, Ibai Llanos was accompanied by part of his team from Ibailand, made up by other Twitch content creators. In contrast to the broadcasts on his own channel, in this case the production and technical resources for the broadcast were those of the Cuatro program and channel themselves. Subsequently, the edited video could also be seen on Ibai Llanos' YouTube profile.

One month later, on 15 March 2021, the second edition of the format "Buscando el amor en IbaiLand" was broadcast. However, the program was not recorded on the First Dates set, but at the streamer's own home. The audience was smaller as it had 117,400 viewers and 152,000 at its peak.

"Charlando tranquilamente" is another example of television content migration to Twitch. This program has the format of interviews carried out by videoconference at a certain time (21:00) on a certain day (Thursdays). The format premiered on 4 February with a two-hour-plus interview with the footballer Gerard Piqué and had a mean audience of 178,599 viewers with 258,432 viewers at its peak minute. Despite having a traditional interview format, Ibai Llanos stressed that it was not an interview as there was no script, the questions had not been prepared and the fact that he was not a journalist. Using the same structure, the streamer carries out weekly interviews of well-known people (sporting figures, singers, youtubers and journalists). This program may be watched again on Twitch but also on other platforms such as YouTube or Spotify.

[3] On the same day, the First Dates program on Cuatro had an audience of 1,054,000 viewers.

5 Conclusions

In the last few years, Twitch has ceased to be a platform linked to gaming and become an entertainment platform with great potential for development due to its diversity of contents. The platform's initial audience was users who played and watched others playing videogames (gamers). However, this original conception of the audience has been surpassed by the great growth of the platform. Young viewers, more distanced from the television medium, are those who have been most attracted by the flexibility of the platform as it offers them the possibility of watching different audiovisual contents in which they are interested, together with other members of the same community at unconventional times.

The Twitchers interact with their audiences in multiple ways in order to create communities. This sense of belonging to a community, thanks to the social intervention of the viewers, is one of the most relevant reasons why the user is prepared to spend so many hours on the platform. The sense of community created on Twitch is the main difference with other platforms such as YouTube, where the level of belonging and permanence is less important.

Streamers such as Ibai Llanos present a solid strategy to gain the loyalty of their public and have developed great complicity with their community which appears to endorse any event or a life program they produce. Proof of this are the viewing figures reached for the channel broadcasts. Additionally, the first examples of synergies between television and Twitch in Spain correspond to their channel.

While it is true that the audience figures for these broadcasts on Twitch are high, at present no strict comparison with the audience figures reached by television can be made. The audience for Twitch is global, and not national, therefore comparisons between the two audiences are not logical.

Twitch is not the new television, but it does present some of the defining characteristics of the television medium such as direct viewing; however, this viewing is much more selective on the part of a predominantly young audience which is also much more active. Each broadcast is a challenge for the streamer and a novelty for the audience who do not know what they are really going to see each time they connect to a broadcast with no prior edition, and so they prefer to enjoy the live experience in the company of other viewers.

References

1. AIMCa. https://www.aimc.es/a1mc-c0nt3nt/uploads/2020/02/2020_02_04_NP_AIMC_Q_Panel_Television_2019.pdf. Accessed 30 March 2021
2. Vázquez-Barrio, T., Torrecillas-Lacave, T., Suárez-Álvarez, R.: Percepción sobre la televisión en el ecosistema audiovisual de la convergencia digital. Profesional de la información **29**(6), e290640 (2020). https://doi.org/10.3145/epi.2020.nov.40
3. González-Neira, A., Quintas-Froufe, N.: Preferencias televisivas de la audiencia española (2005–2019): programas, formatos y cadenas. Estudios sobre el Mensaje Periodístico **26**(2), 583–595 (2020). https://doi.org/10.5209/esmp.67777
4. Buonanno, M.: Editor's introduction the end of television: not yet. Media Commun. **4**(3), 95–98 (2016). https://doi.org/10.17645/mac.v4i3.661

5. Spilker, H.S., Ask, K., Hansen, M.: The new practices and infrastructures of participation: how the popularity of twitch.tv challenges old and new ideas about television viewing. Inf. Commun. Soc. **23**(4), 605–620(2020). https://doi.org/10.1080/1369118X.2018.1529193
6. AIMCb. https://www.aimc.es/a1mc-c0nt3nt/uploads/2021/02/marco2021.pdf. Accessed 30 March 2021
7. AIMCc. http://download.aimc.es/aimc/cc8ke5T/naveg2020_principales_resultados.pdf. Accessed 29 March 2021
8. Barlovento Comunicación. https://www.barloventocomunicacion.es/wp-content/uploads/2021/01/Audiencias_Campanadas_2020_Barlovento-2.pdf. Accessed 27 March 2021
9. Barlovento Comunicación. https://www.barloventocomunicacion.es/informes-barlovento/balance-del-total-consumo-de-la-television-en-el-primer-ano-covid/. Accessed 28 March 2021
10. Capapé, E.: Nuevas formas de consumo de contenidos televisivos en España: una revisión histórica (2006–2019). Estudios del Mensaje Periodístico **26**(2), 451–459 (2020). https://doi.org/10.5209/esmp.67733
11. Lotz, A.: The Television will be Revolutionized, 2nd edn. NYU, New York (2014)
12. Polo-López, M., Miotto, G., Fondevila-Gascón, J.F.: My time: incidencia de la televisión a la carta en la evolución del prime time en España. Revista Latina de Comunicación Social **73**, 208–227 (2018). https://doi.org/10.4185/RLCS-2018-1253
13. Cha, M., Kwak, H., Rodriguez, P., Ahn, Y.Y., Moon, S.: I tube, you tube, everybody tubes: analyzing the world's largest user generated content video system. In: Proceedings of the 7th ACM SIGCOMM Conference on Internet Measurement 2007, 24–26 October 2007. San Diego, California, USA, pp 1–14 (2007). https://doi.org/10.1145/1298306.1298309
14. Sjöblom, M., Hamari, J.: Why do people watch others play video games? An empirical study on the motivations of Twitch users. Comput. Hum. Behav. **75**, 985–996 (2017). https://doi.org/10.1016/j.chb.2016.10.019
15. Woodcock, J., Johnson, M.R.: Live streamers on twitch.tv as social media influencers: chances and challenges for strategic communication. Int. J. Strateg. Commun. **13**(4), 321–335 (2019). https://doi.org/10.1080/1553118X.2019.1630412
16. Taylor, T.L.: Watch Me Play: Twitch and the Rise of Game Live Streaming. Princeton University Press, New Jersey (2018)
17. Pires, K., Simon, G.: YouTube live and twitch: a tour of user-generated live streaming systems. In: Proceedings of the 6th ACM Multimedia Systems Conference, pp. 225–230 (2015). https://doi.org/10.1145/2713168.2713195
18. Streamelements. https://blog.streamelements.com/state-of-the-stream-december-and-2020-year-in-review-aa4146f074be. Accessed 30 March 2021
19. Twitch. https://brand.twitch.tv. Accessed 30 March 2021
20. Sjöblom, M., Törhönen, M., Hamari, J., Macey, J.: Content structure is king: An empirical study on gratifications, game genres and content type on Twitch. Comput. Hum. Behav. **73**, 161–171 (2017). https://doi.org/10.1016/j.chb.2017.03.036
21. Gutiérrez-Lozano, J.F., Cuartero, A.: El auge de Twitch: nuevas ofertas audiovisuales y cambios del consumo televisivo entre la audiencia juvenil. Ámbitos. Revista Internacional de Comunicación **50**, 159–175 (2020). https://doi.org/10.12795/Ambitos.2020.i50.11
22. Hilvert-Bruce, Z., Neill, J.T., Sjöblom, M., Hamari, J.: Social motivations of live-streaming viewer engagement on Twitch. Comput. Hum. Behav. **84**, 58–67 (2018). https://doi.org/10.1016/j.chb.2018.02.013
23. Siutila, M.: The gamification of gaming streams. In: CEUR Workshop Proceedings, pp. 131–140 (2018)

24. Hamilton, W. A., Garretson, O., Kerne, A.: Streaming on twitch: fostering participatory communities of play within live mixed media. In: Proceedings of the SIGCHI Conference on Human Factors in Computing Systems, pp. 1315–1324. https://doi.org/10.1145/2556288.2557048
25. Gandolfi, E.: To watch or to play, it is in the game: the game culture on Twitch.tv among performers, plays and audiences. J. Gaming Virtual Worlds **8**(1), 63–82 (2016). https://doi.org/10.1386/jgvw.8.1.63_1
26. Wulf, T., Schneider, F.M., Beckert, S.: Watching players: an exploration of media enjoyment on twitch. Games C. **15**(3), 328–346 (2018)
27. Hu, M., Zhang, M., Wang, Y.: Why do audiences choose to keep watching on live video streaming platforms? An explanation of dual identification framework. Comput. Hum. Behav. **75**, 594–606 (2017). https://doi.org/10.1016/j.chb.2017.06.006
28. Hamari, J., Keronen, L.: Why do people play games? A meta-analysis. Int. J. Inf. Manage. **37**(3), 125–141 (2017)
29. Zhao, Q., Chen, H.-W., Cheng, J.-L., Wang, J.-L.: Determinants of live streamers' continuance broadcasting intentions on Twitch: a self-determination theory perspective. Telemat. Inform. **35**(2), 406–420 (2018). https://doi.org/10.1016/j.tele.2017.12.018
30. Churchill, B.C., Xu, W.: The modem nation: a first study on Twitch.tv social structure and player/game relationships. In: 2016 IEEE International Conferences on BDCloud, SocialCom., SustainCom., Atlanta (2016). https://doi.org/10.1109/BDCloud-SocialCom-SustainCom.2016.43
31. Payne, K., Keith, M.J., Schuetzler, R.M., Giboney, J.S.: Examining the learning effects of live streaming video game instruction over Twitch. Comput. Hum. Behav. **77**, 95–109 (2017). https://doi.org/10.1016/j.chb.2017.08.029

Twenty-First Century Trends and International Cross-Cultural Perspective: Cultural Hybridizations and Narrative-Dramatic-Cinematographic Fusions Between Europe and Latin America. The Case of Kiro Russo (Cinematography) and Rodrigo García (Literature)

Miguel A. Orosa, Daqui Lema, and Viviana Galarza-Ligña(✉)

Pontificia Universidad Católica del Ecuador, Ibarra, Ecuador
{maorosa1,cdlema,vngalarza}@pucesi.edu.ec

Abstract. In a century where diverse group identities surpass any kind of frontier and seem to be reflected ever more in the mirror of a clawing cultural selfhood, we are going to make an analysis of the archetype and artistic patterns of two authors of recognized prestige and, undoubtedly, excellent aesthetic practice: the Bolivian Kiro Russo (in the field of cinematography) and the acclaimed literary author Rodrigo García, of Spanish-Argentine origin. For this purpose, we will make use of a series of models in the scientific field related to the indigenous culture of Latin American (considered from a post-dramatic perspective), secondly to the culture that has been developing in the internal flow of the Spanish language and, finally, to the European post-drama of aesthetic bias (literary and cinematic). We will also delve into the technical and cultural influences of narrativity and post-drama in the artists mentioned above and we will design the conceptual theoretical maps of these productions within the Spanish language and indigenous Latin American culture. The technical fusions just mentioned and the cultural hybridizations of international stamp lead us to a summation where the intensive components of narrative character, the libertarian forms typical of the Spanish culture and the metamodern mentality of our century open the doors to an inquiry about the future of literature and cinematography through the patterns of cultural hybridization.

Keywords: (Post-)dramatic trends of the twenty-first century in film and literature · Cultural hybridizations between Europe and Latin America · Narrative-dramatic-cinematographic technical fusions

1 Introduction

Law is becoming a privileged channel and instrument for cross-cultural hybridizations built on the reciprocal recognition of the common value of what it is to be human, leading

© The Author(s), under exclusive license to Springer Nature Singapore Pte Ltd. 2022
Á. Rocha et al. (Eds.): ICOMTA 2021, SIST 259, pp. 374–383, 2022.
https://doi.org/10.1007/978-981-16-5792-4_37

to the construction of shared spaces even at the global level. Throughout and within these processes, the narratives of literature, dramaturgy and cinematography are faced with the challenge of being able to translate what the law establishes as a global aspiration for equality.

This fact has triggered a debate that opens a reflection on colonial practices aimed at ignoring the knowledge of so many human groups alien to what we understand as the West, whether in their epistemological production, in their collective existence and even in terms of limiting their exercise of self-determination, all in order to create homogeneous identities, governable and consistent with the official and dominant narrative.

On these bases, interesting processes have been opened that have been fundamental for the construction of societies for peace, where cultural production finds sufficient space for its development and dissemination. Especially in the Latin American context, we can say that these processes have opened a window to the future, also providing new debates around an even deeper recognition of diversities, as in the case of the Plurinational States of Ecuador and Bolivia or, to give another example, the central axis of Neoconstitutionalism as a mechanism that attributes a determining role to the State in terms of its obligations regarding Human Rights. These mechanisms define an agenda that is important for civil society to promote for peaceful coexistence among diverse identities. The role of the media and languages, in this sense, should be nurtured by those different meanings that build spaces of exchange for understanding and reciprocal knowledge [1].

2 Methodology

The present work, of mixed approach with predominance of the qualitative paradigm, has as its object of study the cultural hybridizations and narrative-dramatic-cinematographic fusions between Europe and Latin America and based on certain models included in this article, then move on to the case studies of two artists: Kiro Russo and Rodrigo García. For this purpose, the analytical-synthetic method will be used: first, there is a decomposition of the works in several of their constituent parts and, subsequently, the common characteristics are synthesized in order to be able to draw relevant conclusions.

This is not a mere description or theoretical exposition of the state of contemporary literature or of current narrative trends, be they cinematic or post-dramatic, and how they are interconnected between Latin America and Europe. An authentic scientific framework has been developed, consisting of four empirical models that describe the variables of our research in an exhaustive manner in the fields of indigenism, metamodern culture, Spanish-language drama and contemporary audiovisual language (studies that do not exist to date, as far as we have been able to verify). From here, it is possible to open the great questions of the investigation, namely: if cultural alliances of identity character are opened beyond the mere geographical limits already outdated of the old nationalities and, later, from very representative authors of two arts and continents, to see in what way the variables of the mentioned models are fulfilled to see if the initial premise is accomplished: contemporary aesthetic hybridizations between Europe and Latin America beyond the artificial borders of nations and continents, which is indeed fulfilled in the present article.

3 Theoretical Framework

The following panel depicts the most representative characteristics and patterns of Latin American Indigenous culture as seen from a post-dramatic perspective. It is a vision very different from the European one that has never been studied from an aesthetic-post-dramatic point of view until today, as far as we know. For the elaboration of this Table 1, we have observed Latin American plays of indigenous influence in countries such as Ecuador, Bolivia, Peru and Colombia. A canonical play has been the basis for us to cipher the patterns of this culture, La flor de la Chukirawa, by Patricio Vallejo Aristizábal, although we have also carried out doctrinal studies, some of which we cite in references [2–7].

Table 1. Latin American indigenous post-dramatic panel

	Category	Component
1	Systemic or organic vision Atmospheres Environments	Post-dramatic pariverse or duoverse (or multiverse) versus western artistic universe (unity) Truth as a dramatic parity. Complementary dramatic duality "Greek" (Native)-Andean heavy liturgies Refusal of homocentrism Harmonies and structures proper to the entire Nature
2	Conflict Complementary forces Post-dramatic organization Denouement	Conflict understood as vital tension, not in a destructive way It is not necessary for one dramatic force to confront and defeat another Unsolved conflict Complementary pairs versus opposite and excluding pairs There is no denouement or resolution
3	Time Post-dramatic tension	There is no vision of dramatic tension understood as attention or interest without cracks in the dramatic play "Dramatic tension" is understood as the intensity of the present, regardless of the past or the future Timelessness or non-existence of time
4	Type of story Narrative and Post-drama	Narrative-dramatic organization linked to the narrative cosmovision It is in the interest of the "author" to tell a (narrative) story (not a plot) within a conceptual space proper to the cultural cosmovision
5	Pariverse Technical-formal organization	Repetitive ties Parity and cosmic bonding Formal organizations do not pursue the same aims as in the West: the thematic and unitary focus of the play

Source: Orosa [8, 9]

We have already carried out some studies on the analysis of this post-dramatic culture, such as those just cited at the base of Table 1. However, it may be useful to emphasize and reiterate the basic aesthetic idea of the indigenous Latin American post-drama, which revolves around the concept of pariverse or multiverse (as opposed to the universe, so typical of the Western conception: unity, composition) from which two fundamental concepts spring in this aesthetic manifestation: the dual, bicephalic organization (not around a single idea that rules the whole composition), and the system of complementary pairs, which modifies the Western concept of dramatic organization (setup, confrontation and resolution) because there is no destructive confrontation and therefore the notion of conflict changes and, consequently, there is no (post-)dramatic resolution.

Table 2 above shows some of the most important patterns of Western post-drama of our times. In the sphere of post-drama, clearly unlike performance attitudes, there is or should be some kind of internal reason (of sense, of order) that justifies that some things are next to others (post-dramatic juxtaposition), because mere chaos in its pure state, without any sense, does not seem to be a sufficient argument to speak of art or about spectacle. In the performance it seems that this reason could be external to the play, having a political, social, ethical, personal, etc. character. But in the post-drama scene, we must assume that there must be an internal (il-)logical reason of an aesthetic, architectural or organizational nature (apart from the extrinsic motivations proper to artivism). We have already referred to this issue in scientific works cited in this article and previously.

As we see it, in contemporary narrative movements, and in particular within the trends we have been referring to at this point, there are two chronotopes (or points of view) from which the action is narrated: one with a mystical stamp (beyond the mind, from a place and time in consciousness) and another linked to the historical origin of post-drama: the Spanish-language culture, anti-dogmatic, libertarian, highly narrative, driven by desire, improvisation, festive liturgy. Within the (post-)dramatic culture in the Spanish language (we also witness this phenomenon in the Latin American indigenous post-drama) the staging arises around a celebration, the people join the party with that pretext and, without norms or prefixed rules, join the event with joy or festive crying, in the company of the crowd but alone, maintaining their freedom and their individualistic spirit. Multiple themes or manifestations are developed here and there within the party, some people sing, others cry, their theme is one and that of other groups is another: freedom. It is precisely from this libertarian and festive, anti-normative and anti-classical chronotope and history that we can understand the characteristics and patterns that we observe in Table 2 [11–13]: the absence of linear times, the feeling of the present, the fragmentation, the rejection of a textual autarchy, the denial of a univocal concept of reality and the conditionalization of events; or also the multiperspectivisms, the multiplane techniques (simultaneisms), the rhizomatic relations, the juxtaposition of ideas, the texts understood as voices and not as characters; and, finally, all the patterns described in the categories 4 Scenes, 5 Dialogues and languages, 6 Participation and result.

Precisely, the (post-)dramatic culture in the Spanish language, to some of whose deep patterns we have just referred, would be characterized by the notions shown in Table 3, below.

Table 2. West post-dramatic and metamodern panel

	Category	Component
1	Time and reality	Absence of chronological or linear time Fragmentation of characters, of architectures… "Kairos" or present time Disregard or controversy over the concept of "reality" Positions in conditional or go to potential ones
2	Theme and text	Textual autarchy (the predominance of the text is denied) Visuality and multi-disciplinarity of the show besides the text. Thematic fragmentation or dramatic fragmentation of actions on stage. Juxtaposition of ideas against organic unity Apparent irrationality, self-referentiality. Collage. Multiplicity and multi-perspectivism. Repeating the opposite of what it looked like before. Many rhizomatic relationships that prevent synthesis. The dramatic conflict and the conversational character of the theatre disappears
3	Characters	Constitution of characters tends to fragmentation or puppets in the hands of the author. Breakthrough of the real: the characters become actors. Texts with voices, more than characters
4	Scenes	Inconsistency of disciplines and events Non-hierarchical (horizontality) of topics or speeches Sensory communication with the viewer. Relations between text and scenes are autonomous and noninterpretive. Reiterations of scenes. Micro-scenes Daily routines and micro-stories. Post-drama, self-fiction. Exploration of the body and the dance
5	Dialogues and language	Organizations and non-logical provisions The truth and the exclusivity of the word are questioned No causal logic. Use of the virtual realities (especially screens), documentary language. Symbols, signifiers (as opposed to meanings). Gimmicky rhetoric, dissolution of the text into textuality. An anecdote becomes the subject of a play. The sense is placed in the atmosphere of the language. Marginal speech is mixed with lyrical language. Rhythm of words and silences, the value of the ineffable is up to the reader to reveal
6	Participation and result	Sensitive and emotional communication with the viewer Reflection on the world. No interpretation, no immediate understanding, open reflection. Physical presence and visuality. Performative dimension (some signs do not explain others). The result is not contained in the text but does not reject the text: it is a stage practice

Source: Orosa, M.A. and López-López, P.C. [10]

Table 3. (Post-)dramatic culture in the Spanish language panel

	Category	Component
1	Plot	The play does not necessarily work with a plot, but with a story or a motive within which there are not or need not be opposing forces
	Characters	The constitution of the characters seems somewhat in the hands of the author (puppets), and perhaps serves different purposes other than those that could claim their own identity
	Dialogues	The dialogues do not follow a logical-causative line, in addition there is a certain liturgical look at the scene
2	Dramatic organization	The dramatic organization may respect, in its historical evolution, certain structural components such as conflict among others, but its dispositions and architectures are much freer, more seductive and narrative than the classical ones The festival and freedom predominate
3	Dramatic tension	The play may respect, in its historical evolution, the fundamental components or columns of the dramatic tension, but the intensity of the narrative and the lengthening of the narrative phases within drama may dispense with the intense use of dramatic attention on the altar of the festive celebration and what is happening within it The collage originated by multiplane techniques, simultaneities and narrative multiperspectivisms is predominant, the festive freedom and participation of the audience is prevalent
4	Narrative organization within drama Type of narrative organization	The narrative component is very strong, as opposed to the dramatic one. The play is not based on the Greek agon and its dramatic technique by virtue of which actors are placed on stage motivated by the confrontation of forces. The narrativity of the situations is predominant
5	Technical-formal organization	The work tends more to juxtapositions, to narrative organizations (much more descriptive and loose) than to other more intellectual or dogmatic dispositions and architectures such as those of the form, etcetera

Source: Orosa

Another scientific model and conceptual map that we would like to show in this Theoretical Framework (Table 4, below) refers to the audiovisual post-dramatic narrative panel of our days.

Table 4. Analysis panel of the post-dramatic audiovisual narrative

	Category	Component
1	Point of view	+ From the use of the image (camera): subjective shooting, multifragmentation of shooting in the scene, change from the subjective shoot to the objective one in the same shot, rupture of the fourth wall, dream sequences + From the use of sound (linked to impossible or innovative chronotopes): voice off or voice over (to express the character's thoughts), prolonged silences, sound suspension, change from extradiegetic sound to diegetic sound
2	Dynamism	+ Camera movements: tendency to subjective audiovisual and emotional organicism + Editing: multifragmentation, variation in the speed of the sequences (acceleration, slowdown) for reasons linked to the post-dramatic chronotope + Dynamic sound treatment: music, fluency in the dialogues
3	Postproduction	+ Rupture of the technique of invisible assembly and of the splices + Fragmentation of the chronological line abruptly, associated with a sensation of present time: ellipsis, flashback, flashforward by cut, intentional crossing the action lines, jump cut, internal rhythm of the shoot, sequence shot and non-academic narratives
4	Image	Horizontality of the disciplines of image and text Importance of an anti-classical aesthetic in the composition of the shoots, in the lighting
5	Genders	Hybridization of genres, tendency to self-referentiality, intertextuality and referential citations to other works and disciplines (amateur cinema, avant-garde movies, video clips, TV, literature, etc.), mix of formats, creativity, not copy
6	Reception	The spectator as an autonomous and active subject that gives meaning to the images and interprets the story. Participation of the public in the creation of the work

Source: Orosa and Fernández-Holgado [14]

4 Results and Conclusions

We will now discuss the results analysis and conclusions of the two authors who are the subject of this study: Kiro Russo, in the cinematographic field, and Rodrigo García, in the literary one. Both embody the cultural hybridizations to which we have been referring and also the technical fusions of narrative, (post-)dramatic and cinematographic character, development and trend of the twenty-first century.

4.1 Kiro Russo (Cinematography)

Kiro Russo is a Bolivian film director whose production is cited in references below so that his works can be followed by the scholar in this field [15–20]. Viejo Calavera is an 80-min feature film that depicts a tragedy of Andean components with a marked narrative structure of travel and learning. The intense use within the drama of this type of organization is very specific to Spanish-language discourse and indigenous culture too, as well as mixing or blending of narrative, dramatic and cinematographic techniques very pertinent to twenty-first century trends.

Clearly, it is not in a rational and logical-causative world where the story unfolds but in a mythical-magical one, very proper of the Western and Andean metamodern and post-dramatic discourse, where the constant temporal and spatial displacements and the collage technique (simultaneity of planes) seek a juxtaposition of scenes and sequences so characteristic of the contemporary European discourse.

Latin America and Europe, Spanish and Andean culture, (post-)dramatic and cinematographic techniques, as well as narrative ones, meet in a work in which the identity tradition of a people punished by history and the most electrifying post-modernity are enjoyed.

The story, because we cannot properly speak of a plot (in the Andean world the conflict is not made up of opposing forces, but complementary ones), offers us an apparent motive (the work of a boy in the mine because as a human being he does not fit into society), but also a real one: a previous world in the hero's life, the door, the descent into hell, the road, the forest, the search for the father, that is, the narrative of the European bildungsroman in an Andean setting where Western techniques of dramatic tension are disregarded in order to live a present that so often seems to us millenarian and full of emptiness. Mirrors and narrative duplications so common to novelistic techniques show up within the (post-)drama, and the appeal to a personal imaginary that sometimes leaves us with the sensation that the story is quite simple and routine, as befits the tendencies of our days.

The streams of consciousness, the subjective points of view, the multi-fragmentation of shots in the sequences, the dreamlike scenes and the prolonged silences speak to us of an extraordinary mixture between a magical Latin American and Andean world and the more common but sophisticated techniques of Western cult drama. We hope that Kiro Russo's next feature-length work, The Great Movement, that homage to the city of La Paz and its inhabitants (the story of a madman whom no one believes and who apparently ends up performing a miracle), will be as attractive and innovative in its look as are his recent and still young efforts.

The work of his short films (Enterprisse, Juku, La Bestia, Materiales and Nueva Vida) runs between the European signs dissolved in the textuality and narrative vitalisms of Spanish culture or the organizations of the pariverse so appropriate to the mythical indigenism. The small everyday narratives, in accordance with post-dramatic postmodernity, are merged with the absence of resolving contexts as befits the philosophy of complementary pairs in indigenous Latin America.

We are witnessing a mosaic of apparent improvisations where the hybridization of European and Latin American cultures as well as the fusion of narrative techniques are confused with those designed for the stage, be it post-theatrical or cinematographic. An experience, without a doubt, for peace and cultural understanding.

4.2 Rodrigo García (Literature)

The Spanish-Argentine writer Rodrigo García stands for similar values to those of the Bolivian filmmaker, but in the field of literature precisely where popular, festive and anti-dogmatic Spanish and Latin culture marries European structural and architectural cultism.

The sense of improvisation in Golgota Picnic, the aroma of the street (the feast that liturgically celebrates this play: the fundamental event that is only discovered at the end), the descriptive narrations of all the events of this joyous gathering which definitely characterize the heart of the spirit of the dramatization in Spanish and Latin American language: anyway, we are at the very heart of the post-dramatic core in the culture of Spain and Latin America, which is essentially popular in character; and, on the other hand, European intellectual cultism (not only stylistic, but also architectural) is also present in García's artwork, so loose, so fragmentary, so unreal and conditional, so full of apparently irrational juxtapositions, so rhizomatic and contradictory, so sensitive and reiterative, so untrue and illogical, so lyrical, so in the atmosphere of language, in short, so European, Western and metamodern.

It would be difficult to find two authors, Rodrigo García and Kiro Russo, who better represent the current tendencies for the hybridization of cultures between Europe and Latin America as well as the fusion of narrative and dramatic-cinematographic techniques in line with our aspirations for an understanding of different and harmonious identities.

References

1. Hooker-Blandford, A.S.: Contribución de la Universidad de las Regiones Autónomas de la Costa Caribe Nicaragüense (URACCAN) al proceso de construcción de un modelo de desarrollo intercultural, equitativo, autonómico e integrador. In: Mato, D. (coord.) Diversidad cultural e intercultural en educación superior: Experiencias en América Latina. UNESCO: IESALC, Caracas (2008)
2. Vallejo, P.: La flor de la Chukirawa. In: Antología de teatro ecuatoriano contemporáneo, pp. 71–88 (2007)
3. Vallejo, P.: La flor de la Chukirawa 1ª parte (2007). https://www.youtube.com/watch?v=ftzNL4mXtkA
4. Vallejo, P.: La flor de la Chukirawa 2ª parte (2007). https://www.youtube.com/watch?v=ZPY6ZuhbQ10
5. Francés, C.: La fanesca. Teatro Malayerba, Quito (2009)
6. Gallegos, C.: Barrio Caleidoscopio. Fundación Teatro Nacional Sucre, Quito (2010)
7. De la Torre, L.M., Peralta, C.S.: La reciprocidad en el mundo andino: el caso del pueblo de Otavalo. Runapura makipurarinamanta, otavalokunapak kawsaymanta. Editorial Abya Yala, Quito (2004)

8. Orosa, M.A., Galarza-Ligña, V.: Latin American indigenous post-drama architectures from an andean perspective revisited. In: Rocha, Á., Ferrás, C., Montenegro Marin, C.E., Medina García, V.H. (eds.) ICITS 2020. AISC, vol. 1137, pp. 693–702. Springer, Cham (2020). https://doi.org/10.1007/978-3-030-40690-5_66
9. Orosa, M.Á., Lema, D., Galarza-Ligña, V., Culqui, A.: Ecuador: the popular liturgical and festive origins of the Latin American indigenous post-drama and its specific conflict. Comparisons with the Spanish and European post-drama. In: 15ª Iberian Conference on Information Systems and Technologies, pp. 279–288. Springer, Heidelberg (2020)
10. Orosa, M.A., López-López, P.C.: Postdrama culture in Ecuador and Spain: Methodological framework and comparative study. Comunicar **57**(XXVI), 39–47 (2018)
11. Orosa, M.A., Galarza-Ligña, V., Culqui, A.: Postdrama communication in Spanish language: Ecuador and Spain. Origins and current scene. The indigenous postdrama. (La flor de la Chukirawa, by Patricio Vallejo Aristizábal, and Gólgota Picnic, by Rodrigo García.). RISTI, N.° E20, 05/2019, pp. 350–363 (2019)
12. Pérez Priego, M.Á.: El auto de los Reyes Magos. Arbor **177**(699/700), 611–621 (2004)
13. Poza Diéguez, M.: El Concepto de Teatralidad en el Teatro Medieval Castellano. Espéculo nº 26 (UCM) (2015)
14. Orosa, M.Á., Romero-Espinosa, S.F., Fernández-Holgado, J.A.: Transformation of Andean cinema in Latin America: identity and prostdrama. In: Rocha, Á., Ferrás, C., Paredes, M. (eds.) ICITS 2019. AISC, vol. 918, pp. 944–953. Springer, Cham (2019). https://doi.org/10.1007/978-3-030-11890-7_88
15. Russo, K.: Viejo Calavera [Video file] (2016). https://mega.nz/#!NUlDSKyb!dLyYnN5sfqjQoNSczzmyaGm_hJcOP0LHJrbiY9U0DpU
16. Russo, K.: Enterprisse [Video file] (2010). https://vimeo.com/47093230 pass: EulogioCuevas
17. Russo, K.: Juku [Video file] (2012). https://vimeo.com/47058431
18. Russo, K.: La Bestia [Video file] (2015). https://vimeo.com/118579245 pass: bestia
19. Russo, K.: Materiales [Video file] (2015). https://vimeo.com/160706499 pass: Materiales
20. Russo, K.: Nueva vida [Video file] (2015). https://vimeo.com/127053679 pass: NuevaVida
21. García, R.: Gólgota picnic. Centro Dramático Nacional, Madrid (2011)
22. García, R.: Cenizas escogidas. Ediciones la uña rota, Segovia (2011)

Coronavirus on Iberic Digital Media. The Most Consumed News by Spanish and Portuguese Readers

Bruno Carriço Reis[1,2](✉), Nuno Amaral Jerónimo[2,3](✉), and Sheila Liberal Ormaechea[4](✉)

[1] Universidade Autónoma de Lisboa – OBSERVARE, Lisbon, Portugal
breis@autonoma.pt

[2] Vilniaus Gedimino Technikos Universitetas, Vilnius, Lithuania
nunoaj@ubi.pt

[3] Universidade da Beira Interior – LabCom, Covilhã, Portugal

[4] Universidad Francisco de Vitoria, Madrid, Spain
s.liberal.prof@ufv.es

Abstract. In this preliminary research, we try to understand the major characteristics of the news coverage of the Covid-19 pandemics in Spanish and Portuguese digital media, during the first period of lockdown of 2020. Following the trend previously observed in traditional media and about other issues, digital news coverage of Covid-19 assumed a single-dimension point of view, a patronising and moralist tone, an emotional alarmist discourse, and a strongly polarised interpretation. Journalist coverage also opted to highlight the official speeches and the nearby dramatic situations, and disregard alternative speeches and different dimensions of this social phenomenon.

Keywords: Digital media · Coronavirus · Information · Audiences

1 News Consumption in Pandemic Times

Nowadays, a bundle of factors related to technological expansion and daily life digitalisation (Bossio 2017) resulted in an increasing spread of information within daily life. The consumption of information answers to the socialising configurations performed from instantaneity, from the fluidness of mobile phones' technological portability, and from the multiplicity of devices used from information consumption (Culver and Jacobson 2012). This procedure amplifies the circulation of contents among the platforms and channels diversity that people use in real time (Hernández-Pérez and Mateos 2016).

The search for information intensifies even more when exceptional situations occur (Grossi 1981), especially events that invade the society risking the lives of its citizens. Covid-19 pandemics seems to fit into this category. In a recent study about the pandemics, Casero-Ripollés (2020) registered an accentuated search for information, made in particular by audiences usually less interested in news.

© The Author(s), under exclusive license to Springer Nature Singapore Pte Ltd. 2022
Á. Rocha et al. (Eds.): ICOMTA 2021, SIST 259, pp. 384–391, 2022.
https://doi.org/10.1007/978-981-16-5792-4_38

This evidence was registered in the beginning of the pandemics, in Spain, when the media reported the first cases of Covid-19, on January 31, 2020. On this day, there was an increase of 252% on digital information searches for "coronavirus", according to IPG Mediabrands (2020). With the compulsory lockdown on March 14, 2020, Comscore (2020) registered an increase of digital news consumption of 59% more than the previous months. In Portugal, the same increase happened (Carriço Reis et al. 2021). A research made by Group M (2020) shows that the main digital headlines of Portuguese media doubled the number of views after the first reported cases in Portugal, on February, 4th, 2020. This search increase was mainly for general news, but also for economic information.

Consuming news about the pandemics was decisively supported by digital ecosystem, where networks and websites accolated to traditional media amplify the spread of information (Newman et al. 2019). Sharing information registered a huge spike, towards a model of involvement that predisposes people to share information from a process of relational involvement with information (Dessart 2017). The main point is to understand what kind of content draws digital audiences' attention. This paper focuses on a longitudinal analysis of the most read news headlines during the first period of the pandemics (March and April of 2020), in Portugal and Spain. More properly, our goal is to analyse the news headlines of the digital media with more audience reaching and involvement.

We intend to:

- Profile the actors invoked by digital media in news coverage
- Analyse the news and establish a theme and discourse typology
- Understand how media position themselves interpreting the pandemics.
- According with these goals, our main question is to know which news framedid the news about the pandemics with higher reaching and involvement correspond to.

2 Methodological Protocol and Data Analysis

We suggested a longitudinal (from March 8 to April 27, 2020)[1] to the news that appeared on digital news portals of Spain (.es) and Portugal (.pt). For the research, the ten news with more reaching and involvement of each medium were considered, using a software that allows ranking such criteria. We adopted a comparative perspective to understand how countries with similar social, political and media traits, following Hallin e Mancini (2004), report the issue of the pandemics.

To extract information, we used the software for content analysis for web, *Buzzsumo*, using geographical (Spain and Portugal), time (March and April) and semantic (Covid-19 and Coronavirus) filters. The purpose was to learn the tone or the leaning of the news headlines with higher reaching and involvement. From this procedure, we got a sample of 200 news in Spain (graph 1) and 90 in Portugal (graph 2) (Fig. 1).

Based on this methodological procedure, a system of categories was created – consisting in categorise information within the news according to criteria previously defined

[1] On March 11, 2020, the World Health Organisation decreed the pandemic state – this is an important date to determine the time span of this research, which tries to cover the most consumed digital news in the first days of this global phenomena.

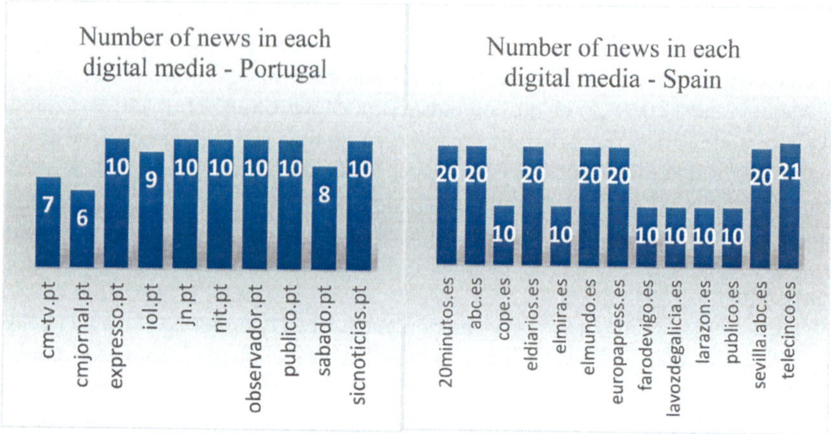

Fig. 1. Number of news in each digital media – Portugal/Spain. Source: own construction

in an analysis grid[2] (Carriço Reis 2017). In an exploratory study like this, given the contingencies of space, we will present, for the comparative study, the aspects that seem to be more relevant to frame the choices made by Portuguese and Spanish, regarding the research period.

Table 1 shows the issues of the headlines that raised more interest by the readers. It is possible to notice that the most common issue is health, by far than politics or economics. This importance given to news concerning health issues seems to correspond to the feature of information as a familiar mechanism towards a current social phenomenon (Matthes 2006). The breaking emergence of a pandemics that brought into daily life a huge amount of new health related issues was the starting point to a single-issue journalist approach, which looks at the pandemics from a unidimensional angle, underlighting the understanding of the phenomenon in other variables or social implications arising from the pandemics.

The understanding of this issue takes on greater meaning when we look at the pitch or direction of headline news, coded with a predominance of positive, negative or neutral headlines about the Covid-19 pandemics. On Table 2, we can see a certain appetite for a polarization of the news coverage, more significant in the Spanish context than in the Portuguese, a structural hallmark of the media landscape in Spain, where extremely polarised views prevail (Masip et al. 2020). The increase in polarisation responds to how

[2] News was codified according to six variables: 1) Original site of the information media; 2) Social networks where the news circulated, to know the media with more reaching and involvement: Facebook, Twitter, Pinterest, Redditt. To get the information we have relied on big data tools offered by the web content analysis application *Buzzsumo* from the search algorithm and web analytics. 3) Main issue: Politics, Economics, Employment, International, Health, Education, European Union, Environment, Energy, Sports, Industry, Social Welfare. 4) Information actor: institutional, politician, economic, alternative, social society, media system, cultural realm. 5) Information space: Spain, Portugal, World reference, United States. European Union, Rest of Europe, Russia, Asia, Latin America, Middle East and Magrebe, Sub-Saharian Africa. 6) Headline's tone: positive, negative and neutral.

Table 1. Description of the main issue on Spanish and Portuguese headlines

Spain	Frequency	%
Welfare (social policies)	4	2,0
Sport	1	0,5
Economics	22	11,0
Employment	6	3,0
Industry	3	1,5
International	1	0,5
Environment	2	1,0
Monarchy	1	0,5
Law	3	1,5
Politics	33	16,5
Religion	1	0,5
Health	123	61,5
Total	200	100,0

Portugal	Frequency	%
Welfare (social policies)	1	1,1
Economics	3	3,3
Education	1	1,1
Environment	3	3,3
Others	1	1,1
Politics	2	2,2
Health	79	87,8
Total	90	100,0

Source: own making

media build the perception of the phenomenon itself, configured in an "apocalyptic construction" of reality, as Berardi (2020), Agamben (2020), Levy (2020) and Carriço Reis (2021) have sharply observed. The background tone of the news was clearly underlined by an alarmist speech.

Table 2. Tone used on headlines in Spain and Portugal

Spain	Frequency	%
Negative	71	35,5%
Neutral	58	29,0%
Positive	71	35,5%
Total	200	100,0%

Portugal	Frequency	%
Negative	33	36,7
Neutral	33	36,7
Positive	24	26,7
Total	90	100,0

Source: own making

Inseparable from how media build journalistic discourse are the main characters brought in to personify the events interpretation. On Table 3, it is possible to observe that in both countries the actors (individual or collective) with higher visibility are the civil society members, those in charge with healthcare, and institutional actors.

This trend reproduces a classical typology, long ago identified by the studies of political communication. The digital news frame follows the same patterns identified in classical mass media: it privileges the elitist approach, amplifying the voices of those who already embody the official agenda (Sampedro and Martínez-Avidad 2018). In this study, the political actors, under the soft power of healthcare agents, were the privileged speakers heard by journalists, who brought a highly biased reading, towards a sanitary interpretation of the issue.

Simultaneously, it is possible to understand, from the analysis, a highly significant number of news pieces that frame the pandemics from stories of common people, echoing traumatic experiences with the disease and testimonies reporting the loss of loved ones. This trend towards an emotionally shaped news coverage, intensified by sensationalist headlines, shows a distinctive and increasingly present trait on digital information, which answers to a business model highly orientated towards a cyber-bait strategy. This model transformed the processes of producing and consuming news (Medina et al. 2018).

Table 3. Main actor of the news in Spain and Portugal

Spain	Frequency	%
Cultural	2	1,0
Economical	18	9,0
Institutional/ Official	41	20,5
Media	3	1,5
Other actors	24	12,0
Political	19	9,5
Religious	1	0,5
Healthcare	36	18,0
Civil Society	56	28,0
Total	200	100,0

Portugal	Frequency	%
Cultural	2	2,2
Economical	3	3,3
Institutional/ Official	14	15,6
Media	1	1,1
Healthcare	23	25,6
Civil society	47	52,2
Total	90	100,0

Source: own making

Table 4 largely reinforces the emotional statement described in the previous paragraph. News consumers came to build a preferential relation with the "geographical nearby" value of the news. The pandemics as a social and health phenomenon at a global scale is regarded by journalists from a strongly local point of view, allowing them operating within emotional strategies previously descripted.

Table 4. News headlines by geography in Spain and Portugal

Spain	Frequency	%
Asia	5	2,5
Spain (national, regional, local)	161	80,5
United States	7	3,5
Middle East and North Africa	1	0,5
Worlwide/global	19	9,5
European Union	7	3,5
Total	200	100,0

Portugal	Frequency	%
Asia	4	4,4
United States	1	1,1
Middle East and North Africa	1	1,1
Portugal (national, regional, local)	46	51,1
Worldwide/global	22	24,4
European Union	16	17,8
Total	90	100,0

Source: own making

3 Final Considerations

From the analysed news, it is possible to understand a strong similarity in the informative process regarding the pandemics by Spanish and Portuguese digital media. We will try to present a typology towards the answer to our initial question and the intended goals drawn at the beginning of this study.

We understand that it is possible to draw these enunciations:

a) Headlines about the pandemic crisis gravitated, almost exclusively, around the health issues, in a minimalist media agenda, centred on the sanitary dimensions of the pandemics, and disregarding complementary readings and interpretations of the phenomenon. The news approach combined three main strategies on its readings of the pandemics: 1) official speakers' reports about the statistics of the pandemics and the procedures that the population should abide; 2) alarmist speeches about the official data, emphasising the critical situations and deaths, and adopting a moralising and patronising discourse towards citizens' behaviour (more expressively and repeatedly in Portugal); 3) news stories that privilege emotional testimonies, highlighting the dramatic aspects of the pandemic phenomenon.

b) The information framework followed the trend of a polarised coverage, placing the speeches in very distant and almost opposite interpretations of the sanitary crisis raised by Covid-19. Due to this exceptional event, journalists gave up on the neutrality of the informative build up, balancing between the hashtag "everything will be fine" and a predominantly pessimistic discourse. The topics that gathered the higher number of both negative and positive headlines were Health and Politics (govern actions), issues about which the most different interpretations could be found. In the Spanish media, these interpretations mostly followed an ideological path, according to each medium stance.

c) Civil society was the collective actor that generated more attention from the digital media, as a protagonist of this health crisis. More than Governments and even healthcare workers. This informative frame is very orientated towards the daily effects of the pandemics on the population, where testimonies and reports about the difficulties of dealing with the disease and its sanitary effects.
d) Following the previous argument, it is not strange that digital media would focus essentially on the national, regional and local levels of the crisis, and in a very limited way, on the events in China, United States and European Union (Italy and Spain, mainly).

References

Agamben, G.: Reflexiones sobre la peste. In: Amadeo, P. (ed.) Sopa de Wuhan, pp. 135–138. Editorial ASPO (2020)

Berardi, F.: Crónica de la psicodeflácion. In: Amadeo, P. (ed.) Sopa de Wuhan, pp. 35–54. Editorial ASPO (2020)

Bossio, D.: Journalism and Social Media. Palgrave Macmillan, London (2017)

Carriço Reis, B.: Os conteúdos em análise - teoria e práticas da análise de conteúdo. In: Feijó, J. (Coord.) Metodologias de investigação em Ciências Sociais, pp. 205–236. Editora Escolar, Lisboa (2017)

Carriço Reis, B.: Empestados. In: Carriço Reis, B. (Coord.). Um mundo de incertezas; as leituras possíveis de um tempo pandémico, pp. 7–9. NIP-C@M & UAL, Lisboa (2021). https://doi.org/10.26619/978-972-8191-54-2.01

Carriço Reis, B., Sierra, J., Vences, N.: A cobertura mediática da Pandemia pelos órgãos de informação digitais portugueses: uma leitura das notícias mais consumidas. In: Carriço Reis, B. (Coord.) Um mundo de incertezas; as leituras possíveis de um tempo pandémico, pp. 50–71. NIP-C@M & UAL, Lisboa (2021). https://doi.org/10.26619/978-972-8191-54-2.3

Casero-Ripollés, A.: Impacto del Covid-19 en el sistema de medios. Consecuencias comunicativas y democráticas del consumo de noticias durante el brote. El Profesional de la Información **29**(2) (2020)

Culver, S., Jacobson, T.: Alfabetización mediática como método para fomentar la participación cívica. Comunicar: Revista científica iberoamericana de comunicación y educación (39), 73–80 (2012)

Dessart, L.: Social media engagement: a model of antecedents and relational outcomes. J. Mark. Manag. **33**(5–6), 375–399 (2017)

Grossi, G.: Professionalità e casi eccezionali. Problemi dell'Informazione **VI**(1) (1981)

Hallin, D., Mancini, P.: Comparing Media Systems. Cambridge University Press, Cambridge (2004)

Hernández-Pérez, T., Rodríguez Mateos, D.: Medición integral de las audiencias: sobre los cambios en el consumo de información y la necesidad de nuevas métricas en medios digitales. Hipertext.net 14 (2016)

Lévy, B.-H.: Este Vírus que Nos Enlouquece. Guerra & Paz, Lisboa (2020)

Masip, P., Suau, J., Ruiz-Caballero, C.: Percepciones sobre medios de comunicación y desinformación: ideología y polarización en el sistema mediático español. Profesional De La Información **29**(5) (2020)

Matthes, J.: The need for orientation towards news media: revising and validating a classic concept. Int. J. Public Opin. Res. **18**, 422–444 (2006)

Medina, F.J., Proust, V., Núñez-Mussa, E.: Consumo incidental de noticias en un contexto de redes sociales y múltiples pantallas. Revista Ibérica de Sistemas e Tecnologias de Informação (E16), 308–320 (2018)
Newman, N., Fletcher, R., Kalogeropoulos, A., Nielsen, R.: Reuters institute digital news report 2019. Reuters Institute for the Study of Journalism (2019)
Sampedro, V., Martínez-Avidad, M.: The digital public sphere: an alternative and counterhegemonic space? The case of Spain. Int. J. Commun. **12**, 23–44 (2018)

Broadcast Journalism Education Through Quality Parameters in the Information on Television's Technology System

Joaquín Sotelo-González[1](✉), Francisco Cabezuelo-Lorenzo[1], and Sheila Liberal-Ormaechea[2]

[1] Complutense University, Madrid, Spain
joaquin.sotelo@ccinf.ucm.es, fcabezue@ucm.es
[2] Francisco de Vitoria University, Madrid, Spain
s.liberal.prof@ufv.es

Abstract. The Observatorio de la Calidad de la Información en Televisión (Observatory for the Quality of Information on Television, OCITV) is a research and teaching innovation project that aims to study news programs and compare them with quality parameters (research) and instruct Journalism students in the technique of analyzing these programs (teaching). The project, which has been running since 2014, has created a database that shows the evolution over time of the contents and the informative treatment of news broadcasts. This work describes the operation of the information system that the project has required to create, supported by different technological platforms and in which teachers and students participate. The documentary evinces that this system raises and the solutions adopted are also exposed. Throughout the project, students acquire, in addition to other skills and further knowledge, academic and professional competencies around the topic of television information. Participants recognize this teaching and learning initiative as highly satisfactory and beneficial.

Keywords: Teaching innovation · Journalism · Newscasts

1 Introduction

During the 2013–2014 academic year, the Faculty of Information Sciences at the Complutense University of Madrid (UCM) launched an experimental research and teaching project on the study of television news programmes in Spain, a model for analysing news programmes [1] under the name Observatory for the Quality of Information on Television (Observatorio de la Calidad de la Información en Televisión, OCITV).

The scientific and academic study of this subject has declined in recent years, as many researchers have focused their interest on the new cybermedia. We understand that television and, more specifically, its news programmes are essential factors for democratic life [2] and their study must therefore be kept up to date.

News programmes are a powerful way of representing the world through images and sounds. In the current digital environment, they no longer have the monopoly on

© The Author(s), under exclusive license to Springer Nature Singapore Pte Ltd. 2022
Á. Rocha et al. (Eds.): ICOMTA 2021, SIST 259, pp. 392–402, 2022.
https://doi.org/10.1007/978-981-16-5792-4_39

the construction of socio-political reality, but they continue to be the medium through which most people are informed in Spain [3] and, in many countries, citizens have a high degree of confidence in this source of information [4].

The OCITV has analysed more than 6,000 pieces from more than 130 TV newspapers until 2021. These analyses are carried out by the students of the subject Television Information, in the 4th year of the Journalism Degree, with the assistance of their professors. An entire information system has been created around this vast work, within which numerous processes, tasks and platforms are managed. It is a model of content analysis shared by teachers and students in a collaborative and interactive learning environment in which the technological platforms created ad hoc are of great importance and in which the documentary implications of the project are also of notable relevance.

2 The Methodology of the Quality Parameters in Television Information

The OCITV proposes a continuous monitoring of the quality of television information in Spain and, to this end, it establishes quality parameters that, in simplified terms, can be summarised in two parts: pluralism [5] and professional treatment of information [6]. Pluralism includes the diversity of locations, news agents and themes, while professional treatment refers to the use of sources, news balance, genres and formats, and the use of hard/soft information [7].

Journalism as a public good must serve the formation of the voice of different groups beyond the place they occupy in the social structure and in the power structure. Pluralism is the basic guiding principle of communicative relations [8] that guarantees a balance between the different subjects involved in the information relationship. In Europe, two different discourses lead to consider pluralism as an essential principle that should govern the information ecosystem [9]: 1) the neoliberal logic of the free market of ideas, which emphasizes competition and freedom of choice; and 2) the Habermasian logic of the public sphere, which is committed to the expression of society in its multiplicity of voices and values.

From the professional point of view, we take as a reference the set of values traditionally linked to the objectivist professional current [10], beyond its questioning from scientific and even professional positions [11], and other concepts such as impartiality, rigor and honesty [12]. We follow in the footsteps of works such as those of Esser and Umbrich [13], who apply certain variables to the analysis of objectivity, such as points of view, expert sources, data-centered structure and formal separation between facts and opinions. And we are also inspired by Anderson and Egglestone [11], who measure news quality by means of a qualitative matrix that takes into account the criteria of selection (news values), assessment (hierarchy), sources, context, depth and formal quality.

Our study universe is daily television news programmes. At the beginning of the project, the sample was limited to the news programmes from the five most popular national generalist channels (TVE1, Antena 3, Cuatro, Telecinco and La Sexta). Cuatro stopped broadcasting daily news programmes -as such- during the second half of the 2018–2019 academic year, and was therefore excluded from our sample from that moment onwards. The samples are made up of daily news programmes, including weekends. The sample is constructed in two annual waves: 1) March and April and 2) October and November. The midday and evening editions are taken into account, excluding morning and early morning slots, which have a lower audience and, in general, are dependent on the content of the main news programmes. The complete news programmes are analysed, from the incoming headline to the outgoing headline, excluding advertising blocks, autonomous sports programmes (except in the case of TVE, which has integrated sports information in the news programme itself) and the weather-logical programmes. The unit of analysis is the news item, understood as individualised information in a specific presentation format.

The presentation of information in television news is basically done from the studio, connecting with the outside and using pre-edited video. This gives rise to the formats commonly used in news programmes: on-camera presentation; edited video (VTR); queues (presenter covered by video) and live. An event can give rise to one or several news pieces, depending on its importance and the different news aspects it presents. This fragmentation of the discourse, which, on the other hand, responds to production routines, is the most effective way of recording the prominence of places, characters and themes in a differentiated way.

Once the universe, the sample and the unit of analysis have been established, a coding sheet has to be drawn up with the variables to be studied and their possible values. Our coding sheet, inspired by the work of Galtung and Ruge [14] and Fernández del Moral [15], has between 30 and 36 variables (some are dependent on others) and each variable has multiple values of different natures. Our method of analysis allows us to systematically assign the contents of the communication to categories, using statistical methods, while at the same time allowing us to attend to both the "meanings" (thematic analysis) and the "signifiers" (analysis of procedures, conventions, formal features) of any text.

For each piece of information, a file with the different variables and their corresponding values is filled out in the Analysis Tool (AT), a permanent platform of the OCITV. The analysis variables are organised around the scope and location of the information (places); "who is talking" (sources); "who is being talked about"; "what is being talked about" and "treatment" (type of sources, images, rhetorical treatment, balance, contextualisation, relationship with the chain). Variables can be free text (e.g. headline); closed list or controlled language (e.g. Autonomous Communities); tag cloud or free language (e.g. localities) or numerical scale (e.g. rating, balance, number of times). In addition to detecting the presence of variables, countries, Autonomous Communities, news agents and people spoken about and thematic categories and labels are rated on a scale of 1 to 5 (1, very negative; 2, negative; 3, neutral; 4, positive; 5, very positive). It should be noted that these ratings respond to the subjective impression that the analyst perceives, as opposed to the (totally objective) recording of data, such as, for example, the number of times a character speaks. This subjective perception of the assessment is formed from the statements, the informative locutions and the images and sounds of the piece.

Our analyses have yielded basically quantitative results. As is well known, quantitative research in the social sciences has limitations and shortcomings and must therefore be complemented by qualitative research. However, quantitative results provide clues for the subsequent development of qualitative and more specific studies based on the information collected, which generally allows us to unravel the meaning hidden in a text, i.e., an uncovering or revelation of the expression, where it is of interest to investigate the hidden, latent, non-apparent, potential, unpublished (unsaid) aspects of any message [16].

3 The OCITV as an Information System

The coding cards of each piece of information analysed must be grouped in a database, in which each variable is a field, to which control fields are added. The quantitative results of the cross-checking of variables must then be obtained and statistically analysed. In addition, the documents (the recordings of the news programmes) must be kept in order first to verify the analysis and then to carry out qualitative analyses on the basis of the results obtained.

In our case, the work is not done individually, not even by a small number of researchers, but by a research community made up of student analysts, teachers who direct and verify the students' work, project administrators and researchers who exploit the data. This requires the use of shared, interactive online platforms that are easy and intuitive to use, and which all members of the community can access with different powers, according to their respective profiles. The information system that is the OCITV manages the five processes shown in Fig. 1 (participant management, analysis, exploitation, documentation and dissemination).

Processes 2, 3 and 5 (analysis, exploitation and dissemination) are consecutive and are repeated every six months, while processes 1 and 4 (participant management and documentation) are developed and maintained on an ongoing basis. Figure 1 shows in detail the different functions involved in each of these processes. All of these functions involve, in one way or another, creating shared information items.

In any content analysis project, the essential processes are the analysis and collection of data and its subsequent exploitation. In our case, as it is a collaborative project between teachers and students, the management of the participants takes on special importance. In the work of content analysis, as in any research, the basic documentation (standards, protocols, tables) must be managed, but in OCITV, an essential part also consists of constituting a repository of the videos of the news programmes analysed. It should be noted that in Spain there is no public database or repository of the news programmes of the different channels, except in the case of TVE, which has had the news programmes online on its Televisión a la Carta since 2014, so it is particularly important to set up this repository, which not only safeguards the sample of our research, but can also be the starting point for further qualitative research. And, like any research project, the ultimate goal is the publication of results, but at the OCTIV, in addition to the publication of our studies in academic journals, we also want to maintain a regular dissemination of our general results through various online platforms.

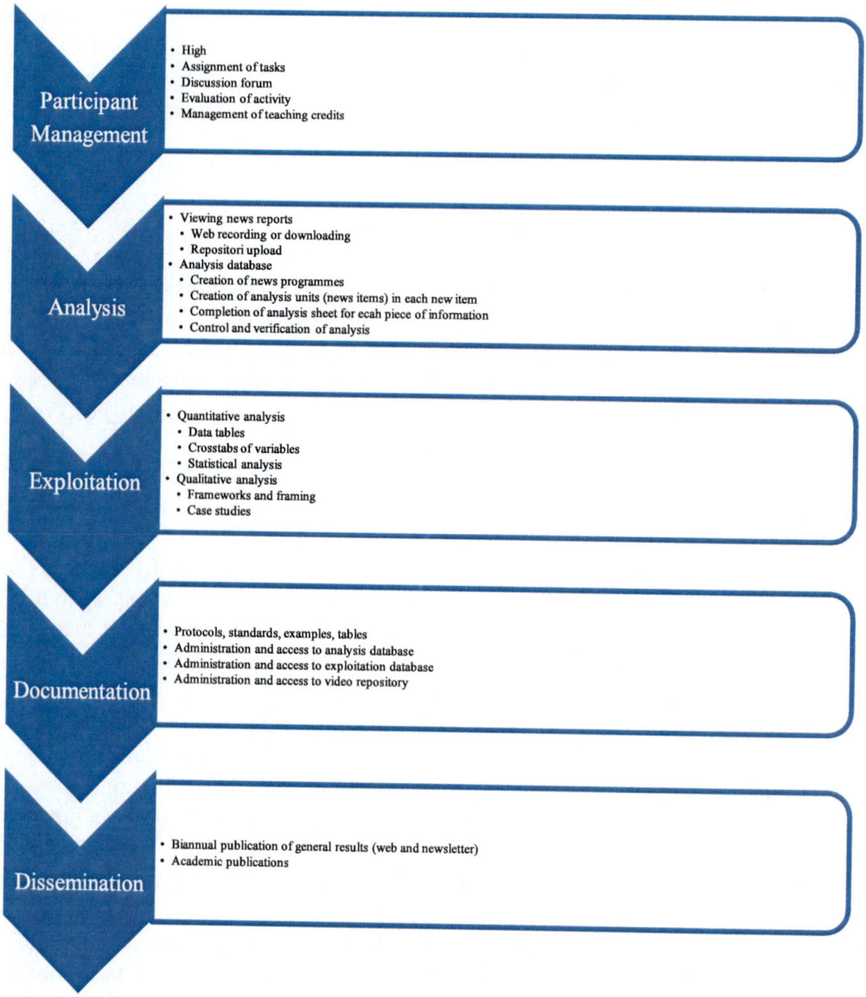

Fig. 1. Processes of the OCITV

A series of tasks (Fig. 2), usually consecutive, have to be performed on a semi-annual basis. These tasks are performed by administrators (teachers), analysts (students), verifiers (teachers) and researchers (teachers). These are the twelve tasks and their performers:

These tasks have a strict implementation schedule, so that they are implemented successively throughout the semester. Tasks 7 and 8 (evaluation of the activity by students and management of teaching credits) have their own development, which is not a prerequisite for the execution of tasks 9, 10 and 11 (cleaning of the analysis base, updating of the exploitation base and publication of results every semester). Task 12 (publication of research papers) is obviously not subject to the half-yearly rhythm, as statistical checks

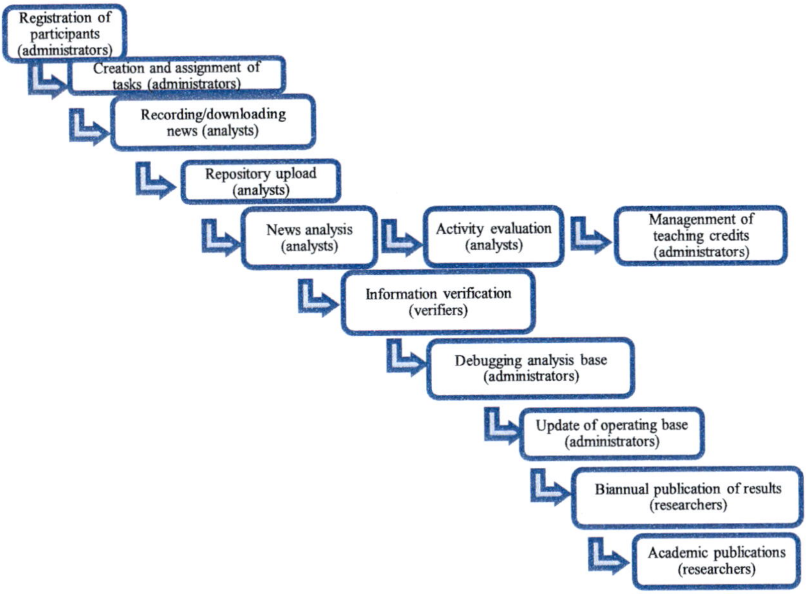

Fig. 2. Task flow of the OCITV

and qualitative analyses (e.g. examination of communicative frameworks) on specific aspects of the general parameters obtained have to be carried out on the basis of the basic data.

Managing all these information flows and sharing them among the participants, a community of ten teachers and fifty students each semester, would have required the construction of an integrated platform, but the group's economic resources are limited, so it has been necessary to use free tools and platforms - with the consequent limitations - and to develop other smaller ones on our own and integrate them with the free ones (Fig. 3). It has been a process in which progress has been slow, awaiting the arrival of more economic funds, gradually incorporating what has been learned at each stage and developed largely thanks to altruistic collaborations. Professor Díaz Arias, the first principal investigator of this project, developed in each of these stages the necessary functional analysis in dialogue with the different specialists who have collaborated in the development of the tools.

Since the start of this project, the Virtual Campus of the UCM, mounted on Moodle, has been used as a reference and meeting place for the community participating in the OCITV. For this purpose, a common work space is created each semester for the four teaching groups of the subject Television Information. In this common space, the participating students are recruited; all the updated documentation is made available; a discussion forum is maintained, where guidelines are given for the analysis of current events; doubts are solved and the tasks assigned to students and teachers are assigned and controlled. This requires up-to-date forms and tables, but instead of using Moodle's own resources, Google Drive forms and tables are used because of their power, capacity

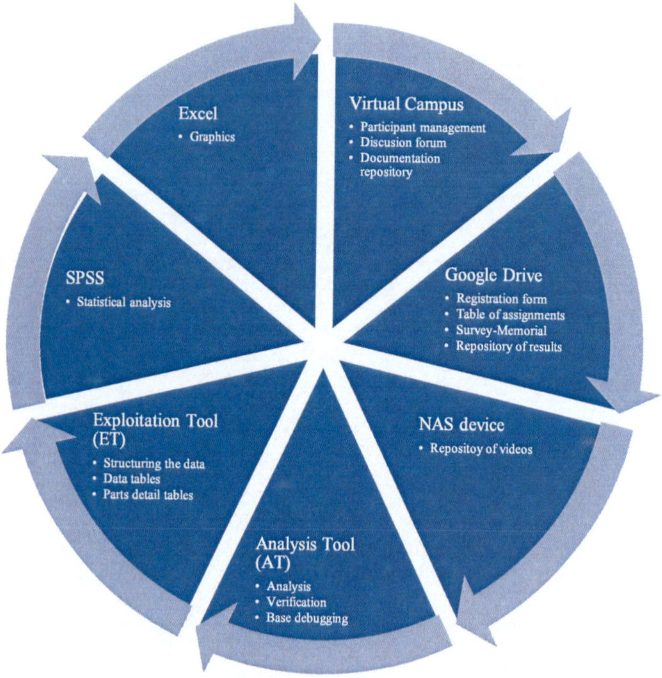

Fig. 3. Platforms and functions of the OCITV

for updating and levels of collaboration and, above all, because they are accessible both inside and outside the Virtual Campus and can be integrated into any web page.

In the first semester of the 2013–2014 academic year, a first analysis tool (AT) was developed using the Google Drive Form function. This solution was very agile for data collection, but not for the review, verification and processing of the data. Nevertheless, it was a first step to refine the analysis and find procedures for the exploitation of the data collected. In the second semester of the 2013–2014 academic year, a new AT was developed on Xolomon, an online database software designed for clinical analysis, available at that time at UCM. The non-renewal of the agreement between UCM and Xolomon forced the analysis to stop in the 2016–2017 academic year. In this first stage, the collaboration of Carmen Bravo Llatas, from the UCM research support staff, was very important. She helped us to understand the characteristics that the database should have for its subsequent statistical exploitation and carried out statistical analyses for us, which allowed us to produce the first academic publication based on our data [17].

In the 2017–2018 academic year, an external computer scientist, Alex Floquet, developed his own AT using the limited financial resources of the OCITV. It is a NoSQL database whose code is developed in the GitHub repository, using the Angular language and is mounted on Google's FireBase application platform. It is an interactive tool that is very intuitive to use. Students register directly as analysts with the requirement to use their UCM institutional email as a username. The data collection process is very simple by means of drop-down lists and has a very useful function, such as showing the definitions of each variable in a pop-up window (tooltip), which makes the coding protocol accessible from the data collection page, field by field. In addition to data collection, the application allows the management of users and their profiles (student, teacher, administrator) and the updating of the values of closed fields and tag clouds. Data is exported as a.csv file, one for each grouping of fields. The analysis file for each of the items can be accessed directly from the AT.

In the academic year 2019–2020, a new results exploitation tool (ET) developed by Professor Félix Hernando Mansilla was launched. The unstructured data collected in the AT are converted in this new application into a structured database. To do this, a JSON file from the AT database is exported from Firebase to an intermediate application that structures the data and finally gives rise to a structured SQL database, the basis of the ET.

At the same time, from the beginning of the project, another one of the objectives has been to establish a repository of the videos of the news programmes analysed to allow the verification of the work and subsequent research, especially qualitative and on specific topics. As we pointed out above, there is no public database that allows access to a significant set of news programmes (except in the case of RTVE since 2014), so this repository can be a very important resource for researchers. The news programmes are recorded or downloaded from the channel's website and uploaded to the Repository by the student analysts themselves. The repository should be accessible to participants, according to their profile (student, teacher, administrator). Given the limitations of uploading large videos (an average of 650 Mb per news item) on free cloud platforms, the most appropriate solution was the installation of a Synology networked NAS disk with two mirrored disks of 4 Tb each. It collects 180 videos of news programmes from the five statewide channels. The capacities of the NAS disk were also used as a server to set up the projects website in Wordpress.

4 Results and Discussion

By participating in the OCITV, students:

- dissect news programs to study their contents, observe their degree of pluralism, and understand the processes used to edit pieces of news in different formats and genres. These are fundamental competencies for their training as future television information professionals;
- input information in a database, which allows them to learn the use of these information sorting and classification tools. In addition to this, while performing these tasks, students categorize information events according to general labels. These skills are useful for information management purposes;
- get exposed for the first time to one of the most widely used research techniques in the communication field, content analysis, which they can later on harness to complete their Graduation Dissertations and during a subsequent academic career.

In their project summary reports, students rate this teaching-learning experience as being positive or very positive. Virtually all of them stress the fact that, although they are close to graduation, they had never approached TV news programs from such professional and academic perspectives. They admit to being, until now, passive spectators uneducated to appreciate content diversity, sequencing and editorial treatment. Several students are surprised that they have not been exposed to similar exercises until now, and they acknowledge that this project has helped them to find a purpose for previously acquired knowledge. The following three quotes taken from project summaries reports are testament to these views:

"I have learned, first of all, how to put four years of theory of journalism genres into practice. This has allowed me to see what goes into creating a headline, to look for the use of the 5 W's, to tell a piece of news apart from a feature story, and to analyze what information news anchors should provide to not overlap the information provided by reporters, and vice versa. I have also learned how to structure a news program, the types of pieces of news included in them, and how they work."

"The Observatorio has allowed be to build a mental picture of the running order of a news program, of the production process behind the program, and of the elements that shape the program."

"We get to practice everything that we have learned, thus helping us to single out our weaknesses and areas for improvement, while allowing us to see the reality behind news programs and appreciate the amount of work that goes into them. I feel it would be beneficial to develop similar projects for other course dealing with other media such as the radio or written press."

A number of students confess their initial reservations towards group work. While some studies analyze student profiles in order to build ideal groups and improve group performance [18], and others issue recommendations based on different variables [19], our project decided to charge professors with assembling work pairs rather randomly, instead of having students deciding who they would like to work with. In general, participants report good group coordination and a good experience in this regard too.

Based on project results, it can be said that the predefined analysis rules are clear, and that the category definitions included in the database facilitate work. The students appreciate the guidance received through the (Virtual Campus) forum, despite some complaints about people disrupting the forum operation by making personal queries (e.g., questions about lost access credentials). For some students, the project was 'enjoyable', while for others it was overly thorough.

5 Conclusions

A content analysis project is a system of input and output information flows aimed at extracting the most significant elements from the mass of information that constitutes the discourse under analysis. Ideally, these information flows should be integrated into a single tool for data collection, administration, processing, analysis and exploitation. In the case of the OCITV this has not been possible, but it has been possible to integrate free tools and others created specifically through the establishment of operational and analysis protocols.

Document analysis and content analysis share techniques, although their objectives are different (to obtain relevant information in the case of document analysis, to establish the relevant elements of discourse in content analysis). They are complementary processes that can support each other. Thus, a content analysis will often start from a documentary search or refine its results by retrieving information that presents the relevant discourse variables, while documentary analysis, for example, in order to construct a controlled language tool such as a thesaurus, may start from the results and categorisations obtained in a content analysis.

Finally, the OCITV demonstrates that teaching and research can be successfully linked in a direct way to introduce students to the pursuit of enquiry. As teachers, we have undertaken fruitful research work on our own teaching practice ("research for teaching") and we also understand that we have developed a "research as teaching" project, motivating students to do research and breaking with their passivity in the reconstruction of knowledge. It has also shown that the theoretical and practical dimensions of teaching a university subject can be effectively integrated. The creation of a collaborative and interactive environment beyond the class group makes practical training and skills acquisition more homogeneous and coherent. Students develop a teamwork experience using different technological platforms.

References

1. Díaz, R., González, J., Aparicio, D.: Parámetros de calidad en la información de televisión. La metodología del Observatorio de la Calidad de la Información en Televisión. Ámbitos. Revista Internacional de Comunicación **30**, 20–45 (2015)
2. Mazzoleni, G., Schulz, W.: Mediatizacion of politics: a challenge for democracy? Polit. Commun. **16**, 247–261 (1999)
3. CIS: Study nº 3277. March barometer (2020). http://www.cis.es/cis/export/sites/default/-Archivos/Marginales/3260_3279/3277/es3277mar.pdf
4. Newman, N., Fletcher, R., Schulz, A., Andi, S., Kleis-Nielsen, R.: Digital News Report 2020. Reuters Institute for the Study of Journalism. https://www.digitalnewsreport.org/. Accessed 17 Jan 2021
5. Zeller, C.: Los medios y la formación de la voz en una sociedad democrática. Anàlisi: Quaderns de Comunicació i Cultura **26**, 121–144 (2001)
6. Beder, S.: Moulding and manipulating the news. In: White, R. (ed.) Controversies in Environmental Sociology, pp. 204–220. Cambridge University Press, Melbourne (2004)
7. Sparks, C., Tulloch, J. (eds.): Tabloid Tales: Global Debates Over Media Standards. Rowman and Littlefield, Nueva York and Oxford (2000)
8. Díaz, R.: La libertad de programación en radiodifusión. Un desarrollo del art. 20 de la Constitución Española, Madrid (2000). https://eprints.ucm.es/id/eprint/2227/. Accessed 26 May 2021
9. K.U. Leuven-ICRI; Central European University-CMCS; Jönköping International Business School-MMTC and Ernst & Young Consultancy Belgium. Independent Study on Indicators for Media Pluralism in the Member States – Towards a Risk-Based Approach. K.U. Leuven, Leuven (2009). http://ec.europa.eu/information_society/media_taskforce/doc/pluralism/pfr_report.pdf. Accessed 27 May 2021
10. Schudson, M.: Discovering the News. Basic Books, New York (1978)
11. Anderson, P.J., Egglestone, P.: The development of effective quality measures relevant to the future practice of BBC news journalism online. Journalism **13**(7), 923–941 (2012)
12. Consejo Audiovisual de Andalucía: Indicadores y metodología para evaluar la imparcialidad informativa de los medios audiovisuales de titularidad pública. Andalucía (2014). http://www.consejoaudiovisualdeandalucia.es/sites/default/files/informe/pdf/1501/imparcialidad._indicadores_para_evaluar_la_imparcialidad_informativa_141217.pdf. Accessed 26 May 2021

13. Esser, F., Umbricht, A.: Competing models of journalism? Political affairs coverage in US, British, German, Swiss French and Italian newspapers. Journalism **14**(8), 987–1007 (2013)
14. Galtung, J., Ruge, M.H.: The structure of foreign news. J. Peace Res. **2**(1), 64–90 (1965)
15. Fernández del Moral, J. (ed.): El análisis de la información televisiva: hacia una medida de la calidad periodística. Dosat, Madrid (2007)
16. Krippendorff, K.: Metodología del análisis de contenido. Teoría y Práctica. Paidós, Barcelona (1990)
17. Aparicio, D., Salgado, C., Díaz, R.: Los agentes informativos en los telediarios: reforzamiento del statu quo y cambio sociopolítico. El análisis del OCITV. In: Libro de Comunicaciones del V Congreso Iberoamericano de Comunicación 'Comunicación, Cultura y Cooperación'. AE-IC, Madrid (2016). https://eprints.ucm.es/40476/. Accessed 18 Feb 2021
18. Duran, E.B.: Modelo del alumno para sistemas de aprendizaje colaborativo. In: Actas del Workshop de Inteligencia Artificial en Educación, Mendoza, Buenos Aires, pp. 11–15 (2006)
19. Haller, C.R., Gallagher, V.J., Weldon, T.L., Felder, R.M.: Dynamics of peer education in cooperative learning workgroups. J. Eng. Educ. **89**(3), 285–293 (2000)

The Tone in Media Coverage of Women Politicians. Comparative Analysis of the Polarity of Journalistic Texts in Spain, France and the United Kingdom

Cristina Fernández-Rovira[1] (✉) and Santiago Giraldo-Luque[2]

[1] University of Vic-Central University of Catalonia, 08500 Vic, Spain
cristina.fernandez1@uvic.cat
[2] Autonomous University of Barcelona, 08193 Bellaterra, Spain

Abstract. Women in public office have been treated differently in the media than their male counterparts, as they have been discriminated under stereotypical media coverage. The article proposes an analysis of the treatment given by the digital media to female political leaders of different parties in three countries. The aim of the research is to identify the polarity of the information published about them. The text focuses on the cases of Anne Hidalgo and Marine Le Pen (France) Nicola Sturgeon and Theresa May, (United Kingdom); and Ada Colau and Inés Arrimadas (Spain). The study develops a computerised sentiment analysis of the information published in two main digital newspapers in each country during November 2019. The research, based on the analysis of 1100 journalistic pieces, shows that the polarity of the women analysed is predominantly neutral and positive, and that journalistic genres do not determine the media representation of the women analysed. On the contrary, the country of study has a predominant incidence on the tone used to depict women politicians in media.

Keywords: Media representation · Women · Sentiment analysis · Journalism

1 Introduction

Female politicians have been questioned because of their gender and criticised for aspects that go beyond their political management. Despite this, women in different European countries are important cases of political leadership and have assumed the highest positions of responsibility as prime ministers, mayors of large European capitals or leaders of political parties. The tendency to eliminate barriers to the entry of women into politics has also been driven by more egalitarian coverage in the media.

The study proposes a systematic and exploratory analysis of the treatment that different media in Spain, France and the United Kingdom give to six female political leaders from different parties: Ada Colau and Inés Arrimadas (Spain); Anne Hidalgo and Marine Le Pen (France), and Nicola Sturgeon and Theresa May (United Kingdom) [12, 18].

© The Author(s), under exclusive license to Springer Nature Singapore Pte Ltd. 2022
Á. Rocha et al. (Eds.): ICOMTA 2021, SIST 259, pp. 403–413, 2022.
https://doi.org/10.1007/978-981-16-5792-4_40

The research carried out aims to identify and analyse the polarity (positive, neutral or negative) of the information published about these leaders in two media of the countries observed, to characterise the validity of the journalistic coverage. In order to achieve this objective, the article implements a quantitative methodology that has been operationalized through the technique of computerized sentiment analysis on 1100 journalistic pieces collected in November 2019. Based on the identification of the polarity of the units of analysis on the six women studied, it is possible to answer the following three research questions:

- **RQ1.** What is the predominant polarity of media coverage of female politicians in the media analysed?
- **RQ2.** Does the journalistic genre determine the validity of women politicians' representation in the media analysed?
- **RQ3.** Does the country and the ideological positioning of the media determine the validity of women politicians' representation in the media analysed?

The data obtained provide relevant conclusions on the media treatment of the cases studied and show a trend of change in the coverage of female politicians. Specific differences can be found in each of the countries or media observed, defined by contextual ideological structures.

1.1 Women Politicians and Media

The media coverage of women politicians has been studied from the perspective of gender bias. The under-representation of women is reflected in a triple dimension: that of the media, that of public opinion and of politics itself. Aaldering and Van der Pas [1, 23] explain that gender differentiation in media coverage contributes to the under-representation of women in politics. Barnes, Jinhyeok, and Jaehoo [5] noted that less than ten percent of heads of state in the world were women and that they occupied around twenty percent of the seats in parliaments around the world. Media coverage can have electoral consequences given the great influence of the media in society.

Although in the past gender discrimination in media coverage of female politicians was notorious, some research suggests that this is no longer the case [10]. According to Bystrom and Dimitrova [6], women were often portrayed with an emphasis on traditional gender roles, focusing on appearance or their perceived lack of worth as candidates. As stated by Banwart, Bystrom, and Robertson [4] what is found in current media coverage are more subtle forms of gender discrimination. According to Johnstonbaugh [11], the under-representation of women in the media is due to their under-representation in public office and she points out that the probably most difficult challenge is to get more women into these positions.

Over time, Norris [15] pointed out that instead of using strong stereotypes, coverage had been transformed towards the use of finer frames: the frame of first woman, a pioneer whose leadership is presented as an advance for all women, and as something anomalous [8]; the frame of outsider or newcomer character, and the frame of leaders as agents of change.

O'Neill, Savigny and Cann [16] have researched the ways in which women politicians are constructed as "others" as opposed to the norm of male politicians and found that media coverage emphasizes their appearance or femininity; however, less research has been done on the visibility of women in the media. In the case of the United Kingdom, Ross et al. [17] found that women appeared less in the news, and when they did, it was more often in gender-related feature articles. Comparing media coverage between British Prime Ministers Margaret Thatcher and Theresa May, Williams [24] observed that more attention was paid to May's gender roles, particularly in the conservative press. In the French case, Achin and Lévêque [2] saw the presidential elections as a key moment for the politicization of sex and gender. In analysing the case of Marine Le Pen, Snipes and Mudde [21] found that the prevailing media coverage framework was that of the radical right-wing populist, as opposed to a softer gender framework. From an intersectional perspective, Galy-Badenas and Gray [9] found that traditional gender roles are reinforced by the main French newspapers, but there are other factors besides gender that can affect media coverage. In the Spanish case, Fernández-Garcia [8] maintains that the media coverage received by male and female ministers is different, but that gender is not the only explanation. It also seems to influence the distribution of ministries between the sexes.

Van der Pas and Aaldering [23] found that a gender bias exists in the coverage of politicians in proportional electoral systems, where women receive less media attention, but not in majority electoral systems. Similarly, the authors findings suggest that different types of electoral systems and their characteristics can influence media coverage of women politicians. Other studies also point out that the political bias of the media can condition the representation of female political leaders depending on the party they belong to. According to Shor [19, 20], there is some support for the idea that relatively liberal newspapers are more likely to cover women's issues in a positive way. The political affiliation of the media may be one factor in understanding the differences between male and female politicians' media coverage, but Shor [19, 20], Ward, and Skiena (2014) found that both conservative and liberal newspapers are more likely to cover men.

As for the tone of media coverage, the existing literature uses the categories "positive", "negative" and "neutral" to observe the evaluative tone of the news [25], as this factor provides a fundamental evaluative component of the information provided. According to the theory of asymmetry bias [22], due to different psychological factors, negative information has a deeper impact than positive information. In this way, the positive or negative tone of news related to female politicians can have electoral effects in relation with visibility and influence, and even professional and personal consequences for their protagonists. This is an element which is less analysed and for which there is less evidence in studies on the media and female politicians in Spain, France and the United Kingdom.

2 Material and Methods

The research presented is developed through an exploratory methodology. This is operationalised in Natural Language Processing (NLP) [7] to describe the type of treatment (positive, neutral or negative) that the subjects analysed receive in the media of the different countries. This is applied to a body of textual analysis using the sentiment analysis method [3].

Sentiment analysis has been identified as a technique that allows the identification of the polarity (positive, neutral or negative) of a large set of texts using programming techniques. In the research about communication discourses, sentiment analysis has been used to identify the polarity in discussion on social media networks [12, 18]. Similarly, studies by Leavy [13, 14] have used these techniques in the study of media portrayal of women.

Sentiment analysis is used to find out whether the media's treatment of women politicians is positive, neutral or negative and whether there are significant differences between countries and media within the same country. The sentiment analysis was carried out on six European female politicians representing three countries: United Kingdom, France and Spain. The study uses all the articles found in one month (from the 1st to the 30th of November 2019) in two media (defined as ideologically opposed), that refer to the political leaders observed. The sample analysis is described in the Table 1:

Table 1. Sample of analysis.

Country	Politician analysed	Media analysed (Articles)
Spain	Ada Colau: Mayor of Barcelona and President of Barcelona en Comú, a left-wing party	El País (69) & ABC (43)
	Inés Arrimadas: Member of the Spanish Congress and President of Ciudadanos, a liberal party	El País (63) & ABC (54)
France	Anne Hidalgo: Mayor of Paris and member of the Socialist Party	Le Figaro (23) & Le Monde (23)
	Marine Le Pen: Member of the National Assembly and President of Rassemblement national, a conservative nationalist party	Le Figaro (39) & Le Monde (24)
United Kingdom	Theresa May: former prime minister and former leader of the conservative party	The Guardian (185) & The Times (278)
	Nicola Sturgeon: Chief Minister of Scotland and Leader of the Scottish National Party (Nationalist and Social Democrat)	The Guardian (106) & The times (193)
Total	6 female politicians	6 media (1.100)

The study analyses 1100 articles. The journalistic pieces were collected through a simple search in FACTIVA software in each of the selected media. For each woman, her full name (first and last name) was used as a search word. The selected media were chosen according to two criteria. The first was the importance of the medium in the national context in terms of reach and circulation, and the second was that they represented distant ideological positions with the aim of comparing the media tone given to women within a specific territorial context.

Once the articles were stored, duplicates were eliminated, and their format was adapted to be entered into an appropriate database to do the sentiment analysis. The figure of 1100 articles analysed corresponds to the final database. In this database, each article was categorized under the genre: information or opinion, and each one was considered as an independent unit of analysis.

The sentiment analysis process of the MeaningCloud platform [3] was applied to the databases created, one for each female politician studied, as an API extension of the Microsoft Excel software. This allowed us to identify the local polarity of the different sentences in the text—using the natural language processing—and the relationship between them evaluated, resulting in a global polarity value for the whole text. The confidence level of the sentiment analysis, according to the values of the study, was 86.1, on a scale of 0–100.

The results of the processing carried out allow us to account for three variables:

1. Polarity obtained by each female politician and by each media according to the percentage of news items analysed.
2. Polarity obtained according to the genre of the articles by media.
3. Polarity obtained according to the countries studied.

The data obtained offers a description of the news' polarity to characterise the tone of media's treatment of female politicians. Moreover, it allows to determine two types of comparison on the variables mentioned. Firstly, comparisons are presented between the media by country (according to the ideology of the politicians analysed). Secondly, it is possible to compare the results between different media and countries, which also provides information about the media system.

3 Results

Of the total articles analysed (1100), 226 (20.5%) indicate a negative polarity, 431 (39.1) a positive polarity and 438 (39.8%) a neutral polarity. Only two articles (0.18%) were identified as very positive. The results of the sample show that the polarity of the media representation of the analysed women is mostly neutral and positive (78.9%).

In total, the sample yielded 911 informative pieces and 189 opinion pieces. The difference between the polarity of information and opinion is reflected in the Table 2:

Table 2. Polarity of media representation of women politicians by journalistic genre.

Polarity	Information	Opinion	Total
Negative	175 (19,2%)	51 (26,9%)	226 (20,5%)
Neutral	356 (39%)	82 (42,3%)	438 (39,8%)
Not identified	2 (0,2%)	1 (0,5%)	3 (0,2%)
Positive	376 (41,2%)	55 (29,1%)	431 (39,1%)
Very positive	2 (0,2%)	0	2 (0,1%)
Total	911 (100%)	189 (100%)	1100 (100%)

In a comparative perspective the results show greater differences than those found in journalistic genres. Spain has the highest percentage of articles with negative polarity (27%), while France (14.6%) and the United Kingdom (19.4%) are below the average of the study. Likewise, the positive or very positive value shows distances between the countries analysed. France has the best rates, with 61.4% of articles with a positive polarity, while the United Kingdom has a 38.1% and Spain, a 31.8%.

3.1 Spain: The Media Tone Defined by Ideology

Data related to Ada Colau and Inés Arrimadas in their coverage by the newspapers ABC and El País show significant differences in how each media treats them (See Table 3). Ada Colau receives more negative coverage, but it is noticeable that in each media the politicians receive different treatment. While the negative polarity of Colau in ABC is 37.2%, that of Arrimadas is 20.4%.

Table 3. Polarity of media representation of Ada Colau and Inés Arrimadas

Polarity	Ada Colau			Inés Arrimadas		
	ABC	El País	Total	ABC	El País	Total
Negative	37,2%	24,6%	29,5%	20,4%	28,6%	24,8%
Neutral	37,2%	36,2%	36,6%	42,6%	46,0%	44,4%
Not identified	2,3%	0,0%	0,9%	0,0%	0,0%	0,0%
Positive	23,3%	39,1%	33,0%	37,0%	25,4%	30,8%

The polarity analysed in terms of journalistic genres increases the distance between the two media analysed. In Ada Colau's case, her media treatment in the opinion genre in ABC reaches 50%, being the only majority case of negative treatment of the sample. In the opposite case, Colau only obtains 11% positive treatment in the ABC, also in opinion genre. In the case of El País, the opinion expressed does not have a negative polarity and the articles of the informative genre reach 40%, 8 points more than the representation of Colau made by the ABC (32%).

In the case of Inés Arrimadas, neutral polarity is more predominant, both in opinion and information, in media studied. The negative value of the opinion genre in El País is also notable, exceeding 42%, a figure which is close to the negative value of the opinion genre in the ABC (40%). The distance of the negative treatment in the informative genre is also significant. In the case of El País, the data indicate a negative assessment of 26.8%, while in the ABC this indicator is reduced to 15.9%. Regarding the positive polarity, Arrimadas obtained almost 16 points more in the ABC than in El País.

3.2 France: The Most Positive Treatment for Female Politicians

The French case is remarkable for being the one that represents the most positive polarity (See Table 4). Anne Hidalgo stands out with a positive evaluation in 76.1% of the articles. Although the treatment received by Marine Le Pen does not have such high values and, in fact, marks a difference with Hidalgo of more than 25%, she receives the second highest positive valuation among the six women analysed (50.8%). In the French case there is a difference in the tone used on each woman analysed, without a political alignment of the media with a specific politician.

Table 4. Polarity of media representation of Anne Hidalgo and Marine Le Pen

Polarity	Anne Hidalgo			Marine Le Pen		
	Le Figaro	Le Monde	Total	Le Figaro	Le Monde	Total
Negative	4,3%	8,7%	6,5%	17,9%	25,0%	20,6%
Neutral	8,7%	17,4%	13,0%	23,1%	33,3%	27,0%
Not identified	4,3%	0,0%	2,2%	2,6%	0,0%	1,6%
Positive	82,6%	69,6%	76,1%	56,4%	41,7%	50,8%
Very positive	0,0%	4,3%	2,2%	0,0%	0,0%	0,0%

Results also clarifies that the percentage of information with positive valence is higher in Le Figaro than in Le Monde, for the two politicians studied. The neutral and negative values are, on the contrary, higher in Le Monde but the differences between the two media remain similar for each polarity in the two cases. In both media the positive values fall in the case of Le Pen.

In the specific case of Anne Hidalgo, results show her high positive media coverage. For her, in the period of analysis, no opinion articles were found in Le Monde and only one in Le Figaro. This article determines a slight percentage of negative polarity in the total observed for Le Figaro, since in this medium there is no information representing Anne Hidalgo with a negative valence in the information genre. The positive polarity of the Mayor of Paris is 86.4%.

In Le Monde, Hidalgo obtains some negative representation (which does not exceed 9%) and the number of neutral pieces also increases (17.4% compared with 9.1% in Le

Figaro), but positive valence also predominates with 69.6%. Anne Hidalgo's treatment is mainly positive in the two media studied. The case of Marine Le Pen is different, although positive valences predominate in both media. In Le Figaro, opinion appears for Le Pen, nevertheless it maintains almost the same percentages of negative assessment as the information genre, 16.7% and 18.2%, respectively. The important differences between genres appear in the neutral polarity. It increases in opinion (from 21.2% to 33.3%) and in the positive polarity. The total for Marine Le Pen shows a positive polarity (56%) in Le Figaro.

3.3 United Kingdom: The Position of Women Defines Coverage

In the case of the journalistic coverage by The Guardian and The Times of the Theresa May and Nicola Sturgeon, there are two different results according to the politician analysed. Referring to Theresa May, the main difference is in the positive valence. While the information with positive polarity is around 30% in the case of The Guardian, for The Times it is over 40% (see Table 5).

Table 5. Polarity of media representation of Theresa May and Nicola Sturgeon

Polarity	Theresa May			Nicola Sturgeon		
	The Guardian	The Times	Total	The Guardian	The Times	Total
Negative	21,6%	18,7%	19,9%	18,9%	18,7%	18,7%
Neutral	49,2%	41,0%	44,3%	37,7%	39,9%	39,1%
Positive	29,2%	40,3%	35,9%	42,5%	41,5%	41,8%
Very positive	0,0%	0,0%	0,0%	0,9%	0,0%	0,3%

In the case of Nicola Sturgeon, the similarity of results in the two media analysed is striking. There are no important differences in any of the polarities. Sturgeon reaches a significant value in its positive valence (41.8%), six points higher than May and more than ten points ahead of Arrimadas (30.8%), although below the French female politicians, who are the best rated in the analysis carried out.

Results show that The Times maintains a consistency in the percentage of news and opinion pieces according to their polarity when either Theresa May or Nicola Sturgeon are mentioned. In fact, the treatment given to the two women in the two journalistic genres is like the general values already mentioned. In The Guardian, the incidence of opinion genre is representative when analysing the tone used for Theresa May. Opinion distances itself from average values and from the information genre. In opinion articles, the increase in May's negative polarity stands out, reaching 28.9%. There is also an increase in the neutral values (55.6%) and a decrease in the positive valence (15.6%), the second lowest value obtained by the female politicians analysed in the sample, which is only ahead of the positive tone given to Ada Colau in ABC (11.1%).

In the case of Nicola Sturgeon, her treatment in The Guardian and The Times is homogeneous, without any major differences depending on the genre analysed.

4 Discussion and Conclusions

The study confirms the importance of the tone of the news (Zunino, 2016) by finding that most of the journalistic pieces analysed from all countries contain a value (positive or negative). The tone of the pieces shows that the negative polarity is lower than what could be ventured based on the results of previous research. Thus, the preponderance of a polarity, which is mostly neutral or positive deepens the change of trend towards a less discriminatory media coverage of women who participate in politics. In this way, the presence of more subtle forms of gender discrimination tends to diminish in women's media representation, such as those studied by Banwart et al. [4].

With regard to media coverage and its possible influence on electoral success, the fact that the majority of the media analysed are positive or neutral towards women suggests that the possibility of accessing public posts is increasingly greater for women, as is shown by the cases of Anne Hidalgo and Ada Colau. The cases of Inés Arrimadas, Marine Le Pen and Nicola Sturgeon, as leaders of their parties, are also representative.

In contrast to Johnstonbaugh's [11] statement, the women analysed report progress in both media representation of women and in holding important public positions. Under the theory of asymmetry bias [22], it can be inferred that greater positive coverage of women politicians could give them greater visibility and influence. However, there is still a manifest inequality in public life between men and women [1].

Regarding the Spanish case, the political affiliation of the media can be a factor which determines its tone of journalistic coverage with regard to the women politicians analysed [19]. In the French media studied, the high positive polarity found follows the line of previous studies [21]. This situation is particularly true in the case of Marine Le Pen, where the positive tone was found even in the most progressive media, Le Monde. In contrast to previous research, the results for the United Kingdom show consistent coverage of May and Sturgeon, which is not focused on gender but on their role as high-level political representatives.

On an ideological level, contrary to Shor's studies [20], the data indicate that the highest percentages of positive polarity are found in conservative newspapers, with the exception of the Spanish case, with a partisan and polarised trend.

The sentiment analysis carried out on the media coverage female politicians in three European countries provides specific and comparative data on the treatment of female politicians in the media. Firstly, the study shows that the polarity or validity of the women analysed is not negative. Secondly, the data collected shows that the journalistic genre does not determine the tone used in the coverage of the women analysed. In general, the incidence of journalistic genre in the treatment of women is scarce, except for the Spanish newspapers (El País and ABC). Thirdly, the country of study does have a greater impact on the way in which women politicians are treated in the media. While in Spain the distance and the indirectly proportional relationship between the media and its representation of the two female politicians studied is evident, under a very well-defined ideological and polarised position, in France and the United Kingdom the behaviours of the women studied are less differentiated.

Future studies can use sentiment analysis, accompanied by detailed information on each case of media coverage, to identify the specific treatments and tones that each media provides of female politicians. At the same time, a future line of research could be to carry out longitudinal, comparative and trend studies on samples of constant analysis to determine whether differences in media treatment of female politicians compared to men persist or whether, on the opposite, the struggle for media equality for women has borne some valuable fruits in recent years.

References

1. Aaldering, L., Van Der Pas, D.J.: Political leadership in the media: gender bias in leader stereotypes during campaign and routine times. Brit. J. Polit. Sci. **50**(3), 911–931 (2018)
2. Achin, C., Lévêque, S.: Jupiter is back: gender in the 2017 French presidential campaign. French Polit. **15**(3), 279–289 (2017)
3. Arcila-Calderón, C., Barbosa-Caro, E., Cabezuelo-Lorenzo, F.: Big data techniques: large-scale text analysis for scientific and journalistic research. El profesional de la información **25**(4), 623–631 (2016)
4. Banwart, M.C., Bystrom, D.G., Robertson, T.: From the primary to the general election. Am. Behav. Sci. **46**(5), 658–676 (2003)
5. Barnes, T.D., Jinhyeok, J., Jaehoo, P.: Gender stereotypes and election coverage in South Korea. An exploratory analysis in presidential and Seoul mayoral elections. Rev. Korean Stud. **19**(2), 165–193 (2016)
6. Bystrom, D., Dimitrova, D.V.: Migraines, marriage, and mascara. Am. Behav. Sci. **58**(9), 1169–1182 (2014)
7. Eisenstein, J.: Introduction to Natural Language Processing. MIT Press, Cambridge (2019)
8. Fernandez Garcia, N.: Framing Hillary Clinton En La Prensa Española: "Candidata o Mujer". Observatorio (OBS*) J. **4**(3), 209–228 (2010)
9. Galy-Badenas, F., Gray, F.E.: Media Coverage of Rachida Dati and Najat Vallaud-Belkacem: an intersectional analysis of representations of minority women in the French political context. Women's Stud. Commun. **43**(2), 181–201 (2020)
10. Hayes, D., Lawless, J.: Women On the Run: Gender, Media, and Political Campaigns in a Polarized Era. Cambridge University Press, Cambridge (2016)
11. Johnstonbaugh, M.: Where are all of the women? Untangling the effects of representation, participation, and preferences on gender differences in political press coverage. Socius **4**, 1–12 (2018)
12. Kumar, A., Jaiswal, A.: Systematic literature review of sentiment analysis on twitter using soft computing techniques. Concurr. Comput. Pract. Exp. **32**, e5107 (2020)
13. Leavy, S.: Uncovering gender bias in newspaper coverage of Irish politicians using machine learning. Digit. Scholarsh. Humanit. **34**, 48–63 (2019)
14. Leavy, S.: Uncovering gender bias in media coverage of politicians with machine learning. arXiv:2005.07734 (2020)
15. Norris, P.: Women, Media and Politics. Oxford University Press, New York (1997)
16. O'Neill, D., Heather, S., Victoria, C.: Women politicians in the UK press: not seen and not heard? Fem. Media Stud. **16**(2), 293–307 (2016)
17. Ross, K., Evans, E., Harrison, L., Shears, M., Wadia, K.: The gender of news and news of gender: a study of sex, politics, and press coverage of the 2010 British general election. Int. J. Press/Polit. **18**(1), 3–20 (2013)
18. Sandoval-Almazan, R., Valle-Cruz, D.: Sentiment analysis of facebook users reacting to political campaign posts. Dl.Acm.Org **1**(2), 1–13 (2020)
19. Shor, E.: Political leaning and coverage sentiment: are conservative newspapers more negative toward women? Soc. Sci. Q. **100**(1), 307–319 (2019)

20. Shor, E., Ward, C., Skiena, S.: Is there a political bias? A computational analysis of female subjects' coverage in liberal and conservative newspapers. Wiley Online Libr. **95**(5), 1213–1229 (2014)
21. Snipes, A., Mudde, C.: France's (kinder, gentler) extremist: Marine Le Pen, intersectionality, and media framing of female populist radical right leaders. Polit. Gend. **16**(2), 438–470 (2020)
22. Soroka, S., McAdams, S.: News, politics, and negativity. Polit. Commun. **32**(1), 1–22 (2015)
23. Van der Pas, D., Aaldering, L.: Gender differences in political media coverage: a meta-analysis. J. Commun. **70**(1), 114–143 (2020)
24. Williams, B.: A tale of two women: a comparative gendered media analysis of UK Prime Ministers Margaret Thatcher and Theresa May. Parliam. Aff. **74**, 398–420 (2020). https://doi.org/10.1093/pa/gsaa008
25. Zunino, E.: La valoración de las noticias políticas en la agenda mediática: Una propuesta metodológica para el análisis de contenido. Comunicación y Sociedad **29**(4), 235–254 (2016)

Creation and Development of a Sports Cyber-Media: The Adrenalina Deportiva Case

Diego Bustamante Bustamante(✉) and Gabriela Coronel-Salas(✉)

Department of Communication Sciences, Universidad Técnica Particular de Loja, (UTPL), Loja 110107, Ecuador
{dfbustamante3,glcoronel}@utpl.edu.ec

Abstract. Currently, sports communication is gaining more space at local, national, and international levels, as a result of the multiple digital tools that are available on the Web. It is common to find spaces where only information related to the sports world is disseminated in traditional and digital media. However, locally there has been no such communication innovation so imperative in the digital era, so this study seeks to highlight the experience of the creation and development of the sports cyber-media www.adrenalinadeportiva.ec, a journalistic proposal that swims from the academy to society. The development of six migrant and native sports communication media was analyzed, from their architecture, design, narrative, resources, and media used, to content dissemination techniques and, based on this, the site www.adrenalinadeportiva.ec was created. As a result, a comprehensive proposal for the sports cyber-media was obtained, that is, the creation and development of the digital media with all its key elements: identity and image, style and writing manual, newsroom, journalistic routines, and content dissemination, thus revolutionizing sports journalism in Loja, Ecuador.

Keywords: Sports cyber-media · Sports journalism · Digital journalism

1 Introduction

Journalism, as technology evolves, is undergoing changes. This technological evolution also allows communication and journalism to undergo a metamorphosis of its form and substance, considering important the migration of traditional media to digital media or innovation in the management of essentially native media on the Web. The arrival of the Internet meant a major breakthrough for journalism in general, which is based on fundamental tools such as multimedia, interactivity, and hypertextuality [1]. The creation of the website www.adrenalinadeportiva.ec as part of the research and experimentation work had greater validity as a result of the COVID-19 pandemic, the reality established that remote work would be a tool to keep alive several traditional media and, on the contrary, the gateway for digital native media.

© The Author(s), under exclusive license to Springer Nature Singapore Pte Ltd. 2022
Á. Rocha et al. (Eds.): ICOMTA 2021, SIST 259, pp. 414–423, 2022.
https://doi.org/10.1007/978-981-16-5792-4_41

1.1 Evolution from Media to Cyber-Media

The presence and development of the Internet has changed the business or financing model of traditional media and marks a difference between them and cyber-media or digital media. The Internet is the space of the definitive digital convergence in which the exercise of incessant communication between cultures is possible; the Internet is what Humanity has been dreaming of for a long time [2]. The future of the media seems to be uncertain. Audiences or consumers move more and more and in less time towards digital platforms and social media, this has a direct impact on the business model of conventional media: print media print less and fewer copies, advertisers decrease their advertising budgets for traditional media and the media try to figure out a business model that allows them to survive. The business model used by the traditional media has been based, in the case of print media, on the financing of the medium through advertising and copies sold, today the trend is that the public adapts to a digital payment model or simply does not pay for information that can be found on the Internet. On the other hand, in television, the sale of spaces and advertising have been the main sources of income for decades, taking into account that several authors point out that this business model would not survive for many years [3], however, the current model tends to digital broadcasting through the Internet, but without stripping in its entirety of the essence of the medium and what it intends to show to its audience. In the case of radio, a particular situation can be distinguished. The business model of traditional radio can be replicated on the Web with the same gratuity, but the profitability and sustainability over time of online radio are characteristics that are still under development [4].

The answer to the traditional media's problem is that the Internet offers exclusive content of interest to the consumer. New technological developments, increased access to the Web, and the human need to have as much information as possible in the shortest time possible are some of the reasons to understand the new scenario of traditional media facing the possibility of being born or migrating to digital media. The Internet has revolutionized the communication industry, being yet another tool to reach new consumers, as information can be accessed anytime, anywhere. "All this is causing, since about 1995, a profound transformation of journalism and the way in which humans communicate and exchange information in general" [5]. The trend announces that in the future there will be a greater amount of digital content, with new journalistic formats on the Web and probably with greater advertising guidelines on digital platforms, in addition to finding tools to improve on the Web what has already been done in traditional media. "Traditional media will not survive if they don't adapt to the Internet." [6].

1.2 New Journalistic Languages on the Web

Journalism, like technology, is constantly undergoing change and innovation. One of the main ones in the communications industry is new narratives. The way stories are constructed, told, and disseminated are fundamental factors of change in current communication models. This metamorphosis in communication aims towards the search for new ways of approaching the reader, especially transmedia [7]. The emergence of new social media platforms has brought with it more changes, not only in the news, entertainment, or opinion content but also in the way it is presented to the public. In this digital environment and in the face of the economic crisis that several traditional media are going through, interesting characteristics stand out, such as the development of new narratives on the Internet by these media, which have adopted new formats that influence their traditional format [8]. The user or consumer shows the behavior and the need to obtain information quickly, with quality and in a somewhat different way from what he/she has already used for several years, which is why the media also adapt to these needs demanded by their audience and also present their final products based on innovation.

2 Methodology

In studies on the teaching of cyberjournalism, the reference literature evidences a diversity of methodologies adopted in research: case studies, survey, essay, literature review, experiment, quasi-experiment, content analysis, historical account and applied research. There are, in the field of communication, qualitative, quantitative, and experimental research techniques of proven validity that can be applied with a renewed perspective in the study of Internet genres, starting first of all with the development of a content analysis of the alternating pieces of information. This type of examination makes it possible to recognize the formal and textual characteristics or elements inherent to the cyber-media and is valid for a first approach to the issue. Although the essence of the present work lies in experimentation, previous processes/methods are needed for the development of the www.adrenalinadeportiva.ec sports cyber-media and, subsequently, to enrich the research from experimentation.

2.1 Qualitative Method

This method is used to obtain information from the people who are in charge and up to date of the digital native sports media and nationally recognized sports journalists, chosen according to the researcher's criteria, and to know thoroughly how each media is developed. Here the key is the collection of data through qualitative techniques such as interviews, focus groups, observation, document collection, web ethnography, etc. The media Bendito Fútbol, FutbolRed, El Deportivo, and renowned journalists in this field have been considered to develop this research method.

2.2 Quasi-experimental Method

The quasi-experimental method is considered an experiment because an action is taken and the effects are measured while assessments are made [17]. By means of this research, the results of an experimental research can be approximated to situations in which it is not possible to control or completely manipulate all the variables involved. According to Monje Álvarez [18], some of the characteristics of quasi-experimental research are: to be appropriate in natural situations in which not all-important variables can be controlled; its difference with experimental research is the degree due to the fact that not all requirements are satisfied just because of not having total and rigorous control of all the factors that can affect in practice (experiment). For this reason, the study is quasi-experimental, since a group of people and media chosen at the discretion of the researcher and already mentioned above will provide information on a particular topic, in this case, the creation of a sports cyber-media, so that opinions can be known and suggestions can be applied in the experiment. Being a cyber-journalistic product, the research will be conducted in three phases: Phase 1: Pre-production. Phase 2: Production. Phase 3: Post-production. This type of methodological design (applied research and in phases), will allow the development of the sports cyber-media in a planned and strategic manner, whose purpose is to deliver a journalistic product according to the demands of the public, awakening in the reader/consumer/user the need to consume this type of information. Clarifying the idea of where you want to go and what it will take to get there, then leading to action and finally presenting a quality product.

3 Results

The creation of the sports cyber-media www.adrenalinadeportiva.ec arose from the need to have an essential web element that contains the information published on the *Adrenalina Deportiva* Fanpage (Facebook), a site where local, national, and international sports information has been updated for more than 3 years. In addition to having a website that allows for the storage of information, it works as an archive or repository whose purpose is to organize, preserve and disseminate the information freely. For the creation of the website www.adrenalinadeportiva.ec, the Spanish newspaper Diario Marca was taken as a reference for its trajectory, information management, and successful journalistic practices focused on sports, and a sketch was prepared on paper as a proposal to then, together with the design team, transfer it to the website as such.

3.1 Pre-production

The research and literature review on sports cyber-media yielded fundamental information for the creation of the website www.adrenalinadeportiva.ec, among which the design of the website, the information architecture, identity and image, as well as key elements for the proper development of a digital media stand out taking as a reference *Diario Olé, Diario Marca, Futbol Red, and Bendito Fútbol* because, according to the researcher, these are the digital media that have achieved a greater and better staging of a cyber-media focused on the dissemination of sports information. The participation of the members of *Adrenalina Deportiva* was essential to build the outline of the site, that is, all participants gathered as many ideas as possible and wrote them down on paper, trying to adapt what was observed in the aforementioned digital media. Leonardo Lima [19], as founder and editor of the media, stated that "we need the site to be easy to use, for the user's navigation to be intuitive and, above all, for the user to find what he/she came looking for". For his part, Calderón [20] expressed that "the first impression counts a lot, so the website must be impressive from the beginning". These criteria, reinforced with the observation of the researched cyber-media and all captured on paper, were the basis for the creation of the web page. *NODORED* also played an important role in the creation of the web page for *Adrenalina Deportiva*, since from a technical point of view they were able to design a site with very similar characteristics to the sketch shown in

Fig. 1. It is important to mention that *Adrenalina Deportiva*, having more than a decade in traditional media and having social networks since 2017, already had a logo and colors that identified it, which would facilitate the construction of the website.

3.2 Production

As a result of the SARS-COV-2 pandemic, many media changed their way of transmitting the news as remote work was here to stay for quite some time worldwide. The confinement was so strict that many people had to stay at home, which led media editors -mainly traditional media- to rethink the methods and perhaps the content. Adrenalina Deportiva also underwent changes as a result of this situation. The program, which was broadcasted for more than ten years on radio, had to change the transmission channel and migrate to digital because, since it no longer had the revenue from advertising sales due to the economic crisis, the program could no longer pay the lease (air time) on the broadcasting radio station. This would be the first big step into the digital world. Since 2017, the program already had social networks such as Facebook, Instagram, and Twitter, however, these did not have any major activity since Adrenalina Deportiva's audience identified themselves with the more traditional channel. On Monday, July 13, 2020, *Adrenalina Deportiva*, thanks to the *Streamyard* platform, broadcasted for the first time on its fanpage, *YouTube* channel, and *Twitter* account the program that used to regularly broadcast on Satellite Radio 100.9 FM in Loja, Ecuador, Monday to Friday from 1:30 pm to 3:00 pm, now in a 100% digital format. From that date on, *Adrenalina Deportiva* became a digital project in its entirety, since its daily broadcast and all the information generated in the program was broadcasted through social networks. However, it was not yet consolidated as digital media. The creation of the website www.adrenalinadeportiva.ec, which began its pre-production phase in May 2020, generated a great deal of expectation among the group's members. Pineda Marín [21] states that having its own website improves the quality of the communication project since it would no longer be a sports program with social networks, but a digital media. The creation and development of the sports cyber-media requires a number of tasks to be carried out, which is why these were gradually planned and executed as the development of the site as such progressed.

3.3 Creation and Development

After conducting research on how cyber-media develops and how they create content for their audience, the website www.adrenalinadeportiva.ec was created, where the main objective is to inform about the different sporting events that occur around the world and also to offer opinion papers, chronicles, and reports, covering a need found in the media.

3.4 Creation of the 360° Newsroom

From the creation of the cyber-media, the newsroom was built with the members of the *Adrenalina Deportiva* media. Editors, authors, designers, and *community managers* are some of the roles that were born along with the newsroom, since being a digital media and no longer just a *Facebook* page, demands greater organization and planning when creating news content (Fig. 2).

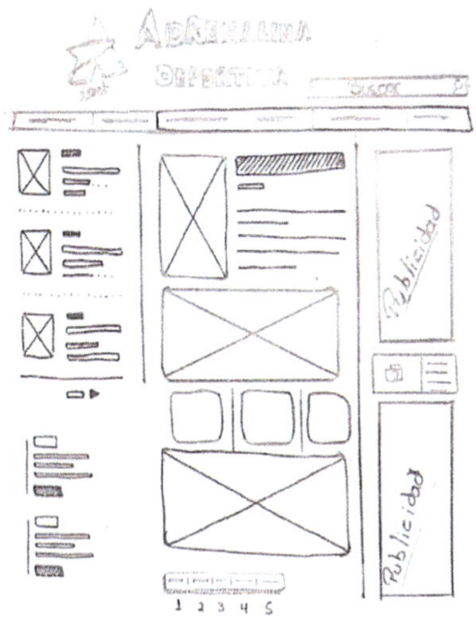

Fig. 1. Website sketch for www.adrenalinadeportiva.ec.

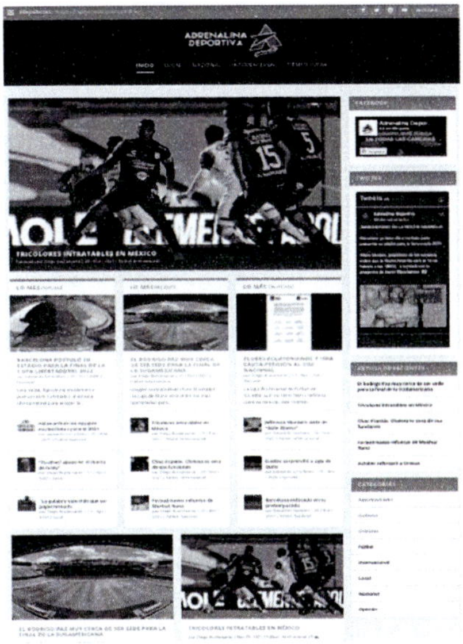

Fig. 2. Screenshot of the Adrenalina Deportiva website already developed.

3.5 Development of Journalistic Routines

The responsibility of creating and developing a digital media demands the creation of journalistic routines within the media, thus ensuring consistency and organization in publications, as well as always having sports information both in social networks and on the website (Table 1).

3.6 Hypermedia Management

Based on the new journalistic trends studied and researched, news content was generated that integrates media such as text, audio, video, infographics, photographs, and more, thus providing the user with a better communication experience. One of them is to embed tweets from official publications in the notes written with the intention of presenting verified and contrasted information, and thus generate the necessary credibility in users so that they continue to consume information from the website.

3.7 Innovation in the Broadcasting of Sports Information

What characterizes the sports media is that they offer their audiences the most up-to-date information, however, Arcos [22] states that when a digital media is taking its first

Table 1. Schedule of activities for the *Adrenalina Deportiva* media.

Responsible	Director	Editor	Author	Designer	Community Manager
Diego Bustamante	Oversee that everyone fulfills their roles		Text on irregularities in Second Category		
Nelson Calderón		Review all notes and articles			
Freddy Cabrera			Pro League in its final stage/daily news		
Pablo Rodríguez			Text on Libertad FC (2020 analysis and 2021 projection)		
Sebastián Guevara			Daily notes		
Leonardo Lima			Text about Gustavo Alfaro/Daily Notes		
Fabricio Cadme				Design of all the visual pieces for its dissemination	
Sebastián Guevara					Social media management

steps on the web, what will differentiate it from the rest is the information that can be generated from this media, that is, that it is this media the one in charge of finding and telling an unpublished story. On the other hand, Castro [23] ratifies what Arcos said, because for him "general" information is in every media, not so the stories that can be discovered, but he also stresses that it is important to have daily information on the website, since the initial *Adrenalina Deportiva* format was to report daily sports events locally, nationally and internationally. Another of the innovations we worked on for the broadcasting of sports information was the podcast. Given the changes in the way of consuming different communicative products and with the aim of adapting to this audience, *Adrenalina Deportiva* developed a podcast called "Tiempo Fuera" (Time Out) in which, within a talk of no more than 40 min, a specific topic is analyzed with members of the media and guests. As this is a digital publication hosted on the website and on popular platforms such as *YouTube, Spotify and Ivoox*, this allows *Adrenalina Deportiva*'s audience to download this communicative product and listen to it whenever and wherever they want, thus allowing for a greater presence on the Internet. This podcast is published periodically, every Tuesday, with the varied participation of its members, as it is a medium formed by ten people, it is important to have everyone's participation.

3.8 Post-production

After going through the pre-production and production phases during the period from October 2019 to October 2020, several results were obtained, gathered with the *Google Analytics* tool, based on the content made on the website www.adrenalinadeportiva.ec. From October 19, 2020, to January 30, 2021, the *Adrenalina Deportiva* media website registered a total of 2629 users with an average time of 01:54 min per session, the first day having the highest impact with a total of 301 online users. After four months of having published and disseminated the first informative note in the media, the audience of *Adrenalina Deportiva* became mostly people between 18 and 34 years old, surpassing 60% of the total number of joint sessions and being mostly men with a total of 54.15% over 45.85% of women. Having a presence on the web makes it possible for any person in the world with an Internet connection to access the site. Therefore, during the aforementioned period, Adrenalina Deportiva had visitors from 25 different countries. As of the cut-off date (from October 19th, 2020 to January 30th, 2021), 122 news stories were published, including briefing notes, chronicles, reports, and op-eds, the latter being the most popular among the media audience during the four months in which the site was being developed, so it was decided to give the latter more regularity. Three of the four most-read articles during this period were "Crisis en Libertad FC" (Crisis at Libertad FC), "El tan manoseado torneo de segunda categoría" (The much-talked-about second-tier tournament), and "Libertad FC se queda sin gerente deportivo" (Libertad FC is left without a sports manager), all of which are related to local soccer and the bad moment that this young team went through in the Second Category tournament. This reading and interpretation of the results shows that Adrenalina Deportiva's target audience prefers local content (Table 2).

The creation of the *Adrenalina Deportiva* sports cyber-media during the COVID-19 pandemic was a challenge due to the difficult circumstances that the members of the media had to go through, but at the same time it was an experiment that leaves, as a result, the first digital sports media in Loja that, in addition to publishing daily information on sports events locally, nationally and internationally, is characterized by being the pioneer in this field when it comes to publishing op-eds, soccer broadcasts and being a multiplatform media, that is, it is not only present in social networks but also consolidated as a specialized sports media that has several communication channels: Website, *Facebook, Instagram, Twitter, YouTube, Spotify, and Ivoox.*

Table 2. Posts with more visits in the Adrenalina Deportiva website.

N°	Headline	Genre	# Visits	Link
1	Crisis en Libertad FC (Crisis at Libertad FC)	Op-eds	368	https://bit.ly/39GB1wV
2	El tan manoseado torneo de segunda categoría (The much-talked-about second-tier tournament)	Op-eds	235	https://bit.ly/3tqs4Qf
3	Mushuc Runa premiará a sus jugadores por ganar a Barcelona (Mushuc Runa will reward its players for beating Barcelona)	Information note	205	https://bit.ly/3j6oHZX
4	Libertad FC se queda sin gerente deportivo (Libertad FC is left without a sports manager)	Information note	201	https://bit.ly/3pHW73n

4 Conclusions

In this type of study in which the experimentation from the creation and development of a sports cyber-media stands out we can highlight:

- It is possible to create cyber-media with a global vision, that is, to think globally and act locally, based on the knowledge acquired in academia and put into practice in the journalistic practice.
- Expert opinion is needed when creating websites. They are the ones who help us improve things like: design, color, information architecture, and even the cyber-media background in which the content to be published is highlighted.
- It is essential to research national and international media trends and innovations and adapt them to the new media. Audience/users should be offered what they want to consume and anticipate their information needs through analytics and constant monitoring of social media audiences.
- It is necessary to have a multidisciplinary team (newsroom) for the correct development of a digital media, because for the organization, planning and execution of the activities that a website demands, the presence of a specialized work team is imperative, both journalistically and in different roles: SEO, networks, analytics, video, graphics, etc.
- It is important to know the audience to which the digital media is addressed, this will allow to generate content more focused on the needs of that audience.
- The research was made possible thanks to the First Call for Research Works of the Universidad Técnica Particular de Loja, UTPL (Private Technical University of Loja).

References

1. Salaverría, R.: Approach to the multimedia concept from the communicative and instrumental planes Studies on the journalistic message, p. 393 (2001)
2. Barbero, J.M.: Cultural diversity and digital convergence. IC Sci. J. Inf. Commun. 12–13 (2008)
3. Vinader, R., Abuín, N.: Digital strategies of television operators: new business models and the Internet. Ámbitos: Int. J. Commun. 1–11 (2013)
4. García, A., Román, M.: On new business models in radio activities. Span. J. Span. Assoc. Commun. Res. 40–45 (2017)
5. Díaz-Noci, J.: Internet media: some trends. Inf. Prof. 562 (2010)
6. Bilton, N.: Traditional media will not survive if they don't adapt to the Internet. La Vanguardia. (M. Martínez, Interviewer), 11 July 2011
7. Irala, P. (2014). New narratives in today's journalism. Transmedia journalism. Studies on the Journalistic Message, 147–158.
8. Cabrera, M.Á.: Coexistence of print media and online press in their transition to the multimedia communication model. Studies on the journalistic message, pp. 71–78
9. Hernández, R., Fernández, C., Baptista, P.: Research Methodology (2004). https://n9.cl/ya4dj. Accessed May 2020
10. Monje Álvarez, C.: Quantitative and Qualitative Research Methodology Teaching Guide (2011). https://cutt.ly/ayE3dWM. Accessed 3 May 2020
11. Lima, L.: Outline of the Adrenalina Deportiva website. (D. Bustamante, Interviewer), May 2020
12. Calderón, N.: Outline of the Adrenalina Deportiva website. (D. Bustamante, Interviewer), May 2020
13. Pineda Marín, D.: Website creation for Adrenalina Deportiva. (D. Bustamante, Interviewer), May 2020
14. Arcos, D.: Testing of the Adrenalina Deportiva website. (D. Bustamante, Interviewer), September 2020
15. Castro, R.: Testing of the Adrenalina Deportiva website. (D. Bustamante, Interviewer), September 2020

Interactive Documentary as a Narrative Form of Expression. Towards a Second Birth and Institutionalization

Arnau Gifreu-Castells(✉)

ERAM-Universitat de Girona, Girona, Spain
arnau.gifreu@eram.cat

Abstract. This work analyses the evolution of the documentary genre in the new media by characterizing four periods: appearance, emergence and experimentation, consolidation and diversification. First, we define the range of new media applied to the documentary genre based on theories that propose certain important milestones in the evolution of digital interactive documentary. Second, we present an original proposal for a chronological evolution divided into four stages or specific periods, in which we outline the main elements that constitute each stage and that have made the next stage possible. We believe that this format is experiencing a second birth and moving towards institutionalisation with the aim of differentiating itself from its audiovisual counterpart and becoming a narrative form of expression with its own identity.

Keywords: Documentary · New media · Interactive storytelling · Historical evolution · Double birth

1 Introduction

Over recent years, the way we produce, teach and research new media has dramatically changed. The interactive non-fiction narratives have transformed the processes of producing, distributing and showing documentaries, and especially the processes involved in how the viewer relates to the text. One of these new media forms of narrative expression is "interactive documentary". As a new media object, interactive documentary challenges traditional methods of study and dissemination. Textual analysis, which has been a key method of documentary research since the 1970s [1], is difficult when there are several potential ways of relating to the documentary text. This new phenomenon needs to be studied from global, multidimensional and complementary perspectives, taking into account, for example, aesthetics, economics, sociology, technology, etc.

© The Author(s), under exclusive license to Springer Nature Singapore Pte Ltd. 2022
Á. Rocha et al. (Eds.): ICOMTA 2021, SIST 259, pp. 424–434, 2022.
https://doi.org/10.1007/978-981-16-5792-4_42

The interactive documentary form needs its own space (a definition and description) in a complex borderline region (it is both a documentary and interactive) as well as stability and consolidation in its organisation and production. It is also undergoing constant reformulation because it lies between two powerful opposing forces: narrative and interactivity. Interactive documentary proposes a challenge (encourages, motivates, stimulates), provides data to make decisions (informs, complements, experiments) and forces the brain to retain the data to make sense of the story and connect knowledge (learning).

Defining what is documentary has never been an easy task. Today, defining the possible intertwining of narration and interaction is even more complex (interactive documentary), not to mention when we add new media and platforms to the equation and user participation becomes essential (transmedia documentary). Interactive and transmedia documentary lies in an area where documentary and the so-called new media intersect, composed of many different media and platforms for production, distribution and exhibition, such as the web (webdocumentary), hardware (installation), visual media (film and television), virtual, augmented and extended reality and multiplatform (transmedia documentary), among others.

We are in a fertile moment for determining a provisional definition when several theories on the concept, production strategies for designing these works and their relations with other forms of audiovisual, interactive and transmedia expressions have emerged. Some of the most widely accepted classifications of the documentary genre were proposed in the last century [2–6], and a group of new media researchers have added a growing number of academic works in recent years [7–12], in order to define the interactive field. Even more recently, some other authors have started to characterise transmedia documentary [13, 14] and the concept of expanded and New Media documentary [15, 16]. In terms of a possible functional definition, Galloway et al. [17] consider an interactive documentary any film of the genre that uses interactivity as a core part of its relational mechanism. Aston and Gaudenzi [18] define interactive documentary as “any project that starts with an intention to document the ‘real’ and that does so by using digital interactive technology”.

2 Theoretical Framework

We believe it is justified to divide up the brief history of the interactive documentary based on various theories, such as the concept of “intermediality” [19, 20], the theory of the “double birth of the media” [21, 22], Altman’s model applied to cinema [23, 24] and the study on the modalities of interaction made by Sandra Gaudenzi [8].

Presented by Jürgen E. Müller in 1987, the concept of "intermediality" refers to a specific question: the identity of the media and therefore of their historical development with their reciprocal interferences [24]. Müller created the hypothesis that television should be considered a hybrid and intermediate device meeting in complex interactions with other devices. In treating the media in terms of identity rather than specificity, this approach considers them to be processes [25]. The concept of intermediality has been taken up recently by cinema researchers in an attempt to show that the identity of cinema as a new media has gone through a long period of constitution. According to the definition of Rick Altman, intermediality denotes a historical period of transition during which a form that will eventually be a separate media is still divided into various existing media to the extent that its own identity is suspended.

André Gaudreault and Philippe Marion developed the model of "double birth" based on a detailed analysis of the consolidation of cinema, applying it also to photography and comics, among others [21]. To demonstrate how it functions and how the case of the interactive documentary adapts to the model, we will apply this concept referring specifically to cinema and offline supports (CD ROM), which can be considered to be two of the basic pillars on which the interactive documentary is built. Of particular interest is the relationship between the new form and the preexisting media in the three phases of the model, since this will reveal the situation of the new emerging media or form.

The "double birth" theory of Gaudreault and Marion states that a media is born in the first place as a prolongation of practices that occur before its appearance and in which it was integrated in its first phase. It is re-born when it establishes its own route through which the media that it has developed acquire the institutional legitimacy that recognizes their specificity [22]. From this initial hypothesis, Gaudreault and Marion then replaced the ambivalent term 'birth' by three other terms to refer to the gestation and development of a media: the appearance (of a technology), the emergence (of a device), and the advent (of an institution). The model is called "double birth" because it concentrates on two stages and/or processes: the process between the appearance of the technology and the constitution of the media, and the process between its re-birth and its real consolidation. This transition is divided into three phases, "appearance", "emergence" and "constitution" which are characterized in various ways according to the agents that are involved at different moments.

In the case of the beginnings of cinema, Altman incorporates into his analysis the roles of the agents involved in each phase (for example, inventors, camera operators and directors), the production processes, and the relationship with the institutional surroundings and the established related media. In the phase of appearance, or new use of technology, the media remains subordinated to the pre-existing conventions (media, genres, etc.). In this phase, the new media "cites" other media to disguise its "bastardy" or lack of identity. During the phase of emergence, a group of proceedings or discursive practices appear that differentiate the new media. This new media continues to evoke the other media but now it is often in order to show its superiority, though in some disguise or other. The constitution phase takes place when these new practices rebel and the discourses are clearly differentiated from other media and the new media acquires its own identity.

However, for the media to be consolidated, an institutionalization is necessary, which is the result of the relationship between all the agents and factors involved. From this point, the media gains autonomy and an identity, which Gaudreault calls a "second birth" or consolidation: "Its second birth, or constitution, will appear when its quest for identity and autonomy coincides with institutional recognition and a decisive improvement in the economic resources devoted to its production" [26]. The digital media gradually became aware that they could contain traditional audiovisual genres, but now with interactivity as a new and emerging key factor.

Gaudenzi, in her doctoral research [8], proposes a focus on the description of some important milestones in the evolution of the digital interactive documentary genre. Important moments that, in her view, also coincide with major changes in the notion of interactivity. She selected for this purpose a limited set of examples that show how the evolution of the so-called new media has created new opportunities for the representation of reality. Gaudenzi offers different modes of interaction –conversational, hitchhiking/hypertextual, participatory and experiential– to illustrate ways that authors communicate with their audience in interactive documentary forms.

3 Period Division

Interactive and transmedia documentary originates in digital media, which gave the traditional audiovisual genres the possibility of interactivity. The desire to take documentary beyond simply providing information has made creators and authors "test and experiment" with interaction with works mainly financed by museums and other cultural areas.

According to Gaudreault, the appearance of technology is the appearance of the digital media, characterized by optical offline supports and the Internet. The emergence of a specific device occurred when interactive documentary parted company from its lineal audiovisual homonym and offered the alternative, and/or possibility, of narrating in a different way. This ran parallel with an explosion of formats, supports and platforms at the beginning of this century. Finally, the advent of an institution began in the second decade of this century with a group of organizations dedicated to the study, analysis and production of new media. Specific examples of the development of interactive documentary are: production companies and agencies involved (Upian, Honkytonk Films, Submarine Channel, Helios Design Labs, Barret Films, etc.), digital newspapers (Le Monde, The New York Times, The Guardian, etc.), festivals and conferences (IDFA Doclab, i-Docs conference, interDocsBarcelona), research labs (MIT Open Documentary Lab), platforms and initiatives (interDOC, Tribeca Sandbox), interactive and transmedia markets (Cross Video Days, Sunny Side of the Doc, Sheffield DocFest, etc.), private funding (Tribeca Film Institute, Sundance Institute, etc.), project indexes (MIT Docubase, Docshift Summit), etc.

In accordance with the double birth theory, the process that took place between the appearance of the technology and the constitution of the media occurred between 1980 and the beginnings of the 21st century. Today we are immersed in the process between its second birth, which was the explosion of the form during the years 2009–2010, and its real consolidation, which is yet to come. It is in this transition that we can see the three main phases that we are using in our division into periods or stages, the "appearance", the "emergence" and the "constitution", with the addition of "diversification/institutionalization".

In the appearance phase or new use of the technology, the interactive documentary remained clearly subordinated to the pre-existing conventions (media, genres, etc.). In this phase, the new media "cited" other media in order to hide its "bastardy". Its lack of identity is evident in the fact that nobody called it by its name nor took into account that the documentary could come to be part of interactive digital media. This is the "citation" phase, to use Altman's term [27]. During the "emergence" phase, a series of procedures or discursive practices appeared that differed from earlier ones, as experimentation led to the exploiting and enriching of certain aspects of the interactive discourse and created a divergence from its predecessor, the digital media. The media continued to evoke other media but often to show, more or less discreetly, its superiority; the interactive documentary began to demonstrate that it was ideal for telling stories in an entertaining and original way, very different from the web of hypertexts that was rigid and difficult to access and understand. The constitution of the media takes place when practices become insubordinate, when discourses are clearly differentiated from those of other media and when the media acquires its own identity, all of which is beginning to happen at the present time. We are now, according to Altman, in the "separation" phase, which we call "diversification". But the consolidation of the media needs institutionalization, the result of a relationship between all the agents and factors involved. This would give the media the autonomy and identity that Gaudreault called the "second birth" (or consolidation). But this will only be possible if a solid profitable business model is built up.

Based on the above theories and models, we have concentrated on a group of projects that marked a tendency with their impact, thematic and formal innovation, with the aim of analysing the period in which they were conceived. The result has been the definition of four key stages or decades which constitute the brief chronological history of this specific format. These stages correspond to stages of production: at the end of 1979, the first simulation that is a clear precedent of this format was produced, at the same time as various games developed during the 1980s. At the end of the eighties, the first application named as such was created, and the following decade saw experimentation with formats for more than one support, mainly offline – CD-ROM and DVD-ROM, online and for interactive installation. All this innovation was consolidated with the production at the beginning, and mainly at the end, of the first decade of the 21st century, and has continued up to the present where new tendencies are diversifying and examples of each existing category are increasing in number. Although the definition of the periods is debatable, we have tried to offer a simple linear chronology in order to facilitate the description, selection and classification of the examples. Each stage is named according to the "double birth" theory of Gaudreault and Marion: appearance, emergence and experimentation, constitution and consolidation and a last stage which we have named "diversification", which comes immediately before the phase of institutionalization that precedes the "second birth".

During the years 1980–1990 a small number of precedents and antecedents led to the birth, at the end of this decade, of the interactive documentary. It appeared in the audiovisual stage, some years after a period of increasing awareness of the possibilities of the digital media and the computer. The last decade of the 20th century saw the beginning of a second, very intense, period of experimentation in which the interactive documentary used different supports, taking advantage of the appearance of the web. This was the phase of emergence that led to its constitution in the third period as an autonomous form and its consolidation as an interactive audiovisual format during approximately the following ten years (2000–2010). At present, we are immersed in the fourth period of development, in which production has increased considerably. We can begin to cautiously talk of a certain diversification of projects, platforms, practitioners, companies and, in general, of the constitution of a mature format with its own specific characteristics. This is the ideal situation for the second birth, in an institutional sphere that is beginning to be solid and stable. It must be pointed out that our division into decades should not be taken as exact or definitive, but only as a starting point for the theoretical and applied research that with time will fine tune it.

3.1 The Appearance of Interactive Documentary (1980–1990)

During this first phase, several antecedents and precedents showed key aspects that would lead to the future constitution of interactive documentary as a non-fiction expression form. Ten years after the appearance of the *Aspen Movie Map* (MIT Media Lab, 1980), the technology evolved and the introduction of personal computers as an object of mass consumption allowed *Moss Landing* to become probably the first digitally-produced piece officially called an "interactive documentary". In 1989, the Apple Multimedia Lab, a leading research group in electronic media created by Apple Computer and founded in 1987 by cognitive psychologist Kristina Hooper Woolsey, organized a one-day session in the small American town of Moss Landing. That day, several cameras simultaneously recorded the lives of people in the Port of Moss Landing. During this first period, the element that made the gestation of the second period possible was the interest and investment of several laboratories (MIT, Apple, etc.), which led to a new research experimentation stage. In Table 1 we summarize the main contributions to the first phase described.

3.2 Emergence and Experimentation (1990–2000)

The appearance of this narrative expression form led to the emergence of authors and companies interested in experimenting in this area. During the early 80s, only laboratories with high budgets could experiment with mixing documentary and new technologies. In this second stage, the birth of the web was the milestone that fostered a period of intense experimentation with online documentary. We would like to highlight in particular, along with the birth of the web, the contributions from countries like France and the United States, which promoted cultural and informative projects using optical discs

Table 1. Characterization of the first period

Phase stage period	Technology media platforms	Key elements	Actors and authors	Examples	Modes of interaction/processes
Appearance Precedents and antecedents. Birth of the interactive documentary	Videodisc Optical supports Installation	Academic labs Multimedia companies Pioneer researchers	MIT Media Lab Apple Multimedia Lab Glorianna Davenport Mike Murtaugh	*Aspen Movie Map* (1980) *Sim City* (1980) *Moss Landing* (1989) etc.	Conversational mode (world building with rules) View/interpret Play

and offline supports halfway between interactive essay, documentary and art. In Table 2 we summarize some of the main key elements of the period studied.

Table 2. Characterization of the second period

Phase stage period	Technology media platforms	Key elements	Actors and authors	Examples	Modes of interaction/processes
Emergency and experimentation (with the interactive documentary for different supports)	Optical supports Web 1.0 Installation	Birth of the web Interactive essays Narrative experiments	Hypercard System Voyager company Reunion Museux Nationaux French museums Chris Marker Director (Macromedia)	*Boston Renewed Vistas* (1995–2004) *Rehearsal of Memory* (1995) *Dans un quartier de Paris* (1996) *Inmemory* (1997) etc.	Hitchhiking /Hypertext (design patterns and possibility of choose between them) Previous one View/interpret Play Learn Share

3.3 Constitution and Consolidation (2000–2010)

After several years of experimentation, the early 21st century is a time in which the format has experienced a certain degree of constitution. This led, at the end of the first decade, to interactive documentary being considered as a consolidated interactive non-fiction form due to an explosion of activity and work (projects, companies, researchers, softwares, etc.). The consolidation was possible thanks to digitalisation and media convergence processes that allowed significant multimedia and transmedia works to be produced. In Table 3 we summarize the main contributions to the third phase described.

Table 3. Characterization of the third period

Phase stage period	Technology media platforms	Key elements	Actors and authors	Examples	Modes of interaction/ processes
Constitution and consolidation (expansion of the exhibition supports)	Web 2.0 Installation Cinema TV Mobile devices Multiplatform	High band increase Digitalization Media convergence New visual and programming languages	Flash HTML Korsakow Florian Thalhofer NFB Arte Upian Honkytonk Films	*Filmmaker-in-residence* (2006) *Rider Spoke* (2007) *Gaza Sderot* (2008) *The Big Issue* (2009)	Participatory mode (add content to a database) Previous ones View/interpret Play Learn Share

3.4 Diversification and (Possible) Institutionalisation

We are currently in the period in which the format has experienced, to a certain degree, a second birth. If some key issues are solved, this could lead to the institutionalisation of the form. However, there are some major issues that this format has to overcome: the problem with the narrative voice (author's role), the business model (strategies and financing models), the language (interaction, user experience, usability, etc.), the new models of producing, distributing and exhibition (change of dynamics and logics), and the role of the interactor in the story (audience position). As of 2017, a certain loss of interest in the study and production of this form of narrative expression can be perceived in key producers, such as the NFB and Arte, due to doubts about the progress of certain central aspects (audience, business model, technological complexity, etc.) and especially due to the emergence and advances in immersive narrative and virtual reality (technological giants are making large investments in this field). This deviates the focus of attention from the interactive towards the immersive, and interactive documentary is one of the formats most affected by this change in trend. In parallel, certain Latin American countries (mainly Colombia, Argentina and Mexico) are leading the exploration in the new avenues of documentary as they represent innovation and visibility in this region. These Latin countries have reached this point of experimentation with the new narratives a few years later in a process similar to that followed by certain European countries and Canada in approximately 2013–2014 (Table 4).

Table 4. Characterization of the fourth period

Phase stage period	Technology media platforms	Key elements	Actors and authors	Examples	Modes of interaction/ processes
Diversification (Diversified production. Towards a possible institutionalization)	Web 2.0/ 3.0 Installation Cinema TV Virtual Reality Mobile devices Transmedia Crossmedia Multiplatform	High budgets Transmedia projects RV techniques New media actors entering the field etc.	Digital newspapers Festivals Research labs Platforms Markets Private funding NGO'S Academia	*Prison Valley* (2010) *Highrise* (2009–2015) *Fort McMoney* (2014) *Do not track* (2016) etc.	Experiential mode (dynamic environment) Previous ones View/ interpret Play Learn Share

4 Conclusion

In this article we have analysed the short history and evolution of interactive documentary and have named each period following the double birth of media theory of Gaudreault and Marion. We believe that, due to various initiatives in this field, we are at an early stage where the second birth of this field will culminate with a final institutionalization as a specific area. Interactive documentary is currently in a transition phase where traditional ways of producing and distributing documentary films coexist with new forms of expression and intervention that have been made possible by digital media, such as open and generative systems, the new generation of multimedia programming languages, the refinement of the narrative and aesthetic resources and the innovation in the business models of the interactive industry.

The first phase or model of documentary production lasted from the beginning of the genre to the last decades of the 20th Century. In the late 1980s, the second phase or model emerged: the interactive documentary across several media and/or platforms. It currently coexists with the first model. We are witnessing the birth of immersive and generative documentary. In this phase, which is beginning now, the documentary is generated from the decisions of the interactors and their contributions of related content through the Internet. It is now, in this third stage that, thanks to interactive communication, when we will begin to exploit the true potential of the format. This is determined by the confluence of several factors, such as the enhancement of open and generative systems and the semantic web, the use of the HTML5 language and gamification components (fiction).

The interactive documentary form has gone through the phases of birth, emergence and experimentation, constitution and consolidation and is now in the initial process of institutionalization. The diversification phase has occurred, but it has not been completed and culminated with the institutionalization process. For this to occur, the most advanced European and North American countries in the study and production of this type of non-fiction narrative (France, Canada, the United States and the United Kingdom) must establish synergies, dialogue and work together with Latin countries (Colombia, Argentina, Chile, Brazil and Mexico), so that this fusion can take place effectively in this third decade of the 21st century and the interactive documentary format can be established as an autonomous form. If that does not happen, the interest will decrease and interactive documentary will remain in the media ecosystem but as a marginal and complementary form of the audiovisual and other nascent forms of narrative expression.

References

1. Corner, J.: Perils of Everyday Spaces. Lexington Books, Lanham (2008)
2. Barnouw, E.: Documentary: A History of the Non-fiction Film. Oxford University Press, Oxford (1983)
3. Meran Barsam, R.: Nonfiction Film: A Critical History. Indiana University Press, Bloomington (1992)
4. Nichols, B.: Representing Reality: Issues and Concepts in Documentary. University of Indiana Press, Indiana (1991)
5. Plantinga, C.: Rhetoric and Representation in Nonfiction Film. Cambridge University Press, Cambridge (1997)
6. Renov, M.: Theorizing Documentary. Routledge, New York (1993)
7. Davenport, G., Murtaugh, M.: ConText: towards the evolving documentary. In: Electronic Proceedings of ACM Multimedia 1995, San Francisco (1995)
8. Gaudenzi, S.: The living documentary: from representing reality to co-creating reality in digital interactive documentary. Ph.D., University of Goldsmiths, Centre for Cultural Studies, London (2012)
9. Author: El documental interactiu com a nou gènere audiovisual. Estudi de l'aparició del nou gènere, aproximació a la seva definició i proposta de taxonomia i d'un model d'anàlisi a efectes d'avaluació, disseny i producción. Ph.D., Universitat Pompeu Fabra, Departament de Comunicació, Barcelona (2013)
10. Nash, K., Hight, C., Summerhayes, C.: New Documentary Ecologies. Emerging Platforms, Practices and Discourses. Palgrave Macmillan, London (2014)
11. MIT Open Documentary Lab, John, D., MacArthur, C.T.: Mapping the Intersection of Two Cultures: Interactive Documentary and Digital Journalism (2016). http://opendoclab.mit.edu/interactivejournalism/
12. Aston, J., Gaudenzi, S., Rose, M.: i-Docs: The Evolving Practices of Interactive Documentary. Columbia University Press, New York (2017)
13. Author, Moreno, V.: Estrategias y modelos de financiación del documental interactivo y transmedia. Fonseca J. Commun. (9), 41–63 (2014)
14. Scolari, C.A.: Narrativas transmedia. Cuando todos los medios cuentan. Deusto, Barcelona (2013)
15. Sucari, J.: El documental expandido: pantalla y espacio. UOC Press, Editorial UOC, Barcelona (2012)
16. Ocak, E.: New media documentary: playing with documentary film within the database logic and culture. In: Moser, D., Dun, S. (eds.) A Digital Janus: Looking Forward, Looking Back. Inter-Disciplinary Press, Oxford (2014)
17. Galloway, D., McAlpine, K.B., Harris, P.: From Michael Moore to JFK reloaded: towards a working model of interactive documentary. J. Media Pract. **8**(3), 325–339 (2007)
18. Aston, J., Gaudenzi, S.: Interactive documentary: setting the field. Stud. Doc. Film **6**(2), 125–139 (2012)

19. Müller, J.E.: Intermedialität. Formen moderner kultureller Kommunikation. Nodus, Münster (1996)
20. Müller, J.E.: Mediengeschichte intermedial: Perspektiven, Postulate, Prognosen. In: Furtwängler, F., et al. (eds.) Zwischen-Bilanz. Eine Festschrift zum 60. Geburtstagvon Joachim Paech (2002)
21. Gaudreault, A., Marion, P.: The cinema as a model for the genealogy of media. Convergence **8**(4), 12–18 (2002)
22. Gaudreault, A., Marion, P.: A medium is always born twice. Early Pop. Vis. Cult. **3**(1), 3–15 (2005)
23. Altman, R.: De l'intermédialité au multimédia: cinéma, média, et l'avènement du son. Cinémas J. Film Stud. **10**, 1, 37–53 (1999)
24. Altman, R.: Los géneros cinematográficos. Ediciones Paidós Ibérica, Madrid (2000)
25. Lancien, T., et al.: La investigación sobre la comunicación en Francia. Tendencias y carencias, Comunicación y Sociedad, no. 2, p. 59. Universidad de Guadalajara, Mexico (2004)
26. Gaudreault, A., Marion, P.: op.cit (2002)
27. Altman, R.: op.cit (1999)

Web Experience Effects on Online Purchase Intention by Millennials on Retail Websites in Lima Metropolitan: An Application with Regression Analysis

Stephanie Matilde Briceño Yañez, Alexandra Cabezas Navarro, and Hernán Talledo Flores(✉)

Universidad Peruana de Ciencias Aplicadas, San Isidro, Lima 15076, Peru

Abstract. The current context shows an increase in the attraction to online purchases on retail websites. Hence, there is a change in the behavior of millennial users and the factors that seek their purchase intention. Therefore, the objective of this study is to analyze the effect of WE factors (usability, interactivity, trust and aesthetics) on the OPI of users on retail websites, specifically in the clothing category, in Lima Metropolitan. The study's findings would aid retailers in designing more effective websites. From 486 questionnaires distributed to millennials in Lima Metropolitan, 400 effective responses were obtained. Likewise, non-probability sampling was used with a convenience sampling technique. The collected data was processed using SPSS. Cronbach's Alpha was used to check the reliability of the scales. An exploratory factor analysis was performed for data reduction that allowed exploring the variables under study. Finally, a multiple linear regression was performed to determine the relationship structure between the variables. The results show that usability, interactivity, trust and aesthetics are the WE factors that positively and significantly affect online purchase intention in millennial users in Lima Metropolitan. 4 hypotheses were proposed which were fully accepted. This research shares relevant information about the effects of WE factors on OPI. It expands the knowledge regarding the importance of effective website design by integrating the most relevant factors such as usability, interactivity, trust and aesthetics to improve the WE.

Keywords: Web experience · Online purchase intention · Millennials · Online retail

1 Introduction

The use of the internet has increased the attraction to online shopping among consumers and has led retailers to adapt their offer in digital environments [3, 16]. Also, E-Commerce has generated opportunities for companies from different sectors and has allowed them to have a greater reach and direct relationship with buyers [11, 17, 30]. Likewise, electronic commerce has become an essential strategy for retailers due to the

© The Author(s), under exclusive license to Springer Nature Singapore Pte Ltd. 2022
Á. Rocha et al. (Eds.): ICOMTA 2021, SIST 259, pp. 435–445, 2022.
https://doi.org/10.1007/978-981-16-5792-4_43

change in consumer behavior and has generated attraction between consumers, migrating from purchases in physical stores to websites [3, 6, 9, 33]. Authors have investigated the factors that generate the consumer's online purchase intention (OPI); and include topics such as the web experience (WE) [6, 23, 32]. One of the leading categories and that generates the largest transactions in retail electronic commerce worldwide is clothing [26, 33, 38]. Therefore, the objective of this study is to analyze the effect of WE factors on the OPI of users on retail websites, specifically in the clothing category, in Metropolitan Lima. WE factors have been identify as functional factors (usability and interactivity); psychological factors (trust) and content factors (aesthetics) [3, 6, 23, 32]. The existence of a positive relationship between usability, interactivity, and trust with the OPI has been demonstrated [32]. In addition, usability and aesthetics are relevant factors that positively influence OPI [17]. There is evidence of the scarcity of scientific research on WE factors and their possible impact on the OPI of Lima users on retail websites. Millennials are a population group that is changing traditional purchasing models. They tend to do a lot of shopping online and seek to establish links with them. The browsing experiences are in line with their attitude towards the web, influencing their purchase intention [39]. This research will contribute to the retail sector, providing comprehensive knowledge about the elements that would motivate users to make purchases on these websites. Also, a more effective retail web environment would increase the profitability of businesses, attracting new customers and increasing website transactions [38].

2 Literature Review

2.1 Online Purchase Intention

OPI is the probability of purchase of an item made by a consumer [35, 37]. It refers to the predisposition that a client presents to acquire a product and make the purchase in the future [1, 3, 8, 12, 16]. In a digital environment, it is the consumer's desire to purchase a product through a web platform [1, 17]. Some authors state that OPI would be significantly affected by certain WE factors that would motivate consumers to make an online purchase [1, 3, 5, 8, 10–12, 16–18, 20, 27, 32]. Therefore, it is important to understand the motivations of users that would drive a purchase on a retail e-commerce site [35].

2.2 Web Experience

WE is defined as consumer experiences while visiting a website [23], and includes elements such as search, navigation and evaluation of the information found on the website [6]. It has been proven that WE facilitates online shopping through different elements that promote visits and digital transactions [1, 32]. A model of three groups that make up the WE factors was proposed: functional factors, psychological factors and content factors, which present four dimensions: usability, interactivity, trust and aesthetics. which would affect the OPI [32].

Functional Factors. A set of important characteristics of a website that meet the needs of users when performing a specific task online [1, 33]. It presents elements that promote good operation in the interface. Factors such as usability and interactivity are included on the website [6, 23, 32].

Usability. This term refers to the functionality and utility of a website and it includes elements such as convenience, ease of search, navigation and access to information on the website [4, 5, 8, 18, 28, 32]. The design of an easy-to-use interface reduces the time and effort of the users, which allows them to make online purchases in an effective and autonomous way [5, 8, 14, 15, 18, 25, 33]. Studies show that this factor would have a positive and significant effect on the consumer's OPI on a website [5, 6, 32]. Therefore, the following hypothesis is proposed:

H1: Usability significantly and positively affects OPI on a retail website.

Interactivity. It is the degree to which consumers can communicate with online sellers to solve their doubts and problems on the website [16]. It includes elements such as easy two-way communication, personalization in the search, product evaluation, and recommendations from customers who contribute to the WE [16, 24, 32]. Studies support that interactivity would positively and significantly affect OPI [32, 35]. As a result, the following hypothesis is proposed:

H2: Interactivity positively and significantly affects OPI on a retail website.

Psychological Factors. It includes the elements that improve the credibility of the website, reducing uncertainty and guaranteeing the security of customer information in online transactions [6, 23, 32].

Trust. It is defined as a factor that improves the credibility of the online store, providing accurate information to reduce uncertainty, facilitate the purchase on the website and guarantees security in transactions [6, 31, 32, 36]. Various authors confirm that trust allows the development of B2C relationships in online shopping channels; therefore, retailers must provide better web security for consumers [5, 22, 30, 34]. Studies show that trust would positively affect OPI and define the success of e-business [2, 5, 13, 17, 18, 21, 28–30, 32]. The following hypothesis is proposed:

H3: Trust positively and significantly affects OPI on a retail website.

Content Factors. They are defined as the set of characteristics that allow the website to be displayed in a more attractive way [6]. They improve WE, including aesthetics as its main dimension [6, 23].

Aesthetics. It is defined as a set of visual elements, including the design, presentation quality and the environment of the website [6, 32]. It is important in the WE, since if the offer is displayed in an attractive way, the online purchase process would be more pleasant [19]. This factor would allow consumers to be retained on the website [6, 17, 25, 35] found that aesthetics positively and significantly impacts OPI. In contrast, [32] mention that, although aesthetics is an important factor, it would have a negative relationship in OPI because consumers will perceive aesthetic design as a way to cover deficiencies. The following hypothesis is proposed:

H4: Aesthetics significantly and positively affects OPI on a retail website.

3 Research Model

(See Table 1 and Fig. 1).

Table 1. Variables, dimensions and sources

Variables	Dimensions	Authors
Web experience factors	Usability	[1, 5, 6, 23, 32]
	Interactivity	[6, 23, 32, 35]
	Trust	[2, 5, 6, 13, 17, 18, 23, 29, 32, 36]
	Aesthetics	[6, 17, 23, 32, 35]
Purchase intention	Online purchase intention	[1, 3, 11, 17, 18, 27, 32]: [5, 8, 10, 12, 16, 29]

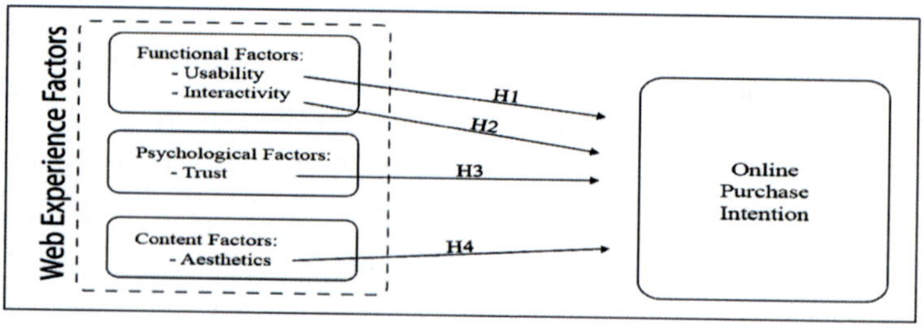

Fig. 1. Proposed research model

4 Methodology

This quantitative study collected data from an online questionnaire distributed to 400 men (45%) and women (55%) belonging to the millennial generation (1985–1999) [1]. Previously, users had to buy at least one item from the clothing category, at least once in the last three months on a website of a department store in Metropolitan Lima. A non-probability sampling was carried out due to the lack of access to the sampling frame with a convenience sampling. The field work was carried out between the first week of September and the first week of October 2020, during the SARS-CoV-2 pandemic context. The indicators were measured using a 5-point Likert scale, where 1 is totally disagree and 5 is totally agree. In addition, an exploratory factor analysis (EFA) was used as a technique for data reduction that allowed the indicators to be grouped. Cronbach's alpha was used to check the reliability of the scales under study. Finally, a multiple linear regression was performed to determine the structure of the relationship between the factors found with the EFA (independent variables) and the intention to buy online (Table 2).

Table 2. Indicators used for the study

Indicators	Description
*Functional Factors (*Adapted from [32]*)*	
H1: Usability (1 - totally disagree and 5 - totally agree)	
Usab1	Convenience
Usab2	Shopping navigation is simple
Usab3	I found the online store with little effort
Usab4	The ordering process is simple
Usab5	The website offers good internal search services
Usab6	Website pages load very fast
Usab7	The website is easily accessible
H2: Interactivity (1 - totally disagree and 5 - totally agree)	
Interact1	The website offers excellent online customer service
Interact2	Interacting with store staff on the website is easy
Interact3	The website offers an excellent personalized search
Interact4	The website offers access for other consumers to incorporate their experiences (product ratings, customer reviews, testimonials and chat boxes)
*Psychological Factors (*Adapted from [32]*)*	
H3: Trust (1 - totally disagree and 5 - totally agree)	
Tru1	The website offers adequate guarantees for the security of online transactions
Tru2	The website offers guarantees against the misuse of customer personal information
Tru3	The website offers adequate guarantees for the protection of the client's personal data
Tru4	The website features seals or logos of organizations that guarantee safe shopping
Tru5	The website has a transparent warranty policy
*Content Factors (*Adapted from [32]*)*	
H4: Aesthetics (1 - totally disagree and 5 - totally agree)	
Aes1	The website design is attractive
Aes2	The presentation quality of the website is of a high level
Aes3	The website design is unique
Aes4	The atmosphere (navigation structure, product presentation, sound, etc.) of the website is very good
*Online Purchase Intention (*Adapted from [5]*)*	
(1 - totally disagree and 5 - totally agree)	
PI1	I would be willing to purchase a product on the website

5 Results

The online questionnaires (Google Forms) were distributed to 486 surveyed. 400 effective responses were received (response rate of 82.3%). The gender distribution shows that 45.0% are men and 55.0% are women. The majority (62.3%) of those surveyed belong to the age range of 21 to 25 years, 28.5% of 26 to 30 years and 9.25% of 31 to 35 years. The total of surveyed stated that they habitually reside in Metropolitan Lima and have made at least one purchase on a department store website. 45.0% of the sample indicated that they had made their last purchase on a department store website a month ago, while 40.8% a week ago, and 14.25% three months ago. Also, they indicated having made their last purchase on the website of Saga Falabella (71.0%), Ripley (22.8%), Oechsle (2.8%) and Estilos (1.5%), all having acquired at least one item from the clothing category. The collected data were entered into SPSS. Cronbach's alpha was used to check the reliability of the scales, obtaining a value of 0.868 for factor 1, factor 2 (0.859), factor 3 (0.789) and factor 4 (0.689). Based on Cronbach's theory (1951), the excellent internal consistency and reliability of the scales for research is demonstrated [7]. To verify the degree of joint relationship between the variables, the KMO test was performed, obtaining a value of 0.954. Based on Kaiser's theory (1970), it is confirmed that the data found is appropriate for factor analysis. Similarly, the Bartlett sphericity test was performed, obtaining a significance of 0.000, showing that the model is suitable for factor analysis. An exploratory factor analysis was carried out in the present study in order to reduce the number of indicators and analyze the structure of the interrelationships. As a first result, 3 factors were obtained; however, the first factor was very broad and encompassed multiple indicators that belonged to different independent variables; therefore, it prevented the dimensions from being explained correctly. It was decided to perform a factor analysis again, adding a factor to better identify the dimensions and determine the degree to which each variable is justified by dimension. Therefore, a principal axis factor analysis with orthogonal rotation (varimax) was performed. The first factor obtained shows a variance of 20.8%; the second 15.8%; the third 7.8% and the fourth 7.6%. All 4 factors explained 51.982% of the variance (Table 3).

Factor 1: Usability (Total Variance Explained 20.844%). The first factor found "Usability" contains 9 indicators in total, of which 7 correspond to the research variable "usability", 1 refers to the variable under study "interactivity", and 1 indicator represents the variable "aesthetics". This factor refers to the functionality and usefulness of the website of a department store, meaning it has an easy-to-navigate and convenient interface, as well as a correct structure and high quality of the information that allows the consumer to find with the product easily and continues browsing the website.

Factor 2: Trust (Total Variance Explained 15.806%). The second factor obtained "Trust" is made up of 6 indicators in total, of which 5 correspond to the research variable "trust" and 1 indicator is part of the variable under study "interactivity". However, the essence of this factor indicates a greater similarity with the variable studied "trust". It refers to the security perceived by the consumer while browsing a website of a department store, having elements such as truthful and transparent information and seals or logos of organizations that guarantee the protection and security of the client's personal data during transactions.

Table 3. Factor load

Factor Load	
Usability	*1*
Navigation on the website was easy	0.721
The ordering process was straightforward	0.645
The website is easily accessible	0.593
I found the online store with little effort	0.553
The website offers good internal search services	0.530
The website offered access to other consumers to incorporate their experiences. (product score, customer review, testimonials and chat boxes)	0.511
The website was convenient	0.510
The website design is attractive	0.489
Website pages were loading very fast	0.448
Trust	*2*
The website offered adequate guarantees against the misuse of customer's personal information	0.745
The website has a transparent guarantee	0.615
The website offered adequate guarantees for the security of online transactions	0.609
The website offered an excellent personalized search	0.514
The website prominently featured seals or logos of organizations that ensure safe online shopping	0.503
The website offered adequate guarantees for the protection of client's personal data	0.490
Aesthetics	*3*
The website design is unique due to the innovation of elements	0.635
The atmosphere (navigation structure, product presentation, sound, etc.) of the website was very good	0.495
The presentation quality of the website is of a high level	0.485
Interactivity	4
The website offered excellent online customer service	0.665
Interacting with the store staff on the website was easy	0.658

Factor 3: Aesthetics (Total Variance Explained 7.765%). The third factor identified "Aesthetics" is fully comprised by 3 indicators that correspond to the research variable "Aesthetics". This refers to innovative and high-quality elements such as the attractive presentation of the product, as well as the composition of images, colors, typography and iconography that, in harmony, generate in the consumer the perception of a nicer online environment when browsing the website of a department store.

Factor 4: Interactivity (Total Variance Explained 7.568%). The fourth factor obtained "Interactivity" is composed of 2 indicators, which are part of the research variable under the same name "Interactivity". Indeed, this dimension represents the ease of interaction with the online store that users perceive while browsing the website. In this sense, it has elements that facilitate communication and assistance to users such as a chatbox, a question and answer section that in turn improve the quality of online customer service.

A multiple linear regression was carried out, in order to explore the relationship between the dependent variable (OPI) and the four dimensions obtained in the factor analysis. An adjusted R squared of 0.419 (41.9% of explained variance) was obtained, which indicates that the model does manage to explain, acceptably, the variability of the data. The explained variance is not greater than that found, since not all possible indicators have been considered in the model, or at least a greater number of indicators from other authors. The ANOVA test was administered, obtaining a significance of 0.000. This result explains that it is possible to build a linear regression model. The regression's results analysis provide evidence that the 4 dimensions obtained present statistical significance $p < 0.05$. Usability, trust, and aesthetics of the website have a statistical significance of $p = 0.000$, and the interactivity of $p = 0.001$. It indicates that the 4 dimensions contribute to the OPI of millennial users on department store websites. The values of B obtained in the 4 dimensions are positive. Statistics indicate that usability receives the highest score of 0.336 (with 95% of confidence interval, lower limit 4,384 and upper limit 4,481). The B score obtained for trust is 0.215 (2,80 and 3,93 confidence interval below and higher than 95%), followed by aesthetics and interactivity with scores of 0.127 (lower limit 0,062 and upper limit 0,191, with 95% of the confidence interval) and 0.104 (0,043 and 0,166, lower and upper limit with 95% of the confidence interval respectively. The initial results show that usability is the most important factor among all. Also, it suggests that OPI is positively affected by the usability, trust, aesthetics and interactivity. Finally, the regressions are significant and positive for the four factors in the study of the WE: usability, trust, aesthetics and interactivity; therefore, the hypotheses are validated.

6 Discussion

The present study shows evidence that the factors of the WE that positively and significantly affect the OPI of young millennials in a department store site in Metropolitan Lima are: usability, trust, aesthetics and interactivity. In the first place, usability shows to be the most important factor among all the factors of the WE, since it shows a greater positive and significant effect with the OPI, which is consistent with what was found [6, 23, 32]. It can be concluded that department stores that offer a website with great ease of search and navigation increase the perception of usefulness and functionality for the user. They allow the creation of a better WE that motivates the consumer to continue browsing the website during the purchase intention process. Secondly, trust also shows a positive and significant effect on OPI, which is consistent with what is proposed by [17, 32]. Department stores should consider that building credibility and trust on the website is necessary and important, since consumers take into account the information provided through the online store to make purchasing decisions. Those online stores that provide truthful, precise, and transparent information, manage to reduce uncertainty, and increase the possibility that the user uses the website and intends to purchase a product. The WE must generate trust in the user to be able to persuade them with elements that guarantee the security of personal information and during transactions to generate OPI in an online department store. In third place, aesthetics is another important factor that positively and significantly affects OPI, which is consistent with what is proposed by [17, 35]. It was identified that the visual elements stimulate consumers to have an initial impression of liking and attractiveness towards the website. Retailers should verify the visual design of the website to optimize the WE [17]. In contrast, [32] mention that aesthetics is an important factor that encourages OPI but has a negative relationship. This is because aesthetics would generate different moods in each consumer, so those consumers who consider the visual appearance irrelevant will have less affinity with the website. According to the evidence provided in this study, this factor provides attractiveness to consumers towards the website, promoting greater OPI. In fourth place, interactivity is a factor obtained that positively and significantly affects, on a smaller scale, the OPI, which is consistent with what is proposed by [32, 35]. The importance of effective and rapid communication by the department store with the online user is evident [32]. It is important to emphasize that users seek a quick and immediate response to their online queries, an argument supported by [21, 24], which indicates that, with good online customer service, it would increase the consumer's OPI.

7 Conclusions

This research provides evidence on the different effects of the WE factors on the purchase intention of Millennials on department store websites in Metropolitan Lima. In this sense, the factor with the greatest positive and significant effect on purchase intention is usability, followed by trust, aesthetics and interactivity in that order. Indeed, it is indicated that the online purchase intention of consumers depends, in different measures, on usability (usefulness and functionality of the website), trust (credibility and security of the website), aesthetics and interactivity between retailers with online users.

8 Limitations

On the one hand, there was no access to a representative sampling frame, so the data collected is not completely representative of the young millennials of Metropolitan Lima and the findings presented correspond to a non-probabilistic sample. On the other hand, it was not possible to know the impact of the Covid-19 pandemic on online shopping, since this type of purchase increased without knowing exactly its size, nor how much buyers, in total, stopped buying due to the economic uncertainty generated.

9 Future Investigations

Future research is encouraged on the effects of WE factors in the decision to buy online or in the repurchase. First, authors could carry out the study with a probabilistic sampling frame to obtain precise data that allows the effects of WE factors to be analyzed more accurately. Secondly, the hypotheses presented offer researchers from Metropolitan Lima a terrain for future empirical tests and model validation. Additionally, studies on WE factors that affect OPI between generations (generation X and Z), by gender or intercultural aspects could be carried out in the future to identify the existence of possible differences in users' WE. Finally, it will be important to delve into the analysis, using PLS-SEM to know if the variables used in the model can predict the effects of the WE on online shopping, even knowing the possible different effects that the variables could have on a segmentation, made with PLS.

References

1. Anaya, R., Castro, J., González, E.: Millennial consumer preferences in social commerce web design. Revista Brasileira de Gestão De Negócios **22**(1), 123–139 (2019)
2. Athapaththu, J., Kulathunga, D.: Factors affecting online purchase intention: effects of technology and social commerce. Int. Bus. Res. **11**(10) (2018)
3. Bebber, S., Sperandio, G., De Toni, D., Eberle, L., Slongo, L.: Antecedents of Purchase intention in the online context. J. Relat. Mark. **16**(1), 82–98 (2017)
4. Changchit, C., Cutshall, R., Lonkani, R., Phowaln, K., Pongwiritthon, R.: Determinants of online shopping influencing Thai consumer buying choices. J. Internet Commer. 1–23 (2018)
5. Chen, Y., Hsu, I., Lin, C.: Website attributes that increase consumer purchase intention: a conjoint analysis. J. Bus. Res. **63**(9–10), 1007–1014 (2010)
6. Constantinides, E., Lorenzo-Romero, C., Gómez, M.: Effects of web experience on consumer choice: a multicultural approach. Internet Res. **20**(2), 188–209 (2010)
7. Cronbach, L.J.: Coefficient alpha and the internal structure of test. Psychometrika **16**(3), 297–334 (1951)
8. Dakduk, S., Horst, E., Santalla, S., Molina, G., Malavé, J.: Customer behavior in electronic commerce: bayesian approach. J. Theor. Appl. Electron. Commer. Res. **12**(2), 1–20 (2018)
9. Freitas, A., Santos, A.: Using a multicriteria approach to identify factors that influence e-tailing service quality. Int. J. Electron. Mark. Retail. **10**(1), 1 (2019)
10. Frik, A., Mittone, L.: Factors influencing the perception of website privacy trustworthiness and users' purchasing intentions. J. Theor. Appl. Electron. Commer. Res. **14**(3), 89 (2019)
11. Gautam, V., Sharma, V.: Mediating role of company information in the relationships among perceived risks and purchase intentions in an online retailing. J. Relat. Mark. **18**(1), 1–9 (2019)
12. Huseynov, F., Yıldırım, S.: Internet users' attitudes toward business-to-consumer online shopping. Inf. Dev. **32**(3), 452–465 (2014)
13. Hsin Chang, H., Wen Chen, S.: The impact of online store environment cues on purchase intention. Online Inf. Rev. **32**(6), 818–841 (2008)
14. Inegbedion, H., Obadiaru, D., Bello, V.: Factors that influence consumers' attitudes toward internet buying in Nigeria. J. Internet Commer. **15**(4), 353–375 (2016)
15. Khare, A., Khare, A., Singh, S.: Attracting shoppers to shop online—challenges and opportunities for the Indian. J. Internet Commer. **11**(2), 161–185 (2012)
16. Kim, D., Ammeter, A.: Shifts in online consumer behavior: a preliminary investigation of the net generation. J. Theor. Appl. Electron. Commer. Res. **13**(1), 1–25 (2017)
17. Kühn, S., Petzer, D.: Fostering purchase intentions toward online retailer websites in an emerging market: an S-O-R perspective. J. Internet Commer. **17**(3), 255–282 (2018)
18. Liew, Y.S., Falahat, M.: Factors influencing consumers' purchase intention towards online group buying in Malaysia. Int. J. Electron. Mark. Retail. **10**(1), 60 (2019)
19. Liu, F., Xiao, B., Lim, E., Tan, C.: The art of appeal in electronic commerce. Internet Res. **27**(4), 752–771 (2017)

20. Lee, T.S., Ariff, M.S.M., Zakuan, N., Sulaiman, Z., Saman, M.Z.M.: Online sellers' website quality influencing online buyers' purchase intention. In: IOP Conference Series: Materials Science and Engineering, vol. 131, no. 1, p. 012014 (2016)
21. Lee, G., Lin, H.: Customer perceptions of e-service quality in online shopping. Int. J. Retail Distrib. Manag. **33**(2), 161–176 (2005)
22. Lu, B., Fan, W., Zhou, M.: Social presence, trust, and social commerce purchase intention: an empirical research. Comput. Hum. Behav. **56**, 225–237 (2016)
23. Lorenzo, C., Constantinides, E., Gómez, M., Geurts, P.: Análisis del consumo virtual bajo la influencia de las dimensiones constituyentes de la experiencia web. Estudios sobre consumo **84**, 53–65 (2008)
24. Merrilees, B.: Interactivity design as the key to managing customer relations in e-commerce. J. Relat. Mark. **1**(3–4), 111–126 (2002)
25. Molinillo, S., Cabanillas, F., Sánchez, R.: A social commerce intention model for traditional e- commerce sites. J. Theor. Appl. Electron. Commer. Res. **13**(2), 80–93 (2018)
26. Pandey, S., Chawla, D.: Online customer experience (OCE) in clothing e-retail. Int. J. Retail Distrib. Manag. **46**(3), 323–346 (2018)
27. Prashar, S., Sai-Vijay, T., Parsad, C.: Effects of online shopping values and website cues on purchase behaviour: a study using S-O-R framework. Vikalpa **42**(1), 1–18 (2017)
28. Raman, P.: Understanding female consumers' intention to shop online: the role of trust, convenience and customer service. Asia Pac. J. Mark. Logist. **31**(4), 1138–1160 (2019)
29. Rishi, B., Al-Khasawneh, A.: Determinants of online purchase intention: a study of Emirati consumers. Int. J. Islamic Mark. Branding **2**(3), 200–214 (2017)
30. Rosmayani, Mardhatillah, A.: Model of intention to behave in online product purchase for Muslim fashion in Pekanbaru, Indonesia. J. Islamic Mark. **1759** (2020)
31. Rose, S., Clark, M., Samouel, P., Hair, N.: Online customer experience in e-Retailing: an empirical model of antecedents and outcomes. J. Retail. **88**(2), 308–322 (2012)
32. Salleh, N., Ha, N., Kitchen, P., Any, A.: Online purchasing: the role of web experience factors. Int. J. Electron. Mark. Retail. **10**(3), 260 (2019)
33. Strähle, J.: Online fashion shopping: mystery shopping-based evaluation of online German fashion stores. J. Glob. Fash. Market. **4**(3), 193–210 (2013)
34. Tandon, U., Kiran, R., Sah, A.: Customer satisfaction using website functionality, perceived usability and perceived usefulness towards online shopping in India. Inf. Dev. **32**(5), 1657 (2016)
35. Teng, H., Ni, J., Chen, H.: Relationship between e-servicescape and purchase intention among heavy and light internet users. Internet Res. **28**(2), 333–350 (2018)
36. Torres, J., Cañada, F., Berrio, S., Pinzón, O., Cerpa, W.: The Colombian electronic consumer: analysis of the leading factors of e-commerce use. Int. J. Electron. Mark. Retail. **10**(3), 283 (2019)
37. Wang, O., Somogyi, S.: Consumer adoption of online food shopping in China. Br. Food J. **120**(12), 2868–2884 (2018)
38. Young Kim, E., Kim, Y.: Predicting online purchase intentions for clothing products. Eur. J. Mark. **38**(7), 883–897 (2004)
39. Moreno, F.M., Lafuente, J.G., Carreon, F.A., Moreno, S.M.: The characterization of the millennials and their buying behavior. Int. J. Mark. Stud. **9**(5), 135–144 (2017)

Perceived Quality, Brand Image and Brand Loyalty in the Purchase Intent of Smartphones in College Students

Daniela Zaharia Seinfeld and Hernán Talledo Flores(✉)

Universidad Peruana de Ciencias Aplicadas, Lima, Peru

Abstract. This research seeks to examine the relationship between perceived quality, brand loyalty and brand image with respect to the purchase intent in an audience of young Lima college students who are between 17 and 24 years old. As a result, it was obtained that brand loyalty and image are fundamental to generate a purchase intent in this public; however, Perceived Quality as an influencing factor of purchase intent was eliminated and Brand Confidence was added, since a relationship with the dependent variable was found. In the same way, 261 surveys were conducted with the target audience through an online questionnaire. The study developed was quantitative correlational, focusing on non-probabilistic convenience sampling. To obtain the results, there were made two Confirmatory Factor Analysis, an Exploratory Factor Analysis and a Monotonic Regression, in addition to performing two times the Cronbach's Alpha and using the item-Factor correlation to eliminate the least influential indicators.

Keywords: Brand equity · Brand loyalty · Brand image · Perceived quality · Brand trust · Purchase intention

1 Introduction

This research focuses on perceived quality, image and loyalty, which are dimensions of brand equity. These terms are the reasons why consumers are willing to buy cell phone equipment and become loyal to a brand [1, 32, 57]. Many authors relate these three terms to purchase intention, which is based on the consumer's willingness to choose the product of one brand over another [20, 36]. This study focuses on the university audience in Lima, Peru, for whom the smartphone is an essential tool for their studies and social life. It seeks to find out what is the quality standard demanded by young people, the loyalty they have towards a particular brand and the importance they give to the image of this brand in such a way that it generates a positive influence on the intention to purchase such smartphones [32].

2 Theoretical Framework

2.1 Brand Equity

According to Veríssimo et al. (2017), brand equity is a broad term that includes brand liabilities and assets, which include the name, logo, symbols and letters, among others.

© The Author(s), under exclusive license to Springer Nature Singapore Pte Ltd. 2022
Á. Rocha et al. (Eds.): ICOMTA 2021, SIST 259, pp. 446–457, 2022.
https://doi.org/10.1007/978-981-16-5792-4_44

Furthermore, Moslehpour et al., (2019) add that these elements allow the value of a brand to be increased or decreased. However, Keller (1993) defines the concept as people's response to brand marketing in the face of the distinctive effect of brand awareness. On the other hand, Gunawardane (2015) presents a different perspective by focusing on brand equity as an indispensable tool at the time of purchase, since it contributes to customer decision-making. In addition, other authors refer to brand equity as the learning that the customer has and whose brand knowledge allows generating various attitudes towards the brand [16, 41].

2.2 Perceived Quality

Perceived quality refers to people's perception of the quality of a certain product (Shin, 2017). It goes beyond quality itself as it involves each customer's judgment about the superiority of a brand and thus positively or negatively influences the overall value [24, 42]. In addition, the result of productivity, which includes customization and lack of defects, allows customers to trust these and the expectations they have about the product [7, 24]. It is a fundamental dimension of brand equity, which applies across all product categories. On the other hand, quality always involves a comparison between two or more brands [1]. Perceived quality has two categories: intrinsic and extrinsic [66]. Appearance and performance are also added to them [9].

2.3 Brand Loyalty

Brand loyalty is the nexus that the consumer has with this brand and makes that people want to continue buying it [54, 55]. In this case, thanks to loyalty, consumers generate a connection with the smartphone brands. According to Buil et al. (2013), loyalty is the total commitment that consumers have with a brand. For other authors, loyalty refers to the adequate security and trust that consumers have for a specific brand or product [43]. There is further research that associates loyalty and brand preference; in this association, the level of loyalty is the predilection one has about a smartphone brand [52]. On the other hand, the more satisfied a person is with a brand's smartphone equipment, the more loyal he or she will be to it [18].

2.4 Brand Image

Image refers to some word or symbol that allows differentiating and recognizing the products of a brand from the rest of the competition [43]. There are authors who see image as the various connections that people have in their minds related to a particular brand [20]. On the other hand, brand image is also seen as the appreciation that consumers have for a brand, which allows its association [43, 71]; that is, it is what consumers believe about a particular brand [43]. Thus, this can influence people in such a way that they decide to buy a product from one smartphone brand or another [52]. In addition, brand image enables different decisions about promotions, plans, strategies and prices [71] used by smartphone brands.

2.5 Purchase Intent

Perceived quality, image and brand loyalty are related and have a direct impact on purchase intention [5, 32]. However, other studies have determined that purchase intention is influenced by customer satisfaction towards the brand, and, at the same time, this satisfaction is related to perceived quality and brand loyalty [59]. Finally, there are authors who have defined that the purchase intention in categories such as cell phones is different in each country depending on the conditions, needs and socioeconomic and cultural differences of its citizens [5, 37].

3 Hypothesis and Model

- **H1: Perceived quality positively influences purchase intention for smartphones.** This relationship has been analyzed by other authors, such as: [20, 28, 64, 72].
- **H2: Brand image positively influences the purchase intention of smartphones.** This relationship has been analyzed by other authors, such as: [6, 10, 20, 28].
- **H3: Brand loyalty positively influences purchase intention for smartphones.** This relationship has been analyzed by other authors, such as: [20, 28, 59, 64].

4 Methodology

Study was conducted, where an online survey was developed through the Ligthouse Studio version 9.8 program to 261 young people between 17 and 24 years old, undergraduate university students who have had smartphones for at least 3 years, since they have more experience and knowledge about them. A non-probabilistic sampling was used, since there is no adequate sampling frame, and the type of sampling was by convenience. The methodology used was CFA, EFA, Monotonic Regression and Cronbach's Alpha.

Measuring instrument support: Perceived Quality [36]: Good value for money (PC1), Superior quality for higher price (PC2), Brand durability (PC3), Better image quality (PC4), Excellent functional characteristics (PC5) and Visibly attractive and favorable brand (PC6). Brand loyalty [36], Brand preference (BL1), Brand recommendation (BL2), Future brand consideration (BL3), Brand trust (BL4), Low probability of change (BL5), First choice (BL6). Brand image [10]: Brand reference (BI1), Good brand reputation (BI2), Fulfillment of needs (BI3), Reliability in brand promises (BI4). Purchase intention [10]: Purchase in the near future (PI1), Purchase intention (PI2).

5 Results

In total, 261 surveys were obtained, in which most of the young Peruvian respondents were female (71.3%), aged between 23 and 24 years (57.1%), have their current smartphone 1 year ago (30.7%) and use smartphones 7–8 years ago (36.4%). In addition, the activities they do most with the smartphone are leisure (68.2%), while, in COVID-19 times, the activity they do most are virtual meetings with friends (34.5%).

5.1 Cronbach's Alpha

The reliability of the data according to the value obtained in Cronbach's Alpha is 0.866. the values obtained ranging between 0.7 and 0.9 point to internal consistency. In addition, split-half reliability was identified, where the proposed indicators are distributed in two halves and the highest ratings of each half are correlated. The values obtained in both halves were 0.707 and 0.799. Reliability was found by obtaining Cronbach's Alpha for each of the research indicators if an item has been deleted. In this case, all the indicators have a value greater than or equal to 0.853 [39].

5.2 Confirmatory Factor Analysis

The significance level of the Chi-square statistic is 0.000 and the RMSEA value is 0.120, which is high, the value should be between 0.05 and 0.06 [34]; however, there are other authors such as Ruiz et al. (2010) who corroborate that the data fit the model if an RMSEA of up to 0.08 is obtained.

5.3 Re-specification of the Model

The model was re-specified using the two-half reliability analysis to find the Item-Factor Correlation through the corrected total item correlation (corrected homogeneity coefficient), where items 1 (Good value for money) and 3 (Greater durability) were discarded, since they obtained the two lowest values, 0.218 and 0.233, respectively [51].

Corrected total item correlation: PC1 (0.218), PC2 (0.536), PC3 (0.233), PC4 (0.441), PC5 (0.545), PC6 (0.597), BL1 (0.583), BL2 (0.595), BL3 (0.643), BL4 (0.580), BL5 (0.502), BL6 (0.606), BI1 (0.434), BI2 (0.507), BI3 (0.559), BI4 (0.557).

5.4 Cronbach's Alpha After Model Re-specification

Once the suppressed values were obtained, Cronbach's Alpha 0.881, so it is observed that the value is higher once the two indicators were eliminated through the corrected total item correlation. Therefore, the indicators used maintain a correlation among themselves and a construct that is considered valid [56]. The split-half reliability was then performed, where the values obtained were as follows: 0.791 and 0.763. This indicates that both halves achieve a correlation between the indicators [39]. Reliability was also obtained with Cronbach's alpha for each of the indicators if an item was deleted. All the indicators have a value greater than or equal to 0.869 [56].

5.5 Exploratory Factor Analysis

Taking into account the 14 indicators of the model. The main axis factorization extraction method and the Varimax rotation method with Kaiser normalization were used. The Chi-square statistic had a value of 0.000; therefore, according to Kerlinger and Lee Howard [39] and Ferrando and Lorenzo-Seva [27] (2014), the model is proven to be linear. The Kaiser-Meyer-Olkin measure was 0,889. Three dimensions were found, the Perceived Quality factor was eliminated, and the Brand Trust factor was incorporated.

- Factor 1: Brand loyalty (20.678% of variance explained). Strongest preference for the smartphone brand. It their first choice when they plan to change their phone, even if it has a higher price. It is the brand that has the highest quality and always covers all their needs. They would never choose another brand. It is the brand they would always consider in the future. Indicators represent what Brand Loyalty is. Factor Load Brand Loyalty: BL1 (0.709), BL6 (0.794), BL5 (0.642), PC2 (0.411), BI3 (0.410) and PC6 (0.747)
- Factor 2: Brand satisfaction (16.780% variance explained), Users are willing to recommend the brand and trust it and the promise it has given them. They find the functional features. Factorial Load Brand Trust: BL2 (0.614), BI4 (0.615), PC5 (0.653), BI4 (0.632).
- Factor 3: Brand image (10.816% of variance explained). Their smartphone brand has the best quality image. It is their major reference for future purchases, as it has a good reputation. The Factorial Load Brand image: BI1 (0.678), PC4 (0.599), BI2 (0.424).

5.6 Confirmatory Factor Analysis

The model re-specification in EFA fit the model, a new CFA was developed. The Chi-square $p = 0.000$ [34] and the RMSEA value is 0.08, which is an acceptable value [58], the model is approved if the RMSEA obtains a value greater than or equal to 0.05 and less than or equal to 0.08. GFI value of 0.892, close to 0.9, was obtained. Otherwise, the TLI value is 0.861, which is close to 0.9. The CFI is 0.887 [17, 22].

5.7 Monotonic Regression

The dependent variable is ordered and fits the model better, since it is ordinal and nonlinear when a Likert scale is used [47]. In contrast, linear regression should be used if the scale is linear [27, 39].

Two different monotonic regressions were performed. With the first indicator (habitual brand purchase in the future), we obtained a monotonic R^2 (goodness of fit) of 0.434 (43.4% of explanation), while with the second indicator (habitual brand purchase intention), we obtained a value of 0.664 (66.4% of explanation). This indicates that the most appropriate item to be used in the Monotonic Regression is the second one, since it reached a higher goodness-of-fit value [15, 47]. The p-value was <0.05, so it is verified that the dependent variable of the model is ordinal [15, 47]. The three factors (Loyalty, Satisfaction and Brand Image) have a significance level of p-value <0.05, so the three factors positively influence the dependent variable "habitual brand purchase intention" [15, 47].

According to Bernstein et al. (2002), Exp(Beta) should be as isolated as possible from the value 1, since it allows the dependent variable to be explained and related more closely to the independent variable. Brand Loyalty obtained an Exp(Beta) value of 9.22 and was the factor that had the greatest weight in the explanation in relation to the dependent variable, followed by Brand Satisfaction which had a value of 2.09 and Brand Image with a value of 1.67. On the other hand, the Beta statistic explains the consideration of the effect for each of the factors added to the model [47]. In this case, brand loyalty has a 2.22 times greater chance of generating a purchase intention, a value that decreases in the case of trust and brand image, which have a chance of 0.74 and 0.51, respectively [47].

- Brand Loyalty: $\beta = 2{,}22$ ($p = 0{,}001$), Exp(Beta) = 9,22. Perceived Quality: $\beta = 0{,}74$ ($p = 0{,}001$), Exp(Beta) = 2,99.
- Brand Image: $\beta = 0{,}51$ ($p = 0{,}0018$), Exp(Beta) = 1,67.

As shown in Fig. 1, the dotted curved line obtained in Monotonic Regression manages to explain and capture the values obtained on the Likert scale better than the straight line obtained in Linear Regression [47].

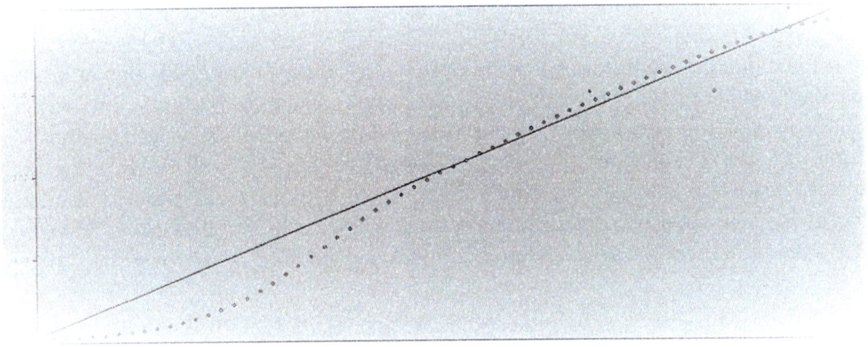

Fig. 1. Dotted curved line obtained

6 Discussion

The research framework was developed to identify the relationships between perceived quality, brand loyalty and brand image related to the purchase intention of smartphones. The initial model, which takes into account what was done by the authors, was not tested through Confirmatory Factor Analysis. The hypotheses are not fulfilled in the same way as in the proposed model, because, due to the data obtained, the research has changed and the composition of the factors has been transformed along the way.

By eliminating the two indicators (good value for money and greater durability) with the corrected total correlation of elements, the model was re-specified by performing the Exploratory Factor Analysis, where the results obtained were different and had a vision, concepts and results different from the initial ones. Therefore, the hypotheses obtained are fulfilled in a different way, since the factors are composed of a similar, but not identical structure. The initial starting concept of the starting factors is different from the one achieved with the data obtained.

The composition of the factors and the results obtained will be explained in greater detail below: Several authors [11, 25, 31, 35, 46] have used CFA to corroborate the proposed models; however, when performed to validate the models used by authors Hossain et al. (2018) and Ali et al. (2020), the model was not corroborated. When the first CFA was performed to validate the initial model, the applied data did not fit the aforementioned models, as the RMSEA was 0.120 [34]. This could be due to the fact that the research has been conducted in a different context, country and culture and the items used in the Ali et al. (2020) research do not focus on the smartphone category, while the items used by the authors Hossain et al. (2018) are focused on that category. Another influential factor may be the effect caused by the COVID-19 pandemic. All this may influence the lack of adaptability of the data in the initial proposed model; however, once the re-specification of the model was done and the new grouping of the indicators was verified with the Exploratory Factor Analysis, a value of 0.8 was obtained after checking it, so it was confirmed that the data were adapted to the new proposed model [58].

On the other hand, authors such as [35, 36, 67], used the EFA to find the correlations and covariances between the factors [45]. The initial model proposed had three factors (perceived quality, brand loyalty and brand image); however, when the model was re-specified and the EFA was performed, three factors were obtained, which were given the following names: Brand Loyalty, Brand Trust and Brand Image. Perceived Quality was eliminated from the new proposed model Several authors [14, 35, 37, 40, 60] have used Linear Regression with a Likert scale to verify their hypotheses. However, Monotonic Regression has better adaptability for ordinal scales such as Likert [47]. Therefore, Monotonic Regression was taken into account to test the proposed hypotheses.

- Factor 1 (brand loyalty): it was initially composed of six indicators [36]; however, brand recommendation and brand trustworthiness were deleted, since they did not have a higher correlation with the other indicators of the dimension. This factor finally consists of the following seven items: brand preference, first option chosen, low probability of change and consideration of the brand in the future, in addition to those that were added, which are the coverage of needs with respect to the competition, higher quality for a higher price and visibly attractive and favorable brand.
- Factor 2 (brand trust): this factor was not included in the initial model; however, the indicators found in the AFE are related to those used by authors such as [5, 10, 12, 71]. It is made up of the following four items: brand recommendation, excellent functional characteristics, brand reliability, and brand promise reliability.
- Factor 3 (brand image): it was initially composed of four indicators [10]; however, the need fulfillment with respect to competition and brand trust were deleted, as they did not have a strong correlation with the other indicators of the dimension. This factor is finally composed of the following three items: brand reference and good brand reputation, in addition to the image of better quality, an item that was added.

The results obtained with the modification of the factor structure were as follows: Brand Loyalty, Brand Trust, and Brand Image positively influence smartphone Purchase Intention. All three hypotheses were partially corroborated. As mentioned above, due to the change in the structure of the factors and their regrouping, the hypotheses were partially corroborated. Therefore, the new proposed model was presented, in which the Perceived Quality variable was eliminated, and Brand Trust was added.

Showed that Perceived Quality and Brand Loyalty positively influenced purchase intention. However, for Falahat et al. (2018), Brand Image had no influence on Purchase Intention, whereas, for Chi et al. (2019), Brand Image does have influence on Purchase Intention. Roozy et al. (2014) verified that Brand Loyalty has influence on Purchase Intention, but Perceived Quality does not. Ali et al. (2020) verified that Brand Loyalty, Brand Image, Brand Quality and Brand Trust have a positive influence on Purchase Intention. With the results obtained, it was found that Brand Loyalty, Brand Trust and Brand Image, with the modifications made, have a positive influence on purchase intention. However, quality was eliminated from the final proposed model due to the regrouping obtained from the indicators.

Loyalty, Trust and previous Image that young Peruvians have had with smartphone brands are essential to generate a Purchase Intention. However, Perceived Quality was eliminated from the re-specified model, which may be due to the fact that, being loyal to a brand and already having a good image of it, a person does not consider that the brand may have a poor quality. Compared to the other factors studied, Perceived Quality does not work in conjunction with the other dimensions. Brand loyalty is the most predominant factor and the one to be guided the most.

7 Limitations

Initially, the research focused on the population of socioeconomic level D. However, the greatest limitation that has been encountered throughout the research is focused on the lack of internet coverage in the cones located in Metropolitan Lima. On the other hand, in certain areas of the capital, the equipment required to answer the surveys virtually is not sufficient.

References

1. Aaker, D.A.: Measuring brand equity across products and markets. Calif. Manag. Rev. **38**, 3 (1996)
2. Adekunle, S.A., Ejechi, J.O.: Modelling repurchase intention among smartphones users in Nigeria. J. Model. Manag. **13**(4), 794–814 (2018). https://doi.org/10.1108/JM2-12-2017-0138
3. Adhikari, K., Panda, R.K.: The role of consumer-brand engagement towards driving brand loyalty. J. Model. Manag. **14**(4), 987–1005 (2019). https://doi.org/10.1108/JM2-03-2019-0067
4. Agrebi, S., Jallais, J.: Explain the intention to use smartphones for mobile shopping. J. Retail. Consum. Serv. **22**, 16–23 (2015). https://doi.org/10.1016/j.jretconser.2014.09.003
5. Akinbode, M., Adegbuyi, O., Kehinde, O.J., Agboola, M.G., Olokundun, A.M.: Percieved value dimensions on online shopping intention: the role of trust and culture. Acad. Strateg. Manag. J. **18**(1) (2010)
6. Akram, U., Ansari, A.R., Fu, G., Junaid, M.: Feeling hungry? Let's order through mobile! examining the fast food mobile commerce in China. J. Retail. Consum. Serv. **56**, 102–142 (2020). https://doi.org/10.1016/j.jretconser.2020.102142

7. Al-Arafati, A., Kadir, K.A., Al-Haderi, S.: The mediating effect of output quality on the relationship between top management support and customer satisfaction on the implementation of customer relationship management system in public sector. Acad. Strateg. Manag. J. **18**(2) (2019)
8. Algharabat, R., Rana, N.P., Alalwan, A.A., Baabdullah, A., Gupta, A.: Investigating the antecedents of customer brand engagement and consumer-based brand equity in social media. J. Retail. Consum. Serv. **53** (2020). https://doi.org/10.15640/jmm.v3n1a10
9. Alhaddad, A.: Perceived quality, brand image and brand trust as determinants of brand loyalty. J. Res. Bus. Manag. **3**(4), 01–08 (2015)
10. Ali, A., Sherwani, M., Ali, A., Ali, Z., Sherwani, M.: Investigating the antecedents of halal brand product purchase intention: an empirical investigation. J. Islamic Mark. ahead-of-print No. ahead-of-print (2020). https://doi.org/10.1108/JIMA-03-2019-0063
11. Alić, A., Činjarević, M., Agić, E.: The role of brand image in consumer-brand relationships: similarities and differences between national and private label brands. Manag. Mark. **15**(1), 1–16 (2020). https://doi.org/10.2478/mmcks-2020-0001
12. Al-Msallam, S., Alhaddad, A.: Customer satisfaction and loyalty in the hotel industry: the mediating role of relationship marketing (PLS approach). J. Res. Bus. Manag. **4**(5), 32–42 (2016)
13. Aziz, S.A.: Does fear of new car technologies influence brand loyalty relationship. J. Mark. Manag. **4**(1), 125–136 (2016). https://doi.org/10.15640/jmm.v4n1a12
14. Baloglu, S., Henthorne, T.L., Sahin, S.: Destination image and brand personality of Jamaica: a model of tourist behavior. J. Travel Tourism Mark. **31**(8), 1057–1070 (2014). https://doi.org/10.1080/10548408.2014.892468
15. Bernstein, L., Bradley, K., Zarich, S.: GOLDmineR: improving models for classifying patients with chest pain. Yale J. Biol. Med. **75**(4), 183 (2002)
16. Buil, I., Martínez, E., De Chernatony, L.: The influence of brand equity on consumer responses. J. Consum. Mark. **30**(1), 62–74 (2013). https://doi.org/10.1108/07363761311290849
17. Cea D'ancona, M.A.: Análisis multivariable. Teoría y práctica en la investigación social. Síntesis. Madrid (España) (2002)
18. Chen, C.M., Ann, B.Y.: Efficiencies vs. importance-performance analysis for the leading smartphone brands of Apple, Samsung and HTC. Total Qual. Manag. Bus. Excellence **27**(3–4), 227–249 (2016). https://doi.org/10.1080/14783363.2014.976937
19. Chen, Y.S., Huang, A.F., Wang, T.Y., Chen, Y.R.: Greenwash and green purchase behaviour: the mediation of green brand image and green brand loyalty. Total Qual. Manag. Bus. Excellence **31**(1–2), 194–209 (2018). https://doi.org/10.1080/14783363.2018.1426450
20. Chi, H.K., Huang, K.C., Nguyen, H.M.: Elements of destination brand equity and destination familiarity regarding travel intention. J. Retail. Consum. Serv. **52** (2019). https://doi.org/10.1016/j.jretconser.2018.12.012
21. Crescitelli, E., Figueiredo, J.B.: Brand equity evolution: a system dynamics model. BAR-Braz. Adm. Rev. **6**(2), 101–117 (2009). https://doi.org/10.1590/S1807-76922009000200003
22. Cuervo, A.A.V., Vázquez, F.I.G., Acuña, G.M.T., Murrieta, M.U.: Medición en Investigación Educativa con Apoyo del SPSS y el AMOS. CONACyT, México (2019)
23. Danish, M., Ali, S., Ahmad, M.A., Zahid, H.: The influencing factors on choice behavior regarding green electronic products: based on the green perceived value model. Economies **7**(4), 99 (2019). https://doi.org/10.3390/economies7040099
24. Dib, H., Al-Msallam, S.: The effect of the determinanats of customer satisfaction on brand loyalty. J. Res. Bus. Manag. **3**(3), 01–12 (2015)
25. Dwivedi, A., Miles, M., Oczkowski, E., Weerawardena, J., Johnson, L.W., Wilkie, D.: Buyer–seller relational engagement and seller brand equity. J. Bus. Ind. Mark. ahead-of-print No. ahead-of-print (2019). https://doi.org/10.1108/JBIM-01-2019-0062

26. Falahat, M., Chuan, C.S., Kai, S.B.: Brand loyalty and determinates of perceived quality and willingness to order. Acad. Strateg. Manag. J. **17**(4) (2018)
27. Ferrando, P.J., Lorenzo-Seva, U.: El análisis factorial exploratorio de los ítems: algunas consideraciones adicionales. Anales De Psicología/Ann. Psychol. **30**(3), 1170–1175 (2014)
28. Fong, C.H., Goh, Y.N.: Why brand equity is so important for private healthcare? View from an emerging market. Int. J. Healthcare Manag. 1–8 (2020). https://doi.org/10.1080/20479700.2020.1755811
29. Gomez, M., Lopez, C., Molina, A.: A model of tourism destination brand equity: the case of wine tourism destinations in Spain. Tourism Manag. **51**, 210–222 (2015). https://doi.org/10.1016/j.tourman.2015.05.019
30. González, E., Orozco, M., Barrios, A.: El valor de la marca desde la perspectiva del consumidor. Revista Contaduría y Administración **235**, 217–239 (2010)
31. González-Mansilla, Ó., Berenguer-Contrí, G., Serra-Cantallops, A.: The impact of value co-creation on hotel brand equity and customer satisfaction. Tourism Manag. **75**, 51–65 (2019). https://doi.org/10.1016/j.tourman.2019.04.024
32. Gunawardane, N.R.: Impact of brand equity towards purchasing desition: a situation on mobile telecommunication services of Sri Lanka. J. Mark. Manag. **3**(1), 100–117 (2015). https://doi.org/10.15640/jmm.v3n1a10
33. Hepola, J., Karjaluoto, H., Hintikka, A.: The effect of sensory brand experience and involvement on brand equity directly and indirectly through consumer brand engagement. J. Product Brand Manag. **26**(3), 282–293 (2017). https://doi.org/10.1108/JPBM-10-2016-1348
34. Hirschfeld, G., Von Brachel, R.: Improving multiple-group confirmatory factor analysis in R-A tutorial in measurement invariance with continuous and ordinal indicators. Pract. Assess. Res. Eval. **19**(1), 7 (2014)
35. Ho, T.N., Wu, W.Y., Nguyen, P.T., Chen, H.C.: The moderating effects for the relationships between green customer value, green brand equity and behavioral intention. Acad. Strateg. Manag. J. **18**(4) (2019)
36. Hossain, M., Ahmed, K.F.: Impact of brand equity on the buying behaviour of Millennials towards smartphones in Bangladesh. Int. J. Bus. Manag. Invention **7**(8), 47–54 (2018)
37. Karunanayake, R.T., Wanninayake, W.B.: Impact of key purchasing determinants on purchase intention of hybrid vehicle brands in Sri Lanka, an empirical study. J. Mark. Manag. **3**(1), 40–52 (2015). https://doi.org/10.15640/jmm.v3n1a4
38. Keller, K.L.: Conceptualizing, measuring, and managing customer-based brand equity. J. Mark. **57**(1), 1–22 (1993). https://doi.org/10.1177/002224299305700101
39. Kerlinger, F.N., Lee Howard, B.: Investigación del Comportamiento. Cuarta edición. México: Ed (2002)
40. Khan, M.N., Rizwan, M., Islam, F., Zain-Ul-Aabdeen, Rehman, M.: The effect of brand equity of mobile phones on customer satisfaction: an empirical evidence from Pakistan. Am. J. Bus. Soci. **1**(1), 1–7 (2016)
41. Konecnik, M., Gartner, W.C.: Customer-based brand equity for a destination. Ann. Tour. Res. **34**(2), 400–421 (2007)
42. Lee, S.H., Lee, S.H.: A scale development of retailer equity. Sustainability **10**(11), 3924 (2018). https://doi.org/10.3390/su10113924
43. Lin, Y., Li, Y., Tsay, C.: An investigation of the relationship between customer satisfaction and loyalty on the brand image of Taiyen's products-a case study of the customer in Pingtung área. J. Mark. Manag. **3**(1), 53–63 (2015). https://doi.org/10.15640/jmm.v3n1a5
44. Lloret, S., Ferreres, A., Hernández, A., Tomás, I.: The exploratory factor analysis of items: guided analysis based on empirical data and software. Anales de Psicología **33**(2), 417–432 (2017)

45. Lloret-Segura, S., Ferreres-Traver, A., Hernández-Baeza, A., Tomás-Marco, I.: El análisis factorial exploratorio de los ítems: una guía práctica, revisada y actualizada. Anales de Psicología/Annals of Psychology **30**(3), 1151–1169 (2014)
46. Macías, W., Cerviño, J.: Unauthorized use of famous brands and its impact on brand equity dimensions. Rev. Mark. Sci. **16**(1), 1–24 (2019). https://doi.org/10.1515/roms-2019-0005
47. Magidson, J.: GOLDMiner 2.0: User's Guide. SPSS Incorporated (1998)
48. Malhotra, N.: Investigación de mercado. 5ª ed. Pearson, México DF, México (2008)
49. Mardhatillah, A.: Model of intention to behave in online product purchase for Muslim fashion in Pekanbaru, Indonesia. J. Islamic Mark. ahead-of-print No. ahead-of-print (2020). https://doi.org/10.1108/JIMA-09-2018-0159
50. Mitra, S., Jenamani, M.: OBIM: a computational model to estimate brand image from online consumer review. J. Bus. Res. **114**, 213–226 (2020). https://doi.org/10.1016/j.jbusres.2020.04.003
51. Morales Vallejo, P., Urosa Sanz, B., Blanco Blanco, Á.: Construcciones de escalas de actitudes tipo likert: una guía práctica. Construcciones de escalas de actitudes tipo likert: una guía práctica (2003)
52. Moslehpour, M., Chau, K.Y., Dadvari, A., Do, B.R., Seitz, V.: What killed HTC and kept apple alive? Brand sustainability comparison of two Asian countries. Sustainability **11**(24), 6973 (2019). https://doi.org/10.3390/su11246973
53. Nikabadi, M.S., Safui, M.A., Agheshlouei, H.: Role of advertising and promotion in brand equity creation. J. Promotion Manag. **21**(1), 13–32 (2015). https://doi.org/10.1080/10496491.2014.946208
54. Ogunnaike, O., Kehinde, O.M., Omoyayi, O.O., Popoola, O.O., Amoruwa, A.: Conceptualization of the relationship between brand equity and purchase behavior. Int. Rev. Manag. Mark. **7**(2), 403–408 (2017)
55. Ortegón, L.: Panorama actual de los métodos de medición de marcas y valor de marca desde la orientación al consumidor. Poliantea (Bogotá) **6**(11), 171–187 (2010)
56. Oviedo, H.C., Arias, A.C.: Aproximación al uso del coeficiente alfa de Cronbach. Revista colombiana de psiquiatría **34**(4), 572–580 (2005)
57. Roozy, E.S.S.M.A.E.E.L., Arastoo, M.A., Vazifehdust, H.O.S.S.E.I.N.: Effect of brand equity on consumer purchase intention. Indian J. Sci. Res. **6**(1), 212–217 (2014)
58. Ruiz, M.A., Pardo, A., San Martín, R.: Modelos de ecuaciones estructurales. Papeles del psicólogo **31**(1), 34–45 (2010)
59. Rungsrisawa, Sirinapatpokin: Impact of brand equity on consumer purchase intent. Utopía y Praxis Latinoamericana **24**(6) (2019)
60. Shahzad, M.F., Bilal, M., Xiao, J., Yousaf, T.: Impact of smartphone brand experience on brand equity. J. Islamic Mark. **10**(2), 440–464 (2019). https://doi.org/10.1108/JIMA-04-2017-0045
61. Shin, D.H.: Conceptualizing and measuring quality of experience of the internet of things: Exploring how quality is perceived by users. Inf. Manag. **54**(8), 998–1011 (2017). https://doi.org/10.1016/j.im.2017.02.006
62. Soedarto, T., Kurniawan, G.S.A., Sunarsono, R.J.: The parceling of loyalty: brand quality, brand affect, and brand trust effect on attitudinal loyalty and behavioral loyalty. Acad. Strateg. Manag. J. **18**(1) (2019)
63. Souki, G.Q., Oliveira, R.L.P.D., Isabella, G., Silva, J.T.M.: The impact of global perceived quality on the behaviour of automobile's consumers. Revista Brasileira de Marketing **17**(3), 444–458 (2018). https://doi.org/10.5585/remark.v17i3.3843
64. Susilowati, E., Sari, A.N.: The influence of brand awareness, bran association and perceived quality toward consumers purchase intention: a case of Richeese Factory, Jakarta. Independent J. Manag. Prod. **11**(1) (2019). https://doi.org/10.14807/ijmp.v11i1.981
65. Su, J.: Examining the relationships among the brand equity dimensions. Asia Pac. J. Mark. Logist. **28**(3), 464–480 (2015). https://doi.org/10.1108/APJML-01-2015-0004

66. Tharmi, U., Senthilnathan, S.: The relationship of brand equity to purchase intention. IUP J. Mark. Manag. ahead-of-print No. ahead-of-print (2011). https://doi.org/10.2139/ssrn.1935740
67. Tu, J.C., Zhang, X.Y., Huang, S.Y.: Key factors of sustainability for smartphones based on taiwanese consumers' perceived values. Sustainability **10**(12), 4446 (2018). https://doi.org/10.3390/su10124446
68. Veríssimo, J.M.C., Tiago, M.T.B., Tiago, F.G., Jardim, J.S.: Tourism destination brand dimensions: an exploratory approach. Tourism Manag. Stud. **13**(4), 1–8 (2017). https://doi.org/10.18089/tms.2017.13401
69. Virla, M.Q.: Confiabilidad y coeficiente Alpha de Cronbach. Telos **12**(2), 248–252 (2010)
70. Wasaya, Ahmad, Malik, Ali: The antecedents of customer loyalty: insights from a developing country. J. Res. Bus. Manag. **4**(5), 01–09 (2016)
71. Xu, F., Bai, Y., Li, S.: Examining the antecedents of brand engagement of tourists based on the theory of value co-creation. Sustainability **12**(5), 1958 (2020). https://doi.org/10.3390/su12051958
72. Yusof, Y.L.M., Jusoh, W.J.W., Maulan, S.: Perceived quality association as determinant to re-patronise Shariah-compliant brand restaurants. J. Islamic Mark. ahead-of-print No. ahead-of-print (2020). https://doi.org/10.1108/JIMA-10-2018-0190

Affective Support Mediated by an On-Line Constructivist Environment in Times of Covid-19

Olger Gutiérrez-Aguilar[1](✉), Aleixandre Duche-Pérez[2], and Osbaldo Turpo-Gebera[1]

[1] Universidad Nacional de San Agustín, Arequipa, Perú
{ogutierrez,oturpo}@unsa.edu.pe
[2] Universidad Católica de Santa María, Arequipa, Perú
aduche@ucsm.edu.pe

Abstract. The main objective is to know the level of influence of the factors that make up the Constructivist On-Line Learning Environment Survey (COLLES) questionnaire, on affective support, mediated through the LMS Blackboard Learn, in engineering students at the level of undergraduate degree at a private university in Peru in times of Covid-19, using the PLS-SEM methodology, which is a multivariate method called Modeling of Structural Equations with Partial Least Squares. The results obtained from the exploratory and confirmatory factorial analysis, has allowed to corroborate that the most important factor in collaboration as a basis for meaningful learning is affective support, in which affective/cognitive mediations are established between students.

Keywords: Collaborative learning · Affective support · COLLES · Blackboard learn · PLS-SEM

1 Introduction

Social isolation as a consequence of Covid-19, has forced educational institutions of different levels and modalities in Peru as in other countries [1], to implement contingency measures and adaptation of educational models based on face-to-face to eminently virtual or online systems. Thus, overnight, universities, in order not to suspend their academic teaching activities, implement various teaching-learning strategies, based on virtual environments for learning, in such a way that the Learning Management System (LMS) are no longer seen as an alternative option for incorporation into educational models, but rather as an imperative need demanded by SUNEDU, as the supervisory body of the University System in Peru.

From these measures of exceptionality, the development of educational strategies based on collaboration, with synchronous and asynchronous activities is the main frame of reference for this study. The effectiveness of the use of digital tools in the academic development of university students, especially multimedia technologies, will make it

© The Author(s), under exclusive license to Springer Nature Singapore Pte Ltd. 2022
Á. Rocha et al. (Eds.): ICOMTA 2021, SIST 259, pp. 458–468, 2022.
https://doi.org/10.1007/978-981-16-5792-4_45

possible to improve work in the classroom and from these experiences the construction of collaborative learning [2].

An online learning environment not only promotes collaboration and participation among its participants, it improves from interaction, communication between students and professors, a proactive attitude, feedback within groups. [3] and an improvement in student grades.

The structure of LMS such as Blackboard Learn and its Mobile mode are designed to promote collaborative learning anytime, anywhere [4], in the same way, social networks, WhatsApp and other communication-based tools are included. [5], and within these ecosystems mediated for collaboration, it will be the «digitally competent» professor who will implement didactic strategies to teach and students will develop strategies to learn, taking into account social and cultural conditions, from the constructivist approach [6].

On the other hand, the level of adaptation of students in university life implies the identification of internal and external factors for a successful transition from secondary education to university, especially in professional architecture and engineering careers [7].

In this process of adapting from school to university, the management of various online learning situations is very important, this from the construction of meanings through 4 key elements in a constructivist virtual environment, such as the "situation", "cooperation", "conversation" and "construction of meanings" [8], based on this concept, Taylor and Maor [9] devised a survey to obtain data about experiences in an online learning environment based on constructivist theories: Constructivist On-Line Learning Environment Survey (COLLES). The 24-item Likert-type instrument allows examining the quality of learning experiences in 6 factors: Relevance, which allows highlighting the importance of online learning in professional practices [10]; Reflective Thinking, stimulates critical and reflective thinking through online learning; Interactivity, which allows participation, dialogue, feedback and interactivity with available technological resources; Tutor Support, allows evaluating how well tutors or professors participate actively in the generation of meaningful learning for students; The Interpretation explains how students and professors or tutors, understand the online communications of others and Affective Support, is the most important factor that supports the constructivist dimension of education for online learning, based on a sensitive and encouraging support [11].

Interactivity, for its part, is one of the key success factors in the teaching-learning process in distance education, undoubtedly interactivity is seen as a variable that influences motivation and with it the commitment of students towards the study [12], thus, improving digital skills that allow educational socialization [13]. Interpretation from an approach centered on constructivist epistemology requires taking into account five levels of learning: learning, learning to learn, learning to unlearn, learning to relearn and learning new ways of learning.[14]. The development of social skills and critical-reflective thinking, a key and fundamental aspect, can be generated from different teaching and learning strategies, one of them with an emphasis on collaboration is artistic education that promotes social integration based on artistic narratives [15]. The relevance that allows highlighting the importance and meaning of online learning, experiences such as teaching in the times of Covid-19, allows new formats of social interaction, based on protocols that specify the available communication channels, connection times synchronous and any other relevant information, activity or learning situation [16]. Socio-educational practices constitute one of the axes of collaborative learning, where the exchange of knowledge of the members invites them to build a series of actions that allow achieving the established goals [17], therefore, the support of the tutor plays a determining role as a mediator and facilitator of the different learning situations. Regarding peer support, it is the central axis of affective/cognitive mediations in educational constructivism mediated by ICT.

Taking the previous considerations, the following hypotheses are formulated:

- **H1.** Interactivity has a positive effect on affective support
- **H2.** Interpretation has a positive effect on affective support
- **H3.** Reflective thinking has a positive effect on affective support
- **H4.** Relevance has a positive effect on affective support
- **H5.** Tutor support has a positive effect on affective support.

2 Methodology

The objective of the research was to determine the influence of the different factors of the COLLES [18] with Affective Support (AC), using Blackboard Learn, which is an LMS environment that enables the development of educational activities for collaborative learning, thus, the COLLES dimensions are based on the social aspects of the collaborative dimension of constructivist thought, these are: Relevance (RE); Reflective Thinking (PR); Interactivity (INT); Tutor Support (AT) and Interpretation (INT_PRE).

The study was carried out with 200 students from the professional careers of Mechanical, Electrical, Civil, Mechatronic and Commercial engineering of the Catholic University of Santa María in the Arequipa region in Peru, being 69% men and 31% women, whose ages are between 16 and 22 years old. The total mean was 18,685 (SD = 1,561). The instrument was applied in September 2020 in a state of health emergency.

3 Results

The research is causal that will allow to establish the influence of the factors: Relevance, Reflective Thinking, Interactivity, Tutor Support and Interpretation, with Affective Support this because this factor determines the support and collaboration between the agents of education involved as they are the students and professors.

Within the initial exploratory analysis, the internal consistency of the instrument was evaluated for this, the data were processed in the IBM-SPSS, of the instrument with the 24 items, whose reliability result is expressed in Crombach's Alpha and was 0.928 i.e. excellent.

As part of the procedure used, the Confirmatory Factor Analysis (CFA) was used to establish the coupling level of the factors, the KMO test and the Bartlett sphericity test were used, through the Rotated Component Analysis. (ACR) in order to analyze the correlations between the different variables observed with the instrument. The KMO and Bartlett test yielded a Kaiser-Meyer-Olkin measure of sampling adequacy of 0.906, which is a very acceptable sampling adequacy for factor analysis. After checking the sample adequacy, the communalities were evaluated, which are the sum of the factorial weights squared for each of the rows, these indicate the proportion of the variance explained by the common factors for each variable. From the analysis, it is observed that the different exogenous latent factors or variables present communalities that oscillate between 0.566 and 0.817, which means that in the worst case the observed items would explain the model in 56.6% and in the best of 81.7% of the cases would explain the model.

Regarding Table 1, the rotated component matrix is presented, it is also noted that the items are grouped into six factors according to the theoretical construct that is based on the COLLES, while the accumulated variance would be explained by 72.101%.

Table 1. Rotated component matrix [A].

	Components					
	1	2	3	4	5	6
RE_01				0.662		
RE_02				0.801		
RE_03				0.737		
RE_04				0.705		
PR_01					0.665	
PR_02					0.797	
PR_03						0.567
PR_04					0.764	
INT_01			0.777			
INT_02			0.845			
INT_03			0.763			
INT_04			0.701			
AT_01		0.751				
AT_02		0.775				
AT_03		0.795				
AT_04		0.816				
AC_01	0.783					
AC_02	0.826					
AC_03	0.845					
AC_04	0.777					
INT_PRE_01	0.563					

(*continued*)

Table 1. (*continued*)

	Components					
	1	2	3	4	5	6
INT_PRE_02	0.634					
INT_PRE_03		0.730				
INT_PRE_04		0.707				

TO Rotation method: Varimax with Kaiser normalization

For validation of the structural model, the PLS-SEM was used, not only because it is appropriate for exploratory research, but also for confirmatory [19]. The PLS-SEM mainly focuses on the interaction between prediction and theoretical tests, and the results must be validated [20]. The SmartPLS (v.3.3.3) was used to evaluate the structural model, that is, if all the required criteria are met.

To determine the assessment of the measurement model for common factor reflective constructs, the criterion of individual reliability of the indicator was used, accepting as the desired threshold in external loads values equal to or greater than $\lambda \geq 0.707$, this indicates that the construct explains more than 50 percent of the variance of the indicator, thus providing an acceptable reliability of the item [21]. Table 2 shows the values obtained, and it is observed that the items INT_PRE_03 and INT_PRE_04 would not meet the desired threshold, the others are reliable.

Table 2. External loads - smart PLS.

	AC	AT	INT	INT_PRE	PR	RE
AC_01	0.834					
AC_02	0.906					
AC_03	0.914					
AC_04	0.886					
AT_01		0.889				
AT_02		0.868				
AT_03		0.863				
AT_04		0.889				
INT_01			0.852			
INT_02			0.845			
INT_03			0.871			
INT_04			0.905			
INT_PRE_01				0.824		
INT_PRE_02				0.878		

(*continued*)

Table 2. (*continued*)

	AC	AT	INT	INT_PRE	PR	RE
INT_PRE_03				**0.55**		
INT_PRE_04				**0.573**		
PR_01					0.768	
PR_02					0.738	
PR_03					0.748	
PR_04					0.742	
RE_01						0.704
RE_02						0.789
RE_03						0.861
RE_04						0.84

In the analysis of construct reliability or internal consistency, this is performed through Cronbach's Alpha ≥ 0.7, Composite Reliability (ρc) ≥ 0.7 and Dijkstra-Henseler's (ρA) ≥ 0.7 [22]. Regarding the Convergent Validity criterion, the Average Extracted Variance (AVE) was used, the values should be ≥ 0.5, this indicates that the construct explains at least 50% of the variance of its elements, as shown in Table 3; therefore, the result is satisfactory. However, the discussion today around the application of the PLS, it is recommended to use the coefficient (rho_A) to verify the reliability of the values obtained in the construction and design of the PLS-SEM.[23], the results obtained in (rho_A) should have values of 0.7 or higher to demonstrate compound reliability, the results obtained are between 0.783 and 0.915.

Table 3. Assessment of the measurement model for reflective constructs.

	Cronbach's alpha	rho_A	Composite reliability	Mean extracted variance (AVE)
Affective Support	0.908	0.915	0.936	0.784
Interactivity	0.892	0.907	0.925	0.755
Interpretation	0.719	0.811	0.806	0.52
Reflective Thinking	0.756	0.783	0.836	0.561
Relevance	0.816	0.854	0.877	0.641
Tutor Support	0.901	0.909	0.93	0.77

For the Discriminant Validity criterion of the model, which will allow to know to what extent the construct is different from other constructs or measures different things. In Table 4, according to the Fornell-Larcker criterion, there is discriminant validity [24].

Table 4. Fornell-Larcker criterion

	AC	IN	INT_PRE	PR	RE	AT
Affective Support	**0.886**					
Interactivity	0.671	**0.869**				
Interpretation	0.621	0.531	**0.721**			
Reflective Thinking	0.38	0.414	0.53	**0.749**		
Relevance	0.339	0.331	0.439	0.559	0.801	
Tutor Support	0.394	0.334	0.533	0.498	0.544	0.877

Another criterion to know the Discriminant Validity in reflective models is the so-called Heterotrait-Monotrait (HTMT) [25] and is defined as the mean value of the correlations of the elements between the constructs in relation to the (geometric) mean of the average correlations for the elements that measure the same construct [21]. The acceptance threshold should be in the following ratios $\leq 0.85 \leq\ 0.9$ Table 5.

Table 5. Heterotrait Criterion - Monotrait –HTMT.

	AC	IN	INT_PRE	PR	RE	AT
Affective Support						
Interactivity	0.734					
Interpretation	0.673	0.587				
Reflective Thinking	0.413	0.452	0.767			
Relevance	0.369	0.376	0.621	0.72		
Tutor Support	0.43	0.365	0.787	0.593	0.628	

For the evaluation of the structural model, the standard evaluation criteria such as Crombach's alpha and the coefficient of determination (R^2) were used, therefore, the coefficients of the structural model for the relationships between the constructions are derived from the estimation of a series of regression equations.

Crombach's alpha, which ensures that the sample studied adequately interpreted the items of the questionnaire. The reliability and internal consistency of the measured factors should express values greater than 0.7 to be considered acceptable. Figure 1 presents the results of the internal consistency of the model.

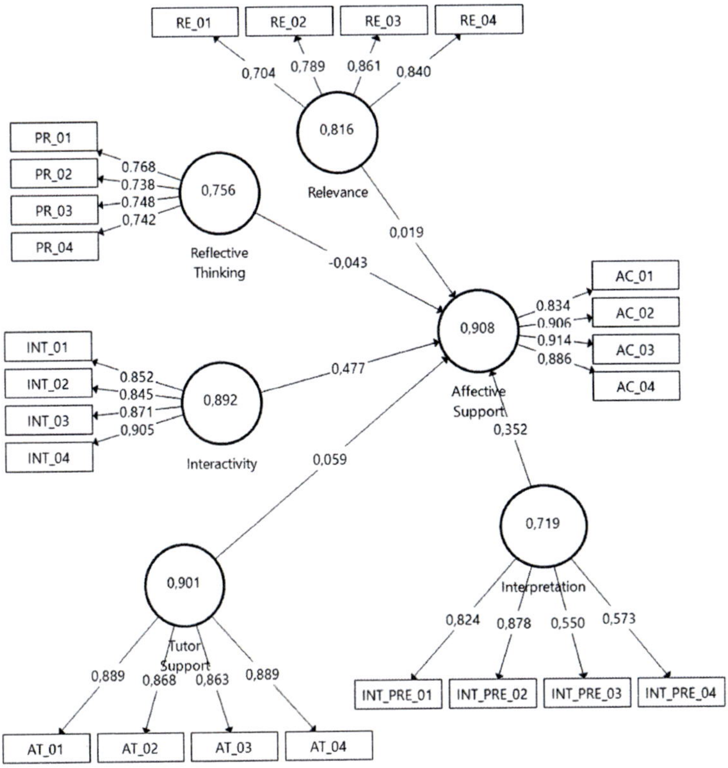

Fig. 1. Model Crombach alpha - Smartpls.

Figure 2 is a graphic representation of the reliability and validity analysis of the model, based on the R2 (determination coefficient), for the Affective Support (AC) variable, according to the data obtained, the R2 has a value of 0.552 which shows that 55.2% of the variance is explained by the proposed model.

This study focused especially on the level of influence of the COLLES questionnaire factors on the Affective Support factor, the latter acting as an endogenous or dependent variable, in such a way that the model would test the influence of latent variables: Interactivity, Interpretation, Reflective Thinking, Relevance and Tutor Support. Table 6 shows the results of the Bootstrapping, and how the model variables were hypothesized, therefore, considering the P Value ($p < 0.05$), the hypotheses H1 and H2 are admitted and the H3, H4 and H5 hypotheses are rejected.

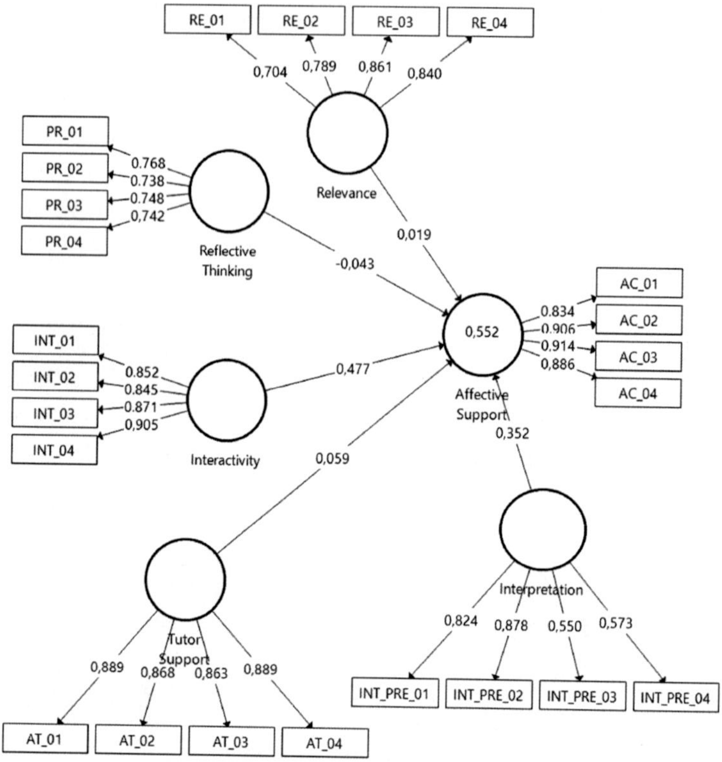

Fig. 2. Model R^2 - SmartPLS.

Table 6. Bootstrapping test results.

	Original sample (O)	Sample mean (M)	Standard deviation (STDEV)	Statistics t (| O/STDEV |)	P Value
(H1) Interactivity - > Affective Support	0.477	0.475	0.066	7,241	0.000
(H2) Interpretation - > Affective Support	0.352	0.354	0.07	5,047	0.000
(H3) Reflective Thinking - > Affective Support	−0.043	−0.036	0.063	0.686	**0.493**
(H4) Relevance - > Affective Support	0.019	0.02	0.062	0.301	**0.764**
(H5) Tutor Support - > Affective Support	0.059	0.058	0.062	0.944	**0.345**

4 Conclusions

The results obtained from the exploratory and confirmatory factor analysis, applying the PLS-SEM methodology, in the homologation and validation of the Constructivist On-Line Learning Environment Survey (COLLES), in the use of the LMS Blackboard Learn as an online learning environment in engineering students, has corroborated that the most important factor in collaboration as the basis of meaning learning is peer support, in which affective/cognitive mediations are established between students. The research model allowed to verify the influence of the interactivity factor and the interpretation in the support factor for classmates, however, the reflective thinking factors, relevance and the support of the tutor do not influence Peer Support from learning experiences in a virtual environment, based on theories of social constructivism. The designed model taking into account the determination coefficient, based on the variance, would explain by 55.2% the relationship of the latent variables and their level of influence on the endogenous variable, such as the Peer Support factor, which is the one that It can better explain the dimension of collaborative learning, as an essential foundation in the different learning situations based on e-learning.

References

1. Shrestha, R., Shrestha, S., Acharya, A., Gupta, A.: Online Education Status at Dental Colleges During COVID-19 Pandemic in Nepal. Kathmandu Univ Med J, 15–20 (2020)
2. Álvarez-Flores, E., Núñez Gómez, P.: Efectividad del USO de herramientas digitales en el desarrollo académico de estudiantes universitarios. Alfabetización Informacional para la gestión del conocimiento en la Universidad Universidad Estatal de Sonora, México DF (2019)
3. Almenara, J.C., Del Prete, A., Muñoz, M.L.A.: Percepciones de estudiantes universitarios chilenos sobre uso de redes sociales y trabajo colaborativo. RIED. Rev. Iberoamericana de Educación a Distancia; Vol. 22, Núm. 2 (2019): Monográfico. Las redes sociales en educación: desde la innovación a la investigación educativaDO (2019). https://doi.org/10.5944/ried.22.2.22847
4. Li, X.: Students' acceptance of mobile learning: an empirical study based on blackboard mobile learn. In: Mobile Devices in Education: Breakthroughs in Research and Practice. IGI Global, pp. 354–373 (2020)
5. Padrón, C.J.: Teaching strate gies based on what sapp instant messaging applicati ons only for phones (mobile learning) and its use to promote collaborative learning. EDUWEB-Revista de Tecnología de Información y Comunicación en Educación **7**(2) (2013)
6. Engen, B.: Understanding social and cultural aspects of teachers' digital competencies. Comunicar **61**, 9–19 (2019). https://doi.org/10.3916/C61-2019-01
7. Duche-Perez, A.B., Paredes-Quispe, F.M., Gutierrez-Aguilar, O.A.: The transition from high school to university: identifying internal and external factors for a successful transition in peruvian students of architecture and engineering. In: EDUNINE 2019 - 3rd IEEE World Engineering Education Conference: Modern Educational Paradigms for Computer and Engineering Career, Proceedings 2019 (2019)
8. Li, O., Li, X.: On line teaching mode of college english based on smart classroom in epidemic situation. In: 2020 International Conference on Big Data and Informatization Education (ICBDIE), 23–25 April 2020, pp. 302–305 (2020)
9. Taylor, P.C., Maor, D.: The Constructivist On-Line Learning Environment Survey (COLLES). Curtin University of Technology, Perth, Western Australia. In (2009)

10. Azhari, F.A., Jasmi, N.N., Abd Wahab, M.S., Jofrry, S.M., Lee, S., Ming, L.C.: Students' perceptions about social constructivist learning environment in e-learning. Indian J. Pharmaceutical Educ. **54**(2), 271–278 (2020)
11. Taylor, P.C., Maor, D.: The Constructivist On-Line Learning Environment Survey (COLLES). Curtin University of Technology, Pert, Australia (2000)
12. Rodríguez, N.D.A., Osuna, J.M.B.: La interactividad en la educación a distancia: un instrumento para su diagnóstico. Rev. Fuentes **22**(2), 190–202 (2020)
13. Gutiérrez-Aguilar, O., Salas-Valdivia, L.: Collaborative learning: the educational perspective of facebook. In: Proceedings - 14th Latin American Conference on Learning Technologies, LACLO 2019, pp. 348–352 (2019)
14. Levy, A.: La construcción del conocimiento y las decisiones estratégicas: Un enfoque constructivista de la dinámica estratégica-operacional. Rev. de Investigación en Modelos Financieros **1**, 1–17 (2020)
15. Solier, P.M.S., Arenas, B.S.S.: Desarrollo de habilidades sociales y pensamiento crítico-reflexivo a través de la perfomance, instalación artística y vídeo-creación en el grado de educación primaria. In: Congreso Internacional de Investigación e innovación en educación infantil y primaria (2020)
16. Rapoport, S., Tablado, M.S.R., Bressanello, M.: Enseñar en tiempos de COVID-19: una guía teórico-práctica para docentes. In. UNESCO (2020)
17. Silvestrini, M.P., Barragán, P., Sánchez, D., Marín, G.H.: Percepción de los estudiantes sobre las prácticas socioeducativas en un curso de Medicina UNICEN. In: III Jornadas sobre las Prácticas Docentes en la Universidad Pública (Edición en línea, junio de 2020) (2020)
18. Baker, J.: Constructivist online learning environment survey. In: Handbook of Research on Electronic Surveys and Measurements. IGI Global, pp. 299–301 (2007)
19. Hair Jr, J.F., Sarstedt, M., Ringle, C.M., Gudergan, S.P.: Advanced issues in partial least squares structural equation modeling. saGe publications (2017)
20. Shmueli, G.: To explain or to predict? Stat. Sci. **25**(3), 289–310 (2010)
21. Joseph, F.H., Jeffrey, J.R., Sarstedt, M., Christian, M.R.: When to use and how to report the results of PLS-SEM. Eur. Bus. Rev. **31**(1), 2–24 (2019). https://doi.org/10.1108/EBR-11-2018-0203
22. Hair, J.F., Hult, G.T.M., Ringle, C.M., Sarstedt, M., Apraiz, J.C., Carrión, G.C., Roldán, J.L.: Manual de partial least squares structural equation modeling (pls-sem). OmniaScience Scholar, España (2019)
23. Dijkstra, T.K., Henseler, J.: Consistent partial least squares path modeling. MIS quarterly 39(2) (2015)
24. Fornell, C., Larcker, D.F.: Evaluating structural equation models with unobservable variables and measurement error. J. Mark. Res. **18**(1), 39–50 (1981)
25. Henseler, J., Ringle, C.M., Sarstedt, M.: A new criterion for assessing discriminant validity in variance-based structural equation modeling. J. Acad. Mark. Sci. **43**(1), 115–135 (2014). https://doi.org/10.1007/s11747-014-0403-8

Factors that Influence Media Competence of Female Streamers Audiences During the Covid-19 Pandemic

Valeria Smilzinia Párraga Chávez(✉) and Victor Omar Vite León

Universidad Peruana de Ciencias Aplicadas, Lima 15023, Peru
{u201411588,pcavvvit}@upc.edu.pe

Abstract. With the arrival of the pandemic, people of all ages have found an alternative in video games to distract themselves. Additionally, streaming (live streaming of game sessions) became a way to earn income from home for creators. This type of content became part of the digital media diet of video game fans, who established a close relationship with streamers and generated different dynamics ranging from the publication of positive comments to strong rejection. Despite the implementation of rules regulating the behavior of streamers on platforms such as Twitch and Facebook, they are not able to control some irregularities, like monitoring negative comments or sexual innuendo during live streams. This has initiated various debates about the correct use of these media that gather people of all ages, from children to adults. In order to know consumers' points of view, two focus groups were carried out (one with 8 women and another with 14 men) in order to find out the factors that influence the media competence of female streamers' audience. The study addresses two dimensions: languages and ideology and values. In the languages dimension, although women are aware of harassment, they consider that a person has freedom of behavior during a stream. Men, meanwhile, consider that the way women show themselves in front of the camera allows them to generate money. In the ideology and values dimension, women believe that a female streamer's behavior should not be questioned or criticized as long as it respects the rules of the community. On the other hand, men consider that the rules are interpreted subjectively, but they are aware that without these practices, the Facebook Gaming platform would not have economic income. To sum up, women take more into account the human side of people who stream while men view these behaviors as a business.

Keywords: Communication · Media competence · Video game · Streaming

1 Introduction

1.1 Media Competence

Audiovisual communication, currently, has a much greater relevance because it is part of people's daily lives; it is present in cell phones, televisions, computers, video games, etc. [1].

© The Author(s), under exclusive license to Springer Nature Singapore Pte Ltd. 2022
Á. Rocha et al. (Eds.): ICOMTA 2021, SIST 259, pp. 469–478, 2022.
https://doi.org/10.1007/978-981-16-5792-4_46

Umberto Eco said, in 1977, that "a democratic civilization will save itself only if it makes the language of the image into a stimulus for critical reflection and not an invitation for hypnosis" In other words, if a person simply consumes content without really understanding what they are witnessing, they will be unaware of the message that is trying to be delivered, which would be a symptom of an absence of digital and media literacy [10].

The definition of competence was, from the beginning, related to the business world. It gradually became a concept used in education and is now part of the vocabulary of all humans. Competence is the combination of knowledge, skills and attitudes that are necessary in a specific context [5].

In the case of the term *dimension*, it is defined as "each of the magnitudes of a set that serves to define a phenomenon" (Diccionario de la Real Academia Española, n.d).

Media communication does not only occur through the delivery of a message from a sender to a receiver, but through a chain complemented by dimensions [5]. Therefore, media competence is the ability to consume and produce media content from a critical, analytical and responsible point of view, in which we will perceive whether what we see and do is ethically correct [5]. In addition, media competence helps to perceive, analyze and enjoy the power of messages, images, stimuli and sounds perceived from the media [3]. This competence has six dimensions from the field of expression and analysis: languages, technology, interaction processes, production and diffusion processes, ideology and values, and aesthetics [5].

The language dimension includes knowledge of codes, ability to use them and to analyze written and audiovisual messages from the perspective of sense and meaning, narrative structures, and categories and genres. The ideology and values dimension includes the capacity for comprehensive and critical reading, critical analysis and an attitude to select media messages, as representations of reality [6].

1.2 Video Games

The isolation generated by the COVID-19 pandemic has increased the consumption of video game streaming at home, due to the fact that health authorities do not advise outdoor physical activities [8]. However, with more options to be distracted at home, the number of people playing and consuming media content has increased exponentially [9].

According to Esports Charts, Twitch had an increase of almost 100%, with an average of 2.2 million viewers just a few days after the lockdown began. Not only did viewers increase, but also stream viewing hours increased by 37%, live streaming hours increased by 26.1% and the percentage of new streamers increased by 29.3%. [2] Although they were platforms with a predominantly male presence, this new situation increased the presence of women [4].

In 2017, a female young streamer named Nyakkj was banned on Twitch for masturbating in front of millions of spectators [12]. Since then, the platform has tried to tighten its rules to avoid similar situations. However, it was not until April 2020, when the presence of female streamers increased, that the rules against sexual content were tightened. Twitch threatened mass bans if its terms and conditions, including dress and behavior codes, were ignored [16].

"Sexually Suggestive Content: To maintain the health of our community and promote content that is appropriate for a diverse audience, sexually suggestive content is prohibited on Twitch. Evaluations on the sexual suggestiveness of a behavior or activity are independent of user attire and are instead based on the overall surrounding framing and context. This policy also applies to embedded media, augmented reality, creative broadcasts, and channel content—such as banners, profile images, emotes, and panels—that are focused on provocative images or video. Content that is considered to be sexually suggestive includes, but is not limited to: Content or camera focus on breasts, buttocks, or pelvic region, including poses that deliberately highlight these elements." [16].

Consequently, consumers of this type of content migrated to the Facebook Gaming application, in order not to lose contact with these creators.

In 2020, Facebook Gaming reached 439 million hours of streaming and 201 million hours seen by viewers [7]. Although they implemented rules against sexual content, from the point of view of its consumers, Facebook has not been so strict, thus this type of content has been normalized and cases of harassment by anonymous users towards female streamers did not disappear completely. A remarkable fact is the increase of investment or donations from the audience to these streamers, who have taken advantage of the lockdown to profit from their hobby. Nevertheless, this content is not always socially accepted. On Facebook Gaming, women usually get more attention than men, either negatively or positively. This includes the imminent image people may have of a female streamer, as it comes to sexualize her and creates doubts about her abilities as a gamer [11].

Male Gaze on Streaming: There is a term called "male gaze". This concept was proposed by Laura Mulvey, who commented that cinema determined the erotic as patriarchal [14] In other words, certain acts performed by women, but not by men, could be seen as sexy, turning them into sexual objects. She also explained the "role" of men in women's lives. She commented that they become heroes in a woman's life and that she has enough power to cause anxiety in a man's life, leading him to do things that satisfy or save a woman [14]. For the purposes of this study, men would be considered to make monetary transactions to these female streamers who would recognize them as their heroes, since they are being saved from the misery that has led them to look for a way to generate income through live video game streaming. Added to this are certain attitudes so that the viewer cannot resist the visual treatment, such as placing the camera 50% higher than men [15] to, most times, show their pronounced breast cleavage and generate sexual attraction [13]. In reward for the transaction, they give men a show that may involve sexy dances, suggestive sounds, among other behaviors of sexual connotation. All these attitudes in front of the camera will arouse men who will continue to donate because, as Mulvey herself stated, women see themselves as a sexual object and men always want to see more and receive something in return [14].

2 Methodology

2.1 Type of Research, Techniques and Objectives

This research is qualitative. It sought to find the factors that influence the media competence of female streamers' audience during the COVID-19 pandemic. The technique used was the focus group.

The specific objectives are the following:

- What are the factors that influence the languages dimension?
- What are the factors that influence the ideology and values dimension?

2.2 Object of Study, Interest and Justification

The object of study of this research is media competence. Two focus groups were carried out: one with 8 women and another with 14 men, all of them of legal age, Peruvians, consumers of streams.

1. W1, 24 years old. Bachelor of Engineering
2. W2, 23 years old. Bachelor of Marketing and International Business
3. W3, 24 years old. Bachelor of Advertising
4. W4, 23 years old. Psychology student
5. W5, 24 years old. Bachelor of Translation
6. W6, 22 years old. Law student
7. W7, 20 years old. Audiovisual Communication and Interactive Media student
8. W8, 19 years old. International Business and Administration student

The men participating in the study were the following:

1. M1, 25 years old. Bachelor of Audiovisual Communication and Interactive Media
2. M2, 25 years old. Bachelor of Psychology
3. 4M3, 24 years old. Systems Engineering student
4. M4, 27 years old. Learning Experience Advisor
5. M5, 24 years old. Manager of a Family-owned Fumigation Company
6. M6, 30 years old. Manager of a Pizza Restaurant
7. M7, 28 years old. Dealer
8. M8, 21 years old. Bachelor of Advertising and Community Manager
9. M9, 22 years old. International Business and Administration student
10. M10, 21 years old. Audiovisual Communication and Interactive Media student
11. M11, 25 years old. Bachelor of Audiovisual Communication and Interactive Media
12. M12, 23 years old. Audiovisual Communication and Interactive Media student
13. M13, 20 years old. Audiovisual Communication and Interactive Media student
14. M14, 19 years old. Audiovisual Communication and Interactive Media student

The units of analysis are the language and ideology and values dimensions of media competence. The unit of observation is the audience of female streamers who engage in sexually connoted behaviors during their streams on Facebook Gaming.

The dimensions and questions addressed in the focus group were the following:

Languages:

- What impression do you think female streamers' followers have of them?
- What do you think of the way female streamers celebrate every time they receive a donation?
- Have you ever seen a stream by the thumbnail? Why?
- What do you think about the framing of the stream? (High-angle, low-angle, close-up, etc.)
- Mention 3 reasons why you think male streamers are watched.
- Mention 3 reasons why you think female streamers are watched.

Ideology and Values:

- Do you know Facebook Gaming rules? What do you think of Facebook Gaming rules? Do you think they are respected?
- According to Facebook Gaming rules, there is a dress code. What do you think about this rule? Why? What would you do to ensure its fulfillment?
- What do you think about female streamers' behavior during their streams?

3 Results

3.1 Languages

Regarding the impression of men and women who follow female streamers, men participating in this research said that viewers' perception of women with sexual behaviors depends on the age and level of maturity of each. Subject M3 mentioned that they are perceived as unattainable people or, mainly, a fantasy. Moreover, subject H8 added that it depends on the subjectivity of each user regarding what he may think of them. He said that sometimes male audience sees these women in a sexy way or with intentions of having something more if money is invested in them. The latter complemented the opinion of women in our focus group, since W3 believed that young men who try to stand out by performing a transaction want, in some cases, to have any sexual relationship with these female streamers. Additionally, most women commented that boys' expectations of female streamers are based on the image they want to project.

W4 and W8 subjects considered the type of content displayed on streams are meant to be commercial. In this category, there are women who decide to profit with their body, since they consider that staying in this area of video games is very difficult when your gameplay does not have a high performance, so entertaining with sexual behaviors becomes a business strategy. On the other side, subjects W1 and W4 commented, from their own experience, that people, at some point, had harassed them during their streams anonymously and for sexual purposes, which is strange for them since, according to them, at no time did they insinuate that their contents were of that type.

Regarding the way female streamers celebrate each time they receive a donation, subject M3 mentioned that people could not be naive. He considered that every action performed in a stream was deliberate. This response was supported by most men during the focus group, as they agreed that every female streamer thinks well when performing their response to any big or small donation and that little things like this are part of a marketing strategy. They did not think it was wrong to do it and in the focus group, they did not express any discomfort. However, women did feel uncomfortable as they considered that consumers of this type of content expect similar celebrations from every girl they can find on the platform.

Subject M8 recognized that, due to the increased presence of women on the platform, the type of streamers is very varied and commented that if there is a "quiet" streamer, she will not attract attention like a young girl who celebrates or behaves in a scandalous way. To reaffirm this idea, M3 recounted the case of a female streamer who claimed that boys are obliged to invest money in her because she is a woman who streams content that a male audience likes.

Regarding whether the participants had seen any video through the thumbnail, M3 commented that he is used to always seeing this kind of thumbnails on Facebook Gaming. In his opinion, such images or misleading titles would cause a child or minor to enter into the stream, because during this phase, people are discovering their own sexuality. M6 mentioned that depending on the thumbnail and how suggestive it could be, the same gamers could detect if it is a girl who really plays or only profits with her body. In the case of M7, he confessed that he had seen some videos through the thumbnail; however, he only needs 10 s in the stream to decide whether to stay or change to another video as he easily detects the content presented.

In the case of women, they mentioned that they had clicked on some videos because of the titles. W3 commented that she had found a video entitled "I play with the same fingers I get rid of boogers", which she thought was fun. Meanwhile, W2 admitted to having watched a streamer that had a very pronounced cleavage during her stream. However, what called her attention was that she was wearing a ski mask because she had had a plastic surgery, but since she was forced to stream, she had to find a way to give a show. W5 said she had watched a streamer because she was dressed up in her favorite cosplay. This confirms that the thumbnail is important to attract the attention of the potential consumer.

Regarding the participants' opinion about the framing used in the streams (High-angle, low-angle, close-up, etc.), men reacted with irony, except for subject M2. He commented that female streamers are aware of their attributes (referring to their body parts that stand out the most, either their butt or breasts); for that reason, these women will try to get attention with their body rather than with their gameplay, thus, it becomes part of the common aesthetics of a female streamer. In the case of women, and relating it to the male gaze, breasts were sexualized so now, these female streamers take advantage of them to turn on or excite men. W7 also mentioned that it is not only the framing that attracts the attention on a live stream, but also the aesthetics behind it, whether it is the clothing, the elements that make up the space or set up and even the same attitude of the female streamer.

Regarding the reasons why the participants in the focus group follow male streamers, they highlighted the skills and sense of humor of male streamers. Thus, M4 commented that male streamers are watched for their gameplay (very good or excellent), because viewers had some encounter with them either in some games or casually on the platforms or because they know them in person (either out of friendship or because he is a mere acquaintance). M13 mentioned that he saw male streamers because they were charismatic, jokers and have skills when playing games. In the case of women, W4 mentioned that male streamers are watched because they play well, they may be famous, so they become streamers, or because they participate in tournaments. W1 mentioned that they are watched for their gameplay, because they are funny, talented and have contact with other famous streamers.

Regarding the reasons why participants consider that female streamers are watched, both for men and women, physical attractiveness (beauty) plays an important role, followed by their talent for the game. M12 said that female streamers are watched because they are beautiful, have a good body, are charismatic, play well and handle sexual attraction as a business model. M1 believed that they have a particular way of celebrating transactions, play well and are charismatic. Meanwhile, W1 commented that she watched them because they are pretty, funny and entertain their audience; for W2, they are sexy, pretty and funny and dress up with cosplay. W4 said they are watched for their clothing, because they are beautiful and may have "extreme" behaviors or rather, with sexual connotations.

3.2 Ideology and Values

They were also asked about their knowledge of Facebook Gaming rules. W3 and W5 mentioned not knowing the rules. W1, meanwhile, considered that the rules are not always respected since the platform is very permissive about sexual behaviors, unlike Twitch where the ban is almost immediate. However, W2 believed that the rules are respected by streamers, but that the euphoria of the moment can cause slips in their behavior. In the case of men, M2 mentioned that Facebook Gaming, more than rules, has terms and conditions that just nobody reads and blindly accepts them without thinking about the consequences. M3 considered that the rules are ambiguous so understanding them will always be subjective. Finally, M7 believed that due to consumer pressure within the platform and the respect expected to have for the community, those who ignore them are starting to be banned.

Regarding the dress code, W1, W7 and W8 considered that these rules are not followed and compared the situation of Twitch where accounts can be suspended at the first violation, regardless of its scope. M13 commented that understanding a dress code is subjective, as each person has a different interpretation of fashion. M3 also agreed and further mentioned that if Facebook Gaming bans many streamers, the platform will be left without brands willing to invest. He explained that it is a business where debauchery and freedom of expression prevail.

Finally, regarding the behavior of female streamers, in the focus group of women, W1 commented that everyone is free to do whatever they want to earn money as long as there is no pressure, and their tactics must depend on the target audience. W2 supported women with this behavior as she knows it is a marketing strategy. She would like that women weren't sexualized, but she also mentioned that each person would face the consequences of their actions. W3 believed that girls' behavior is very ambiguous, it depends on who looks at them to judge whether it is right or wrong, but there must always be a deep respect for the consumer. W4 considered herself neutral, neither in favor nor against these behaviors as long as there is respect for the viewer. W5 considered that she did not judge anyone, but was sure that if a man had this type of behavior, he would not receive as many hateful comments as a woman. Both genres are working, having fun, and should not be underestimated. W6 disagreed with the content. She did not judge, but did not accept it. She considered, for example, that men's curse words are worse, but in girls, it is funny. Despite this, she did not like the content. She felt uncomfortable about the feedback female streamers get from their audience. W7 considered that it is fine that female streamers have the freedom to do what they want, but she found it wrong that harassment is suffered even outside the screen (either in this as in other social networks) and disapproved that there is no regulation, because even children are exposed to this content that would lead them to skip stages in which decency should be important. Finally, W8 mentioned that, due to her upbringing, such content is not to her liking. Even so, she did not despise women who engage in these behaviors with sexual connotation, but considered that these contaminate the platform.

In the case of men, M6 mentioned that these female streamers are business conscious and that if they want to do it through these celebrations and live performances, then they can do it. M6 also considered that if he were given money to show "meat" live for 20 min, he would do so as this money is income. M8 mentioned that anyone could earn money as they want, but they should recognize the way they are doing it, and M2 is neutral on this issue: he did not consider it wrong or right.

4 Conclusions

The isolation generated by the COVID-19 pandemic has increased the consumption of video game streaming at home, due to the fact that health authorities do not advise outdoor physical activities [8]. The findings produced on the dimensions of media competence showed that they could be contrasted and depend on the gender of the groups consulted. We can summarize the findings according to the dimensions of media competence studied (languages and ideology and values) in the following Table 1:

Table 1. Results Comparison. Own Elaboration.

Dimensions	Women	Men
Languages	What women understand about these behaviors with sexual connotations is mostly a free expression of each streamer, but that involves an unfortunate environment of harassment	Men understand that part of a successful business is directly related to how it is presented so visual and sound treatment is very important
Ideology and Values	The behavior that a streamer may have on a platform as large as Facebook Gaming should not be a reason for her to be harassed, nor insulted by anonymous people on the networks. However, it is important to respect the rules of each website and respect the public who tune in to these streams	They comment that Facebook community rules involving clothing, behaviors, among others, are subject to a personal interpretation. Likewise, they consider streaming is more than a form of entertainment, it is a way to generate incomes

To sum up, the study of the dimensions of media competence during the COVID-19 pandemic has exposed the existing prejudices in the gaming community about female streamers. On the one hand, the men interviewed pointed out that women view this type of behavior as personal marketing and a money-making strategy. On the other hand, the women interviewed commented that respect for female streamers depends on themselves and what they wanted to present to each other on a platform as big as Facebook Gaming; however, what is shown in networks should not be an excuse to qualify people or have a bias about who they are.

It remains for the present and future of this research to analyze the factors influencing the dimensions of media competence of female streamers' followers not addressed in this study: technology, interaction processes, production and dissemination processes, and aesthetics.

References

1. Aguaded-Gómez, J.: La competencia mediática, una acción educativa inaplazable. Comunicar, 7–8 (2012)
2. Antón, M.: eSports, 16 de Junio de 2020. Obtained from Marca: https://www.marca.com/esports/otros-juegos/2020/06/16/5ee87a2122601d762c8b458a.html
3. Comisión Europea. Study on the Current Trends and Approaches to Media Literacy in Europe (2010)
4. Cruz, E.: GameLR, 02 de Noviembre de 2020. Obtained from La República: https://larepublica.pe/tendencias/2020/11/02/chicas-gamers-demuestran-que-los-videojuegos-no-son-una-actividad-exclusiva-para-varones/?ref=lre
5. Ferrés, J., Piscitelli, A.: Competencia mediática: Propuesta articulada de dimensiones e indicadores. Comunicar, 75–82 (2012)

6. Mateus, J., Suárez-Guerrero, C.: La competencia TIC en el nuevo currículo peruano desde la perspectiva de la educación mediática. edmetic **6**(2), 129–147 (2017). https://doi.org/10.21071/edmetic.v6i2.6908, E-ISSN 2254-0059
7. Huerta, R.: Qore, 2021 de Marzo de 2021. Obtenido de Yahoo Finanzas: https://es-us.finanzas.yahoo.com/noticias/twitch-facebook-gaming-explotaron-vistas-233500688.html?guce_referrer=aHR0cHM6Ly93d3cuZ29vZ2xlLmNvbS8&guce_referrer_sig=AQAAAIR8jM8Fz6IASO6OOK5cKg6tfsP3vaG6KP_-lH6bwDTedYpqHmoN1uApiBr0vKxu5CZowI3km7hpRAKhWHKpnEYMK
8. Azócar-Gallardo, J., Ojeda-Aravena, A.: US National Library of Medicine, 21 de Enero de 2021. Obtenido de https://www.ncbi.nlm.nih.gov/pmc/articles/PMC7825857/
9. Montaña, M., Ollé, C., Lavilla, M.: Impacto de la pandemia de Covid-19 en el consumo de medios en España. Revista Latina de Comunicación Social, 155–167 (2020)
10. Gutiérrez, A., Tyner, K.: Educación para los medios, alfabetización. Comunicar, 31–39 (2012)
11. Nakandala, S., Luca, G., Makoto, N., Ahn, Y.-Y.: Cornell University, 22 de Noviembre de 2016. Obtenido de https://arxiv.org/abs/1611.06459v2
12. Padilla, L.: MasGamers, 13 de Noviembre de 2017. Obtained from https://www.masgamers.com/twitch-ban-streamer-masturbarse-vivo
13. Sibila, P.: La "pornificación" de la mirada: Una genealogía del pecho desnudo. Cuadernos de Música, Artes Visuales y Artes Escénicas, 35–63 (2015)
14. Mulvey, L.: Placer Visual y Cine Narrativo. Screen, 6–18 (1973)
15. Tifentale, A.: Selfiecity, Febrero de 2014. Obtained from http://selfiecity.net/#theory
16. Twitch. (s.f.). Obtained from https://www.twitch.tv/p/es-mx/legal/community-guidelines/sexualcontent/#:~:text=No%20permitimos%20bajo%20ninguna%20circunstancia,la%20parte%20inferior%20del%20busto

Diagnosis of Digital Teaching Competence: Universidad Viña del Mar

Kathya Oróstica Verdugo(✉) and Sebastián Herrera Peñaloza

Universidad Viña del Mar, Viña del Mar, Chile

Abstract. This article aims to diagnose the level of digital teaching competence of the professors of Universidad Viña de Mar, who develop teaching in various faculties of the institution. The data obtained were collected through a heading to assess the digital competence of university teachers adapted to the Latin American context, an instrument composed of four dimensions, and four indicators on levels of development. Overall results show that teachers with less work experience according to their age show greater mastery of expert and transformative levels. On the other hand, those teachers with more experience in teaching self-evaluate at the middle level and even beginner with respect to the dimensions. Considering that the instrument allows to measure the self-perception of digital competence, it can be concluded that university teachers recognize their lacks in relational, ethical and security dimensions and in personal and professional dimensions, in which the scores are below average. It is also necessary to develop training programs to strengthen digital teaching competences, currently indispensable for university teaching.

Keywords: Digital teaching skills · Evaluation · University teaching · Educational technology

1 Introduction

1.1 Digital Teaching Competition

The development of digital competence is now a necessity in higher education, not only because of the current context in which the Institutions of Higher Education (IES) had to transfer the teaching and learning processes to digital mode due to the massive confinement that affected all Latin American countries; but also because digital competition is key in training 21st century citizens to become personally and professionally part of a “digital society” [16, 17].

Likewise, the Digital Teaching Competence (CDD) transforms into a professional competence that university teachers must incorporate into their work, through the pedagogical, methodological and evaluative use of ICT resources. Because of this, several studies have been developed for more than a decade [5, 6] which express the importance of this topic. As Lazarus and Gisbert [11, 12] CDD argue, it is defined as “the need for teachers to possess a level of digital competence that allows them to use technology effectively, appropriately, adapted to their students and the learnings they must achieve”,

© The Author(s), under exclusive license to Springer Nature Singapore Pte Ltd. 2022
Á. Rocha et al. (Eds.): ICOMTA 2021, SIST 259, pp. 479–486, 2022.
https://doi.org/10.1007/978-981-16-5792-4_47

and Castañeda [2] reaffirms it, considering that "it is what a teacher must know to teach with technologies".

Other researches [5, 6] show the need to train digitally competent teachers for optimal insertion into educational processes and, in this context, frameworks and models are presented to allow us to understand the dimensions to be included in the teaching training, and generate inputs for the implementation plans that each institution requires through its curriculums [12, 14, 15]. Therefore, teachers need to develop a digital teaching competence that allows them to integrate ICTs in an original way, not only of acquiring instrumental knowledge, but also linking content, pedagogies and technologies [1], and allowing to act with responsibility, respecting the socially established standards and taking advantage of these tools to inform, learn, solve problems and communicate in different scenarios of interaction, allowing the teacher to be able to communicate such information through the use of different technological and digital media [15].

For these reasons, it is necessary to diagnose the level of digital teaching competence [9, 10, 12] to identify the level of digital teaching skills presented by academics in higher education. In this sense, it is intended to apply a diagnostic instrument to identify the levels of digital competence of teachers who perform in various random programs of Universidad Viña del Mar, Chile.

For this purpose, it is determined to apply the heading of self-perception of digital teaching competence [12] whose elaboration arises from theoretical references and international standards [8, 13, 16, 17] and, subsequently, adapts to the Latin American context to apply (higher education institutions [3, 4, 14, 15] with the purpose of measuring dimensions of teaching performance focused on digital skills, among which we identify Didactic, curricular and methodological, Planning, organization and management of spaces and digital technological, relational, ethics and security, and personal and professional resources [11].

With regard to the case of this study, which corresponds to Universidad Viña del Mar, private, regional and inclusive, the institution aims to collaborate in the development of the teaching skills of academics in function, since the institution considers it relevant to equip itself with innovative and well-trained teaching teams, so that they can become true drivers of methodological change for the improvement of the learnings of university students. Therefore, the purpose of this research will be to explore the CDD of teachers, through an evaluation rubric of the university teachers [12] to obtain results that allow to develop processes of improvement according to those aspects uneven that teachers present in the face of the dimensions of the digital teaching competence enunciated in the rubric.

2 Method

2.1 Research Design

The research was attached to a descriptive, non-experimental quantitative approach that aims to evaluate the CDD belonging to the faculties of Universidad Viña del Mar. The sample consisted of 50 teachers (55%) women and (45%) men. The majority are teaching in careers (53.1%) (46.9%) in academic units. Teaching experience from 1 to 3 years is (10%), 4 to 10 years (51%) 11 years or older (38.8%). (89%) has developed training or virtual teaching. (81%) respondents are between the age of 30 and 53, one (8.2%) 27 to 29 years old and (11.7%) 54 to 73 years old, with an average of 43.5 and standard deviation of 11.3K.

Therefore, the general objective of this research is to explore the levels of digital competence of the teachers of the Viña del Mar University, and the specific objectives of this research correspond to:

- **Objective 1:** Recognize the level of digital competence of teachers according to age.
- **Objective 2:** Recognize the level of digital competence of teachers according to their teaching experience.
- **Objective 3:** Determine the correlation between the dimensions of digital competence.

2.2 Instruments

The technique used was the survey and the data were collected in the application of an online questionnaire answered voluntarily and anonymously, through an evaluation rubric of the digital competence of university teachers adapted to the Latin American context, instrument composed of four dimensions and four indicators on levels of development. The first part is composed of personal data of teachers, followed by 4 dimensions with a total of 22 items. The dimensions are: Didactic, curricular, and methodological, Planning, organization and management of digital technological spaces and resources, Relational, Ethics and Security and Personal and Professional, with four levels of development from 1 to 4, beginner, medium, expert and transformer.

Various analyses were performed to examine the psychometric properties of the instrument. The internal consistency of the teaching digital competency scale, the Cronbach Alpha was 0.94.9, which indicates that the level of reliability is good. For the validity of construct an exploratory main component analysis was executed with the 22 items of the scale, 4 components were obtained with the varimax rotation. The 4 components account for 74.6% of the variance. THE KMO sample adequacy index was adequate (.824), as well as Bartlett's sphericity test, (153) x 553,949; $p < .000$. Similarly, the Kaiser-Meyer-Olkin (KMO) valued 0.877, the KMO is an indicator of the strength of the relationship between the variables, a value close to one indicates that factor analysis is possible because it indicates the existence of Inter correlation between variables.

3 Data Analysis

The IMB SPSS Statistics v20 software was used for statistical analysis of this study. The techniques used, given the objectives set out, were: descriptive, frequency, percentages, data reduction techniques (factorial analysis) and statistical inference (average comparison and percentages), working with a .0.5.

To begin this analysis, first the results obtained are presented in the following table, with the purpose of explaining how the data of the surveyed teachers were distributed. The indicators in the table correspond to the levels of teaching digital competence: beginner, medium, expert and transformer. The data of the teachers are divided into three groups characterized by the following names (Table 1):

- DJ_ young teacher
- DA adult teacher
- DAM senior adult teacher

Table 1. Distribution of participants by Dimension of Teaching Digital Competence

	Dimension 1 didactics			Dimension 2 planning			Dimension 3 relational			Dimension 4 personal		
	DJ	DA	DAM	DJ	DA	DAM	DJ	DA	DAM	DJ	DA	DAM
Beginner	0	12	1	0	12	3	0	6	2	1	20	2
Half	1	13	3	1	17	2	1	15	3	1	14	3
Expert	1	9	1	3	10	0	2	17	0	1	2	0
Transformer	2	6	0	0	1	0	1	2	0	1	4	0

In this table it can be identified that the highest scores are generated by the rank of adult teachers in the high categories, which can be better recognized in the following graphs (Fig. 1).

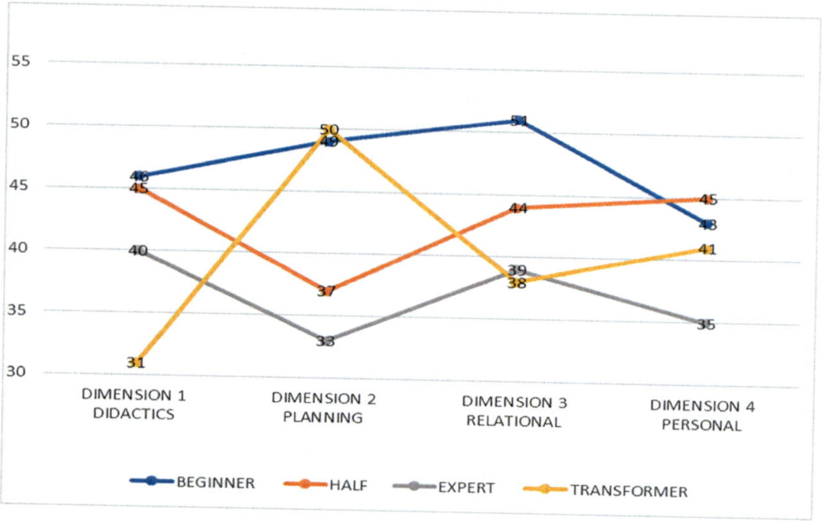

Fig. 1. Teaching digital competence graph by age

The graph identifies as the main variable the age of teachers in the development of digital competence. Regarding the Didactic, curricular and methodological dimension, it is appreciated that, at the youngest age of teachers, whose average is 31 years, achieves the transformative level in digital competence. Then 40-year-old teachers reach expert level and then between 45 and 46 years old are at the middle and beginner levels.

On the Dimension Planning, organization and management of digital technological resource spaces, there is a significant change when comparing with the Didactic dimension, because the predominant age of teachers reaching the transformative level corresponds to 50 years. However, close to that age range is the beginner level of this dimension, with teachers between the ages of 30 and 40 being at the middle and expert levels.

Regarding the Relational Dimension, ethics and digital security, it is identified that the transformative and expert levels are achieved in the range of 38 and 39 years and over 44 the medium and beginner levels are manifested.

Finally, the fourth Personal and Professional dimension shows the levels of achievement between the age of 35 and 45. This is how the transformative level occurs at 43 years old and the expert at 35 (Fig. 2).

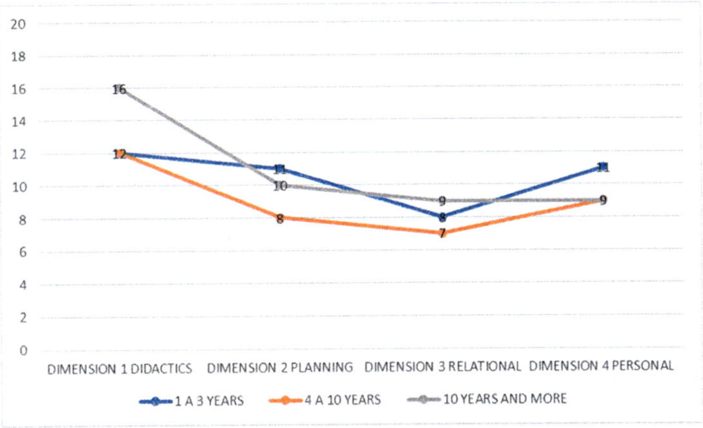

Fig. 2. Teaching digital competence graph by years of teaching

This graph shows the distribution of years of teaching experience and the relationship that exists with the dimensions of the Digital Teaching Competition. If we separate by dimension, it is identified in the didactic, curricular, and methodological dimension, presents the highest score obtained among those evaluated. This is how this dimension states that the score greater than 16 points, and even though it is above average, is the highest value of the analyzed data. In addition, it is distributed in the ranges of 10 to more years of experience, standing out over the other dimensions in more than 50%.

The organizational planning and space management dimension digital technological resources presents a low score but stands out at a point above the average age range between 1 and 3 years (Table 2).

The relational, ethical, and digital security dimension presents all scores below average, being lower than the age range of 4 to 10 years of teachers. Finally, the personal and professional dimension, presents all scores below average and stands out only the age range of 1 to 3 years of teaching, with the highest score in this dimension.

Table 2. Correlation table between dimensions of teacher digital competence

	Dimension 1 didactics	Dimension 2 planning	Dimension 3 relational	Dimension 4 personal
Dimension 1 didactics	1			
Dimension 2 planning	.790**	1		
Dimension 3 relational	.595**	.673**	1	
Dimension 4 personal	.600**	.691**	.847**	1

In this table, we can see that the correlation between dimensions equal to study variables is high. Also, the ratio scores of dimensions 1 and 2 (0.79) are highlighted, in addition to dimensions 3 and 4 (0.87).

Regarding the teaching, curricular and methodological dimensions (d1) and dimension planning, organization, and management (d2), both variables are linked to the pedagogical development of teaching management. At this point, it can be noted that one of the descriptors of dimension 1, corresponding to the applied instrument, is called teaching planning and covers the design of activities and didactic planning, a concept that relates directly to the learning environment descriptor identified in dimension 2. Therefore, both dimensions point to the teaching, learning and evaluation process focused on digital skills, to determine whether teachers have prior knowledge of these statements.

In the case of relational, ethical and security dimensions (d3) and personal and professional dimension (d4), they are linked to the development of indicators, since the first of these dimensions identifies that there are indicators that deal with the same subject matter, but from an institutional perspective (d3) and from a professional perspective (d4). Also, the descriptor on Virtual Learning Communities (d4) relates to Communication, Dissemination and Transfer (d3) and also to Digital Content and Educational Community (d3). Therefore, both dimensions are directly related from the elements of communication and digital identity.

4 Discussion

The results achieved point to three discussion ideas:

First, the age ranges of the teachers surveyed are a major factor in this research, because the data show that older teachers, therefore, with greater experience in teaching, have levels of transformer achievement in the teaching, curriculum and methodological dimensions, related to the planning of the elements that are part of the teaching-learning process [12], and the dimension planning, organization and management of digital technological space resources are directly linked to the teaching process with technologies [11]. This allows to infer that the teaching experience of teachers with years of exercise, considers their skills for the development of pedagogical skills related to the teaching digital competence.

Secondly, it is understood from the data analysis, that those teachers with less work experience, therefore, of lower age range, obtained better scores in the relational, ethical and security dimensions and personal and professional, both dimensions related to communication skills and digital society. This idea makes possible to infer that the management of technologies and the effective use for teaching professional development, allows young teachers to have those more developed capacities with respect to the CDD.

Subsequently, based on correlation results, you can determine the relationship between dimensions that relate to the ideas developed in the preliminary paragraphs. Consequently, the results obtained by the teachers surveyed, exponents that age variables are distributed among the dimensions, segmenting into two groups according to their competencies: those teachers with more age and professional experience dominate the dimensions related to the fields of classroom and educational center [11], and those teachers corresponding to the adult and young teaching rank dominate the dimensions corresponding to the areas of community and professional development [12].

The relational, ethical and security dimensions, and personal and professional, are also recognized with greater complexity when self-perishable, and from that perspective, it is noted that adult and young teachers are considered more experts with respect to the descriptors of these complex dimensions.

5 Conclusions

This diagnosis of the Digital Competence of teachers of Universidad Viña del Mar allowed to explore the level of achievement of digital competence and, according to the results obtained, that relates to the variables of age and teaching experience. The younger older and more experienced, teachers show greater development of the Digital Competence, and those older and experienced teachers focus on beginner and middle levels, i.e. teachers only use technologies to improve learning.

In this context, it would be necessary to train teachers to acquire strategies that allow them to assess the strengthening of digital competence for their academic, teaching and research professional development, understanding that nowadays being a teacher qualified to develop online teaching competently allows, in the reality of remote education, to be able to effectively achieve the learning of students, who must also develop their digital skills. Teachers must anticipate this process to be, in the future, a role model in strengthening teacher digital competence.

This research corresponds to an exploration of the case of Universidad Viña del Mar, therefore, it is intended to further deepen the ideas emanating from this diagnosis, identifying other variables that allow recognizing lines of development to design proposals to improve the digital teaching competence [7].

References

1. Cabero-Almenara, J., Marín-Díaz, V., Riquelme, I.: Uses of ICT tools from the perspective of Chilean University teachers. Sustainability **12**(6134), 2–12 (2020)

2. Castañeda, L.: Inaugural Conference School Ict Congress 2015. Santiago de Compostela (2015)
3. Gisbert, M., Lazarus, J.L: Ongoing training in digital teaching competence and improving the quality of the educational center from the perspective of teachers: a case study. New Approaches Educ. Res. **4**(2), 124–131 (2015). http://naerjournal.ua.es/article/viewFile/v4n2-7/157
4. Gisbert, M., Lazarus, J.L.: Elaboration of a rubric to evaluate the digital competence of the UT teacher. Mag. Cincies de l'Educació 30–47 (2015)
5. Esteve, F., Adell, J., Gisbert, M.: The maze of key competencies and their implications in 21st century education. II International Multidisciplinary Educational Research Congress (2013)
6. Esteve, F.: The digital teaching competence: analysis and evaluation of the performance of university students of education through a 3D environment (2015). http://francescesteve.es/tesis/
7. Falcó, J.M.: Evaluation of digital teaching competence in the autonomous community of Aragon. Electron. J. Educ. Res. **19**(4), 73–83 (2017). https://doi.org/10.24320/redie.2017.19.4.1359
8. Fraser, J., Atkins, L., Richard, H.: DigiLit leicester. Supporting teachers, promoting digital literacy, transforming. Leicester City Council (2013)
9. Gisbert, M., Espuny, C., González, J.: INCOTIC: a tool for the diagnostic assessment of digital competence in the university. Professorship. J. Curric. Teach. Train. **15**(1), 75–90 (2011)
10. Hervás, C., Fernández, E., Rodríguez, M.R., Corujo, M.C.: Validation of the digital teacher competence inventory (ICDD) of teachers in initial training. In: Innovation 2018. IV International Congress on Pedagogical Innovation and Praxis, Seville (2018)
11. Lazaro, J., Gisbert, M.: The development of digital teaching competence from a pilot experience of alternating training in the Degree of Education. Educate **51**(2), 321–348 (2015). https://doi.org/10.5565/rev/educar.725
12. Lazarus-Cantabrana, J., Gisbert-Cervera, M., Silva-Quiroz, J.: A rubric to evaluate the digital competence of the university professor in the Latin American context. Edutec: Electron. J. Educ. Technol. **63**, 1–14 (378) (2018). https://doi.org/10.21556/edutec.2018.63.1091
13. Larraz, V.: The digital competition to the university. Doctoral Tesi Universitat d'Andorra (2013)
14. Lázaro-Cantabrana, J.L., Gisbert-Cervera, M., Silva-Quiroz, J.: A rubric to evaluate the digital competence of the university professor in the Latin American context. EDUTEC Electron. J. Educ. Technol. **63** (2018). https://doi.org/10.21556/edutec.2018.63.1091
15. Silva, J., Morales, M.J., Lázaro, J.L., Gisbert, M.: Digital teaching competence in initial training: study from the cases of Chile and Uruguay. Educ. Policy Anal. Arch. **27**(93) (2019). https://doi.org/10.14507/epaa.27.3822
16. UNESCO: ICT competency standards for teachers (2008). http://www.eduteka.org/EstandaresDocentesUnesco.php
17. UNESCO: 2013/4 Report. Teaching and learning: achieving quality for all (2013). http://unesdoc.unesco.org/images/0022/002261/226159s.pdf

Approach to the Operation and Regulation of Digital Platforms in the Pacific Alliance Countries

Fátima Dávila(✉), Kruzkaya Ordóñez(✉), Abel Suing(✉), and Jorge Cueva(✉)

Universidad Técnica Particular de Loja, San Cayetano Alto, 110107 Loja, Ecuador
{fadavila,kordonez,arsuing,jlcuevaxxx}@utpl.edu.ec

Abstract. Internet is a means of communication of immediate response for users. Some digital platforms operate in this space without setting a regulatory framework, being a pending issue of sectoral policy that in some cases are controversial and legitimate control of them is difficult. Digitalization has allowed these online business models, characterized by the supply of goods, services, information, entertainment using digital platforms with global reach, have merged the digital economy and the traditional economy. These businesses also operate in bilateral and multilateral markets and bring with them a diversification of goods and services. Therefore, this research aims to know how the platforms that introduce new business models focused on entertainment via streaming work and observe their regulation in the countries that make up the Pacific Alliance Chile, Colombia, Mexico, Peru and Ecuador and clear the hypothesis related to the lack of regulation in digital spaces for the promotion of national production and OTTs. The methodology is qualitative and begins with a literature review on the operation of platforms, regional digital market, rules and regulations, in addition to the observation of the existing legal and regulatory frameworks in the region. It is concluded that OTTs should operate under the same rules and conditions, that is, that the entry of international over-the-top and the creation and operation of streaming platforms with local taxation should operate with regulatory frameworks that do not put these initiatives at a disadvantage, as well as traditional and pay TV.

Keywords: Regulation · Digital platforms · Streaming · Internet

1 Introduction

The Digital Platforms ecosystem manages a number of functions and actors that seek to reach diverse audiences by creating spaces that could be start-ups, consolidated technology companies, foundations or even governments [1].

Looking at the classification of various platforms according to how they function, it is analyzed that, according to Wertz and Tran Kingyens [2], the categories of Online Marketplaces Platforms would be:

On-demand online marketplaces: connect consumers with independent contractors who offer on-demand services or products (Uber, Lyft, Upwork).

© The Author(s), under exclusive license to Springer Nature Singapore Pte Ltd. 2022
Á. Rocha et al. (Eds.): ICOMTA 2021, SIST 259, pp. 487–495, 2022.
https://doi.org/10.1007/978-981-16-5792-4_48

Managed online marketplaces: which, in addition to connecting buyers with sellers, take care of other stages of the supply chain to enhance the user experience. An example is Beepi, a car buying and selling platform whose operator reviews the cars offered and provides warranties to sellers.

Online platforms focused on communities: buyers and sellers participate not only to complete transactions, but also for a sense of identity and belonging to a specific community (e.g. Etsy in the communities of artisans and independent sellers).

Online marketplaces enabled by software as a service (SaaS) tools: businesses that offer software as a service tools to consolidate a digital marketplace platform. They attract users through free software tools and thereby motivate them to participate in the online marketplace. An example is OpenTable, which offers reservation management tools to restaurants and, at the same time, has consolidated a related marketplace.

Decentralized online marketplaces: free, non-hierarchical platforms where rules, trust, identity and payments are defined at the user level (OpenBazaar, Lazooz, OpenName, among others) [2].

By obtaining a broad analysis on the various fields of digital platforms, it is possible to create a perspective where it would seem that there is an exact category for each cyberspace, but apparently the audiovisual streaming platforms are not contemplated in a specific addressing. For digital content providers such as DirecTV, Apple iTunes and Netflix operate only as sellers and resellers and not as online marketplaces [3].

Streaming entertainment platforms create spaces for mass consumption and every day the viewer is faced with a streaming offer beyond Netflix. The public also wants or wishes to have access to other platforms such as Amazon Prime Video, Apple 15 TV, Hulu, Peacock, Quibi (a short video service for those who consume on other platforms such as cell phones), Disney+, HBO, Fox Premium, and others; and free platforms that offer their own content such as YouTube TV, Facebook and Google. Thus, today the streaming user is faced with an oversaturation of supply, as there is undoubtedly more content than can be seen. What this reality does show is that the new audiovisual industry stands as one of the great technological and economic revolutions of the 21st century [4].

1.1 The Pacific Alliance and the Regional Digital Marketplace

In Latin American countries there has been a migration of audiences to new on-demand programming platforms that limits or stimulates cultural diversity, according to the strategies of the main players in the Latin American market. With this perspective, it is proposed to identify how open television faces this new context; the approaches of television platforms in Latin America; as well as the changes in formats and which are the most welcomed both in open television and in new television platforms; to finally detect the trends of cultural diversity in this new reality [5].

The Presidents of the Republic of Chile, Sebastián Piñera Echenique; of the Republic of Colombia, Iván Duque Márquez; of the United Mexican States, Andrés Manuel López Obrador; and of the Republic of Peru, Francisco Rafael Sagasti Hochhausler, within the framework of the XV Summit of the Pacific Alliance, held in Santiago, on December 11, 2020; made a Presidential Declaration of the Pacific Alliance on the Development of the Regional Digital Market and the Drive Towards Digital Transformation, which ratified:

> "Full support to continue building competitive markets that preserve the rules and objectives of the World Trade Organization, as well as to maintain the spirit of integration and cooperation demanded by today's globalized world.
>
> Commitment to the transversal importance of digital transformation in our countries and, in particular, of digital trade to promote the economic development and competitiveness of our markets, considering that this will be fundamental to strengthen regional integration and promote the optimal insertion of the Pacific Alliance at the global level in the digital era.
>
> Firm intention to advance in the implementation of a Regional Digital Market within the framework of the Pacific Alliance, to improve access to digital trade; create an enabling environment to promote digital trade and boost the digital economy to generate new sources of growth and productivity.
>
> Willingness to promote a digital trade, through the strengthening of trust and that guarantees the protection of consumers of digital trade in all countries of the Pacific Alliance, through the creation of a secure environment that promotes the protection of personal data and consumer rights" [6].

An instrument could be created similar to the 2016 Communication from the European Commission to the European Parliament (Brussels, 6.4.2016, COM-2016), a document that generates some guidance to support economic development should ensure consumer rights and benefits, such as: stimulating innovation, new business models, flexible jobs or new sources of income. Additionally, the aforementioned European public-policy instrument refers to the identification of possible gray areas that allow the circumvention of rules designed to protect the public interest [7].

As the Internet is an open space where users can access any type of information, it would not be possible to generate a level of control over it, therefore, the computerization of data is essential to be able to observe the behavior of various virtual platforms and understand what is the technical, analytical and dominant development of the same in the face of the demand of its users. Digital marketplace platforms collect large amounts of personal and non-personal data from their users. By using tools for big data analytics, they increase their revenues while enabling their users to generate more value [1].

Within the media ecology, television had marked a territory where its users represented loyalty to its linear programming, which reached everywhere through technology. But now on-demand programming has generated a certain rupture with many users who now opt for Apps to their subscribers to watch their programming everywhere, just as individual channels and services such as Netflix and HBO have done. Existing networks, such as ESPN and HBO, which offer amazing Apps, will have more viewers than in the past, and will have more value. Existing networks that do not develop first-class Apps will lose viewership and revenue, is the issue that is under debate now, where academic research is addressing the future of TV as we know it today [8].

No matter what they do, broadcast TV networks feel the impact of "deprogrammed" forms of audiovisual consumption from platforms such as Netflix, because if there is more demand for online entertainment, advertisers have less interest in paying for advertising spots [9].

2 Methodology

The study on digital platforms and lack of regulation in the countries that make up the Pacific Alliance aims to analyze the normative and regulatory framework that governs the countries of Chile, Colombia, Mexico, Peru and Ecuador. The research hypothesis is that there is still a lack of regulation in digital spaces for the promotion of national production and OTTs.

The methodology used is qualitative and contemplates the bibliographic review on the operation of platforms, regional digital market, topics that make up the state of the art. A second instrument applied for the observation of the legal and regulatory framework of the Pacific Alliance countries is the extended form designed with the following indicators: regulatory quality, regulation of audiovisual services over the Internet, tax reform, promotion of national audiovisual production.

The study sample has focused on the five countries that make up the Pacific Alliance: Chile, Colombia, Mexico, Peru and Ecuador, which joined the regional bloc at the end of 2019. Among the issues that drive the alliance is the progress towards a regional digital market because:

> the digital economy in Latin America and the Caribbean lags behind other areas of the world. Despite regional and sub regional efforts, considerable fragmentation, duplication of activities and inefficient coordination persist, resulting in a patchwork of legal and regulatory environments and underutilization of resources. In this scenario, the formulation and implementation of a common strategy that progressively integrates the different legal and regulatory frameworks would boost investments in the digital economy, with positive effects on growth, productivity and employment for the regional economy as a whole [10].

The observation period included two periods: the second quarter of 2020 (April, May, June) and the first quarter of 2021 (January, February, March).

3 Analysis and Discussion

Digitalization has allowed online business models characterized by the supply of goods, services, information and entertainment using digital platforms with global reach to merge the digital economy and the traditional economy. This research focuses on the study of audiovisual platforms known as over-the-top OTTs. The study of the platforms involves, in the first instance, reviewing aspects of the digital economy that emerged from the creation of transnational companies known as GAFA (Google, Apple, Facebook and Amazon) [11] that have generated profits in millions of dollars, but the questionable part is that they have used international structures in order to move profits to places where taxation is zero or minimal [12].

In the case of OTTs such as Netflix, HBO, Amazon Prime, the OECD Center for Tax Policy and Administration has questioned the way in which these platforms operate because it is not known exactly how much revenue is attributed in each of the countries of consumption, since in each country that offers its services it has no physical presence [12]. There are other cases such as Netflix, which as part of its international expansion strategies has offices in several countries that serve as connections with the major film industries.

Faced with the challenging digital scenario, the countries that make up the Pacific Alliance have indicated in the convergence agenda "the formulation and implementation of a common strategy that progressively integrates the different legal and regulatory frameworks" to help regulate the lack of regulation in digital spaces for the promotion of national production and OTTs, a hypothesis raised in this research.

Among the indicators analyzed, the regulatory quality is observed, with Chile being the country that registers the highest value within the average established by the World Bank −2.5 weak; 2.5 strong and the average value −0.17 [13] and the country with a weak value of −0.82 is Ecuador (Tables 1 and 2).

Table 1. Regulatory quality report

	Chile	Colombia	México	Perú	Ecuador
Quality regulatory	1.22	0.40	0.10	0.56	-0.82

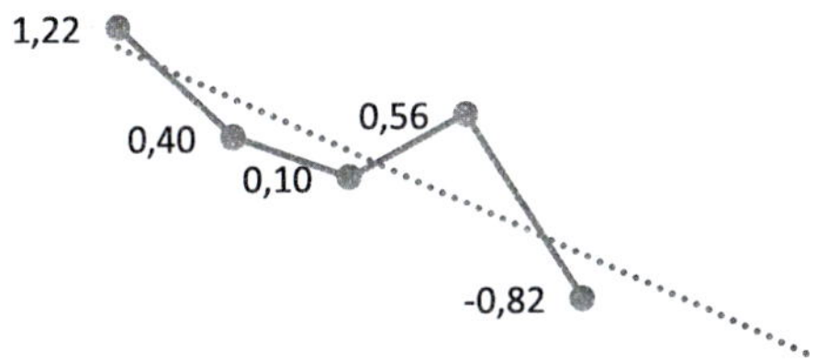

Table 2. Results regulatory frameworks

	Regulation of audiovisual services over the Internet	Tax reform IVA	Promotion of national audiovisual production
Chile	Ley de Reforma Tributaria, approved 2019. For electronic or digital services acquired through foreign suppliers	19%	Política Nacional del Campo Audiovisual 2017–2020, promotes the consolidation of the appropriate legal framework that guarantees copyright, increase and create alliances for the promotion of Chilean cinema at the international level and promotion and consolidation of the national audiovisual industry

(continued)

Table 2. (*continued*)

	Regulation of audiovisual services over the Internet	Tax reform IVA	Promotion of national audiovisual production
Colombia	Approved Plan de Desarrollo 2018–2022 Ley 1955 de 2019 Ley de Reforma Tributaria, approved in 2016. For electronic or digital services acquired through foreign suppliers	19%	For Colombian film co-productions produced between Colombian and foreign companies, with a national economic participation of not less than twenty percent (20%), and with a Colombian artistic participation equivalent to at least 70% of the national economic participation and proving its trajectory or competence in the film sector
México	Ley del impuesto al Valor Agregado, October 31, 2020 There is no specific regulation	16%	Certain provisions of the LIVA are modified to tax certain digital services, including: intermediation between third parties that are suppliers of goods and services and the demanders of these, with the exception of the sale of used personal property [15] Statements by the regulator state that it is not necessary to apply regulatory mechanisms to OTTs, since they are considered to operate efficiently. It is not recognized that they compete head-on with pay Tv*
Perú	Ley de Reforma Tributaria, approved in 2003 Decreto Legislativo N° 970 de diciembre de 2006	18%	"In general and regardless of the nationality or domicile of the parties involved in the operations and the place of execution or performance of the contracts, the following are considered Peruvian source income: i) Income obtained from digital services provided through the Internet or any adaptation or application of the protocols, platforms or technology used by the Internet or any other network through which equivalent services are provided, when the service is economically used, used or consumed in the country" [17]
Ecuador	Servicio de Rentas Internas, RESOLUCIÓN Nro. NAC-DGERCGC20-00000053 Rules for the withholding of Value Added Tax (VAT) (VAT) generated in the importation of digital services	12%	Withholding on the importation of digital services when the provider of the imported digital service is not registered with the Internal Revenue Service, the VAT generated will be withheld by the following parties: 1. Intermediaries in the payment process 2. The importer of the service

* Organization Telecommunications the Iberoamérica

With the above results, Chile, in terms of regulation of the digital ecosystem, concentrates its efforts on reviewing and enhancing coverage by eliminating restrictions and developing a regulatory framework to be able to use public spaces and buildings for the deployment of infrastructure; a second aspect is the leveling of the regulation of traditional services, i.e. to standardize them with the regulation of over-the-top (OTT), which would encourage innovation and regulatory non-discrimination [14]. Regarding the promotion of audiovisual production, Chile's policy proposes to consolidate the national audiovisual industry through sources of financing and thus promote the creation and production of film, television and multimedia, while national works seek to raise international financing and at the same time promote foreign production within the country. In this sense, it is assumed that the regulation of national production issues is defined. However, the regulation for streaming platforms so far has focused, since 2019, on the fact that services provided by foreign providers have to pay 19% of their turnover [15].

In Colombia, the regulation on Internet audiovisual services platforms, included in the National Development Plan 2018–2022, provides that "video on demand services that operate on the Internet must have an accessible section for users in Colombia with audiovisual works of national origin" [16] this decision motivates the Colombian film co-production that has gained momentum presenting hybrid works, produced with Colombian and foreign companies, a requirement demanded by platforms such as Netflix, Amazon, HBO. With regard to tax collection, the Tax Reform Law requires that VoD services acquired from abroad will be taxed at 19% of the Value Added Tax.

In Mexico, regulation does not reach streaming platforms. The regulatory agency "distances itself from the global regulatory trend that seeks to match the competitive terms in the provision of OTT services versus pay TV" [15], because it considers that these streaming services work efficiently and recognizes that they do not compete directly with pay TV. However, there is a discussion about the regulatory obligation, i.e. "the incorporation in the catalog of at least 30% of national production", which may become an over-regulation that may affect these business models and the national production itself.

In Peru, several changes have been made in its regulations regarding Income Tax, which has been in force in this country since 2003. The need to demand a contribution for the use of digital platforms was raised, and so, in 2007 it was established as a Supreme Decree described in Article 9 the collection of the tax to "those who receive digital services provided through the Internet or any adaptation or application of the protocols, platforms or technology used by the Internet or any other network through which equivalent services are provided, when the service is economically used, used or consumed in the country" [17].

In Ecuador the regulation by the Internal Revenue Service was taken for granted on August 22, 2020, with the collection of a charge for the import of Digital Services when the provider of the imported digital service is not registered with the SRI. Then at this point the IVA generated may be retained by:

1. Intermediaries in the payment process, which are companies that work with credit cards, i.e. banks.
2. The importer of the service that in RESOLUTION No. NAC-DGERCGC20-00000053 of the SRI, specified "when the payment is made without an intermediary, the VAT on the import of digital services will be paid by the importer, as a taxpayer, who must also withhold 100% of the VAT generated in the import, as provided in Article 70 of the Internal Tax Regime Law" [17].

This withholding shall be mandatory when importing any type of digital service defined in the tax regulations, even in the case in which the unregistered digital service provider is not included in the registry published by the Internal Revenue Service, being the obligation of the acquirer to identify the nature of the imported service. These collection decisions for foreign services such as streaming platforms fall directly on the users [18].

Regarding the promotion of national production in the reforms to the Organic Law of Communication LOC, the presidential veto presented affects national and independent national production because "by eliminating the mechanisms to promote national production, the government has taken a regressive decision against the communication and information rights of Ecuadorian audiovisual producers" [19].

4 Conclusions

The main objective of this article is to observe the normative and regulatory framework that governs the countries of Chile, Colombia, Mexico, Peru and Ecuador and the conclusion is consistent with the recommendation of the Organization for Economic Cooperation and Development on "technological neutrality; that is, similar services should operate under the same rules and conditions", i.e. the entry of international OTTs and the creation and operation of streaming platforms with local taxation should operate with regulatory frameworks that do not put these initiatives at a disadvantage. This competition also mentions traditional television and pay TV that are competing with on-demand entertainment businesses without regulatory scope. Thus, the hypothesis is confirmed: that there is still a lack of regulation in digital spaces for the promotion of national production and OTTs.

In the digital market, OTTs seek continuous growth. It is necessary to review the regulation in each territory in order to standardize the rules against similar local audiovisual businesses such as national OTTs. On the other hand, the countries that make up the Pacific Alliance have seen the need to demand a contribution for the use of their streaming platforms, through tax collection, which in Chile and Colombia is 19%, in Mexico 16%, in Peru 18% and in Ecuador 12%. These advances in the region show that the strategies of progressive integration of legal and regulatory frameworks are advancing, however, in each territory there is still discussion of national production policies with quality standards that allow the internationalization of audiovisual works that Colombia and Mexico have formalized through the hybrid co-production (national and foreign) required by the platforms.

Finally, as a line of future research, the study of the Data Protection Law in Chile, Colombia, Mexico, Peru and Ecuador is established, considering that every citizen has the freedom to grant his or her personal data, an acquired right in democratic states.

References

1. CEPAL: Datos, algoritmos y políticas: la redefinición del mundo digital. CEPAL (2018)
2. Wertz, B., Tran Kingyens, A.: A Guide to Marketplaces, pp. 35–36. VersionOne. (2015). https://bit.ly/3a1Ozmm
3. Hagiu A., Wright, J.: Multi-sided platforms. Working Paper, Harvard Business School. https://hbs.me/3wN567u
4. Martínez, L.: Una guía para televidentes de streaming en Colombia. Repositorio institucional de la Universidad de Bogotá Jorge Tadeo Lozano (2021). https://bit.ly/3x47ruD

5. Jimenez, C.: La Única Forma De Ser Universal Es Ser Local. El Contenido en Las Plataformas De Distribución Audiovisual Tipo Netflix (2020). https://bit.ly/3aijWcw
6. Alianza del Pacifico, Declaración Presidencial De La Alianza Del Pacífico Sobre El Desarrollo Del Mercado Digital Regional Y El Impulso Hacia La Transformación Digital (2020). https://bit.ly/3x2VVA0
7. Noboa, A. Derecho de la Competencia y plataformas digitales. Derecho y Políticas de Libre Competencia en América Latina (2020). https://bit.ly/3e8duWG
8. Esquivel, J.: Tecnología que está cambiando la televisión. Ciencia UANL (2015). https://bit.ly/3wKrMoG
9. Siri, L.: El rol de Netflix en el ecosistema de medios y telecomunicaciones: "El fin de la televisión y del cine" (2015). https://bit.ly/3sckYNq
10. CEPAL. La convergencia entre la Alianza del Pacífico y el Mercosur. Enfrentando juntos un escenario mundial desafiante. Naciones Unidas (2018). http://bitly.ws/cLcm
11. Ordóñez, K., Suing, A., Ramón, M., Ramírez-Coronel, R.: Conferencia Ibérica sobre Sistemas y Tecnologías de la Información. CISTI (2018)
12. SKATT. Beyond tax advisory. Nuevo regimen fiscal y regulatorio para las Plataformas Digitales en México (2020). http://bitly.ws/cLcs
13. World Bank. The Global Economy. Calidad regulatoria en América Latina (2019). http://bitly.ws/cLcP
14. GSM Association. Claves para la modernización de la regulación del ecosistema digital de Chile (2017). http://bitly.ws/cLdD
15. Organización de Telecomunicaciones de Iberoamerica OTI. Expriencia Regulatoria de Mercado de Contenidos audiovisuales en América Latina (2016). http://bitly.ws/cLdQ
16. MinTic. Proyecto de Decreto. Para establecer las reglas para implementar el artículo 154 de la Ley 1955 de 2019. Bogotá D.C. (2020)
17. Defensa y promoción de la producción audiovisual nacional. https://bit.ly/3ssdlCi. Accesed 14 Apr 2021
18. Asamblea Nacional del Ecuador. https://bit.ly/3e8dN3M. Accesed 13 Apr 2021
19. Plan V. Cine ecuatoriano: "a fojas cero". Publicación del 16 de enero del 2019. https://www.planv.com.ec/culturas/cine/cine-ecuatoriano-fojas-cero

Approach to the Audiovisual Market of the NETFLIX Streaming Platform in Ecuador

Jefferson Ojeda(✉), Jenny Yaguache(✉), and Carlos Ortiz-León(✉)

Universidad Técnica Particular de Loja, Loja, Ecuador
{jjojeda1,jjyaguache,cortiz}@utpl.edu.ec

Abstract. With the fast technologies' growth in the field of production, commercialization, and demand for audiovisual content, rivalry in the video-on-demand market has increased. Netflix is a platform that has international recognition due to its production level, marketing strategies, and alliances. Streaming companies in Ecuador make efforts intending to increase coverage and reach a mass audience with their content, it is for all of this that; in this research, the Netflix panorama was analyzed in comparison with the television companies operating in the national territory, such as CNT, DirecTV, Claro, TV Cable, and Univisa. This study showed that Ecuadorian platforms have advantages and disadvantages compared to Netflix. However, is the customer who decides the best option in a highly competitive market.

Keywords: Streaming · Competition · Audiovisual market

1 Streaming Platforms. A General Overview

1.1 Streaming Platforms and Netflix in Ecuador

Nowadays, there is talk about a digitalized society where the use of technological and alternative media is a priority since they bring variety and speed to internet users. Many companies have decided to change their business model to offer quality products [1]; this results in new consumption trends that move human beings away from traditional television, due to they find in digital platforms a space intended for entertainment, as is Netflix. Its original and acquired productions are of high quality, which is complemented by an attractive and easy-to-navigate interface. These characteristics make it possible that their weekly consumption at a global level states 11 h approximately [2].

Netflix arrived in Ecuador in 2011, becoming a strong rival for some operating companies in the country and offering streaming services. The North American Organization Interactive Advertising Bureau [3], points out that at a national level, there is an increase in this service demand as a result of the use of streaming video platforms. After analyzing the Ecuadorian population, it can be proved that 76% prefer to listen to music, 69% prefer music videos, while 58% decide to watch film products such as movies or series. Similarly, 46% of users access online videos through a smartphone and 16% do so from a computer.

© The Author(s), under exclusive license to Springer Nature Singapore Pte Ltd. 2022
Á. Rocha et al. (Eds.): ICOMTA 2021, SIST 259, pp. 496–504, 2022.
https://doi.org/10.1007/978-981-16-5792-4_49

This article provides an objective and verifiable analysis of the current situation of the streaming television companies station that provides their services nationwide (CNT, DirecTV, Claro, TV Cable, and Univisa). According to data obtained from Arcotel [4], the provinces of Guayas and Pichincha have the highest percentage of people subscribed to pay-TV, with 24.88% and 21.85% respectively, which is related to their population.

These data show that the Ecuadorian population does not have a considerable consumption of pay-TV. Users sign the service to watch exclusive products; however, the pricing policy does not allow many families from accessing content. Information proximity continues to be a consumption factor; though, talking about content supply, this medium has experienced a constant decrease, that is why traditional TV has opted for digital spaces [5]. Streaming is defined as a technology that allows the transmission of data throughout the internet and gives the user access to content without the need for prior downloading. This digital technology gives the viewer the possibility of designing an "a la carta" television because it allows he/she to select what they want to consume.

In the case of Netflix, approximations indicate that in 2018 this streaming giant had nearly half a million subscribers in our country. Netflix's demand percentage increased when the streaming platform began to produce original content in 2011. The 200 million and even more subscribers than the site currently has, can choose from a range of original and acquired movies, series, and documentaries. "Netflix has had a transformative effect in the relationship between customers and content providers in the twenty-first century" [6] (Fig. 1).

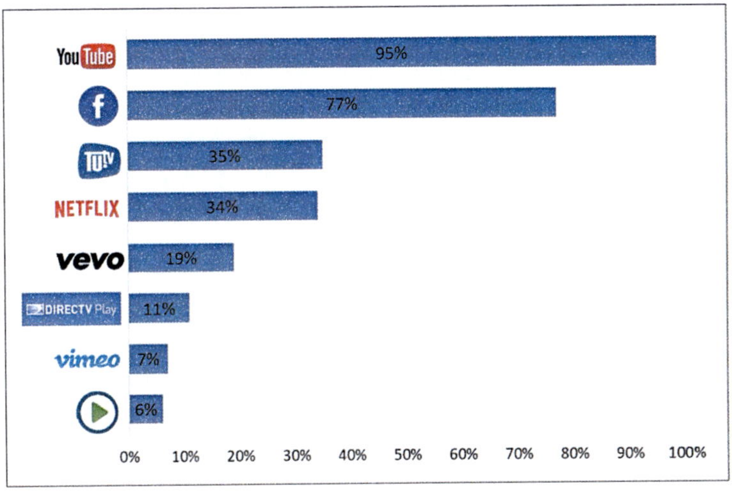

Fig. 1. As YouTube is a free platform, it attracts a larger number of customers [7].

2 Methodological Design

This article aims to describe and characterize the situation of the audiovisual market of the Netflix streaming platform in Ecuador; to know the administrative and economic situation of the streaming agents. Identify Netflix's direct competitors, and describe the alliances with local partners for the production, distribution, or broadcasting of Netflix content in the Ecuadorian market.

The research was divided into three phases, in the first one, a quantitative model was adopted, while in the second and third one a qualitative method was applied. Through these two methodologies it is intended to achieve the general objective: "To describe and characterize the situation of the audiovisual market of the Netflix streaming platform in Ecuador".

The study is conducted under a combined methodology and was executed in the following phases: (Phase 1) Selection and characterization of the media according to their typology (DTT-TV hertziana, CATV, TDH, OTT, IP), administrative and financial data of Ecuadorian television stations was obtained with information from the Telecommunications Regulation and Control Agency (ARCOTEL), Superintendence of Companies, Securities and Insurance (SCVS) and the Internal Revenue Service (SRI), official websites of the analyzed television stations and in their social networks. The data were collected in methodological files validated by the UTPL Communication Observatory [8].

To meet the second objective, (Phase 2), through non-participant observation, the competition was evaluated through a canvas designed for this purpose with variables: similarity, quality, pricing policy, geographical location, innovation and production, bargaining power, and marketing strategies. The third objective (Phase 3) is covered with the application of semi-structured interviews with the managers of CNT, Univisa, TV Cable, DirecTV, and Etapa TV channels, considered competitors of the streaming giant. Not all the companies responded to the research, so interviews with experts from the production companies Filmarte, Touché Films, Levector, Filmeikers, and Octavo Arte, Instituto de Fomento a la Creatividad y la Innovación (IFCI) were included.

Finally, an analysis of the websites and social networks of the five companies evaluated was made, with the aim of identifying possible strategic alliances.

3 Analysis and Results

Administrative Status. After analyzing the selected companies: DirecTV, CNT, Claro, Univisa, and TV Cable, was evident that most of these organizations are Anonymous Corporations (S.A.), except for DirecTV, which is a Private Limited Company (Ltda.). The main buildings of these companies are located in Quito; however, they have an alternate center in Guayaquil. In the particular case of Univisa, it is the only organization that has its main building in Guayas.

Out of the five companies analyzed, CNT is the only public entity. Claro and DirecTV are two multinationals with international coverage, while TV Cable, Univisa, and CNT only reach the national level with their signal. A common factor identified in the studied organizations is that almost all of them have SD and HD video transmission quality, except for DirecTV, which includes 4K quality to provide a greater consumption experience to its subscribers. Regarding the services they offer, CNT, Claro, and TV Cable offer television, internet and telephony, while DirecTV, and Univisa sell only television and internet services.

Economic Status. The research determined that CNT has the largest subscribed capital. According to the Superintendencia de Bacos y Seguros, the subscribed capital is: "something which determines the responsibility of the investors and consists of the part of the authorized capital that each investor agrees to pay at the time of incorporation or with each capital increase made by the institution" [9]. In this sense, CNT has a subscribed a capital of US$245,920,000; followed by DirecTV with US$12,648,510; Claro with US$12,000,000; TV Cable with US$18,825,568; and finally, Univisa with US$7,464,932.

These financial data make evidence that CNT which is a public entity receives full economic support from the State, which allows it to have a higher subscribed capital, meanwhile, the other companies that are private register a lower capital in the Ecuadorian context. According to Bruno and Ruggiero, shareholders and investors determine the difference between the two organizations [10]. In 2017, CNT contributed to the State an amount of $120 million dollars, which makes it a lucrative firm [11]. It is important to remember that, this state-owned company obtains economic benefits for offering fixed Internet services, Pay TV, mobile and fixed telephony.

Next, the values paid by the companies for the item of corporate contributions with cut in 2019 are disclosed. The item of contributions refers to the economic value that domestic companies, branches of foreign companies, and other entities subject to the surveillance and control of the Superintendencia de Compañias, Securities and Insurance (SCV), must pay annually [12]. Therefore, it can be evidenced that Claro reports the highest paid with $1,182,966.14 dollars; after, DirecTV with $65,198.65 dollars; TV Cable with $29,073.34 dollars; and, in the final position is located the Guayaquil's company Univisa with $14,350.29 dollars. In the particular case of CNT, the last report presented was in 2009, where it registered values paid for $682,284.57 dollars. In both analyses, we can see that Univisa registers the lowest financial flow, because it is a company that does not has significant recognition at the national level, which is the reason for the low demand for the service.

Profitability. The monitored companies provide streaming content as an alternative to other main services they offer (TV, Internet, Telephony), otherwise, the business would not be profitable due to quality and market issues. Multinationals such as Claro and DirecTV have a presence in different countries, in this sense, offering streaming can be a sustainable activity.

According to ARCOTEL [13], more than 160,000 subscribers abandoned the paid TV service possibly due to the Covid19 pandemic. In the first quarter of 2020, about 13,000 families canceled this service, in the second quarter there were 87,000 subscribers and in the third quarter approximately 60,000 clients, for such reason, until September 2020 the number of families with pay-TV decreased to 946,962.

Investment. As the graphic shows, Netflix leads the table with a total of $17.3 billion dollars invested in 2020, which is why today it is the leading streaming consumption platform worldwide. The large investments this enterprise makes allow it to be profitable and gain a competitive advantage in the market with successful series such as Narcos and Stranger Things [14] (Fig. 2).

Flores, J.D. [16] states that streaming is costly because the format used is complex. This point of view is shared by Pimentel [17] and Michelet [18] who reaffirm what has

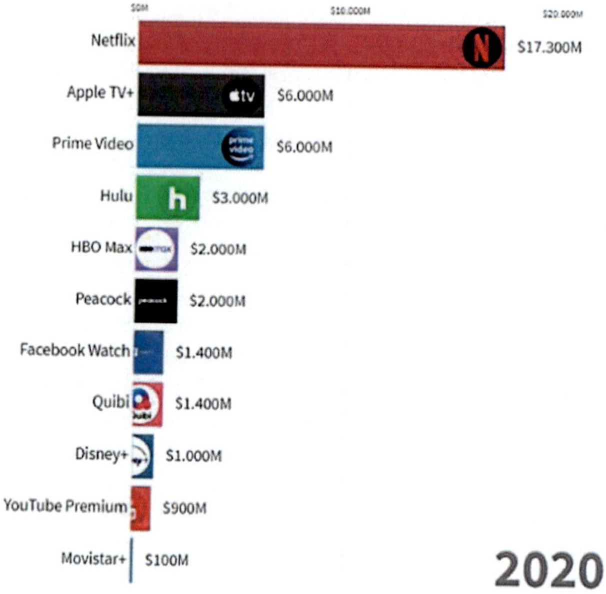

Fig. 2. Annual investment in original content [15].

already been mentioned and comment that to develop this activity it is necessary to have trained personnel. In addition, the acquisition of technological equipment also requires an investment. Regarding financing, Yépez [19] states that the only economic aid that exists in Ecuador for content production is that granted by the Instituto de Fomento a la Creatividad y la Innovación (IFCI), however, the money assigned are very limited and are not enough to cover the expenses of what is planned to be done. According to a study presented by Business and economy [20] worldwide the film industry exceeds US$41 billion per year.

Netflix and Ecuadorian Streaming TV, is There Any Competition?
This platform that operates with fast and reliable speeds [21] arrived in Ecuador on September 9th, 2011 and today ranks among the 15 most visited websites in the country and ranks 7th in downloads [22].

Product
In Ecuador, the streaming service offered by the companies analyzed is similar to Netflix, since these platforms offer a catalog of channels and productions available to subscribers, which can be enjoyed from any technological device, so content is adaptable. Due to the pandemic, several spaces for cultural consumption were opened in the country, which is the case of Choloflix, an online film platform that promotes Ecuadorian audiovisual content. This venture launched on June 7th, 2020 has 14,000 users until this date (October 2020) [23].

Ecuador does have the potential to create audiovisual products for export since the country does have the technological, technical, and human resources equipment necessary for the development of this activity.

Quality

Taking this section into account, Netflix content is offered in SD, HD, Ultra HD, and 4K quality for a greater experience. The subscriber can access these audiovisual products unlimitedly and without commercials.

Streaming companies in Ecuador offer their productions only in SD and HD quality, with DirecTV as the exception. Likewise, by paying for the service, the customer can access all the platform's content from anywhere and anytime without interruption. According to some analysts, streaming contents created by national producers are not of good quality. Yépez [19] mentions that the Ecuadorian public is used to consume unattractive productions, which is the reason why Ecuador is not prepared to face Netflix. Michelet [18] partly contradicts Yépez [19] and argues that there are streaming programs that maintain good quality, however, there are others that do not, due to the fact that some people use their technological devices to create amateur productions.

Price

With the application of the Simplicity Law, some of the foreign platforms that provide digital services in Ecuador must charge the value corresponding to taxes (IVA). In this way, Netflix plans increased in price as follows: the basic plan went from $ 7.99 to $ 8.94; Standard from $ 10.99 to $ 12.30 and Premium from $ 13.99 to $ 15.66. Regarding the approval of the Simplicity Law and Tax Progressivity, Víctor Hugo Albán, vice-president of the Economists Association of Pichincha, states that this kind of taxes applied to platforms, as is the case of Netflix, not only make services more expensive but also low foreign investment in Ecuador, since international companies have fewer incentives to invest in a country that imposes this kind of taxes [24].

DirecTV GO has some of the following TV plans: HD Family Plan: $ 1.07 (per day), HD Gold Plan: $ 39.00, Platinum Plus 4K Plan: $ 85.00. It is important to mention that the streaming content platform is free for users as long as they are customers of the company by having signed any of the services offered, otherwise, they will have to pay a monthly fee of $ 23.00. TV Cable Play has the following TV plans: Basic Plan: $ 20.50, Basic Plus HD Plan: $ 23.00, Premium Plan: $ 27.00. The user can access streaming content free of charge, however, in order to access them, it is necessary to have signed the TV paid service of Grupo TV Cable. As exposed, Ecuadorian television stations maintain higher prices in relation to Netflix, which is the reason why the streaming giant is conquering the public with comfortable prices and variety, quality, and exclusivity in content, as Clinehens (2020) argues.

Coverage

In the case of Netflix, it is marketed throughout Ecuador as long as there is an internet connection to hiring it. The same applies to companies that offer streaming in our country since users must have connectivity to browse the platform. It does not matter the geographical location where subscribers are located, because the service has national coverage, which is mainly due to the accelerated growth of the internet in urban and rural areas. For this reason, both Netflix and streaming companies in Ecuador, have the same coverage. According to a report presented by Ecuador Estado Digital [25], 80% of the population of our country has Internet access, as a result of the pandemic, there was a 30% growth in the demand for this service, with streaming content being the most consumed.

Innovation/Production

Another of Netflix's strengths is the recommendation of content directly from the platform according to subscribers' searches and demand. [26]. The products it sells can be watched up to 4 screens simultaneously and allows the customer to perform some actions such as mute, pause, replay, among others.

The content can be downloaded to the device so that, it can be played without an internet connection. This option also prevents the storage of our device from being affected, since the download is done in the cloud's platform. Finally, Netflix has an application that adapts to different operating systems. The companies that operate in the national territory and offer pay-TV channels can be considered as competition for Netflix because in this analysis parameter they have similar aspects. On the other hand, Yépez [19], states that the issue of production should be seen as an industrial activity and not so much a cultural one, as it has been taken.

Customer's Negation Power

The different subscription plans sold by streaming companies in Ecuador have been created to achieve customer loyalty, since they are shown as the best option compared to the competition, and thus, they establish a direct relationship between quality, satisfaction, and perceived value [27].

In the case of Claro Play, CNT Play, DirecTV GO, TV Cable Play, and Univisa, the customer can pay for the service online or, in some cases by credit or debit card. Flores [16] assures that two barriers limit the entry of Netflix in several sectors in Ecuador. One is internet access and the other one is that consumers do not have a credit or debit card to pay for the service. For either of these two reasons, Netflix loses subscribers. In this sense, streaming platforms in our country could gain some competitive advantage, because users can go directly to pay personally at the offices.

Marketing Strategies

In the case of Netflix, it has short commercials on social media, YouTube, and websites. The company carries out digital campaigns to promote content and its portal web shows the services and plans it offers; it also uses memes, gifts, and dynamic tests on its official sites to create empathy with people. Netflix is supported by mini providers that provide the service. "As a streaming platform, Netflix gives shape and organization to a library of content, similarly to an interactive archive" [28].

Although this platform eliminated the 14 days and the free trial month of the service, Ecuadorian streaming companies continue doing so, that is the case of Claro Video that offers the first month free, DirecTV GO also receives its subscribers with the first 7 days free, as Univisa does with its platform "INTI TV", in addition to having digital spaces where they exhibit the plans, products, and promotions.

Strategic Alliances

It was found in this research that Netflix does not have any strategic alliance in Ecuador, however, it was possible to evidence agreements that national television stations have with local and international companies, to distribute content, provide technology and gain brand positioning. Social networks (Facebook, Instagram, and Twitter) were also monitored, but it was not possible to identify that these companies have published content that evidences any particular strategic alliance, even though they do have.

4 Conclusions

Public companies have fewer possibilities of indebtedness compared to private organizations, because their subscribed capital is higher.

Ecuador does not have audiovisual production at the level of quality standards imposed by Netflix, for this reason, there is a big difference that puts our country at a disadvantage. This is due to the fact that there is no significant economic support for production and television companies. It is the vital importance that the Institute for the Promotion of Creativity and Innovation (IFCI), strengthen economic incentives in the audiovisual sector to produce higher quality products that rise Ecuador as one of the leading content creators in the region, like Colombia, Mexico, and Argentina.

Strategic alliances for the creation of content are very important since they allow to find new markets for the developed pieces. Our country does not have agreements with Netflix or international production companies; therefore, this streaming platform does not buy material developed in Ecuador. To consolidate international alliances, it is convenient to promote the Film Commission, which is in charge of attracting and promoting investments in the audiovisual sector, in order to get foreign producers interested in filming in Ecuador.

Television stations studied in this research offer streaming content as an alternative to other main services they have (TV, Internet, Telephony), because the issue of quality and population quantity (market) is not favorable, however, by having national programming they manage to create proximity with the customer, becoming a competitive advantage for Netflix. For streaming TV stations operating in Ecuador to recover the loss of subscribers caused by the pandemic, it is necessary to modify their pricing policy and strengthen their marketing strategies.

Ecuador has the necessary technological equipment, technical and human resources to create audiovisual products to export, which becomes an advantage for national television stations. In the territory, there are also technology rental houses that offer the equipment required for the development of this activity. With this scenario, institutes can be created to promote the production of local content with an international focus.

References

1. Reuters Institute Homepage. https://cutt.ly/2vbNR1i. Accessed 15 Sept 2020

2. BB-Book Homepage. https://cutt.ly/NlpCOQG. Accessed 15 Apr 2021
3. Interactive Advertising Bureau Homepage https://cutt.ly/pcGHUdE. Accessed 19 Jan 2021
4. Agencia de Regulación y Control de las Telecomunicaciones Homepage. https://cutt.ly/gj81NPX. Accessed 15 Apr 2021
5. Inouye Homepage. https://cutt.ly/nvb9i0E. Accessed 15 Feb 2021
6. McDonald, K., Smith-Rowsey, D.: The Netflix Effect. Technology and Entertainment in the 21st Century, 1st edn. Editorial Bloomsbury, USA (2016)
7. Interactive Advertising Bureau Homepage. https://cutt.ly/pcGHUdE. Accessed 10 Aug 2021
8. Coronel, G.: Yearbook of Communication Companies of Ecuador, 1st edn. Private Technical University of Loja, Ecuador (2012)
9. Telecommunications Regulation and Control Agency Homepage. https://cutt.ly/fko9DuW. Accessed 10 Apr 2021
10. Bruno, S., Ruggiero, E. (eds.): Public Companies and the Role of Shareholders. Kluwer Law International B.V., The Netherlands (2011)
11. El Comercio Homepage. https://cutt.ly/ckV0ZOC. Accessed 04 Jan 2021
12. FIDES Homepage. https://cutt.ly/RkV0Nuk. Accessed 07 Apr 2021
13. Agencia de Regulación y Control de las Telecomunicaciones Homepage. https://cutt.ly/fko9DuW. Accessed 15 Feb 2021
14. Lobato, R.: Netflix nations: the geography of digital distribution (2019)
15. Xataka: Homepage. https://cutt.ly/kkHjJeN. Accessed 23 Mar 2021
16. Flores, J.D.: Personal communication, 15 Mar 2021
17. Pimentel, D.: Personal communication, 16 Apr 2021
18. Michelet, J.P.: Personal communication, 19 Mar 2020
19. Yépez, H.: Personal communication, 17 Apr 2020
20. Business and Economy Homepage. https://cutt.ly/ylpCdg4. Accessed 11 Feb 2020
21. Barker, C., Wiatrowski, M.: The Age of Netflix. McFarland & Company, Inc., North of Carolina USA (2017)
22. Similar Web Homepage. https://cutt.ly/Okx51SB. Accessed 15 Apr 2021
23. Expreso Homepage. https://cutt.ly/ClpGscF. Accessed 29 Oct 2020
24. GK Homepage. https://cutt.ly/Jkx5uA8. Accessed 28 Jan 2021
25. Ecuador Estado Digital Homepage. https://cutt.ly/Xj82Zan. Accessed 17 Nov 2020
26. Diva Homepage. https://cutt.ly/LvbVK7P. Accessed 16 Apr 2021
27. Jahmani, A., Bourini, I., Jawabreh, O.: The relationship between service quality, client satisfaction, perceived value and client loyalty. Tourism Notebooks, 45th edn. Spain (2020)
28. Pallister, K. (ed.): Netflix Nostalgia: Streaming the Past on Demand. Edit. Lexington Books, USA (2019)

Economic Sustainability Models for Alternative and Community Media (ACMs): The Venezuelan Case

Rebeca Sánchez(✉) and Fernando Casado

Universidad Técnica de Manabí, Portoviejo 130105, Ecuador

Abstract. This research suggests three economic sustainability models for Alternative and Community Media (ACMs), based on endogenous, community and exogenous funding, and their joint or mixed combinations, which is what usually is found in practice. This first study deals with the Venezuelan case; however, the researchers expect to test the applicability or functionality of such models in other countries within the region. The methodology is qualitative-quantitative, as it combines data collection from 280 surveys and 25 in-depth telephone and in-person interviews with different ACMs throughout the Venezuelan territory. The research was developed in three stages: 1. identification of funding strategies, 2. classification of economic sustainability models and, 3. assessment of the economic sustainability models employed by Venezuela ACMs. Our results show that as endogenous funding and diversification of sources increase, so does the economic sustainability of the community media; whereas as the exogenous funding and diversification of sources decrease, the potential risks for the economic sustainability of the community media increase.

Keywords: Economic sustainability · Alternative and community media · Funding

1 Introduction

Vast research on Alternative and Community Media (ACMs) was produced during the first decades of the 21th Century, with a preeminence of conceptual and regulatory aspects over other fundamental ones, such as their sustainability [1].

Sustainability, i.e. the ability to overcome internal conflicts and external difficulties [2], is one of the most complex variables in community media management and their study. Many authors go beyond economicist approaches to study sustainability as an interdependent issue, merging social, institutional and economic views [1–5].

Thus, for a community media to be sustainable, it must involve the participation of social actors, but there must also be a legal, regulatory framework, and a set of public policies where it can develop free of censorship or external pressure [3]. All this, notwithstanding the mechanisms and strategies for obtaining essential resources for its operation [2].

© The Author(s), under exclusive license to Springer Nature Singapore Pte Ltd. 2022
Á. Rocha et al. (Eds.): ICOMTA 2021, SIST 259, pp. 505–514, 2022.
https://doi.org/10.1007/978-981-16-5792-4_50

Although the sustainability of community media is a multidimensional variable that does not depend solely on funding, economic concerns are a key factor which has not been fully discussed so far, considering the permanent threats they are prone to, as long as they are, in themselves, no-profit and, therefore, non-capitalist projects inserted in a capitalist economy.

Theorizing about economic issues makes it possible to delve into questions that researchers and social organizations have been posing for a long time about the most viable economic model to ensure their survival, for example: what sort of ownership is the most appropriate, how work and money are internally distributed, how funding should be obtained, or what mechanisms should be implemented to build solidarity economies within an economic system based on selfishness [6].

This study seeks to provide insight into this open topic, based on the identification of funding strategies by Venezuelan ACMs. The obtained information was used to construe three economic sustainability models, respectively including endogenous, community and exogenous funding, and, at the same time, to assess their application to the case study.

We hope that progress in this area will also bear on our knowledge of other dimensions of sustainability, such as the social and institutional ones, which are not to be developed here as yet, though.

2 The Venezuelan Case

During the breakdown of the constitutional order in 2002 in Venezuela, the ACMs played a key role in preventing an absolute information blackout and, since then, this sector has been bolstered up through public legal recognition policies and economic support [7]. It is from that moment that the community media, along with public media, are considered one key stakeholder in the construction of the state "communicational and informational hegemony" [8]. The current political-institutional context has given rise to two stances regarding the role played by ACMs in Venezuela: "on the one hand, those who consider them just another piece in the government media apparatus, and on the other hand, those who see them as tools for the citizenry, as opposed to the different institutions of power, including the government" [7].

According to official data from Conatel[1], between 2002 and 2006, 193 community media were licensed (166 in radio format and 27 TV stations), [9] whereas, in 2018, 598 media were registered nationwide, among which radio stations predominate, with 453 licenses, followed by 67 printed publications, 45 television stations and 33 digital media, according to the Alternative and Community Media Report 2018 [10]. The unprecedented growth of this sector is largely due to the combination of legal-institutional and economic factors.

Specific legal and institutional regulations were created, such as the Organic Telecommunications Law of 2002, which for the first time acknowledged the "legal status" of community media [7], as well as the Regulations for Radio Broadcasting and

[1] The National Telecommunications Commission is an independent Venezuelan regulatory agency that ensures the quality of telecommunication services throughout the country and coordinates national plans and policies for the sector.

Community Open Television of Non-Profit Public Services, that legalizes and protects this historically marginalized and clandestine sector [10]. In the same line, the Popular Power Communication Law was passed in 2015, the expressed purpose of which was "to promote, develop, strengthen and consolidate Popular Communication" (Article 1). Similarly, as of 2003, institutions, such as the MinCI General Directorate for Alternative and Community Media, were created to deal in these issues, in order to "articulate and accompany the ACMs, supporting their political and technical training, and their technological equipment"[2] [10].

A "strong economic investment" was earmarked for training, equipping and improving the infrastructure of this third communication sector [8]. In fact, the budget of the Directorate for Community and Alternative Media includes funds allotted "to strengthen these media and consolidate the National System of Alternative and Community Media" [11]. To mention a few examples, in 2003, former President Chávez announced the allocation of a millionaire sum from the Cooperative Development Fund to finance the community communications network [12]. Subsequently, the 2011 National Budget Law allotted a specific sum to the community media. That same year, the Vice Presidency of the Republic, to which Conatel is attached, granted funding to each the "Consolidation of the Inclusive Communicational Model" and the "Strengthening of Community Media." Likewise, in 2012, Conatel's budget included the line "Strengthening of Community Media within the Framework of Popular Communication" [11].

However, whereas the State became a key (bene)factor in the development of community media, it also conditioned their autonomy and economic sustainability, by favoring their dependence from national funds. The institutional position towards ACMs has dramatically changed, though, after the harsh economic crisis that has been hitting Venezuela since 2015, and State financial support dwindled to virtually nothing.

The crisis has but shown more clearly the great challenges faced by Venezuela ACMs. Confronted with the need for economic self-sustainability due to the loss of State aids, media have been forced to reinvest or disappear, as shown by the documentary review and the 14 interviews carried out throughout this research.

3 Methodology and Analysis of Results

The general purpose of this work is to suggest three economic sustainability models for Alternative and Community Media (ACMs), based on endogenous, community-based, and exogenous funding, and the different combinations thereof. For that purpose, the study methodology combines a quantitative study of Venezuela ACMs funding strategies and a qualitative analysis the data retrieved. This methodology research was developed in three stages: 1. identification of funding strategies, 2. classification of economic sustainability models and, 3. assessment of the economic sustainability models employed by Venezuela ACMs, as described below.

[2] The Ministry of Popular Power for Communication and Information is the body in charge of the communication policy in the Venezuela Government.

3.1 Identification of Funding Strategies

Between January and June 2018, questionnaires were dealt to 280 ACMs, out of a universe of more than 500 media registered in the Conatel and MinCI databases, in order to identify their different forms of funding. The results of this research have already been published [13]. Based on the quantitative data obtained, between March and September 2019, 25 in-depth telephone and in-person interviews were carried out, in order not only to delve into the characteristics of such financing strategies, but also to identify the relevant analysis categories for the present investigation.

3.2 Classification of Economic Sustainability Models

ACMs' economic sustainability depends on their receiving regular long-term incomes which allow them to cope with their operational expenses [14]. In our approach, it is deemed to be configured out of three types of funding: endogenous; community and exogenous, which can and do coexist in practice, so they are not mutually exclusive. Such classification is a mere abstraction to facilitate analysis. The ACMs economic sustainability models based on these three types of funding are defined below.

Endogenous Economic Sustainability. The term "endogenous" is used across different subject fields, denoting something born by and out of itself, because of inner causes, as opposed to "exogenous". In social sciences, it refers to what is born within social, political, and economic organizations [15]. Thus, ACM endogenous sustainability is related to funding generated within the alternative or community medium itself, i.e., through its own productive communication or other activities. In this type of sustainability, the medium produces its own resources, and does not receive funding, as in the case of community or exogenous sustainability. Examples include content production, equipment rental, training activities, such as courses, seminars, or diplomas, or baking, textile, serigraph, or cropping projects.

Community Economic Sustainability. The term "community" is so versatile and polysemous that it can be applied to very different groups of people and to a variety of actions and social configurations [16]. As regards this study, "community" refers to the ACM territory and the people in there. Therefore, Community Economic Sustainability implies contribution from the groups of people living within a community territory, driven by social commitment, community advertising, or volunteering. This category excludes funding either from the community media productive activities themselves or from other sources outside the community.

Exogenous Economic Sustainability. The term "exogenous" can be used in different fields, referring to whatever tangible or intangible means or entities produced or caused to exist from outside the concerned objects or subjects [17]. In Exogenous Economic Sustainability, funding comes neither from the media own sources nor from the community, but from public or private advertising, direct State financial support, international cooperation, or other external sources. This type of sustainability is in contrast with endogenous or community one.

Table 1 below summarizes the sustainability models according to the types of funding.

Table 1. Economic sustainability according to the types of funding

Sustainability model	Type of funding	Category	Subcategory
Endogenous	From the ACMs	Productive activities	Media-related activities (content production, equipment rental, etc.) Educational sector (training courses, seminars, diplomas, etc.) Other sectors (bakeries, textile production, food distribution, etc.)
Community	From the community	Contributions from community members Volunteering Community advertising	
Exogenous	From outside the community	Advertising Direct financial support	Public and private advertising External financing (international cooperation, State or other public aid)

Comparative analyses show that as endogenous funding and diversification of sources increase, so does the economic sustainability of the community media; whereas as the exogenous funding and diversification of sources decrease, the community media economic sustainability is increasingly jeopardized, as shown in the figure below (See Fig. 1).

As it is, whatever the form of funding, whether endogenous, community or exogenous, the diversification of sources will be a key condition for economic sustainability.

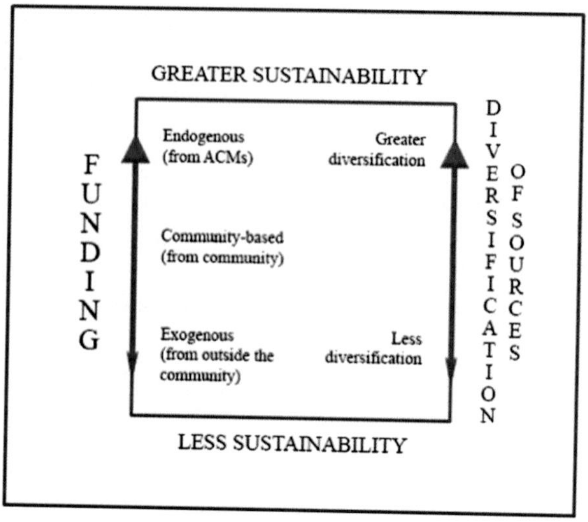

Fig. 1. Qualitative analysis of the economic sustainability for ACMs.

3.3 Analysis of Venezuela ACMs Economic Sustainability Models

According to the results of the 280 survey questionnaires distributed in September 2018, Venezuelan ACMs are funded from mixed sources. One first source involves the commitment of community members, particularly donations by members of the community media themselves (132 cases), and contributions from other community organizations and individuals (69 cases). A second way of funding includes exogenous sources, such as institutional (67 cases) and commercial advertising (53); as well as subsidies from the State (8), NGOs, and foundations (5). In the third place, community media generate endogenous funding from their own productive media-related activities (45) (see Fig. 2).

Community Economic Sustainability. Actually, most funding for ACMs in Venezuela is community-based (53%), that is, it comes from the economic contributions and voluntary work of the ACM community and members, and not from productive activities or external parties. Take, for instance, the case of Radio Llanera Stereo[3], whose eight members are graduates in Communication from Venezuelan public universities, but derive their incomes from the informal trade, be it painting T-shirts, repairing electronic devices, or selling sweets. In a large number of cases, ACMs have found their funding through community advertising or commercial support; some radios even developed an efficient and thorough marketing "department" that helps promote intra-community ventures, as was the case with Radio Ecológica[4], and other radios closely related to the local businesses, such as Santa Barbara Stereo[5].

[3] Radio Llanera Stereo is located in the Francisco Linares Alcántara county (Aragua state), in the north-central part of the country.

[4] Ecological Radio is located in Caracas western area.

[5] Santa Barbara Stereo radio is located in the Tinaquillo county, north of the Cojedes state, in the plain region known as the *llanos*.

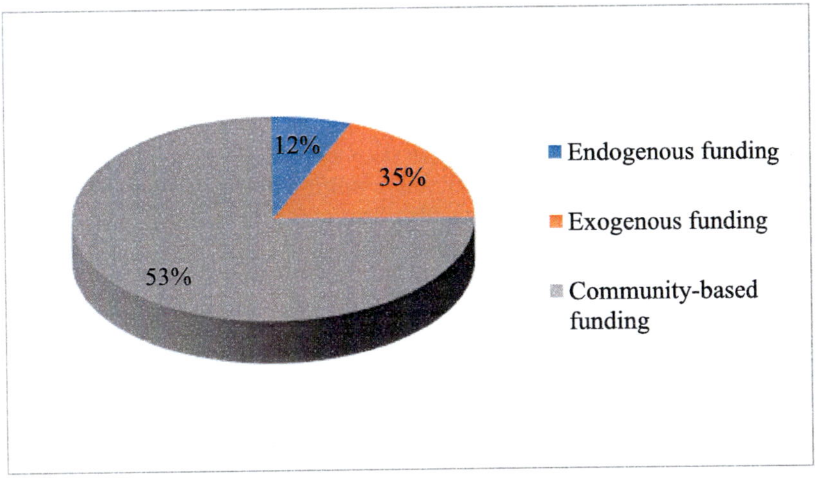

Fig. 2. Source of funding for Venezuelan ACMs

Exogenous Economic Sustainability. Exogenous sources rank second as the funding strategy of ACMs in Venezuela (35%). The State had become the main external source of economic resources and operational support, to the point that three out of four media surveyed in 2018 stated that at some point in their lifespan had received some type of public aid. However, the 2019 interviews show that at present, State financing has shrinked to sheer anecdote in the context of the Venezuelan economic crisis; State advertising –states Antonio Gómez from Radio Libertad de Barquisimeto– "is hardly enough to afford an RCA plus cable" [13].

This situation has jeopardized the economic sustainability of ACMs. The community television channel Catia TV[6] is a good example of how nearly exclusive dependence on exogenous State resources can backfire on ACMs. While in the past it had 50 of its members being publicly paid salaries by the state oil company PDVSA, and received financing from other institutions via advertising or other mechanisms, after the economic debacle that wiped out all public funding, only the 10% of its members remain active, only moved by their militant efforts, with a minimum operational capacity.

Not only are exogenous sources the most unstable and, therefore, risky means of funding for economic sustainability, they can also be expressly or subtly conditioning or clientelistic for the ACMs, threatening their autonomy or even distorting their community identity. In some cases, we found that the frantic search for commercial and state advertising ended up turning the community medium into an entity more similar to a private for-profit company or a public/government medium.

Endogenous Economic Sustainability. Endogenous funding sources account for 12% of the economic strategies of ACMs in Venezuela, in which cases, media embark on

[6] Catia TV is a Caracas-based community TV station, known for the informative role played during the breakdown of constitutional order in April 2002.

different media productive ventures or other economic activities, with a view to self-sustainability. The Coro Televisión y Radio Comunitaria Foundation[7] is financed mainly from its own training courses, for which support it has signed an agreement with the Simón Rodríguez University.

The international community television station Alba TV[8], hit hard by the crisis just like Catia TV, entered a new line of business, creating a production company that either directly works for other media or rents their equipment, and uses the profits from this company to engage in its own productions. This would be the example of endogenous funding derived from a media-related productive venture.

Finally, we find a group of three radio stations, La Minka, Negro Primero and Radio Perola[9], whose main funding mechanisms involve their own productive ventures in non-communication economic sectors. All three developed community semi-industrial bakeries, where they produce different types of bread to be sold at non-speculative prices, even despite hyperinflation. Thanks to these bakeries, the radios help finance their internal expenses, at the same time, creating jobs for people in the community. However, in order to avoid speculation in raw materials, the bread ingredients in these communal bakeries are provided at prices regulated by the State, with which they keep links. The provision of some bread ingredients can sometimes be irregular, though, which forces these bakeries to resort to the informal market.

As the endogenous model has matured, these ventures have expanded and diversified into areas such as, textile, serigraphy, communal crops and food distribution. All three radio stations allot a percentage of the resources obtained from such productive activities to community projects, through initiatives such as the Travesura Vacation Plan, organized online by different community radio stations, which reached more than 1800 children and adolescents from different neighborhoods of the capital Caracas.

4 Conclusions

Although sustainability is a multidimensional variable that integrates economic, social and institutional aspects, we conclude that it is possible to analyze the first of these dimensions in its specificity, in order to provide an insight into its logic, so as to help solve its theoretical, methodological and empirical problems, which would hardly be possible under other conditions.

By abstracting three basic types of funding, i.e., endogenous, community and exogenous, which may be effectively be found jointly or mixed, we have created different economic sustainability models, and arrived to the conclusion that, even though all funding sources contribute to sustainability, not all do it to the same extent.

Our results show that endogenous funding grants ACMs greater economic sustainability compared to community and exogenous funding; indeed, being self-generated,

[7] The Coro Televisión y Radio Comunitaria Foundation is located in the city of Coro, capital of the Falcón state.

[8] AlbaLBA TV is located in the city of Caracas. Even though its facilities are located inside the premises of the Venezuelan public channel Vive Tv, AlbaLBA TV is fully independent from it.

[9] All these radios are located in different neighborhoods of the city of Caracas.

it provides ACMs financial independence to cope with operating expenses and to make different investments, which potentially entails freedom from dependency relationships. However, this type of sustainability will be conditioned not only by the effective functioning of these economic activities, but also by social and institutional sustainability. Endogenous economic sustainability will also result in social sustainability, by stimulating community participation and commitment with local media, as shown in the cases of the Perola, La Minka, and Negro Primero radio stations.

Although providing greater sustainability than exogenous funding, community funding –the most widespread in the Venezuelan ACMs– implies less economic sustainability than endogenous sources, since the resources do not depend on the media themselves but on the community. This type of financing involves a deep connection between the media and the communities on which they depend.

Furthermore, external factors determine the sustainability of exogenously funded community media, configuring a dependency situation which is the counterpart of the potential self-sustainability derived from endogenous financing. Moreover, exogenous funding could be conditioning and jeopardizing for the decision-making autonomy and editorial line independence of the medium.

From a correlational perspective, we can assert that as endogenous funding and diversification of sources increase, so does the economic sustainability of the community media; whereas as the exogenous funding increases and diversification of sources decreases, the economic sustainability of community media is increasingly jeopardized. Furthermore, whatever the form of funding, whether endogenous, community or exogenous, the diversification of resources will be a key condition for economic sustainability.

References

1. Barranquero, A., Candón-Mena, J.: La sostenibilidad del Tercer Sector de la Comunicación en España. Diseño y aplicación de un modelo de análisis al estudio de caso de El Salto y OMC Radio1. REVESCO Revista de Estudios Cooperativos **137**, 1–20 (2021). https://doi.org/10.5209/reve.71863
2. Villagra, E., Traversaro, N.: Medios comunitarios, audiencias y sostenibilidad. El caso de la provincia de Córdoba. Revista Científica de la REDCOM (9), (2019). https://doi.org/10.24215/24517836e024
3. Gumucio-Dagron, A.: Arte de equilibristas: la sostenibilidad de los medios de comunicación comunitarios. Scielo 6–19 (2005)
4. Sáez Baeza, C.: Tercer sector de la comunicación: teoría y praxis de la televisión alternativa. Una mirada a los casos de España, Estados Unidos y Venezuela (Tesis doctoral). UAB (2008)
5. Escobar, R., Salgado, V.: Atrapa sueños. La sostenibilidad en las radios populares y comunitarias. Asociación Latinoamericana de Educación Radiofónica (ALER) y Asociación Mundial de Radios ComunitariasAmérica Latina y el Caribe (AMARC) (2008)
6. Amarc: Dossier Sostenibilidad Económica. Cara y Señal (2008)
7. Gómez, A.: Desarrollo de los medios de comunicación comunitarios en Colombia y Venezuela, convergencias y divergencias. Enfoques de la Comunicación 35–65 (2019)
8. Canelón-Silva, A.: Del Estado comunicador al Estado de los medios. Catorce años de hegemonía comunicacional en Venezuela. Palabra Clave **17**(4), 1243–1278 (2014). https://doi.org/10.5294/pacla.2014.17.4.11

9. Urribarrí, R.: Medios comunitarios: el reto de formar(se) para la inclusión. Comunicación: Estudios venezolanos de comunicación **137**(1), 45–53 (2007)
10. Minci: Informe de Medios Alternativos Comunitarios 2018. Ministerio del Poder Popular para la Comunicación e Información (2018)
11. Bisbal, M.: La comunicación bajo asedio: Balance de 17 años. UCAB Ediciones, Caracas (2017)
12. Rivero, Y.: COMUNICACIONES-VENEZUELA: Chávez financia medios alternativos. Inter Press Services (2003)
13. Casado, F., Sánchez, R.: Logros y desafíos de los medios comunitarios en Venezuela durante la Revolución Bolivariana. Risti 54–65 (2018)
14. Tornay, C.: Creando el derecho a la comunicación desde abajo: radios comunitarias sostenibles en Venezuela, Ecuador y España. COMMONS, Ciencias Sociales y Comunicación **7**(2), 133–163 (2018). https://doi.org/10.25267/COMMONS.2018.v7.i2.05
15. Diccionario De Conceptos en Ciencias Sociales: Endógeno (2021)
16. Úcar, X.: La comunidad como elección: teoría y práctica de la accióncomunitaria. Universidad Autónoma de Barcelona, pp. 1–28 (2009)
17. Diccionario De Conceptos en Ciencias Sociales: Exógeno (2021)

Check for updates

'Quarantine' on Google and YouTube During the Covid-19 Pandemic: United States, United Kingdom, Spain and Italy

Daniel Villa Gracia and Víctor Cerdán Martínez(✉)

Universidad Complutense de Madrid, Madrid, Spain
{daniel.villa,vicerdan}@ucm.es

Abstract. Background: On March 11, 2020, the World Health Organisation (WHO) declared the SARS-CoV-2 virus a pandemic. Spain and Italy decreed a state of emergency, implementing an enforced confinement of citizens. The United States and the United Kingdom took similar steps. Method: This article quantitatively investigates the evolution of the most searched terms on Google and YouTube on 'quarantine'. Google Trends data on the word 'quarantine' was used in the four countries with the highest number of total deaths from Covid-19 disease at the end of May 2020: United States (85,906), United Kingdom United (33,614), Italy (31,368) and Spain (27,459) from February to June 2020. Results: Linear regression analysis show a positive correlation between searches for the word "quarantine" in Italy in relation to those in the United States (R2 = 0.96) and Spain (R2 = 0.96), being able to generate predictive models for the future. Comparison of the data for Italy with the UK is less statistically relevant (R2 = 0.78). Conclusions: There is an increase in the searches for 'quarantine' in Google and YouTube up to June 2020. The citizens of these countries first searched for this concept on Google and later on YouTube. There is a statistical correlation between Google searches in Italy compared separately to the United States and Spain. The quarantine data of interest in Italy generate a prediction pattern in the United States and Spain. However, this phenomenon does not happen between Italy and the UK due to the lack of statistical correlation.

Keywords: Health communication · Science and media · Visual communication · Coronavirus disease · SARS-CoV-2 · Quarantine · Communicable disease control

1 Context

1.1 Pandemic

The Chinese city of Wuhan has become internationally known as the origin of the spread of the SARS-CoV-2 virus, commonly known as coronavirus or Covid-19. In December 2019 appeared the first cases of pneumonia of an unknown cause [16]. Recent reports have considered the clinical repercussions of Covid-19 in Asia [6,7,13,18,29,30], and

© The Author(s), under exclusive license to Springer Nature Singapore Pte Ltd. 2022
Á. Rocha et al. (Eds.): ICOMTA 2021, SIST 259, pp. 515–523, 2022.
https://doi.org/10.1007/978-981-16-5792-4_51

the spread of the virus to Spain [26], and other countries of the European Union [14] and Latin America [8].

On December 31, 2019, the Wuhan Municipal Health Commission reported several cases in the city of the hitherto atypical pneumonia [30]. That day, the World Health Organization alerted health authorities in Hong Kong, Macau, and Taiwan to strengthen its border surveillance. The unknown virus could become a serious threat to public health [31]. Later research proved that a novel coronavirus caused these cases of pneumonia.

On January 10, the World Health Organization published a series of international technical recommendations. The organization's regional emergency managers communicated these recommendations to all representatives of their respective countries [32]. The recommendations were based on other coronavirus epidemics, specifically Severe Acute Respiratory Syndrome (SARS) and Middle East Respiratory Syndrome (MERS), and the transmission routes of other respiratory viruses. The disease spread from a single point to all of China in just 30 days, and in 3 months, cases were identified in over 100 countries.

On January 30, the WHO Director-General declared the Covid-19 outbreak a Public Health Emergency of International Concern (PHEIC). On March 11, the WHO declared a pandemic given the high level of epidemiological instability and ease of movement throughout the world and across international borders [36].

The purpose of a quarantine is to prevent certain organisms from entering or leaving a certain spatial range. Quarantine involves separation and restriction of movement of anyone who might have been exposed to an infectious disease or agent, despite having no symptoms, to observe if they develop the disease [19]. Studies of infectious respiratory diseases state that quarantine can stop the spread of the virus by 80% to 90% [9]. Mandatory confinement occurred in some countries with confirmed cases of coronavirus. Its duration depended on risk assessment made by the authorities and epidemiology of the disease within a country. It is worth noting that measures introduced by each country varied in both severity and enforcement, and that no country fully implemented a quarantine in the strictest sense of the term. Each country implemented varying levels of lockdown, confinement, social distancing and self-isolation, and adapting to the evolving situation over time. However, across all four countries, the most commonly searched term during the first months of the pandemic was for quarantine [11], suggesting a conflation of these different terms and measures among Google and YouTube users across all four study countries. Recent research studied the social aspects of searches of audiovisual content on YouTube [28]. The popular portal has also been covered in research on various pathologies and medical treatments [1, 36]. Other projects have studied the impact of educational public health videos such as vaccination campaigns [2, 3, 20] and the use of YouTube as a public database of patient network behavior [25, 29, 37]. There are just a few studies of the impact of the coronavirus on YouTube [3, 17] and none of them has focused on the impact of the disease on visits to the YouTube platform [35]. Use of the Google search engine has become so widespread that it can be a useful tool to study the behaviour of citizens in modern societies. Through the search data, it is possible to understand the interests and fears of citizens on different matters, such as the Covid-19 health crisis [24]. By studying the frequency of use of certain search terms, economic, social, or health trends can be predicted [15]. Other studies have concluded that Google data shows a correlation between influenza outbreaks and unemployment levels, being able to anticipate other methods such as official reports or surveys [27]. The analysis of searches on YouTube and Google can help us understand the tendency of citizens to different security measures during the first months of the pandemic.

2 Objective

The aim of this study is to examine searches for the term 'quarantine' on Google and YouTube in the United States, the United Kingdom, Spain, and Italy between February and June at the beginning of the pandemic. The secondary objective is to determine the correlation between the Google search data for the word "quarantine" in the first country in the west that suffered a health crisis resulting from Covid-19 compared to countries that were later affected: United States, Spain and the United Kingdom.

3 Method

This study conducts a quantitative analysis of the most searched terms on Google and YouTube using Google Trends data. Recent research [4, 20, 21, 28] uses a similar method to study trends on areas of social interest on Google and YouTube. Several health science investigations compare Google Trends data with the spread of the virus around the world to predict future outbreaks [2,23,24,36].

The data provided by Google Trends is an impartial, anonymous, and categorized sample of search data on the YouTube platform. This makes it possible to measure interest in one or several terms of importance anywhere in the world [28]. The analysis method has two filtering options. Real-time data is a random sample of searches from seven days previous to the search day. Non-real-time random sample groups from the Google data set from 2008 to the last 36 h, allowing comparison between various subjects of interest [12, 13].

Google Trends provides a serial time index of Google search query volume in a geographic area. The query index is based on the total volume of queries for the search term in question within a geographic region divided by the total number of queries in that region during the period examined. The maximum number of queries in the specified period is normalized to 100, and the number of queries on the initial date being analysed is normalized to zero [5]. Google Trends calculates its data using a sampling method. For this reason, the results may vary slightly from one day to the next. Also, because of privacy concerns, only queries with significant volumes are tracked. The data from this query index is available at different geographic levels: countries, states, world level, etc.

For this study, Google Trends data on the word 'quarantine' will be used in the four countries with the highest number of total deaths from Covid-19 disease at the end of May 2020 [22]: United States (85,906), United Kingdom United (33,614), Italy (31,368) and Spain (27,459) from February to June 2020 [33, 34].

If our data are quantitative, we will get the evidence on the biases of the information on a phenomenon in different territories and the measures of agreement between them from a linear regression study that will provide us with the R2 value of the comparison between two groups of data to find out the prediction of one variable regarding another.

Since Italy was the first country in the West with a large-scale COVID-19 infections and deaths, we will use it as variable Y of the study. We will compare it with to United States, Spain and United Kingdom, which will work as X variables. With this research, we will use StatPlus™ statistical software to infer the analysis of the linear regression study in the countries mentioned and during the spread of the pandemic. As this is public data of open access on the Google Trends site, this study does not require the approval of any ethical committee. There is no conflict of interest between the authors and any company mentioned in the article.

4 Results

The results (Fig. 1) of the Google search for 'quarantine' show a maximum peak (100) in the United States, on March 16; in the United Kingdom (100), on March 18; in Spain (100) on March 22; and in Italy (100) on March 19. Also noteworthy are the following peaks of searches: on March 15 (98), on March 28 and 29 (both with 97) in Italy; on March 29 in the United Kingdom (77); on March 20 (73) in the United States; and on March 15 (81) in Spain. Likewise, it it is worth noting in the temporal graph of 'quarantine' in Google on February 23 and 25 in Italy (84) and the United Kingdom (34), as these are the first peaks of interest on the subject in the selected period. The United Kingdom is also the place with the highest peak of interest during the month of May (70).

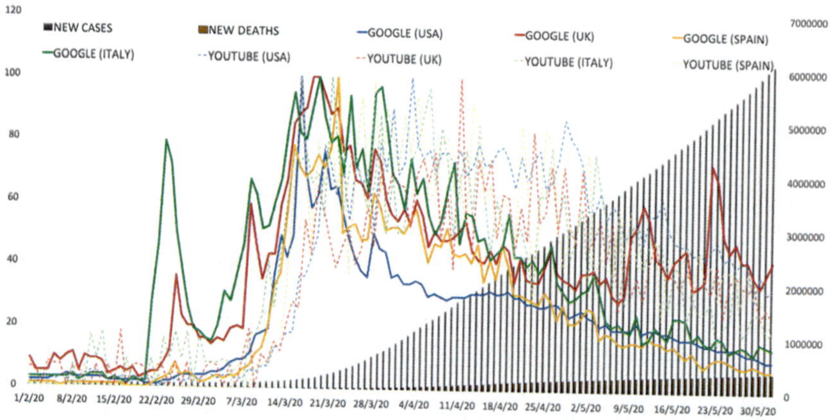

Fig. 1. The interest of searches for the term 'quarantine' on Google and YouTube in the United States, United Kingdom, Spain, and Italy from February to June 2020. The same graph includes the data of infections and deaths from Covid-19 in the world.

On YouTube (Fig. 1), the maximum search peaks are on the following days: April 3 (United States), April 27 (United Kingdom), April 15 (Spain) and April 4 (Italy). The following peaks of interest in searches on audiovisual content of 'quarantine' also stand out: April 26 (89) in Italy; April 11 (94), April 14 (93) and April 19 (92) in the United

Kingdom; April 28 (88) in the United States; and on March 30 (91) and March 14 (85) in Spain.

The contagion and death chart for Covid-19 (Fig. 1) grows from mid-March 2020 and continues at the end of the chosen period. On June 1, 2020, the WHO records the total sum of 6,135,497 confirmed cases since the pandemic began and 373,749 deaths caused by Covid-19. On April 11 the death toll rose to 100,000 people, in a full expansion of the pandemic across the American continent.

A)

Linear Regression

Dependent variable	Quarantine: (Italy)
Independent variables	Quarantine: (Spain)
N	198

Regression Statistics

R	0,98240	***R-Squared***	**0,96511**	*Adjusted R-Squared*	0,96493
MSE	2,96385	***S***	**1,72158**	*MAPE*	58,66782

B)

Linear Regression

Dependent variable	Quarantine: (Italy)
Independent variables	Quarantine: (United States)
N	198

Regression Statistics

R	0,98169	***R-Squared***	**0,96371**	*Adjusted R-Squared*	0,96353
MSE	3,08264	***S***	**1,75574**	*MAPE*	74,17179

C)

Linear Regression

Dependent variable	Quarantine: (Italy)
Independent variables	Quarantine (UK)
N	198

Regression Statistics

R	0,88767	***R-Squared***	**0,78796**	*Adjusted R-Squared*	0,78688
MSE	18,01388	***S***	**4,24428**	*MAPE*	55,37267

Fig. 2. A) Regression analysis between Italy and the United States. B) Regression analysis between Italy and Spain. C) Regression analysis between Italy and the United Kingdom.

The results of the linear regression analysis (Fig. 2) show a positive correlation between searches for the word 'quarantine' in Italy in relation to those in the United States (R2 = 0.96) and those in Spain (R2 = 0.96), being able to generate predictive models for the future. The results of the regression analysis show these prediction formulas of the Italy and United States analyzed data: 'quarantine': (Italy) = −0,82057 + 0,95027 * 'quarantine': (United States). The prediction formula of the variable Italy with Spain is as follows: 'quarantine': (Italy) = −0.21853 + 0.92916 * 'Quarantine': (Spain). The comparison of the data for Italy with the United Kingdom ones is less statistically relevant (R2 = 0.78). In this particularly case we do not value the prediction formula.

5 Discussion and Conclusion

The data in the time chart shows an increase in the interest in the word 'quarantine' in Google and YouTube from mid-February that continues in high levels of searches until June 2020. It also highlights that Italy and the United Kingdom were ahead of the rest of the countries in Google searches and that the highest concentration of searches is found in March and April on both Google and YouTube.

The interest in searches on the audiovisual content portal reached the highest influx of searches a few weeks later than on Google. This leads us to the conclusion that in the case of the term 'quarantine' citizens of the study countries first searched for this concept on Google and later became interested in its content on the audiovisual portal. We also observe in the graph an anticipation of citizen interest in 'quarantine' before the data for victims of Covid-19 shot up in the world to 100,000 deaths. The graph shows that the number of searches for 'quarantine' expects the worst data on deaths from the coronavirus.

Interest in the term 'quarantine' has a statistical correlation between Google searches in Italy compared separately to the United States and Spain during the spread of the Covid-19 pandemic from the first SARS outbreak (2004) to the present day. This shows that the quarantine data of interest in Italy generate a prediction pattern in the United States and Spain (prediction formula). Citizens of the aforementioned countries, regardless of the measures taken by their governments, showed very similar interests through Google searches for 'quarantine'. This positive correlation of the data could reflect on the similarity of the behavior of a several groups of population in Google searches. However, the same similarity does not happen in the comparison between Italy and the UK. Of all studied groups, the UK one shows the most significant differences to Italy due to the lack of statistical correlation.

However, this study has several limitations. Even though Google is the search engine most used by citizens of the countries analysed [10], there are other search engines such as Yahoo, Bing, or Yandex, which were not included in the study. The same happens with searches for audiovisual content, focused solely on YouTube, excluding those from other portals or social networks.

This study provides us with valuable information on the reactions of citizens to health emergencies. It also offers data for prevention strategies and anticipation of future actions in the event that this type of situation occurs successively in the countries studied. By knowing the interest and search patterns of citizens, government and health institutions can act quickly to avoid misinformation, as well as provide clear and consistent messages on prevention and health habits. Given the public's trust in information accessible through Google and YouTube, the use of search engine data has potential to inform effective communication strategies around prevention through promotion of web and audio-visual content.

References

1. Aydin, M.F., Aydin, M.A.: Quality and reliability of information available on YouTube and Google pertaining gastroesophageal reflux disease. Int. J. Med. Inform. **137** (2020). https://doi.org/10.1016/j.ijmedinf.2020.104107
2. Ayyoubzadeh, S.M., Ayyoubzadeh, S.M., Zahedi, H., Ahmadi, M.R., Niakan Kalhori, S.: Predicting COVID-19 incidence through analysis of google trends data in Iran: data mining and deep learning pilot study. JMIR Public Health Surveill **6**(2), e18828 (2020). https://doi.org/10.2196/18828
3. Basch, C., Hillyer, G., Meleo-Erwin, Z., Jaime, C., Mohlman, J., Basch, C.E.: Preventive behaviors conveyed on YouTube to mitigate transmission of COVID-19: cross sectional study. JMIR Public Health Surveill **6**(2) (2020). https://doi.org/10.2196/18807
4. Cerdán Martínez, V., Padilla Castillo, G.: Historia del *fake* audiovisual: *deepfake* y la mujer en un imaginario falsificado y perverso. Historia y Comunicación Soc. **24**(2), 505–520 (2019). https://doi.org/10.5209/hics.66293
5. Choi, H., Varian, H.: Predicting the present with google trends. Econ. Rec. **88**, 2–9 (2012). https://doi.org/10.1111/j.1475-4932.2012.00809.x
6. Corman, V.M., et al.: Detection of 2019 novel coronavirus (2019-nCoV) by real-time RT-PCR. Euro Surveillance **25**(4) (2020). https://doi.org/10.2807/1560-7917.ES.2020.25.3.2000045
7. Dong, Y., et al.: Epidemiological characteristics of 2143 pediatric patients with 2019 coronavirus disease in China. Pediatrics **145**(5) (2020). https://doi.org/10.1542/peds.2020-0702
8. Escalera-Antezana, J.P., et al.: Clinical features of the first cases and a cluster of Coronavirus Disease 2019 (COVID-19) in Bolivia imported from Italy and Spain. Travel Med. Infect. Dis. (2020). https://doi.org/10.1016/j.tmaid.2020.101653
9. Ferguson, N.M., et al.: Strategies for containing an emerging influenza pandemic in Southeast Asia. Nature **437**(7056), 209–214 (2005). https://doi.org/10.1038/nature04017
10. Google: Ver YouTube Originals. https://support.google.com/youtube/answer/6358146?hl=es. Accessed 25 May 2020
11. Google. La cuarentena es la medida de protección más buscada en España (2020). https://trends.google.es/trends/story/US_cu_fPcT5XABAAAfkM_en. Accessed 01 June 2020
12. Google. Google Trends (2020). https://trends.google.es/trends/?geo=ES. Accessed 06 June 2020
13. Guan, W., et al.: Clinical characteristics of coronavirus disease 2019 in China. New Engl. J. Med. **382**, 1708–1720 (2020). https://doi.org/10.1056/NEJMoa2002032
14. Hodcroft, E.B.: Preliminary case report on the SARS-CoV-2 cluster in the UK, France, and Spain. Swiss Med. Weekly **150** (2020). https://doi.org/10.4414/smw.2020.20212
15. Hubbard, D.: Pulse: The New Science of Harnessing Internet Buzz to Track Threats and Opportunities. Wiley, Hoboken (2011)
16. Jin, Z., Du, X., Yang, H., et al.: Structure of M^{pro} from COVID-19 virus and discovery of its inhibitors. Nature **582**, 289–293 (2020). https://doi.org/10.1038/s41586-020-2223-y

17. Khatri, P., et al.: YouTube as source of information on 2019 novel coronavirus outbreak: a cross sectional study of English and Mandarin content. Travel Med. Infect. Dis. **35** (2020). https://doi.org/10.1016/j.tmaid.2020.101636
18. Liu, W., Zhang, Q., Chen, J., et al.: Detection of COVID-19 in children in early January 2020 in Wuhan, China. New Engl. J. Med. **382** (2020). https://doi.org/10.1056/NEJMc2003717
19. Mack, R.N., Simberloff, D., Lonsdale, W.M., Evans, H., Clout, M., Bazzaz, F.A.: Biotic invasions: causes, epidemiology, global consequences, and control. Ecol. Appl. **10**(3), 689–710 (2000). https://doi.org/10.2307/2641039
20. Mahroum, N., et al.: Capturing public interest toward new tools for controlling human immunodeficiency virus (HIV) infection exploiting data from Google Trends. Health Inform. J. **25**(4), 1383–1397 (2018). https://doi.org/10.1177/1460458218766573
21. Quintanilha, L.-F., Souza, L., Sanches, D., Senos-Demarco, R., Ferreira-Fukutani, K.: The impact of cancer campaigns in Brazil: a Google Trends analysis. Ecancer Med. Sci. **13**(963), 1–9 (2019). https://doi.org/10.3332/ecancer.2019.963
22. Ritchie, H.: Coronavirus Source Data. Our World in Data (2020). https://ourworldindata.org/coronavirus-source-data. Accessed 08 June 2020
23. Springer, S., Menzel, L.M., Zieger, M.: Google Trends reveals: focus of interest in the population is on treatment options rather than theories about COVID-19 animal origin. Brain Behav. Immun. **87**, 134–135 (2020). https://doi.org/10.1016/j.bbi.2020.05.005
24. Strzelecki, A.: The second worldwide wave of interest in coronavirus since the COVID-19 outbreaks in South Korea, Italy and Iran: a Google Trends study. Brain Behav. Immun. **86** (2020). https://doi.org/10.1016/j.bbi.2020.04.042
25. Szmuda, T., Rosvall, P., Hetzger, T., Ali, S., Słoniewski, P.: YouTube as a source of patient information for hydrocephalus: a content-quality and optimization analysis. World Neurosurg. (2020). https://doi.org/10.1016/j.wneu.2020.02.149
26. Tagarro, A., Epalza, C., Santos, M., et al.: Screening and severity of coronavirus disease 2019 (COVID-19) in children in Madrid, Spain. JAMA Pediatr. (2020). https://doi.org/10.1001/jamapediatrics.2020.1346
27. Tanz, J.: Soon we won't program computers. We'll train them like dogs. Wired (2016). https://www.wired.com/2016/05/the-end-of-code. Accessed 12 June 2020
28. Villa-Gracia, D., Cerdán, V.: Evolución de la popularidad de Donald Trump y otros mandatarios internacionales en Google Trends (2016–2019). El profesional de la información **29**(1) (2020). https://doi.org/10.3145/epi.2020.ene.12
29. Wang, W., Xu, Y., Gao, R.: Detection of SARS-CoV-2 indifferent types of clinical specimens. JAMA **323**(18), 1843–1844 (2020). https://doi.org/10.1001/jama.2020.3786
30. Wei, M., Yuan, J., Liu, Y., et al.: Novel coronavirus infection in hospitalized infants under 1 year of age in China. JAMA **323**(13) (2020). https://doi.org/10.1001/jama.2020.2131
31. WHO: Neumonía de causa desconocida – China (2020). https://www.who.int/csr/don/05-january-2020-pneumonia-of-unkown-cause-china/es/. Accessed 12 June 2020
32. WHO: La WHO lanza una nueva estrategia mundial contra la gripe (2020). https://www.who.int/es/news-room/detail/11-03-2019-who-launches-new-global-influenza-strategy. Accessed 14 June 2020
33. WHO: COVID-19: cronología de la actuación de la WHO (2020). https://www.who.int/es/news-room/detail/27-04-2020-who-timeline---covid-19. Accessed 14 June 2020
34. WHO: Europe Country report: Italy (2020). https://www.covid19healthsystem.org/countries/italy/countrypage.aspx. Accessed 14 June 2020
35. YouTube: YouTube en cifras (2020). https://www.youtube.com/intl/es/about/press/. Accessed 05 June 2020
36. Yuan, X., Xu, J., Hussain, S., Wang, H., Gao, N., Zhang, L.: Trends and prediction in daily new cases and deaths of COVID-19 in the United States: an internet search-interest based

model. Explor. Res. Hypothesis Med. **5**(2), 41–46 (2020). https://doi.org/10.14218/ERHM.2020.00023

37. Zhang, J., Zheng, Z., Wang, Y. and Zhu, Y.: A study on users' preference towards diabetes-related video clips on YouTube. BMC Med. Inform. Decis. Mak. **20**(1) (2020). https://doi.org/10.1186/s12911-020-1035-1

Influence of Short-Term Study Abroad Program Design in Adjustment Experiences

Ariana Melchor-Bazalar, Jorge Lucas Vargas-Sardon, and Eliana Gallardo-Echenique(✉)

School of Communications, Universidad Peruana de Ciencias Aplicadas, Lima, Peru
{u201410416,pcimjova}@upc.edu.pe, eliana.gallardo@upc.pe

Abstract. The increasingly interconnected world and the demands for internationally educated graduates have had a major impact on higher education and have catalyzed the trend of short-term studies abroad. Differences in the program design- like duration, involvement in cultural integration, support groups and other features- may have varying implications on student learning outcomes. This study aims to analyze the influence of the program design in the adjustment experience of the students from the Iacocca Global Village 2018 edition. A qualitative case study design was chosen and fifteen semi-structured interviews with 19 open-ended questions were conducted followed by thematic analysis. Findings show there is a need for intentional pedagogy focused on intercultural outcomes supported by: (a) ongoing mentoring, (b) mandatory involvement in cultural integration and support groups, (c) pressure for real work and accountability as a prerequisite to leave the comfort zone and foster intercultural encounters and (d) that alumni networks can contribute to keep the sense of belonging developed in the program.

Keywords: Intercultural adjustment · Intercultural communication · Study abroad · Education abroad · Program design

1 Introduction

The last 25 years have seen significant and rapid changes making globalization a word that can no longer be attributed merely to international economic activities since it has created an interconnected, multicultural world having a profound and diverse impact on higher education institutions and the professional sphere [1–4]. Previous studies [5–7] suggest that globalization and the demands for internationally educated graduates have had a major impact on higher education and have catalyzed the trend of short-term studies abroad, directing educators and program administrators efforts to improve support schemes to help students transition and adjust to their new learning environments.

Despite the growing number of students involving in these short-term study abroad programs- particularly those who had no overseas education or lack funds for extended study abroad experiences- research focused on educational outcomes and program efficacy remains in early stages; likewise, a lack of uniformity in their structure troubles

© The Author(s), under exclusive license to Springer Nature Singapore Pte Ltd. 2022
Á. Rocha et al. (Eds.): ICOMTA 2021, SIST 259, pp. 524–533, 2022.
https://doi.org/10.1007/978-981-16-5792-4_52

finding a standardized assessment [6, 8–11]. There is a growing body of literature that recognizes the importance of the emotional and intellectual challenges presented to students during the programs as well as having pedagogical strategies focused on intercultural effectiveness, pointing out how the design and structure of the programs play key role in the different impacts of educational experience on students [9, 12–17].

More recently, researchers obtained contradictory findings about the effectiveness of these programs. Studies that concentrate on understanding intercultural adjustment in students more frequently adopt a quantitative approach relying in measuring tools like the Intercultural Sensitivity Index (IDI) [9, 10, 13, 18, 19] while others opt for mixed methods [5, 6, 17, 20–22]. Such approaches, however, have failed to address "study abroad" as a changeable variable, considering the program design elements as unrelated to the learning gains [8, 14, 22, 23]. Several investigations [6, 9, 17, 19, 24–26] converges and indicates that it is important to (a) study cross-cultural adjustment experiences of specific groups of international students and their coping strategies within their context to enrich the possibilities of improving the programs, (b) recognize specific adjustment experiences of separate groups of international students and then apply differentiated to facilitate the adjustment, (c) focus on the quality of the psychological, socio-cultural and educational experiences of this large com-munity of students, since they are crucial to fostering global intercultural understanding.

Surprisingly, the influence of the program design in the student's adjustment have not been closely examined enough and much uncertainty still exists about the contextual circumstances involved in the student's adjustment experiences. This study attempts to obtain further information from a qualitative view of the participant's experience of the Iacocca Global Village for Future Leaders, an innovative immersive five-week intercultural learning program at Lehigh University (Pennsylvania, United States). Over 30 years, Iacocca Institute programs have hosted participants from more than 150 countries. The Global Village helps bring together university students and professionals from across the globe, from diverse backgrounds (cultural, social, economic, generational, and professional) to educate the next generation of world leaders. In this program, the students have a 5-week immersion experience where they are "hosts" as well as "guests". This study addresses the following research question: In which ways did program design elements influence the students' process of adjustment?

2 Methodology

The study is positioned in the interpretative framework of social constructivism which stresses on developing subjective meanings of human experiences [27]. It was used to develop a pattern of meaning of the students' experience in the program since the case under study is a very complex and multifaceted experience [27, 28]. Qualitative approach has been adopted to understand and value the experience of 15 participants during the five-week immersion experience [27]. A case-study approach [29] was chosen to capture detailed understanding of the programs' design influence in the adjustment of students in the short-term study abroad program: The Global Village for Future Leaders. The study was conducted among students from Global Village 2018 edition [30] which had 61 enrolled participants -who call themselves "Villagers"- from 36 countries and 4 continents aged from 18 to 45 years old [K. Mendez, personal communication, September 29, 2020]. A purposeful sampling size of 15 students was used [27, 29] until theme emergence had reached data saturation [31]. The sample included one respondent per country -Azerbaijan, China, Dominican Republic, France, Greece, Hong Kong, Israel, Italy, Kazakhstan, Morocco, Pakistan, Peru, Puerto Rico, Sierra Leone, and South Africa- and varied across attributes of gender (Female: 9; Male: 6), age (21 to 32 yrs.), and the students' majors ranged from engineering to communications, medicine, accounting, political science, culinary arts and management.

The main qualitative data collection approach was semi-structured interviews with 19 open-ended questions focusing on (a) the student's perception of their experiences during the program, and (b) how the program design elements influenced the process. The interview guide was validated in the field to identify unclear or ambiguous statements [27, 29]. Synchronous online interviews were conducted in English, via computer-mediated communication through a secure online application and took from 30 to 60 min. All participants received an information sheet [32] explaining the purpose of the study and their role within it, as well as the measures taken to preserve the confidentiality of their responses. The rights of individual participants to self-determination, privacy and dignity was always respected [32]. Before the interview, the interviewer thanked each student for his participation and requested his permission to record the interview. An inductive thematic analysis from interview transcripts was used to identify categories and develop 'bottom-up' themes within the data [33]. An alphanumeric code was used to identify participants as follows: Participant Number, Sex, Age, City, Country (P01, Male, 21, Wenzhou, China).

3 Results and Discussion

Four main design elements of the program emerged from the analysis of the responses: (a) extreme diversity, (b) external responsibility, (c) heavily mentored environment and (d) worldwide network. Each of them influenced the final learning outcomes and was reported to support students through the distinct phases of the process of adjusting to the program.

The extreme diversity component refers to the program elements that allowed students to interact constantly with different people within a highly diverse student population from over thirty countries. The main activities were the cultural night and the daily country presentations. In the former, students showcased the traditional culture of their country -like dances, typical clothing, food, etc.- and, in the latter, their business culture. Students answers showcased characteristics alike with healthy generalized ethnocentrism like (a) finding lifestyles in other cultures as valid as in their own; (b) recognizing that they have things to learn from other cultures; (c) respecting values and customs from other cultures; (d) having friends from various cultures; (e) applying different values when judging people who are different; and (f) liking to be involved in interactions with people from other countries [34].

> Both activities [cultural nights and country presentations] were important to me because it shows who we are…The emotional attachment to your culture is important to value what you have... business culture and preference in terms of working

hours as well, then you can easily respect and understand other perspectives while working because [if not understood] you keep arguing about something is wrong without knowing one's culture (…) They showed us the differences and celebrate them. (P13, Male, 23, Chitral, Pakistan).

The extreme diversity component also required students to be involved in extensive direct cultural contact, constant participation in cultural integration, live close quarters, working and learning and planned contrasting "roommates" based on intensive assessment prior to arrival as suggested by previous research as effective to foster intercultural development [12, 23]. Turning now to the experimental evidence on roommates, responses can be classified in three groups: a majority who recognized they had to adjust but finally blended well, some who blended fine without any problems, and only one student who couldn't get along due to strong cultural differences and had to be moved to another room. Over half of those interviewed reported that their roommate experience played a significant role in learning habits from other cultures and diminishing stereotyping as well as adapting and respecting each other, proving its importance as shown by other authors [35–37]. Together these results provide important insights into the importance and influence of the diversity of countries and backgrounds for the success of a short-term program due to its impact in the contrast of ideas of the students and the validation – or not – of stereotypes. Whilst a minority of students mentioned not having stereotypes, the overall response was a sense of surprise for contrasting their ideas about certain nationalities during the program. A common view amongst students was that mass media shapes common beliefs and the importance to contrast them with real people, corroborating earlier findings as to the power of media to shape stereotypes that don't portray the truth of countries [38–43].

My roommate was from Latin America… at the beginning I would walk around naked in the room, but my roommate was not very comfortable with that because you know in Latin America, they have this culture of *machos* (…) Night after night, we shared our life stories, and everything changed for us. We became very good friends and adapted and respected each other. (P3, Male, 31, Foggia, Italy)

As an Asian, I had some knowledge about Hindus… but I must admit I also thought they would eat curry all day (laughs). In the kitchen I discovered my knowledge is limited and they are more than that. I realized they are very generous, warm and with good humor. They are characterized by taking care of who they consider family and this all traces back to their culture and I think that is beautiful. (P01, Male, 21, Wenzhou, China)

The external responsibility element describes the components that moves students out of their comfort zone. The respondents reported to be subject to real work accountability in diverse teams, where they were assigned to a cross-cultural team for an international or U.S. based client and appointed with a mentor, had constant checkups from their Project Mentor for results and continuous communication with the client. All students revealed to have difficulties working with their peers in a higher or lower degree and highlighted (a) how big cultural differences start showing up in small disagreements until they become big; (b) how difficult it is to work with people with completely different worldviews;

and, (c) how guidance was key to connect with the team and see the diversity as a benefit. A common and recurrent topic that emerged in responses under this element was that the main stressors in teamwork were time and punctuality, working styles (high tolerance to ambiguity vs low), leadership styles (individualistic vs collectivistic), time for indulgence vs full time working [44], and language as a stressor [45]. The teams who were able to blend well appointed the following as crucial for them: effective communication, guidance from their project mentor, responsibility, and the urge to get the work done for the external client. Also, students belonging to teams who adjusted, reported to appreciate the difference, and adapted some costumes from other peers. These findings are consistent with that of L. Engle and J. Engle [12] who found that the real power of education abroad comes when students face challenges in the emotional and intellectual sphere. Students faced real-life responsibilities, having to cope with challenges that are not easy or cannot be found in role-plays, case-studies or other programs without the diversity of this one [46]. This view was echoed by another informant who shared his experience as challenging and gave insight on the differences in working styles and the main stressors found as common among the majority of respondents. Overall, these results indicate that the work in diverse teams culturally and professionally while having external responsibility for results, made it necessary to adapt to different working styles and provided an environment for the development of effective intercultural leadership and group communication to deliver results.

> We were so different… maybe too different, we suffered working together but there were constant checkups and we had to deliver the work for the client in a deadline. Without this pressure we would have never finished or get past those discussions. Order and time management were mainly the problems and misunderstandings like… we [Asians] are very private for ourselves but maybe for other people from other countries that may feel like we you are not respectful. (P04, Male, 26, Hong Kong, Hong Kong)
>
> My team had members from Sierra Leone, Peru, Puerto Rico, Greece, and France… me. My mentor was from Azerbaijan. In such a different group from also different careers I felt differences in the way we worked (…) You know in Europe we are used to be on time and for example we would agree to meet at four and the Europeans would be there 10 minutes before, and the others would arrive 10 minutes after pretending to talk about their day… I was like what?! we're supposed to work, you're late! (...) When we solved that and also the language problem everything was fine. (P02, Male, 24, Paris, France)

The third component of Global Village, heavily mentored environment, implies the ongoing mentoring focused on intercultural effectiveness students undergo for the adjustment and development of problem solving and intercultural leadership skills. Since the start of the program, students were assigned to a support group with an appointed mentor (GV Alumni) for personal goals and experiencing bonding activities with peers. Respondents indicated that had to participate in compulsory continuous orientation, mentoring and reflective coaching as part of the program. When being asked about their project mentor students over half of those interviewed felt that their project mentor role was mostly professional and the mentor intervened when necessary, to keep the work moving and, while the rest considered that it was not only a professional mentor but also, personal. The importance of mentors has been recently pointed out to play a critical role in education [47, 48]. Another reported theme was the role of support groups and personal guides. A common view amongst interviewees was that the guide groups helped them to interact – among other things – with people at a human level and provided them with guidance for growth. This is in line with studies [9, 13] using the Intercultural Development Inventory which found it is not enough to send students to study abroad without intentional pedagogy focused on outcomes of intercultural effectiveness. These results suggest that the heavily mentored environment serves as a support scheme to students by providing constant mentorship in cross-cultural leadership, teamwork, and problem-solving skills which the students claim also, to be crucial for the program to succeed. Respondents found student-led bonding activities to be as important as faculty mentoring since they received peer mentoring which further support the idea of mentorship as a support scheme.

> Our project mentor … she was like this glue for us, always giving us direction… if something was not right, she'd make sure it was all right. She already had this experience so suddenly after she spoke everyone was happy and moving forward more than focusing on why it didn't work and it was fundamental for us to have a new perspective. (P12, Female, 22, Lima, Peru)

> I think my group leader was more like an emotional guide and showed me how to accomplish my own goals that I wanted in the program. I think I learned to connect with other people in a more personal and human way in the times we shared together… I think the guide groups made me feel how we are similar but the team for the project made me feel how we are different (laughs) (P10, Female, 24, Santiago, Dominican Republic)

Taken together, these results suggest that there is an association between the mentoring and the successful adjustment of students, as noted in prior studies [14, 45]. The fourth component of the program, worldwide network, refers to the influence of the Alumni Network the students belong after the program ends, and was reported by most respondents to endure the lasting bond with the values acquired in the program. It was found that this network further nurtures the learning and values developed even after the return home, rather than being a momentaneous superficial change. After the program, students shared that they stay connected with friends and also meet new ones from the network. When being asked about the importance to be part of the community responses can be classified into: students who affirm belonging means to be part of a family and community and it's of sum importance to them, students who affirm they do feel the connection but have not explored the specific benefits of the network yet and students who report to keep in touch only with their class but not actively participate in the elections of the board or other Alumni activities. This finding has important implications for developing lasting connection networks for short-term study abroad programs to maximize their impact in line with studies showing their potential utility to the broader public [49, 50].

> It is very important to me to be part of the community it's like … if your aunt lives in another city you have to go see your aunt... for me it's like you are being born in a new family and it is international, and I wear it as something that I'm proud of myself… I'd say again like a last name… GV is like a last name or third name… wherever you go you can say: are you a GVer? (P08, Female, 24, Nakhichevan, Azerbaijan)

> I feel like that network really leads to that that goal of having a peaceful world because then we have a lot of people from different countries and they're doing different projects in their own country and then they are in touch with people from different countries... Whenever I see the WhatsApp group it's just a blessing to me (P13, Male, 23, Chitral, Pakistan)

4 Conclusions

This study has identified four main program components and the evidence suggests that they all influence the adjustment experience of student's in an overall positive way. The current data suggests that the highly diverse environment component provides enough space for excitement and disorientation in students and a valuable space to contrast stereotypes in a safe environment. At the same time, the diversity in the living facilities and the working groups, makes students transition to real-life challenges. The results suggest that without an accountability component, probably the urge to adjust wouldn't be present and the intercultural development in short programs could be undermined. The evidence also indicates that the heavily mentored environment is key to help students navigate through the transition and leads to the integration to a respectful world-wide community which serves as a social support scheme to maintain the values learned upon return to home country.

This study has provided a deeper insight into the contextual implications of program design in student's experience and contributes to the literature on short-term study abroad and intercultural learning by starting to identify best practices in this heterogeneous field and proposes the analysis as related to the program design. The insights gained from this study may be of assistance and can be applied to, and guide, the design of intercultural training programs in universities doing internationalization efforts. The present study lays the groundwork for future research into the influence of program design into the students' experience and has gone some way towards enhancing our understanding of the contextual implications of intercultural adjustment.

Despite its exploratory nature, this study offers important lessons to be considered: (a) attention should be paid to the amount of comfort or ambiguity that is provided to students during their first encounters; (b) there is a need for intentional pedagogy focused on intercultural outcomes supported by ongoing mentoring; (c) it's important to have mandatory involvement in cultural integration and support groups; (d) pressure for real work and accountability is a prerequisite to leave the comfort zone (it can take form of a project or internship); (e) housing arrangements and coexistence of the students undergoing the program is essential for developing strong bonds and have "nowhere to hide" from the interactions; and, (f) alumni networks with representation and active involvement can contribute to maintain the sense of belonging developed in the program.

The study is not without limitations. Being limited to the small sample of Global Village for Future Leaders and its contextual characteristics, this study lacks a wide-ranging review of all the background of students and some predictors for their behavior during the program. There was the possibility that students remember and share their responses with a very strong emotional attachment to the program, making their responses less objective.

References

1. Kim, Y.Y.: Globalization and intercultural personhood. In: Samovar, L.A., Porte, R.E., McDaniel, E.R. (eds.) Intercultural Communication: A Reader, pp. 83–94. Cengage Learning, Boston (2012)
2. Saint-Jacques, B.: Intercultural Communication in a Globalized World. Intercultural Communication. A Reader, 13th edn, vol. 39, pp. 45–56 (2012)
3. Krajewska, A.: Globalization and higher education: the Polish perspective. East. Eur. J. Transnatl. Relat. **4**, 15–31 (2020). https://doi.org/10.15290/eejtr.2020.04.01.01
4. Hajisoteriou, C., Angelides, P.: Examining the nexus of globalisation and intercultural education: theorising the macro-micro integration process. Glob. Soc. Educ. **18**, 149–166 (2020). https://doi.org/10.1080/14767724.2019.1693350
5. Cotton, D.R.E., Morrison, D., Magne, P., Payne, S., Heffernan, T.: Global citizenship and cross-cultural competency: student and expert understandings of internationalization terminology. J. Stud. Int. Educ. **23**, 346–364 (2019). https://doi.org/10.1177/1028315318789337
6. Senyshyn, R.M.: A first-year seminar course that supports the transition of international students to higher education and fosters the development of intercultural communication competence. J. Intercult. Commun. Res. **48**, 150–170 (2019). https://doi.org/10.1080/17475759.2019.1575892
7. Mak, A.S., Bodycott, P., Ramburuth, P.: Beyond host language proficiency: coping resources predicting international students' satisfaction. J. Stud. Int. Educ. **19**, 460–475 (2015). https://doi.org/10.1177/1028315315587109
8. Mule, L., Aloisio, K., Audley, S.: Short-term, faculty-led study abroad and global citizenship identification: insights from a global engagement program. Front. Interdiscip. J. Study Abroad **30**, 20–37 (2018). https://doi.org/10.36366/frontiers.v30i3.425
9. Pedersen, P.J.: Assessing intercultural effectiveness outcomes in a year-long study abroad program. Int. J. Intercult. Relations. **34**, 70–80 (2010). https://doi.org/10.1016/j.ijintrel.2009.09.003
10. Bloom, M., Miranda, A.: Intercultural sensitivity through short-term study abroad. Lang. Intercult. Commun. **15**, 567–580 (2015). https://doi.org/10.1080/14708477.2015.1056795
11. Koyanagi, S.: Impact of intercultural communication during short-term study-abroad of Japanese students: analysis from a perspective of cognitive modification. J. Intercult. Commun. Res. **47**, 105–120 (2018). https://doi.org/10.1080/17475759.2018.1435423
12. Engle, L., Engle, J.: Study abroad levels: toward a classification of program types. Front. Interdiscip. J. Study Abroad **9**, 1–20 (2003). https://doi.org/10.36366/frontiers.v9i1.113
13. Vande Berg, M., Paige, R.M., Lou, K.H.: Student Learning Abroad: What Our Students Are Learning, What They're Not, and What We Can Do About It, vol. 1. Stylus Publishing, Sterling (2012)
14. Hudson, T.D., Tomás Morgan, R.: Examining relationships between education abroad program design and college students' global learning. Front. Interdiscip. J. Study Abroad **31**, 1–31 (2019). https://doi.org/10.36366/frontiers.v31i2.452

15. Orozco-Vargas, P.G., Diaz, C.M.F., Arenas, R.D., Perez, M.A.P., Chota, R.M., Ramirez-Villacorta, Y.: Intercultural competencies in graduate students of a private university in Lima. Int. J. High. Educ. **9**, 59–70 (2020). https://doi.org/10.5430/ijhe.v9n9p59
16. Haas, B.W.: The impact of study abroad on improved cultural awareness: a quantitative review. Intercult. Educ. **29**, 571–588 (2018). https://doi.org/10.1080/14675986.2018.1495319
17. Arseneault, R.: Intercultural adjustment challenges of Korean and Canadian self-initiated expatriates in the workplace: an exploratory bidirectional investigation. Int. J. Cross Cult. Manag. **20**, 181–199 (2020). https://doi.org/10.1177/1470595820915630
18. Barden, S.M., Shannonhouse, L., Mobley, K.: International cultural immersion: assessing the influence of a group intervention on intercultural sensitivity for counselor trainees. J. Spec. Gr. Work. **40**, 117–141 (2015). https://doi.org/10.1080/01933922.2014.992505
19. Delmas, P.: Student Learning Abroad: What Our Students Are Learning, What They're Not, and What We Can Do About. Edited by M. Vande Berg, R. Michael Paige, K. Hemming Lou (review). Rev. High. Educ. **36**, 556–557 (2013). https://doi.org/10.1353/rhe.2013.0039
20. Barker, G.G.: Cross-cultural perspectives on intercultural communication competence. J. Intercult. Commun. Res. **45**, 13–30 (2016). https://doi.org/10.1080/17475759.2015.1104376
21. Lin, C.: Culture shock and social support: an investigation of a Chinese student organization on a US campus. J. Intercult. Commun. Res. **35**, 117–137 (2006). https://doi.org/10.1080/17475750600909279
22. Sobkowiak, P.: The impact of studying abroad on students' intercultural competence: an interview study. Stud. Sec. Lang. Learn. Teach. **9**, 681–710 (2019). https://doi.org/10.14746/ssllt.2019.9.4.6
23. Cubillos, J., Ilvento, T.: Intercultural contact in short-term study abroad programs. Hispania **101**, 249–266 (2018). https://doi.org/10.1353/hpn.2018.0117
24. Urban, E., Orbe, M.P., Lin, C.: Culture shock and social support: an investigation of a Chinese student organization on a US campus. J. Intercult. Commun. Res. **36**, 117–137 (2006). https://doi.org/10.1080/17475750600909279
25. Zhou, Y., Jindal-Snape, D., Topping, K., Todman, J.: Theoretical models of culture shock and adaptation in international students in higher education. Stud. High. Educ. **33**, 63–75 (2008). https://doi.org/10.1080/03075070701794833
26. Terzuolo, E.R.: Intercultural development in study abroad: influence of student and program characteristics. Int. J. Intercult. Relat. **65**, 86–95 (2018). https://doi.org/10.1016/j.ijintrel.2018.05.001
27. Creswell, J.W.: Qualitative Inquiry and Research Design: Choosing Among Five Traditions. SAGE Publications Inc., Thousand Oaks (2013)
28. Saldaña, J.: Fundamentals of Qualitative Research. Oxford University Press, New York (2011)
29. Yin, R.K.: Case Study Research and Applications: Design and Methods. SAGE Publications Inc., Thousand Oaks (2018)
30. Iacocca Institute, Lehigh University: The Global Village Experience (2020). https://global.lehigh.edu/iacocca-institute/global-village/experience
31. Corbin, J., Strauss, A.: Basics of Qualitative Research: Techniques and Procedures for Developing Grounded Theory. Sage, Thousand Oaks (2012).https://doi.org/10.4135/9781452230153
32. Rapley, T.: Los análisis de la conversación, del discurso y de documentos en Investigación Cualitativa. Ediciones Morata, S.L., Madrid, España (2014)
33. Clarke, V., Braun, V.: Thematic Analysis (2014). https://doi.org/10.1007/978-94-007-0753-5_3470
34. Neuliep, J.W.: The relationship among intercultural communication apprehension, ethnocentrism, uncertainty reduction, and communication satisfaction during initial intercultural interaction: an extension of anxiety and uncertainty management (AUM) theory. J. Intercult. Commun. Res. **41**, 1–16 (2012). https://doi.org/10.1080/17475759.2011.623239

35. Tolman, S.: The effects of a roommate-pairing program on international student satisfaction and academic success. J. Int. Stud. **7**, 522–541 (2017). https://doi.org/10.5281/zenodo.570013
36. Yao, C.W.: Unfulfilled expectations: influence of Chinese international students' roommate relationships on sense of belonging. J. Int. Stud. **23**, 43 (2016)
37. Erb, S.E., Renshaw, K.D., Short, J.L., Pollard, J.W.: The importance of college roommate relationships: a review and systemic conceptualization. J. Stud. Aff. Res. Pract. **51**, 43–55 (2014). https://doi.org/10.1515/jsarp-2014-0004
38. Sui, M., Paul, N.: Latino portrayals in local news media: underrepresentation, negative stereotypes, and institutional predictors of coverage. J. Intercult. Commun. Res. (2017). https://doi.org/10.1080/17475759.2017.1322124
39. Erigha, M.: Race, gender, hollywood: representation in cultural production and digital media's potential for change. Sociol. Compass. (2015). https://doi.org/10.1111/soc4.12237
40. Ben Labidi, I.: Representation and emancipation: cinema of the oppressed. Int. J. Cult. Stud. (2020). https://doi.org/10.1177/1367877920959338
41. Gabore, S.M.: Western and Chinese media representation of Africa in COVID-19 news coverage. Asian J. Commun. (2020). https://doi.org/10.1080/01292986.2020.1801781
42. Morgan, M., Shanahan, J., Signorielli, N.: Cultivation theory. Int. Encycl. Commun. Theory Philos. 1–10 (2016). https://doi.org/10.1002/9781118766804.wbiect015
43. Potter, W.J.: A critical analysis of cultivation theory. J. Commun. (2014). https://doi.org/10.1111/jcom.12128
44. Hofstede, G.: Dimensionalizing cultures: the hofstede model in context. Online Read. Psychol. Cult. **2**, 1–26 (2011). https://doi.org/10.9707/2307-0919.1014
45. Interis, M.G., Rezek, J., Bloom, K., Campbell, A.: Assessing the value of short-term study abroad programmes to students. Appl. Econ. **50**, 1919–1933 (2018). https://doi.org/10.1080/00036846.2017.1380292
46. Brislin, R.: Encouraging depth rather than surface processing about cultural differences through critical incidents and role plays. Online Read. Psychol. Cult. **7**, 1–18 (2002). https://doi.org/10.9707/2307-0919.1063
47. Shalka, T.R., Corcoran, C.S., Magee, B.T.: Mentors that matter: international student leadership development and mentor roles. J. Int. Stud. **9**, 97–110 (2019). https://doi.org/10.32674/jis.v9i1.261
48. Clarke, A., Mena, J.: An international comparative study of practicum mentors: learning about ourselves by learning about others. Teach. Teach. Educ. **90** (2020). https://doi.org/10.1016/j.tate.2020.103026
49. Ding, F., Riccucci, N.M.: The value of alumni networks in responding to the public administration theory and practice: evidence from the COVID-19 pandemic in China. Adm. Theory Prax. **42**, 588–603 (2020). https://doi.org/10.1080/10841806.2020.1798694
50. Snijders, I., Wijnia, L., Rikers, R.M.J.P., Loyens, S.M.M.: Alumni loyalty drivers in higher education. Soc. Psychol. Educ. **22**(3), 607–627 (2019). https://doi.org/10.1007/s11218-019-09488-4

Treatment of Gender Violence in Digital Newspapers of the Andean Region

Vanessa Rojas-Fernández(✉), Verónica Altamirano-Benítez(✉), and Diana Gabriela Moreira-Aguirre(✉)

Universidad Técnica Particular de Loja, Loja, Ecuador
{vlrojas1,vpaltamirano,dgmoreira}@utpl.edu.ec

Abstract. The United Nations Organization defines Gender-based violence as any act of violence as any act directed to or applied to what belongs to the female sex sphere that may result in physical, sexual or psychological harm or suffering for women, including threats of such acts, coercion or arbitrary deprivation of liberty, whether they occur in public or private life. During the last decades gender violence against women has marked the political, legislative and social agenda of the countries of the world; Latin America in a special way is one of the most affected by this phenomenon, which is considered a public health problem for the states. Without a doubt, feminicide is the most atrocious manifestation of this violence. Through this research work we try to analyze the phenomenon of gender violence specifically the occurrence of crimes of feminicide through the review of news as published in social media in the periods between March 2018 of some digital newspapers of countries of the Andean Region: Bolivia, Peru, Ecuador and Colombia, accounting for the interactions they have with users.

Keywords: Gender violence · Social media · Media · Femicide · Women · Andean community

1 Introduction and Objective

Every day, newspaper headlines and television news broadcasts information related to cases of violence against women, specifically femicides. Gender-based violence against women is not a recent issue, however it is recently that it has become one of the topics of debate in states worldwide due to the disproportionate increase in relation to reported figures of violence and femicide. Women have historically been restricted in their rights and freedoms by historical discrimination based on gender, that is, on the power relations between men and women. One of the most outrageous manifestation of violence against women is their murder, known as femicide. In some penal systems, the murders of women are named as "feminicide" or "femicide", which is considered the most extreme form of violence. In this sense, it is essential to address and conceptualize the two problems that seriously affect society. The Latin American model protocol for investigating violent deaths of women due to gender which according to reports highlights in some cases of intimate feminicide, that they are committed by the sentimental partner and the death

© The Author(s), under exclusive license to Springer Nature Singapore Pte Ltd. 2022
Á. Rocha et al. (Eds.): ICOMTA 2021, SIST 259, pp. 534–543, 2022.
https://doi.org/10.1007/978-981-16-5792-4_53

of the woman is the consequence or the final act of the violence. The objective of this research work is to know, identify and evaluate the treatment that media, especially digital media, hears to issues related to gender violence, femicide in this case. Mass media, and particularly digital media, bear a great responsibility when choosing the correct language and audiovisual material to be able to disseminate with caution the news that prevent and warn society, especially women gender that fears the most for their integrity. It is also geared to evaluate the impact and reaction of official social media of digital newspapers followers of Andean Community in order to analyze whether the content makes visible violence as stated in the comments issued by the followers.

2 Approach to the Problem

World Health Organization-WHO [16], defines violence as a matter of public health, describing it as the intentional use of physical force, threats against oneself, another person, a group or a community that has as consequence, or is very likely to result in trauma, psychological damage, developmental problems, or death.

Violence means the power that one person imposes unto another, thus violating her rights. Violence in itself is not a natural or normal process for human beings, since it implies causing harm in any of its forms to another person. On the other hand, the term gender has also been defined by the same organization WHO [17], as encompassing the characteristics of women and men as defined by society, in norms, roles and relationships existing between them. What is expected from both genders varies from culture to culture and can change over time. It is also important to recognize identities that do not fit into the binary categories of male and female. Gender norms, relationships and roles also influence health outcomes for transgender or intersex people. The Royal Spanish Academy [20] defines the term gender as "group to which human beings of each sex belong, understood from a sociocultural point of view instead of exclusively biological", from this perspective, each body receives a meaning (feminine or masculine) which will be the distinctive of each being from the personal and social. Hernández [6] considers that gender is "A symbolic construction that contains the set of attributes assigned to people based on sex" (p. 182) [8]. In the current debate it is reviewed how the practices of women and men are not derived from essences but are cultural and psychic constructions related to the order of language and representations [9]. These groups or symbolic constructions create patterns of differentiation, thus establishing a model for each gender (female and male), to which roles and limitations are assigned; and inequality is generated from these characteristics that society tries to make believe is correct for each gender, thus creating a division and therefore a discrimination that is reflected in the inequality that leads to violence. Gender is thus constituted as the result of a process of social construction through which the expectations and values that each culture attributes to its men and women are symbolically assigned (p. 53) [3]. The combination of these two concepts does not define the term gender violence, Moreno [11, 14] thinks that gender violence is "the violence that men exert against women, based on the ideology of the patriarchy or machismo" (p. 49). The idea of patriarchy places the male gender as the dominant figure over the female gender, giving women a secondary place. From this point of view, gender violence is exercised against women when men mistakenly believe that women are not equal as their gender and not only inside the family context, but also in the social and even work context. The United Nations Organization [19] defined the term gender violence as: “Any act of violence based on the, or what is commonly known as female sex environment that has or may result in physical, sexual or psychological harm or suffering for women, including threats of such acts, coercion or arbitrary deprivation of liberty, whether they occur in public or private life” [13], when trying to define the gender violence, refers to “every act of aggression, physical or psychic, based on the superiority of one sex over another.

Data obtained from the World Health Organization [18] show that a third of the female population (35%) has suffered physical and/or sexual violence. A large percentage of women (30%) of the world’s population claim to have been the victim of physical and/or sexual violence by their partner; and even more alarming, 38% of the women murdered in the world do so at the hands of their partners. Violence against women, in all its forms, has detrimental consequences for the physical, psychological, sexual and reproductive health of women, causing psychological disorders, physical injuries, contagion of sexually transmitted diseases, interruptions in pregnancy and even death.

This problem has not only great human costs for the world population, but also produces a direct impact on society, causing high economic and social costs, since these attacks can produce conditions of isolation, disability and annulment of women, preventing them from carrying out daily activities such as themselves care, as well as that of their children and attendance at work [18].

3 Media and Gender Violence

Mass media exert great influence on society and can change their thinking patterns and view and acting, so it is important that the news and information they generate are correctly selected and treated, analyzing, thinking and visualizing about the reaction they may have. Sierra [15] considers that the news is a fact that goes through a selection process; In other words, a specific topic is chosen from among so many that are raised daily and attention is focused on those few. The author also believes that modern journalism “resorts to specific rules, which privilege the violent act over the peaceful one, the exceptional data on the normal, the incident on the process, the individual on the general, the immediate on the mediate” (p. 133).

Media is in search of an extravagant or unusual event to be published and generate expectation and interest in the public. By labeling certain outrageous news items as important, the media are tackling a topic of sensationalism, from which the analysis to be presented in the following pages follows.

Sensationalism is defined by the Royal Spanish Academy as the “tendency to produce sensation, emotion or impression, with news, events, etc.” That is, it addresses the senses of the reader to make an impression on a certain topic. This “feeling” stimulates the readers or recipients of the information to catch their attention because they believe that that is what interests them the most, thus allowing themselves to be carried away by feelings rather than coherence.

4 Methodology

For this research analysis, research methods, techniques and other tools were used which helped to determine the treatment and interaction of each news item analyzed during the four-week period of March 2018. The methods used are the following: qualitative method or non-traditional and quantitative or traditional method.

Quantitative or Traditional Method: The quantitative method, also called traditional method, is derived from an already constructed theory and consists of measuring and contrasting the theories or social phenomena from the hypotheses of said theory, for this it is necessary to obtain a sample that will be the object of study [2]. Within the quantitative method, a social analytics tool was used to determine the number of news published in the month of March 2018 (analysis period). In addition, we worked with the signing technique to count the number of news that had or did not have the parameters that were raised.

Qualitative or Non-traditional Method: This method describes, interprets and deepens the study of specific cases, but not general ones. In this case, the issue of gender violence is very broad and encompasses various classifications; however, the news about femicide has been investigated and analyzed. Within this type of methodology, techniques typical of this classification were used, such as: observation technique, content analysis and documentary review.

Description of the Sample - Selected Media: The digital media chosen for the analysis were determined from the Alexa website, which ranks the websites with the highest number of visits. For this, three media were chosen for each country according to their position in the Alexa ranking [1].

Thus, the chosen media are the following: Bolivia: Diario El Deber, Los Tiempos and Página Siete; Perú: El Comercio Pe – La República Pe – RPP Noticias; Ecuador: El Comercio, El Universo and Teleamazonas and Colombia: Minuto30, Canal RCN and El Tiempo.

4.1 Results and Discussion

This informative treatment aims to generate an impact on the audience through different elements such as inappropriate words, images or videos that generate morbidity in the recipient of the information.

4.2 News Analysis

During the month of March 2018, a total of 123 news items were collected on the Facebook social network divided between the three digital media of the four countries that make up the Andean Community as follows: in Bolivia 30 news were published, in Peru 40 news, in Ecuador 26 news and in Colombia 27 news.

Headline Analysis. On average, 30 news items related to gender violence or femicide are published in each country. Out of the 30 news items published per month, 20 of them do not use headlines that promote morbidity in the countries: Bolivia, Peru and Colombia. On the other hand, Ecuador shows a 50/50 ratio, since 15 of the analyzed headlines use this morbidity promotion while 15 news items do not use the headlines in the remaining. Colombia appears as the country that most avoids morbidity in media headlines, followed by Bolivia.

Avoid Headlines that Encourage Morbidity: That is, headlines that expose unpleasant details but that are attractive to users.

Bolivia: 30 news, from the analyzed sample, it is identified that 21 news items avoid sensational headlines. The news that use headlines that encourage morbid were published in: Page 7 with 5 news, followed by Diario El Deber with 3 and finally Los Tiempos only has one news with these headlines.
Ecuador: 26 news. Out of the total news, 13 avoid headlines that encourage morbid. Of the 13-remaining news (sensationalist), 9 were found in Teleamazonas medium.
Perú: 40 news. Out of the 40 news items collected in the three digital media, 26 of them avoid this type of headline. Out of the 14 remaining news items using striking headlines, 10 of them appear in La República medium, 3 in El Comercio, Peru and finally one is issued by RPP medium.
Colombia: 27 news. Of the total of identified news 26 of them appear in El Minuto 30 medium and the remaining in El Tiempo medium. 20 news items avoid sensational headlines and are published in the Minuto 30 outlet. In the third medium analyzed (Canal RCN), no news related to violence or femicide was found during the selected period. In general, the countries analyzed avoid inappropriate headlines in about 64.95% of news stories.

Informational sensationalism. Informational sensationalism stimulates the senses of the receiver through information which attracts him, producing a sensation of emotion or impression. This parameter aims to determine whether digital media make use of this trend to obtain or attract users.

The country that publishes objectively and avoiding information sensationalism in most news is Colombia, despite the fact that some of its headlines are striking, the writing is impartial, clear and short. Ecuador is the second country that gives adequate treatment to information on violence, portraying Teleamazonas as the medium that has the largest number of sensational news.

Peru and Bolivia, on the other hand, are the countries with the highest percentage of sensational news, with an average of 30 news items per month, these countries publish sensational news by 43.3%.

In the Manual Guidelines for the informative treatment of violence against women in Social Media [7], it was identified that news against women is presented:

With a sensational character, seeking to impact more than to report, sometimes resorting to harassment of the victim to obtain a testimony and invading her privacy by questioning her about morbid details of the violent act, re-victimizing her. It resorts to aesthetic resources and lurid narrative.

Regarding this parameter, digital media of the four countries avoid news sensationalism by 70.8%, thus it is evident that the issues of violence in the Andean Community are treated with some care. However, it is important that this percentage increases, in such a way that media become a fundamental help to, echo this problem and on the other hand for the rest of media to become aware of the treatment and importance emphasizing what to avoid when dealing with news of violence.

Obviously, the issue of respect for people victims of violence should be deepened aiming to avoid morbid details spreading as well as that information that is too abundant, but not really relevant neither objective in aspects that even put dignity and reputation at stake and can even revictimize women.

The morbid detail of the acts of violence must be avoided, since the pain of a person who has been violated in her rights is not a spectacle nor a show. Details of the physical appearance of the victim, her way of dressing and behaving or others that do not contribute to the information and should be avoided in the news about this type of violence but which put their reputation in question, ending up by revictimizing them (p. 39) [10].

Violence Justification. Within this parameter, whether the woman who has been a victim of violence or femicide is blamed directly or indirectly has been analyzed; in most cases the perpetrators mostly their own husbands or partners, in some way argue that they did it because of "jealousy" (Table 1).

Table 1. Analysis of terms that justify the facts. Personal elaboration.

Country	**Use the terms that try to justify the fact** "Crime of passion", "love crime", "victim of jealousy"
Bolivia	30 news: From the news collected, one of them refers to a "Passionate Crime". From the newspaper Diario Siete. In addition three news stories also describe that events were carried out of jealousy
Ecuador	26 news: Five news items from this medium refer that the violent acts against women were provoked out of jealousy and one out of marital infidelity
Perú	40 news: Two acts of violence are justified under the excuse of infidelity, one piece of news mentions shows that leaving the perpetrator forced it and finally one more piece of news is justified for the starting a new relationship
Colombia	Total: 27 news Two news items mention that the act was committed by her former romantic partner

In Bolivia the literal term "crime of passion" was found; however, in other news jealousy is referred as an argument or motive the situation of violence. In Ecuador, Peru and Colombia the argument of "jealousy" was also found to try to justify acts of violence and femicide, in total 14 news items were cited. Information that addresses issues of gender-based violence or femicide published in a media outlet, must take certain care throughout the development of the news (headline, download and body), in such a way that they avoid words and therefore messages that dehumanize readers.

These terms were evaluated due to their wrong use, where by mistake or ignorance an attempt is made to justify the violent fact by indirectly blaming a woman for something that she may or may not have committed (but which was not a reason to attempt against her) and dismissing the person who really tried or in other unfortunate cases, produced woman's decease.

Appropriate Selection of Audiovisual Material. The audiovisual material (videos or photographs) are the complement of the writing. It is important to emphasize at this point that not all the media used videos in their news, in fact most of them only used images. The figures for inappropriate audiovisual content are small, as found: Bolivia uses it in 2 news items, Ecuador in 4, Peru in 5 and finally Colombia in 1 of its news.

The audiovisual material is an element that complements the news, which can be detailed with images and voice, but there must be limits to not show details that violate the right of the victim and those involved in the case. The published material, both written and audiovisual, must be published as a sexist crime, the product of a patriarchal society, where male society enjoys certain privileges. This will be a help in society, by spreading the fact that a problem exists that can be assumed as "a structured and coherent discourse with the fight against violence" (p. 69) [4].

Ecuador and Peru are the countries where more news are recorded with images or sensationalist material. 18% of the images and videos published in the region are bloody or intimate and, therefore, it is verified that no ethical review filters were implemented for the publication of news related to gender violence.

According to the Style Manual for the Treatment of Sexist Violence and Inclusive Language in Media "in informational spaces the use of reconstruction is not advisable", it is better not to reconstruct events that show lurid details or details that encourage morbid (p. 71) [4].

Respect to Victim's Dignity. Frequently media expose women to double victimization by spreading cruel images or simply images of the victim that go viral on social media, generating morbidity among users and violating the privacy of the victim.

Peru is the country with the highest count in this parameter, as it has the highest number of news (17) items that include the image of the victim, followed by Ecuador (8) and Bolivia (2). Finally, the analysis shows that Colombia is the country where no media shows or highlights the image of the victim, the news maintains a lot of objectivity.

Protection of the Identity of Victims. Protecting the identity of the victim is one of the fundamental aspects within the analysis and media are in charge of complying with or exposing information about the victim. Based on the legal framework, names, surnames or extra data of the victim are not public information.

The result show that Peru (24 out of 40 news items) and Ecuador (18 out of 26 stories) are the countries with a higher number of publications that reveal the identity of the victim, followed by Bolivia (9 out of 30 stories) and finally Colombia (4 of 27 news items) with a minimum number of news items that do not protect the victim, unlike in other countries. In the scope of this investigation, out of the 123 news analyzed items, 55 did not fit this parameter; Although this result is not equivalent to the majority, a large number of news items that expose the victim are identified.

Respect the Presumption of Innocence. This parameter focuses on the treatment of perpetrator information of, who also has rights, among them the presumption of innocence. In other words, it cannot be affirmed whether the suspect was the culprit of the fact, "As long as there is no final judgment or confirmation of guilt by the police or judicial sources" (p. 7) [5].

In conclusion, it was determined that the three analyzed media from the four countries under analysis respect the presumption of innocence of the perpetrator; no news items were observed to directly accuse the suspect. "During the development of these cases, it is important to exert social pressure on the authorities who often downplay the investigation and sanctions to take measures and punish these crimes" [12].

Treatment of the Issue as a Social Problem. In this parameter, if the news refers to a social problem or at least if the alarming figures of violence and femicide problems are published it was taken into account, so that the authorities take the pertinent measures and stop these problems that society faces; however, there is little news that address and visualize it.

Peru (11), Ecuador (8) and Bolivia (5) are the countries where there is evidence (although in only in few news) a treatment of social problem, while Colombia completely obviates the problem, because no news address this parameter or concern.

Accusation to Victims. This parameter is very different from the early analyzed codes however, it has been considered within the evaluation because in some cases it blames the victim for various reasons: their way of dressing and look, for going out alone late at night, infidelities among others.

Only two cases were found: one of femicide and the other of physical violence, in both cases the aggressor and/or accomplice blame the woman victim directly. Both cases were reported in Peru, however, the case of physical violence occurred in the same country and the case of femicide was reported in Syria.

Turn Information into Service. Mass media should provide help by disseminating information useful to people who are going through similar situations.

Mass media should not only broadcast the problems that society faces, but also provide possible solutions to them. For this reason, within the parameter's information provided by media such as the assistance provided in these cases is relevant. In other words, if they offer content useful for people who are in similar situations, information such as emergency numbers, names of institutions to which they can contact in case they are suffering these happenings and the like. Very often the victims remain silent for fear. However, no news attempts to turn information into service.

5 Conclusions

It is noteworthy how the media exert an enormous influence on society, even modifying its way of thinking and acting, for this reason it is important that the news and information they generate are selected and treated correctly, evaluating the reaction they could actually cause or promote in relation to exposure to violence against women; it is their function to educate and raise awareness about this issue and treat it ethically and responsibly, seeking to generate social awareness and eradicate the problem by not contributing nor promoting sensationalism and morbidity.

Regarding the studies on the treatment of information in the news media analyzed in this article, it is concluded that they still intend to generate an impact on the public through different elements such as words, images or inappropriate videos that generate morbidity in the receiver of the information. It is also noted that not all digital media have a sensational treatment of news related to violence, out of a total of 123 news stories, 80 avoid sensational treatment in the news.

Digital media publish an average of 30 news items per month regarding femicide issues, at the local, national or international level. In Bolivia, 30 news items referring to femicide were found, 17 of them avoid news sensationalism. In Ecuador, 26 news items with femicide issues were recorded, 13 of them avoid news sensationalism. Peru's digital media have published a total of 40 femicide news, 17 of them do not avoid the sensationalism within the newsroom, finally, Colombia has published 27 news items during the month of March, sensationalism is totally avoided at all.

Despite the fact that Colombia is one of the Latin American countries with the highest rate of murder cases against women, the analyzed media give adequate treatment to these issues, which shows that digital media journalists have a clear objective of informing the country reality, without no need to resort to elements that alter or distort facts in order to increase audiences and their consequent economic income.

It is important that journalists in training, students making up their undergraduated career and, in general, professionals in the branch of social communication have knowledge about the issues they will face in the exercise of their profession, that is why the classrooms should become a laboratory to teach guidelines on Appropriate treatments according to the type of information, this based on a guide or manuals for the correct treatment of information, preventing and avoiding informative sensationalism in media.

References

1. Alexa Internet. https://www.alexa.com/topsites/countries/CO. Accessed 08 Mar 2018
2. Bernal, C.: Investigation Methodology. Pearson, London (2016)
3. Bergalli, R., Bodelón, E.: La Cuestión de las mujeres y el deredcho penal simbólico. Anuario de Filosofía del Derecho IX (1992)
4. Castelló, R., Gimeno, A.: Style manual for the treatment of sexist violence and inclusive language in the media. Union of Valencian Journalist, Valencia (2018)
5. Audiovisual Council of Andalusia (2011). https://bit.ly/2RCiqtv. Accessed 12 Mar 2018
6. Hernández, I.: Gender violence. A look from sociology. In: 9th International Proceedings on Scientific Technical Editorial, Havana (2014)
7. Public Ministry of Peru (2017). https://bit.ly/2EO4XK7. Accessed 01 Apr 2018
8. Lagarde, M.: Gender and Feminism. Horas y Horas, Madrid (1996)
9. Lamas, M.: Género en: Conceptos Claves en Estudios de Género. Universidad Autónoma Nacional de México (2016)
10. Ministry of Women and Social Development. https://bit.ly/2QfBCxg. Accessed 21 May 2018
11. Moreno, A.: Intimate partner violence: from inequalities to abuse. New scenarios of violence (2008). Freire. ISBN 978-984
12. Observatory of Citizen Communication State University of Milagro: Manual for the treatment of information of violence against women (2017)
13. Ramírez, J., Alarcón, R., Ortega, S.: Violencia de género en Latinoamérica: Estrategias para su prevención y erradicación. Revista de Ciencias Sociales (Ve) **XXVI**(4), 260–275 (2020)

14. Rodríguez, L.: Violencia de género. Definición, fundamentación y clasificación de la violencia 1–9 (2013)
15. Sierra, A.: The responsibility of the journalistic investigator of the violence. In: Violence in the Media, News Generation and Citizen Perception, pp. 131–147. Flacso, Ecuador (2005)
16. WHO World Health Organization (2014). https://www.who.int/mediacentre/news/releases/2013/violence_against_women_20130620/en/. Accessed 15 June 2018
17. WHO World Health Organization (2015). https://www.who.int/gender-equity-rights/news/gender-health-sdgs/es/. Accessed 15 June 2018
18. WHO World Health Organization (2017). https://www.who.int/es/news-room/fact-sheets/detail/violence-against-women. Accessed 19 June 2018
19. United Nations. https://www.un.org/. Accessed 07 July 2018
20. Royal Spanish Academy (2018). http://www.rae.es/rae.html. Accessed 10 July 2018

Sizing Up "Media Twitter": Exploring Population Extent, Beats, and Utility of Social Media

John P. Wihbey[1](✉), Kenneth Joseph[2], and Daniela Rincon Reyes[1]

[1] Northeastern University School of Journalism, Boston, MA 02115, USA
j.wihbey@northeastern.edu
[2] University at Buffalo, The State University of New York, Buffalo, NY 14260, USA

Abstract. This mixed-methods study explores which types of journalists are on social media and what forms of knowledge-related utility they find there for their practice. We leverage computational techniques to identify more than 166,000 journalist profiles, in English, on Twitter and to examine their beats, follower counts, and volume of activity. We pair this with findings from an original 2019 survey with policy-oriented journalists (N = 450) who work on a variety of beats. Two-thirds of journalists believe social media tools help them frequently in their reporting work across many dimensions. Regression analysis finds significant associations with the technology and international affairs beats, as well as among younger journalists and those with a national audience. Our Twitter analysis, based on a dataset of 2.5 billion tweets collected in mid-2020, finds that the beats of politics, international affairs, and technology see the highest relative number of journalists on Twitter. The findings furnish a descriptive, quantitative picture of "Media Twitter" and speak to questions about social media's place in journalism.

Keywords: News media · Social media · Twitter · Beats · Reporting · Media identity · Social journalism · Computational social science

1 Introduction

The consequences of widespread adoption of social media by journalists have grown as a major area of study since the social web first began, when Facebook (2004), YouTube (2005), and Twitter (2006), followed by others, exploded on the media scene in rapid succession and began changing the media-communications landscape across many dimensions. Over time, though, the research and journalism worlds have significantly evolved in their understanding of the possibilities and perils of these platforms for facilitating and supporting high-quality journalism.

Optimism about the promises for journalism seen in the early years of this new era – swept along by a certain "liberation technology" narrative more generally about the salutary and democratizing effects of social platforms – has given way to a more guarded, pessimistic, and critical tone inflected by fears over rampant mis- and dis-information, corporate exploitation of users, and the steady weakening of journalism as the traditional

© The Author(s), under exclusive license to Springer Nature Singapore Pte Ltd. 2022
Á. Rocha et al. (Eds.): ICOMTA 2021, SIST 259, pp. 544–563, 2022.
https://doi.org/10.1007/978-981-16-5792-4_54

ad-supported model has evaporated [1, 25]. There remain long-running concerns that, in adopting social media platforms in their work, journalists may be trading accuracy for speed [37]. There is also evidence that social media may make issues such as gender bias, among other pervasive problems, even worse within the context of journalism practice [32].

The downside risks of social media use in journalism are increasingly apparent, but there clearly remains vast professional engagement with these technologies. This paper's primary contribution is an empirical one. It seeks to provide data-driven context to various lines of inquiry by answering several interrelated questions: How do journalists now conceive of social media's utility for their work, conditioned on their area of coverage or beat? How do they understand social media's uses in journalism practice across a variety of dimensions? Further, how might we estimate the general scale and shape of their engagement? We first attempt to answer these questions by examining findings from an original 2019 survey with policy-oriented professional and freelance journalists (N = 450) across a variety of different beats or primary coverage areas. Analysis of the survey findings allows us to understand better the types of journalists who believe social media helps them in their work, both with regard to job functions and in terms of epistemic orientation and conceptualization of stories.

Beyond these self-reported data, we are also interested in how journalists are "voting with their feet," so to speak, or revealed preferences in terms of what kinds of journalists populate social platforms. In mid-2020—15 years into the social web era—how many journalists were on social media? What is the extent of so-called "Media Twitter"—that mini-universe that constitutes a kind of water cooler for the industry? (For more on the origins and traits of Media Twitter see [3, 20]. And which kinds of journalists, specifically—in which beats and coverage areas—are most likely to be using social media? To provide suggestive evidence, we explore the contours of journalistic beats across all of English-language Twitter.

We leverage computational techniques and large-scale sampling from Twitter's decahose API to identify more than 166,000 journalist profiles on Twitter and to examine patterns within that group. This analysis produces a first-of-its-kind total estimate of the number of English-language journalists utilizing this social network, drills down on their articulation of beats, and makes estimates of the kinds of beats that are most heavily represented, as well as of dimensions of their popularity and activity.

Given that scholars have become more interested in questions about how journalists come to know things and how journalism might become more knowledge-based and well-justified—especially given the "post-truth" atmosphere of contemporary online discourse and the public sphere more generally—the survey data importantly also have bearing on questions of social epistemology and journalists' ways of intellectually orienting themselves on issues [26, 38]. How do journalists orient themselves intellectually and make selections with regard to the stories they tell, and how does the social world around them affect these selections? Recent work has suggested that social media shapes news judgment, with younger journalists in particular influenced by Twitter, and that social media are used to gauge public opinion, even when users on platforms may be unrepresentative of the general populace [21, 22]. Because social media platforms leverage algorithmic filtering techniques to control and optimize information flows, and are susceptible to mis- and dis-information campaigns, journalists' reliance on social media raises significant questions.

The results of this study suggest a nuanced picture across the contemporary English-language journalistic landscape as it relates to the utility of social media across beats. Notions of utility and value are consistently high, but also contingent on reporting context. Taken together, the survey and computational analysis align on a number of dimensions and provide complementary perspectives. The findings from both analyses suggest that social media may significantly favor certain kinds of journalistic practice and beats. Overall, we furnish a descriptive, quantitative picture of "Media Twitter" and speak to ongoing questions about social media's place in journalism.

2 Literature Review

Social media platforms have long been touted as democratizing tools with which journalists might access broader views and sources. In the digital era, there has been intensive study of the ways in which technology generally is changing journalism, from its functions and practices to its self-conception. However, predictions of sea changes in practice have not always been confirmed by empirical research [27].

Further, the social web has evolved in such a way as to make it potentially less conducive to diverse ideas and sourcing in journalism: For example, increased algorithmic filtering on social platforms, compounded by journalists' intentional and perhaps unintentional network construction that feeds into so-called "filter bubble" issues [38, 39] the rise of coordinated mis- and dis-information and influencer campaigns; and professional and economic incentives that encourage narrow-casting of content to targeted audiences.

Nevertheless, contemporary journalists report they find social media vital for not only keeping up on stories but taking the temperature of the public (assessing and quoting the vox populi) and following trends [21], although citizens' perceptions and acceptance of the use of social media as public opinion data is still evolving [10]. There may be demographic and geographic differences that explain differing notions of utility and value: Younger journalists, for example, may put higher value in social media's usefulness and believe more in its power to enable the populist-mobilizer and disseminator functions in journalism, per the canonical framework of journalistic roles [36, 37]. In a contemporary context, we might see the populist-mobilizer role involving "motivating people to get involved in public issues, letting them express their views, pointing to possible solutions, and developing cultural interests," whereas the disseminator role involves "getting information to the public quickly, reaching the widest audience, and providing entertainment [36].

Other prior research has found that conceptions of social media utility among journalists are "significantly tied to the platform's use for querying followers, conducting research and activities associated with contacting sources" (p. 400) [28]. Of course, utility may vary according to the platform in question, and Twitter and Facebook have been identified as serving multiple purposes, while YouTube, for example, is often used in more specialized fashion [24]. Questions about how and why journalists use social media have seen different answers over time, and there will likely always be differential uses across beats, reporting functions, and political and cultural contexts [5, 33].

It should be noted that in both of our forms of analysis, a key focus area is the concept of utility, which we conceive primarily in the more general social science/economics terms of usefulness of a service or good, rather than the communications studies framework of informational utility that is often used to study news consumer behavior [4]. We are interested in how social media are used by, and are embedded in and interact with, the profession and the people who practice it. We focus primarily on what might be considered epistemological utility – knowledge-related facets of media work, specifically dimensions of story ideation, reporting, search, and other intellectual aspects of the job. This is a deliberately narrow approach, as it leaves out other important dimensions of journalists' use of social media, such as those of career-building or other gratifications. Recent scholarship has already explored audience cultivation and branding through social media to a great extent, and therefore we leave such questions largely aside [6, 23].

About 55% of U.S. journalists have reported regular use of microblogs [34], while more than half have said they frequently find additional information on social media and locate sources there. News media members have flocked to Twitter, in particular. There, journalists' use of social media has been seen by scholars as a hybrid kind of business-editorial activity, one that involves aspects of branding and marketing as well as functions that practically relate to reporting [31].

Setting aside economic incentives, many reporters, producers, and editors have continued to see promise in using social media as tools for enhancing media practice, e.g., sourcing, story development, engagement with audiences. Yet this capacity to aid practice has become part of a difficult tradeoff, as journalists are frequently attacked or harassed on social media, including by prominent politicians across many societies globally. Given these concerns and others relating to the distorting effects of social platforms (p. 12) [19] have called for a general "reckoning" with regard to how certain assumptions have become embedded in news media research, namely that "(1) that social media would be a net positive; (2) that social media reflects reality; and (3) that social media matters over and above other factors."

We now are now a decade-and-a-half into the social web era, and despite much pessimism and turmoil in recent years, there are few signs that journalists are collectively giving up on social media, even as some are trying to dial back in usage or even leave altogether [20]. Indeed, the year 2020 may have seen the opposite trend at work: As the COVID-19 era has pushed so much of social life online, some journalists have found themselves engaged even more with social media in order to meet the needs of bewildered citizens looking for information and answers.

Journalists may increasingly see this form of audience engagement on social platforms as inextricably bound up with their profession. Polling data suggest that the public broadly accepts and encourages this function and approach, and three-quarters of Americans, for example, think that reporter-audience engagement on social media is a good idea [17]. The journalistic embrace of social media might best be characterized as a form of hybrid normalization, or the "restatement of traditional journalistic practices combined with the adoption – or sometimes the mere exhibition – of the norms and practices typical of the participatory web" (p. 287) [2]. These cross-cutting trends, and the questions and uncertainties they continue to surface, point to the need for continuing inquiry into the general scale and scope of journalistic engagement with social media, of primary coverage areas, and of more precisely delineated characteristics of utility, value, and practice on such platforms.

Additionally, the utility of such media platforms may vary tremendously in other areas of the globe. To take just two examples, consider studies that focus on journalists' use of Twitter in Colombia and Ecuador. The research of [12] finds that journalists on Twitter in Colombia, particularly elite journalists, frequently use the platform to express editorial and partisan opinions. In Colombia, politics and journalism are closely tied in the country, as the majority of Colombian presidents have been directors or owners of newspapers in their previous careers; and influential media outlets have been affiliated with traditional political parties. Research suggests that affiliation with traditional versus non-traditional news outlets has a strong influence on the roles and postures that journalists assume on Twitter [12].

By contrast, the main use of Twitter by Ecuadorian journalists is content curation, according to an examination of the Twitter engagement strategies of the 20 most influential journalists in Ecuador [16]. They primarily used Twitter to share their own content and content from their news organization to promote their personal and institutional branding [16]. In any case, the roles of journalists have been discussed primarily in the academic research literature within a Western framework based on news media's contribution to democracy. Although journalism's realities in a global world is not the primary focus of this study, a new and more inclusive classification of roles is needed whereby journalism's relevance in non-Western contexts is better articulated [15]. We hope this current study can, among other things, serve as one type of model for expanded global inquiries.

Beyond these domain-specific questions about journalism and social media, this paper also bears on methods challenges relevant to computational social science and the use of Twitter data in particular to answer questions about human behavior and patterns in media. To perform computational analysis on our social media dataset, we focus on the data within Twitter accounts' bios, i.e., user descriptions. There is, as it stands, relatively little in the literature about leveraging account bios/descriptions using text-analysis in order to make inferences about populations and identities. More specifically, while scholars have used account bios as features in various machine learning models to, e.g., identify user demographics [40], computational scholars typically focus more heavily on tweet content and/or social networks induced by actions on the site.

A critical exception, however, is the work of [41], who rely heavily on account bios when developing methods to detect journalists during crisis or breaking news situations. Through a series of iterative steps leveraging machine learning techniques, the authors conclude that account bios provide one of the strongest signals for their methods to detect journalists, along with whether a given account is included in the Twitter lists of other accounts (suggesting that account is watched by others and may be a "power user.") We leverage these insights in our work as well, using a simplified approach to identifying journalists using Twitter bios that focuses on accuracy over recall.

3 Data Collection

The data were collected from two sources, distinguished in this study as the "survey analysis" and the "computational analysis." The two combine to provide both internal (self-reported attitudes) and external (behavioral) data on journalism practice. The former provides a fine-grained look at the views of journalists on notions of utility and value with respect to social media; the latter provides a much wider look at the actual usage of social media (specifically, Twitter) by journalists generally and subsets of them.

3.1 Survey Analysis

The survey data were obtained through a journalism support project that has a large media audience. Details of the fielded survey are as follows: An online survey using the Qualtrics platform was sent to 4,956 identified journalists on the mailing list of the Journalist's Resource project at the Shorenstein Center on Media, Politics and Public Policy, a project based at Harvard University that promotes topical, research- and policy-oriented background materials to news media. The first contact was Feb. 4, 2019, which was followed by bi-weekly reminders through March 14. The survey saw responses from 701 full- or part-time journalists, or a 14% response rate. The survey, which was anonymous, was also sent out to educators and other information sector workers, whose responses are not included in this analysis.

The characteristics of the journalist sample roughly conformed to a more general picture of the news profession described in [35], in terms of education levels, estimated age/tenure, and medium of publishing. The sample had the following characteristics: 76% identified as full-time journalists; 74% were based in the United States; 65% reported working for for-profit organizations and 35% for nonprofit news outlets; about 25% said they published work through audio or video frequently or occasionally; and roughly half of respondents said the primary audience of their outlet was national or international. In terms of tenure in the news business, 53% had worked in journalism 20+ years; 21% had worked for 10–19 years; and 26% had worked in news for fewer than 10 years.

Given the origins of the survey and the project mailing list, the online convenience sample produced likely skews toward more policy-oriented journalists, and generalizability would require additional research. That said, the survey captures insights relating to an important and influential group in news media whose attitudes are important to understand; moreover, the computational analysis used in this study attempts to capture a fuller picture of journalists on social media, lending wider perspective to this study overall.

Through the online survey, journalists were asked, "In terms of your professional work, how useful are social media for the following?" Respondents then chose answers across a 5-point Likert-scale, ranging from "always/almost always useful" to "not useful," on eight key topics: "Diversifying the ideas I encounter"; "Exposing me to political views I don't normally hear"; "Identifying voices or perspectives to quote"; "Finding story ideas"; "Finding sources to contact"; "Locating experts"; "Keeping up on a particular issue"; and "Getting audience feedback on stories."

In summary, about half of these functions relate to journalistic search problems (finding sources, ideas, experts), while others represent the utility of platforms to add intellectual value (diversity of ideas and views), allow for maintenance of awareness/attention (keeping up), or mechanisms for judging reactions (feedback). These functions are the primary measures of utility in our survey analysis. As we sought to probe questions about general value of social media and how it might affect practice and epistemic orientation, the questions did not specify a particular social media platform. Further, because prior literature has already extensively studied the use of social media by journalists for audience cultivation and branding, we chose to focus more on reporting and ideation functions and not to explore branding functions for the most part [6, 23]. The answers provide a general and comprehensive picture, rather than a tactical one about specific affordances of individual platforms or comparisons (e.g., how Instagram might be better than Twitter for a given function).

The survey also asked journalists to identify their primary beats, as well as whether their outlet's primary audience was a national, regional, or local one and what their length of tenure in journalism was. Further, journalists were asked to indicate if their primary mode of publication was online/web, in order to identify digital-first respondents as a plausible category that might have special views on social media.

3.2 Computational Analysis

Our computational analysis leveraged access to Twitter's decahose API, which yields a 10% sample of all tweets across that microblogging platform. Our analysis is carried out on all decahose data in June and July of 2020 where Twitter's internal language detection algorithm identified the tweet as being in English. This dataset amounts to approximately 42 million tweets per day, or around 2.5 billion tweets.

3.3 Research Questions

The survey analysis and computational analysis allowed for different research questions to be asked, but the intention was to use the survey findings to motivate the computational analysis.

For the survey analysis, the research questions were:

- **RQ1(a):** What are mean responses for all journalists together across the eight different measures of utility?
- **RQ1(b):** To what extent do the beats of journalists predict the usefulness of social media to them, across the eight different measures of utility?
- **RQ2:** Does length-of-tenure in journalism predict the utility of social media?
- **RQ3:** Does the audience size of a journalist's outlet predict the utility of social media?
- **RQ4:** Does publishing primarily online as a medium (digital-first) predict the utility of social media for journalists?

For the computational analysis, the research questions were:

- **RQ5:** What percent of active Twitter users are journalists?

- **RQ6:** How many English-speaking journalists exist on Twitter?
- **RQ7:** What percentage of all journalists have a given beat?
- **RQ8:** How many accounts have multiple beats?
- **RQ9:** How do journalists with different beats use Twitter?

4 Methods

For the purposes of statistical analysis, we focused on journalists who had primary beats in nine relatively mainstream/traditional, common areas: state/local government; environment; health/medical science; business and economics; politics; criminal justice; education; technology; international affairs. After removing incomplete surveys and narrowing the focus to these major beats, the sample was about (N = 450) across the relevant questions. We first looked at the patterns of means across all journalists for the eight measures of social media utility; for the purposes of descriptive statistics reported in R1(a), we summed the percentages of those journalists saying always/almost always/often for a measure of utility on a frequent basis.

We then treated the beats as independent variables and, using multivariate linear regression, sought to explain the response variable, which was the self-reported attitude of journalists regarding the usefulness of social media across the eight dimensions mentioned. The regression analysis also included as independent variables the length of a journalist's tenure in news media; the size of the audience of the outlet of journalists; and whether the journalist indicated that online/web was the primary mode of output.

With respect to the computational analysis, to address RQ5, we defined an active Twitter user as any individual who tweeted at least once, in English, in our decahose dataset. We randomly subsampled 200 of these users, and then developed a coding task where five graduate students in the School of Journalism at Northeastern University were asked if these users were journalists or not. Coders were trained by instructing each graduate student to review models of known journalist user profiles; they reviewed verified Twitter profiles from leading journalists across 30 outlets, chosen based on a recent, major media-related analysis by the Pew Research Center [18]. Each user was seen by at least two coders; where disagreements arose between coders, the authors of the paper conferred and agreed on a final labeling.

RQ6 differs from RQ5 in that it seeks an estimate of the total number of journalists on Twitter. One means of estimating this is to seek an extrapolation from the percentage calculated for RQ5. However, extrapolations of infrequent events from percentages is known to be difficult [8]. We therefore resort to a second, complementary approach to provide an estimate of the total number of journalists, by simply seeking to count them in the decahose. To do so, we engage in an iterative procedure to identify users who are likely to be journalists, using only their profile descriptions.

We begin by searching the profiles of all users that either sent a tweet or were retweeted in our dataset. We then extract from this set all users whose profiles contain the keywords "journalist," "staff writer," "reporter," "producer," "anchor," "host," or "editor." This collection produces a set of users that we expect to have high recall – that is, to capture most journalists – but low precision – that is, it is likely to also contain a large number of non-journalists. In general, well-documented keyword-based approaches to identifying relevant users and tweets have been shown to be both effective [29] and competitive with machine learning based approaches for similar tasks [14]. To refine and evaluate the keywords used, we select a second set of 500 Twitter accounts containing these keywords for hand-coding by the same five graduate student coders. We asked coders, again, to determine whether or not the account belonged to a journalist. Disagreements are again resolved using the approach described above.

Finally, we used this set of labeled users to refine our keyword search. Our final approach to identifying journalists on Twitter identified any individual with the words "journalist," "staff writer," or "reporter" in their profile. This more-limited set of keywords captured 71% of the accounts that our hand-coders labeled journalists in the set of 500 accounts labeled (i.e. our approaches recall was 71%). And of all the accounts that our method labeled as journalists, 90% of them were actually labeled as journalists by the hand-coders (i.e. our precision was 90%).

For RQ7–9, we also performed a keyword-style analysis to identify beats on all accounts identified using "reporter". The keywords used to identify reporters aligned with each beat are given in Table 1. We leveraged this larger set of accounts labeled with particular beats to explore patterns in how journalists used Twitter. Specifically, we estimate three separate negative binomial regressions where the journalists' beat(s) were the independent variable and a) follower counts, b) following counts, and c) total number of tweets sent were used as dependent variables, respectively.

Table 1. Keywords used to identify reporters in Twitter data aligned with each beat. Note that keyword expressions were identified if they matched anywhere in a bio. For example, a bio stating a user was a "Crime reporter" would match the Crime/Justice beat, because it contained the string "crim".

Beat	Keyword expressions
Local/State Government	local, state, government, capitol, state house
Environmental	environment, climate, energy
Health/Medical	health, medic
Business/Economics	business, economic
Politics	politic
Crime/Justice	crim, justic
Education	education, school
Technology	tech, silicon valley, digital
International Affairs	international, global, latin america, europe, middle east, africa, asia, china

5 Results

For the survey analysis, descriptive statistics suggest important insights into areas of maximum utility for journalists. Multivariate regression analysis indicates statistically significant results for several key independent variables (primary beats), while showing no associations for a variety of other covariates (see Table 1) Computational analysis yielded estimates for journalists on Twitter, distribution of beats, and numbers of followers, followership (accounts journalists follow), and status updates across beats.

RQ1(a): In terms of diversifying ideas encountered, 48.4% of all journalists said social media was always/almost always/often useful (hereafter combined to "frequently"). In terms of exposure to novel political views, 42.5% said it frequently had utility. For identifying voices or perspectives to quote, 38% said it frequently had utility. For finding story ideas, 52.2% agreed social media frequently had utility. In terms of finding sources to contact, 44.8% agreed it frequently had utility. For locating experts, 34.6% said it frequently had utility. For keeping up on a particular issue, 56.8% said social media frequently had utility. Finally, in terms of getting audience feedback on stories, 43.7% said it frequently was useful. Further, at least two-thirds of journalists surveyed said that social media was at least sometimes useful on every question. At most, only 15% agreed that social media was "not useful" on any of the eight measures.

RQ1(b): There was a significant association between covering technology across almost all – seven of eight – measures of social media utility, and, to a more limited extent, covering international affairs was also associated with finding social media useful, particularly for finding sources, locating experts, and getting audience feedback. However, the beat of business/economics journalists was negatively associated with finding utility in social media tools, particularly for identifying voices or perspectives to quote, finding sources to contact, and locating experts. The beats of state/local government, environment, health/medicine, politics, and education were not positively or negatively associated with particular attitudes about social media for the most part. See Table 2.

RQ2: Social media tools seem to be more useful to younger journalists rather than veteran journalists, particularly those with more than 20 years of experience, for whom social media does not appear as useful, at a strongly significant level, across a variety of measures. Those with 10–19 years experience also were less likely to find strong utility in social media ($p < 0.01$).

RQ3: Journalists who work for news outlets with a larger, national audience are significantly more likely to see utility in leveraging social media for a variety of purposes, as compared to those with a regional or local audience. Having a national audience proves to be among the single best predictors of a journalist finding substantial utility in social media, as it has a statistically significant association across five areas: identifying voices or perspectives to quote; finding story ideas; finding sources to contact; locating experts; and keeping up on a particular issue.

RQ4: Being a digital-first journalist (primary publication medium of online/web) did not have significant associations in terms of perceived social media utility.

RQ5: Of the 200 users considered, coders unanimously agreed that 190 of them (95%) were not journalists. Coders also unanimously agreed that two accounts were a journalist. The other nine accounts, however, showed disagreement. Inspection by the authors

Table 2. Associations between journalistic beats and aspects of social media utility (N = 450).

	Dependent variable							
	Diversity	Views	Voices	Finding	Sourcing	Experts	Monitor	Feedback
	(1)	(2)	(3)	(4)	(5)	(6)	(7)	(8)
Independent variables								
Local/State Government	0.067	0.124**	0.020	0.017	0.015	−0.021	0.010	0.065
	(0.054)	(0.054)	(0.052)	(0.049)	(0.051)	(0.052)	(0.049)	(0.056)
Environment	−0.014	−0.014	0.020	0.023	−0.012	−0.025	−0.004	0.020
	(0.049)	(0.048)	(0.048)	(0.045)	(0.046)	(0.047)	(0.045)	(0.050)
Health/Medical	0.049	−0.040	−0.004	0.053	0.021	0.012	0.055	0.070
	(0.046)	(0.046)	(0.045)	(0.043)	(0.044)	(0.045)	(0.043)	(0.048)
Business/Economics	−0.029	0.034	−0.121***	−0.072*	−0.097**	−0.105**	−0.049	0.0002
	(0.044)	(0.043)	(0.043)	(0.040)	(0.041)	(0.043)	(0.040)	(0.045)
Politics	0.009	−0.012	0.014	0.086*	−0.005	0.021	0.062	0.026
	(0.053)	(0.052)	(0.051)	(0.048)	(0.050)	(0.052)	(0.048)	(0.054)
Crime/Justice	0.096*	0.065	0.049	0.058	0.071	0.055	0.075	0.012
	(0.052)	(0.052)	(0.051)	(0.048)	(0.049)	(0.051)	(0.048)	(0.054)
Education	−0.046	0.018	0.031	−0.044	0.003	0.039	−0.051	−0.052
	(0.048)	(0.047)	(0.047)	(0.044)	(0.046)	(0.046)	(0.044)	(0.049)
Technology	0.055	0.097**	0.137***	0.107**	0.113**	0.110**	0.072*	0.106**

(continued)

Table 2. *(continued)*

	Dependent variable							
	Diversity	Views	Voices	Finding	Sourcing	Experts	Monitor	Feedback
	(1)	(2)	(3)	(4)	(5)	(6)	(7)	(8)
	(0.047)	(0.046)	(0.045)	(0.043)	(0.044)	(0.045)	(0.043)	(0.048)
International Affairs	0.054	−0.010	−0.013	0.053	0.097*	0.153***	0.032	0.093*
	(0.053)	(0.053)	(0.052)	(0.049)	(0.050)	(0.052)	(0.049)	(0.055)
Career 5–9 years	−0.449*	0.167	−0.294	−0.100	−0.182	0.012	−0.117	−0.458*
	(0.246)	(0.244)	(0.240)	(0.225)	(0.233)	(0.239)	(0.225)	(0.254)
Career 10–19 years	−0.493**	−0.111	−0.330	−0.340*	−0.435**	−0.122	−0.348*	−0.502**
	(0.219)	(0.216)	(0.213)	(0.201)	(0.207)	(0.212)	(0.200)	(0.226)
Career 20+ years	−0.543***	−0.074	−0.485**	−0.530***	−0.474**	−0.183	−0.696***	−0.587***
	(0.195)	(0.192)	(0.190)	(0.178)	(0.184)	(0.189)	(0.178)	(0.201)

suggested that disagreement was sometimes due to the fact that these accounts, while occasionally tweeting in English, occasionally tweeted in other languages, making annotation difficult; freelance and former journalists often appear to identify themselves in less formal ways, as compared to full-time journalists working at large, mainstream outlets. After more thorough review of these nine accounts, we found only one of them to be a journalist. Consequently, as we find that only 3 out of the 200 users we hand-coded were journalists, we estimate using this method that approximately 1.5% of active, English-language Twitter accounts/profiles to be journalists. Critically, however, while agreement was reasonable as compared to other social media annotation tasks (Krippendorf's alpha of .353; compared to, e.g., .39 for toxic behavior and .60 for identifying memes [9], our work and similar efforts of others [41] reflects the difficulties of performing this kind of annotation work.

RQ6: We find that 137,979 Twitter accounts that were retweeted or that tweeted in June of 2020 contained in their profile description a keyword indicating they were a journalist. This is similar to the amount we found in July (134,483). In total, across both months, we found 166,621 journalists using this method. Note that this value is a lower bound for at least two reasons. First, our keywords likely do not identify all journalists on Twitter. Second, we consider only two months of decahose data. Note, in the latter case, however, that any account who a) tweeted at least 10 times or b) was retweeted at least 10 times will almost certainly appear in the decahose, and therefore this lower bound may be relatively tight. This represents approximately .18% of all worldwide, monthly active Twitter accounts, and around 1.4% of all monthly active U.S. Twitter accounts [30]. Notably, our estimate from RQ5 is approximately the same as the 1.4% estimate, although it asks a slightly different question.

RQ7: Of the 166,621 accounts we identify as journalists, only 27,606 (16.6%) matched one of our beat-based keyword lists. Figure 1 presents the number of those accounts that were assigned to each beat we studied.

RQ8: We find that almost all journalist accounts had either zero or one identified beat. Only 15.1% of accounts listed more than one beat. Using the approach in [7], we further find no significant patterns in the sets of beats listed, when more than one beat is provided. We conclude that there is limited evidence in our sample of beats overlapping in significant ways, either practically or statistically.

RQ9: Figure 2 shows that reporters with the politics beat had significantly more followers than any other beat, with international, technology, and business beats also more slightly ahead of the others. We also see that this cannot be entirely explained by increased numbers of accounts these beats follow, or the activity level of journalists in these beats, as measured by the number of statuses sent, at least for international and business beats. Regardless, results suggest that there is a correlation between beats where journalists are more prevalent (politics, international affairs, and technology) and attention received on the site.

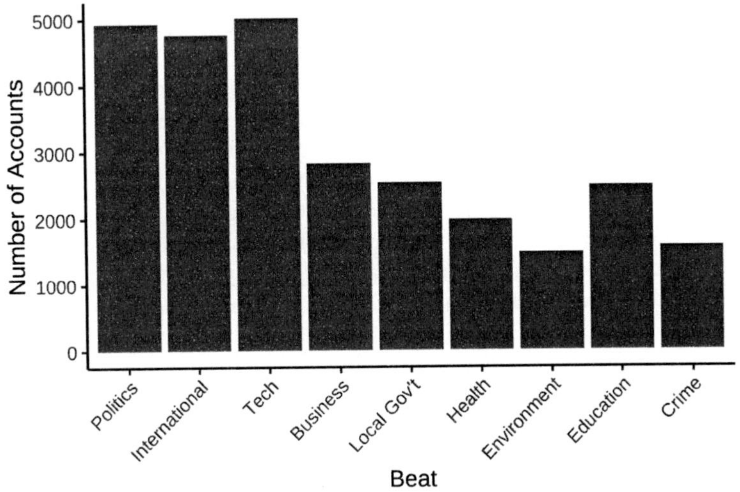

Fig. 1. Number of Twitter accounts that were assigned to each beat studied (n = 27,606).

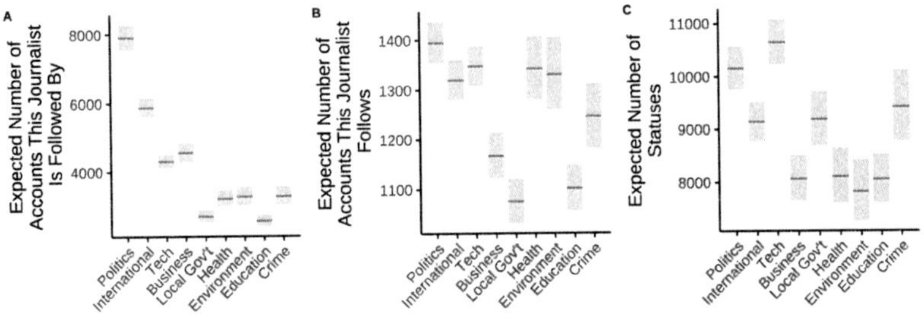

Fig. 2. Output from a negative binomial regression predicting the expected number of Followers (A, left), followership (B, middle), and statuses (tweets) sent (C, left) for journalists across beats studied (n = 27,606).

6 Discussion

Findings from the survey analysis indicate several main points of interest. First, among the journalists surveyed as a whole, social media consistently provided utility for many different functions. Two-thirds or more of respondents said that social media tools were at least "sometimes" useful across all eight measures, and at most 15% said they were "not useful" on any given measure. This level of affirmation for social media is a striking finding, as it suggests the strong value of these digital tools for journalism, even as the problems and many downside risks, mentioned previously, have become salient in discourse about the intersection of social media and news media.

Across all journalists, social media seemed most useful for diversifying ideas encountered, finding story ideas, and keeping up on a particular issue. Nearly half or more of journalists said social media frequently had utility for those purposes. Social media proved to have the least utility, on a relative basis, for locating experts, getting audience feedback on stories, and exposure to novel political views. But even for these functions, more than two-thirds said it was sometimes useful.

These findings contribute to our knowledge of how journalists may understand the world and bring stories into it, deepening our insight into how everything from reporting routines and information-seeking practices to framing and agenda-setting may be viewed. Social media seem to be playing a decisive role in knowledge formation. Scholars have proposed using social epistemology as a new paradigm for journalism studies [13] which would include more attention to the generation of knowledge from technological sources. This study points to the need to evaluate carefully inputs from and interactions with social media by journalists, as these tools are now being used for everything from source- and story-finding to acquisition and maintenance of knowledge about issues. Of course, journalistic roles and the uses of technological sources may vary across news organizations and different types of societies [15].

Further, statistical analysis suggests social media tools seem especially useful for work across the beats of technology and, to some extent, international affairs. Both of these would meet expectations, as the former beat carries with it expectations of high engagement in centers of discourse such as Twitter while the other may require the use of social media tools to span geographies. By contrast, there was a negative association for business/economics journalists, who were more likely to say that social media tools were not as useful. Journalists with longer tenures were also less likely to find utility, while journalists with a national audience were more likely to value social media tools for a variety of functions. Further, there were few significant associations among journalists covering general assignment beats such as municipal affairs/local and state government/politics, as well as specialty beats such as environment, health, and education.

In many ways, the survey findings meet what would likely be the common expectation of even the most casual media industry observer, namely that being a younger journalist with a national audience, and covering technology or international affairs, is highly correlated with finding social media useful. Again, this confirms aspects of prior research showing how age is a predictor in this area [36].

The lack of significant associations with certain beats in the survey analysis are also interesting to note. Among the many common beats such as municipal or state government and crime, and the specialty beats such as education, environment, and health, there are few significant associations in terms of finding more value in social media, and no particular pattern emerges. It is likely that reporters, editors, and producers are heterogeneous in their approach to their beats and coverage areas, and therefore no single view or norm for social media prevails among these journalistic types. The exception is business/economics, where there is a negative association. A plausible hypothesis is that business and economics coverage tends to be highly structured around specific sources of information (markets, agencies, analysts, firms) that are already well defined, and routines have a different character on that beat. Such an explanation, of course, warrants further investigation.

The computational analysis complements the survey picture by, among other things, providing scale and empirical perspective on the world of journalism at its intersection with social media. As mentioned, we identified 166,621 journalists on Twitter, which we believe to be a solid lower bound. (We did not assess nationality given the difficulty of that task, but our coding procedures surfaced many English-language journalist profiles from around the globe, in addition to U.S. and Western journalists.) Although our keywords likely do not identify all journalists and our sampling took place over a given two-month period, any account that tweeted, or was retweeted, at least 10 times during that period would likely have been captured. This relatively tight lower bound allows us to make, to our knowledge, a reliable, first-of-its-kind estimate of the number of journalists with English-language profiles on Twitter. The figure of 166,621 journalists (albeit only English-language accounts) would represent approximately .18% of all worldwide, monthly active Twitter accounts. For a further sense of scale, if compared to all monthly active U.S. Twitter accounts, our figure would represent 1.4% [30], although of course we include English-language journalists from around the world. This was approximately the same number that we identified via manual coding of a small sample (200) active, English-speaking accounts, meaning the estimate is consistent across two different methodological approaches.

Moreover, of the 166,621 accounts we identify as journalists, 27,606 (16.6%) matched one of our beat-based keyword lists, which we attempted to keep concise. Notably, those lists did not include keywords for entertainment, sports, or cultural beats, for example, so our number includes only what might be considered hard news domains. Indeed, our list may be overly narrow on the question of beats. Findings from a study of 384 U.S. journalists on Twitter – whose bios were hand-coded – found that 57% listed a beat or coverage area [23]. The disparity between those findings and ours may be explained by our narrower criteria, which were helpful for computational analysis and purposes of comparison.

Twitter profiles are often highly personalized and idiosyncratic, and prior literature establishes the difficulty of this task of identification; a low percentage of positive matching would therefore meet expectations. Still, we cannot conceive of any a priori reason that this would present a skewed internal distribution, i.e., that any given beat would be harder to identify computationally, or that journalists in a given beat would necessarily make it more obscure in their profile. So the 27,606 subset stands, we believe, as a valid and reasonably large sample of journalists with which to make comparisons and draw analytical insights about beats and behavioral patterns. Among those, journalists on the politics, international, and technology beats alone make up more than half the accounts. Because we did not try to identify journalists from all conceivable beats, we cannot say that these three beats necessarily have the greatest representation overall on Twitter. But on a relative basis, within a set of 9 common, hard news-related beats, these are clear numerical leaders. Further, those same beats are also most likely to have the largest number of followers, and politics and technology are likely to have the most status updates (original tweets), suggesting stronger norms for presence maintenance.

Finally, there was little evidence of journalists covering more than one beat, and only about 15% of accounts listed more than one beat. We could not discern significant patterns even when more than one beat was provided. This lack of explicit or consistent overlap may be explained in a functional way: Journalists' profiles are a way of branding and establishing a presence for an explicit purpose, and perhaps listing multiple beats would confuse/muddy their intention to audiences for purposes such as: gaining followers and gathering particular kinds of information; participating in certain communities; or being known by audiences for a specific information stream. Because of the decline of the number of journalists in countries such as the United States, many journalists may be covering multiple beats in newsrooms and serving in more roving, general assignment roles. However, our data do not capture or speak to those trends necessarily.

7 Conclusion

This mixed-methods study set out to provide perspective based on both internal (survey-based responses) and external (observation of social media platform) data in order to assess journalism practice. By doing this, we believe that we are able to create a unique, in some ways panoramic, picture of the uses of social media in journalism, of Media Twitter, at the end of the second decade of the twenty-first century.

Taken together our survey and computational analysis converge to point to the special role that the technology and, to some extent, international affairs beats may play in social media, and vice versa. More generally, though, we can observe massive participation on the Twitter platform by journalists; and through the survey, we learn that social media tools have significant utility across a variety of knowledge functions, from search problems (finding sources, ideas, experts) to adding intellectual value (diversity of ideas and views) to maintenance of awareness/attention (keeping up on issues) to mechanisms for judging reactions (feedback). The attitudes of journalists about these functions should motivate more research to assess how these technologies may be shaping news agendas and story framings and affecting journalistic epistemic orientation in substantial ways.

Of course, reliance on algorithmically filtered technologies such as social media platforms carries considerable risks for journalistic independence, judgement, and epistemology, as the ordering, ranking, and production of information and trends on social media may distort empirical realities and hide important truths. This is the paradox of greater journalistic engagement with social platforms, which is that there is now the potential to get closer to the democratic public but also the potential to be led further astray from the public interest by disinformation, bots, biased systems, and the general allure of the latest trending topic and hashtag. New tools and training will undoubtedly be necessary to combat the potential problems that come with reliance on social platforms for sources and knowledge [11].

The two main datasets we leverage have limitations. The survey sample is only a snapshot of journalistic practice among one cohort of journalists, one with specific interests in policy issues, and it cannot necessarily be generalized. We have conducted an analytical study that provides important perspective and shows plausible and robust associations internal to the sample. Yet more research is certainly needed to confirm generalizability to the full journalist population – including other geographical areas with different political and cultural contexts. The computational analysis, obviously, focuses on Twitter, and it does not capture important journalistic activity being done on other social media platforms such as Instagram, Facebook, YouTube, and a variety of other platforms and applications. Our sampling techniques and use of text-based analysis through keyword searches, while demonstrated to be useful in the emerging literature in this area, may also omit important classes of accounts and beats, given that we studied the population for only a two-month period and used a discrete set of keywords and search criteria.

Despite these limitations, though, this study provides, to our knowledge, a first-of-its-kind estimate relating to journalists on social media, their beats, and dimensions of their knowledge-related activity. We offer new insights into how journalists see the epistemological utility of social media along a fundamental set of measures that speak to issues of framing, agenda-setting, knowledge formation, and professional norms. The dynamic interaction of news media and social media continues to redefine and influence public information flows across societies in the twenty-first century. More research in the areas we analyze in this study will certainly be required to critically examine how news and public knowledge are being constructed for, and along with, contemporary publics.

References

1. Bell, E, et al.: The Platform Press: How Silicon Valley Reengineered Journalism. Tow Center for Digital Journalism (2017)
2. Bentivegna, S., Marchetti, R.: Journalists at a crossroads: are traditional norms and practices challenged by twitter? Journal. Theory Pract. Crit. **19**(2), 270–290 (2018)
3. Benton, J.: The Fired New Yorker Writer Who Helped Birth Media Twitter Has Died (and I'm Sure He'd Apologize if He Could). Nieman Journalism Lab (2020)
4. Bobkowski, P.: Sharing the news: effects of informational utility and opinion leadership on online news sharing. Journal. Mass Commun. Q. **92**(2), 320–345 (2015)
5. Bodrunova, S., Litvinenko, A., Ivan, B.: Please follow us: media roles in twitter discussions in the United States, Germany, France, and Russia. Journal. Pract. **12**(2), 177–203 (2018)
6. Brems, C., Temmerman, M., Graham, T., Broersmab, M.: Personal branding on twitter. Digit. Journal. **5**(4), 443–459 (2017)
7. Dianati, N.: Unwinding the hairball graph: pruning algorithms for weighted complex networks. Phys. Rev. E **93**(1), 012304 (2016)
8. Dixon, P., Ellison, A., Nicholas, G.: Improving the precision of estimates of the frequency of rare events. Ecology **86**(5), 1114–1123 (2005)
9. Du, Y., Masood, M.A., Joseph, K.: Understanding visual memes: an empirical analysis of text superimposed on memes shared on twitter. In: Proceedings of the International AAAI Conference on Web and Social Media, vol. 14, pp. 153–164 (2020)
10. Dubois, E., Gruzd, A., Jacobson, J.: Journalists' use of social media to infer public opinion: the citizens' perspective. Soc. Sci. Comput. Rev. **38**(1), 57–74 (2020)
11. Fletcher, R., Schifferes, S., Thurman, N.: Building the 'truthmeter': training algorithms to help journalists assess the credibility of social media sources. Convergence **26**(1), 19–34 (2020)
12. García-Perdomo, V.: Colombian journalists on twitter: opinions, gatekeeping, and transparency in political coverage. Int. J. Commun. **11**(2017), 1574–1596 (2017)
13. Godler, Y., Reich, Z., Miller, B.: Social epistemology as a new paradigm for journalism and media studies. New Media Soc. **22**(2), 213–229 (2020)
14. Grinberg, N., Joseph, K., Friedland, L., Swire-Thompson, B., Lazer, D.: Fake news on twitter during the 2016 US presidential election. Science **363**(6425), 374–378 (2019)
15. Hanitzsch, T., Vos, T.: Journalism beyond democracy: a new look into journalistic roles in political and everyday life. Journalism **19**(2), 146–164 (2018)

16. Henríquez-Coronel, P., Roca Guapacasa, G., Valecillos, C.: Engagement strategies of influential journalists on twitter Ecuador. In: 2020 15th Iberian Conference on Information Systems and Technologies (CISTI) (2020)
17. Jones, J.: Americans Endorse Reporter-Audience Social Media Interaction. Gallup Blog (2019)
18. Jukowitz, M., Mitchell, A., Shearer, E., Walker, M.: U.S. media polarization and the 2020 election: a nation divided deep partisan divisions exist in the news sources Americans trust, distrust and rely on. Pew Research Center (2020)
19. Lewis, S., Molyneux, L.: A decade of research on social media and journalism: assumptions, blind spots, and a way forward. Media Commun. **6**(4), 11–23 (2018)
20. Lieberman, M.: A growing group of journalists has cut back on twitter, or abandoned it entirely. Poynter (2020)
21. McGregor, S.: Social media as public opinion: how journalists use social media to represent public opinion. Journalism **20**(8), 1070–1086 (2019)
22. McGregor, S.C., Molyneux, L.: Twitter's influence on news judgment: an experiment among journalists. Journalism **21**(5), 597–613 (2020)
23. Molyneux, L., Lewis, S.C., Holton, A.E.: Media work, identity, and the motivations that shape branding practices among journalists: an explanatory framework. New Media Soc. **21**(4), 836–855 (2019)
24. Neuberger, C., Nuernbergk, C., Langenohl, S.: Journalism as multichannel communication: a newsroom survey on the multiple uses of social media. Journal. Stud. **20**(9), 1260–1280 (2019)
25. Persily, N., Tucker, J.: Social Media and Democracy: The State of the Field, Prospects for Reform. Cambridge University Press, Cambridge (2020)
26. Reich, Z., Lahav, H.: What on earth do journalists know? A new model of knowledge brokers' expertise. Commun. Theory **31**, 1–20 (2020)
27. Reich, Z.: The impact of technology on news reporting: a longitudinal perspective. Journal. Mass Commun. Q. **90**(3), 417–434 (2013)
28. Santana, A., Hopp, T.: Tapping into a new stream of (personal) data: assessing journalists' different use of social media. Journal. Mass Commun. Q. **93**(2), 383–408 (2016)
29. Shugars, S., et al.: Pandemics, protests, and publics: demographic activity and engagement on twitter in 2020. J. Quant. Descr. Digit. Media **1** (2021)
30. Statista: Number of monthly active Twitter users worldwide from 1st quarter 2010 to 1st quarter 2019. https://www.statista.com/statistics/282087/number-of-monthly-active-twitter-users/. Accessed 13 Oct 2020
31. Tandoc, E., Jr., Vos, T.: The journalist is marketing the news: social media in the gatekeeping process. Journal. Pract. **10**(8), 950–966 (2016)
32. Usher, N., Holcomb, J., Littman, J.: Twitter makes it worse: political journalists, gendered echo chambers, and the amplification of gender bias. Int. J. Press/Polit. **23**(3), 324–344 (2018)
33. Vu, H., Le, T., Nguyen, H.: Routinizing facebook: how journalists' role conceptions influence their social media use for professional purposes in a socialist-communist country. Digit. Journal. 1–19 (2020)
34. Weaver, D., Willnat, L.: Changes in US journalism: how do journalists think about social media? Journal. Pract. **10**(7), 844–855 (2016)
35. Willnat, L., Weaver, D.: The American Journalist in the Digital Age: Key Findings. Indiana University, Bloomington (2014). http://news.indiana.edu/releases/iu/2014/05/2013-american-journalist-key-findings.pdf
36. Willnat, L., Weaver, D.: Social media and US journalists: uses and perceived effects on perceived norms and values. Digit. Journal. **6**(7), 889–909 (2018)
37. Weaver, D., Wilhoit, C.: The American Journalist: A Portrait of U.S. News People and Their Work. Indiana University Press, Bloomington (1986)

38. Wihbey, J.P.: The Social Fact: News and Knowledge in a Networked World. MIT Press, Cambridge (2019)
39. Wihbey, J., Joseph, K., Lazer, D.: The social silos of journalism? Twitter, news media and partisan segregation. New Media Soc. **21**(4), 815–835 (2019)
40. Wood-Doughty, Z., Xu, P., Liu, X., Dredze. M.: Using noisy self-reports to predict twitter user demographics. arXiv:2005.00635 (2020)
41. Zeng, L., Dailey, D., Mohamed, O., Starbird, K., Spiro, E.: Detecting journalism in the age of social media: three experiments in classifying journalists on twitter. In: Proceedings of the International AAAI Conference on Web and Social Media, vol. 13, pp. 548–559 (2019)

Analysis of the Publications of the Universities of the South of the Iberian Peninsula on Facebook

Estefanía Cestino-González(✉), Juan José Leiva-Olivencia, and Francisco-Javier Ruiz-del-Olmo

University of Malaga, 29010 Málaga, Spain
ecestino@uma.es

Abstract. The start of the pandemic in the middle of the 2019/20 academic year meant a great change and adaptation for the entire educational community. The objective of this publication is to analyze and compare the evolution of the publications with the greatest interaction that Andalusian universities, public and private, have made on the Facebook social network from the 2018/19 academic year to the 2019/20 academic year. A mixed, quantitative and qualitative methodology is used. The objectives and themes of the publications, the target audience and the elements and formats of the post are analyzed. The results show an increasing trend in publications dealing with human support, research and development issues, the purpose of which is to inform and inspire the entire community.

Keywords: Andalusian universities · COVID-19 · Facebook · Social networks

1 Introduction

The birth of the Facebook social network entailed a series of advantages of interaction with the public that, although at first there was reluctance to incorporate this medium by Higher education institutions [1], universities have gradually incorporated social networks into their communication strategy as another channel for the dissemination and promotion of communication with their audiences [2]. This is due to the main advantages offered by this medium: among others, it allows them to disseminate their contributions to society [3], and transmits messages between users instantly and globally [4]. The official websites of the institutions favor online communication through the information and dissemination of the facts and events that they publish, [5–7], according to strategic lines defined through good management and planning by the communication departments [8, 9]. They are also in charge of avoiding misinformation and, where necessary, provide clarifications against fakes news [10]. According to international rankings [11], the best universities in the world publish their publications on the Facebook social network in order to inform their audiences, highlighting institutional issues that are of general interest to the entire community [12]. Universities take on the challenge of carrying out a social and responsible work in the creation of online content [5, 13] and for this,

© The Author(s), under exclusive license to Springer Nature Singapore Pte Ltd. 2022
Á. Rocha et al. (Eds.): ICOMTA 2021, SIST 259, pp. 564–572, 2022.
https://doi.org/10.1007/978-981-16-5792-4_55

they use communication strategies that increase their visibility and the engagement of the audience they are targeting. Recent research [12] shows that the objective of the message and engagement on Facebook are related, and that the most successful publications are those whose purpose is to promote, in the sense of encouraging the public to take an action, such as for example, enroll in summer courses, participate in competitions, attend events, congresses, conferences, etc. In coherence with the above, the use of social networks in higher education is a new didactic instrument with a community projection, since interpersonal relationships and interactions can be established that allow improvements in learning and in the acquisition of skills of a student body more connected to the university, educational and social reality. In this sense, social networks become devices with which skills and abilities can be cultivated in students related to the search, identification, analysis and critical elaboration of the information shared in the network, the intersubjective construction of new productions and the development of autonomous learning and teamwork skills. In the same way, universities are institutions that are committed to a commitment to responsible and effective communication, which is attractive and encourages participation in a wide amalgam of topics that are of full interest to students and the university community in general. Culture, research, respect for the environment, social and inclusive sensitivity are part of a heterogeneous spectrum of thematic nuclei that are addressed in social networks with a view that synergistically combines ethical and aesthetic aspects of communication. In addition, the competitive aspect between universities, [14] both public and private in nature and their desire to position themselves as benchmarks in the field of research, entrepreneurship, culture or sustainability, among other aspects, cannot be forgotten either, both among his students and future entrants.

2 Objectives

The objectives of this research are three. First, to identify the publications with the greatest interaction from public and private universities in the south of the Iberian Peninsula, the Autonomous Community of Andalusia (Spain) and the Algarve (Portugal) on the Facebook social network for the academic years 2018/19 and 2019/20. Second, analyze the purpose, predominantly topic, and target audience of these posts. Third, to compare and assess the evolution in the communication strategy of the universities of the south of the peninsula.

3 Methodology

The Facebook social network was chosen for this study because it is one of the most widely used social networks in higher education institutions [15, 16]. All the universities analyzed have official Facebook accounts and keep their profiles active.

A methodology consisting of content analysis and automated data collection has been proposed, with the support of code books, analysis files and statistical tests [12]. Content analysis has been used as a research technique as it is the most suitable technique for objective communication studies [17, 18]. The qualitative data has been coded based on the codebook previously prepared and by means of an analysis sheet in the Excel program. Were taken as references Previous investigations [19–21], for the selection of variables and study models [12, 22, 23] for the elaboration of the code book and analysis files, paying special attention to the purpose, thematic and the audience for the publications. The FanPage karma analysis tool has been used to select the publications with the greatest interaction of each of the official Facebook profiles of Andalusian universities for the period from September 1, 2018 to July 31, 2019 and from September 1, 2019 to July 31, 2020. In have been this way, the 100 publications compiled with the greatest interaction from each Andalusian university, obtaining a total of 2,200 publications.

4 Discussion and Results

Table 1 shows the interaction, the number of Likes and the Coments of the publications of the universities of the south of the peninsula in the Facebook social network for the 2018/19 and 2019/20 courses.

The following universities have increased the number of interactions: University of Cádiz (UCA) 0.01%, University of Córdoba (UCO) 0.02%, University of Granada (UGR) 0.03%, University of Jaén (UJA) 0.03%, University of Málaga (UMA) 0.04%, International University of Andalucía (UNIA) 0.03%, University of Algarve (UALG) 0.1%. The University of Almería (UAL) and University of Sevilla (US) universities have remained the same, on the other hand, the universities have fallen: Universidad de Huelva (UHU) 0.05%, Universidad Loyola (ULO) 4% and Universidad Pablo de Olavide (UPO) 0.01%. All universities have increased the number of Likes and of comments except the University of Cádiz which has dropped.

In the following graphs, (Fig. 1 and Fig. 2) the results of the publications are presented in percentages according to their purpose for each university.

The publications with the purpose of informing are present in all the analyzed universities, and with the highest percentages in both academic years. The average for the 2019/20 academic year has increased 1.47% compared to the 2018/19 academic year. The results for each university are as follows: UALG 10%, UAL2%, UCA18.19%; UCO 5%, UGR 40%, UHU 28%, UJA 13%, ULO -37%, UMA 7%, UNIA -25.69%, UPO -26.48% US -24%. The average number of publications with the objective of promoting has decreased -6.1% in the 2019/20 academic year compared to the 2018/19 academic year. The results for each university are as follows: UALG -15%, UAL -11%, UCA 0% has remained constant with the same percentage in both academic years (15.15%), UCO 8%, UGR 1%, UHU -13%, UJA -8%, ULO -14%, UMA-19%, UNIA -5.7%, UPO -6.96%, US -2%. Publications whose purpose is education have increased the average 2.25% in the 2019/20 academic year compared to the 2018/19 academic year. UALG 1%, UAL 1%, UCA -5.05%, UCO 1%, UGR 1% UHU -5%, UJA 0% has remained constant in both courses (2%), ULO 17%, UMA 5%, UNIA 4%, UPO 4.04%, US 3%. The average of the 2019/20 academic year has slightly decreased compared to the 2018/19 academic year in online reaction publications by -0.25%. The results for each university are as follows: UALG 1%, UAL-3%, UCA - 2.02%, UCO has remained constant in both courses 2%, UGR 4%, UHU-4%, UJA 1%, ULO remains 1%, UMA -1%, UNIA has not obtained data among its first 100 publications with the greatest interaction, UPO 1.01%, US 0% has remained constant with the same percentage in both academic years (1%).

Publications whose purpose is to inspire and/or motivate has seen an average increase of 0.94% for the 2019/20 academic year compared to the 2018/19 academic year. The results for each university are as follows: UALG 3%, UAL11%, UCA -11.11%, UCO -14%, UGR remains 7%, UHU-6%, UJA -6%, ULO 34%, UMA 8%, UNIA 15.99% UPO 28.39%, US 23%.

In the following graphs (Fig. 3 and 4) the results of the publications are presented in percentages according to the subject and for each university.

The institutional theme has increased by 2.27% in the 2019/20 academic year compared to the 2018/19 academic year. The increases and decreases of the publications of each of the universities for this subject are detailed below: UALG -3%, UAL -4%, UCA -6.06%, UCO 0% (remains constant with 29%), UGR -10%, UHU -3%, UJA 2%, ULO 9%, UMA 8%, UNIA 11.96%, UPO 18.25%, US 4%.

Publications on Memorial Day have increased by 1.34% the average. The results for each university are as follows: UALG -1%, UAL 4%, UCA 5.05%, UCO -5%, UGR 7%, UHU 0% (remains the same as the previous year without variation at 7%), UJA 4%, ULO -5%, UMA remains at 2%, UNIA 2%, UPO -093%, US 6%.

Publications whose subject is human support have also increased by 13.36%. The results for each university are as follows: UALG 18%, UAL 21%, UCA 10.10%, UCO11%, UGR 3%, UHU 9%, UJA 19%, ULO 25%, UMA 8%, UNIA 14.97%, UPO 12.25%, US 11%.

For the Research theme, the average has increased by 0.08%. The results for each university are as follows: UALG 11%, UAL 1%, UCA -4.04%, UCO -9%, UGR - 4%, UHU -2%, UJA 6%, ULO -5%, UMA 18%, UNIA -0.7%, UPO -7.85%, US -5%. Publications on academic subjects decreased by -5.37% on average. The results for each university are as follows: UALG -8%, UAL -3%, UCA -11.11%, UCO 12%, UGR remains at 10%, UHU -3%, UJA -6%, ULO -2%, UMA -19%, UNIA -8.48%, UPO -1.39%, US -4%.

The average number of publications on mobility fell by -1.50%. The results for each university are as follows: UALG -1%, UAL -1%, UCA remains at 2.02%, UCO 2%, UGR -3%, UHU 3%, UJA -2%, ULO 7%, UMA -6%, UNIA -2.02%, UPO -0.99%, the US has not had publications on this subject. On the other hand, publications on accommodation have increased by 0.92% on average. The results for each university are as follows: UALG -1%, UAL has not had publications on this subject, UCA 1.01%, UCO 2%, UGR 2%, UHU 2%, UJA 1%, ULO UAL has not had publications on this subject, UMA remains the same as the previous year with 1%, UNIA 5%, UPO -1%, the US has not had publications on this subject.

The average number of publications about events has decreased -13.36%. The results for each university are as follows: UALG -15%, UAL -19%, UCA remains at 17.17%, UCO -16%, UGR 3%, UHU -8%, UJA -30%, ULO 7%, UMA -10%, UNIA -25.35%, UPO -12.92%, US -11%.

The average number of Telework publications has increased by 1.76%. The results for each university are as follows: UALG -1%, UAL 1%, UCA 3.03%, UCO 1%, UGR 1%, UHU 2%, UJA 3%, ULO 2%, UMA 3%, UNIA 1%, UPO 5.05%, US has not had publications on this subject. For complaints, the average has increased by 0.34%. The results for each university are as follows: UALG, UAL, UHU, UNIA has not had

Table 1. Interaction, Nº Likes, Nº Coments

Univ	UAL	UCA	UCO	UGR	UHU	UJA	UMA	US	UNIA	ULO	UPO	UALG
Interaction 2018/19	0,0%	0,04%	0,07%	0,06%	0,43%	0,09%	0,05%	0,06%	0,07%	0,56%	0,11%	0,19%
Interaction 2019/20	0,0%	0,05%	0,09%	0,09%	0,38%	0,12%	0,09%	0,06%	0,10%	0,52%	0,10%	0,20%
Nº Likes 2018/19	0	10992	2956	34673	5409	16248	9088	29028	2012	7746	8080	20402
Nº Likes 2019/20	0	9152	9801	40386	7686	32415	19546	37871	3870	9653	12888	26202
Nº Coments 2018/19	0	521	106	2133	185	311	528	1549	53	121	345	749
Nº Coments 2019/20	0	235	209	3085	307	1386	1092	1786	148	276	575	970

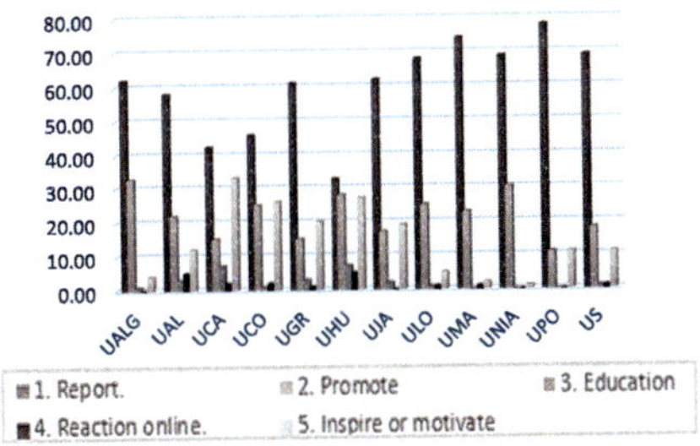

Fig. 1. Purpose posts on Facebook 2018/19

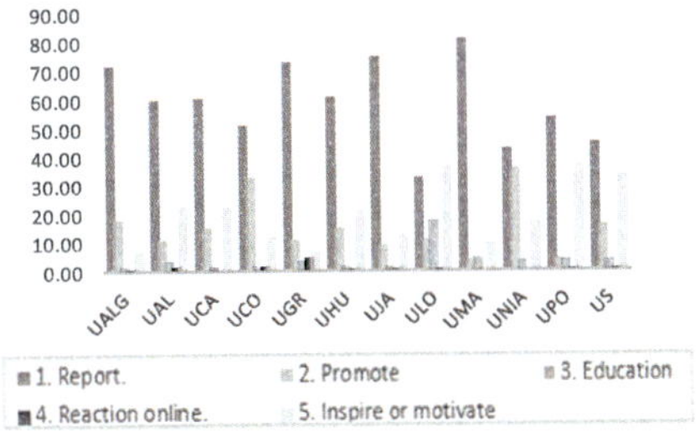

Fig. 2. Purpose posts on Facebook 2019/20

publications on this subject, UCA 2.02%, UCO 1%, UGR 1%, UJA 2%, ULO -1%, UMA 0% (remains the same as the previous year 1%), UPO 1.02%, US -1%. Also, fake new publications have increased by 0.33%. The results for each university are as follows: UCO 1%, UJA 2%, UPO 1.01%. The UALG, UAL, UCA, UGR, UHU, ULO, UMA, UNIA and US universities have not had publications on this subject.

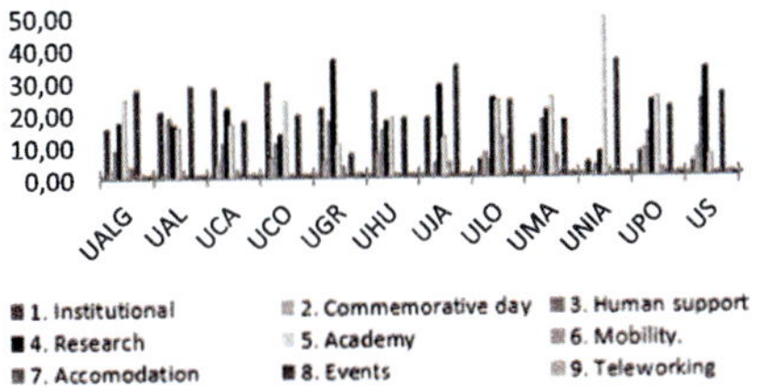

Fig. 3. Theme of the 2018/19 publications

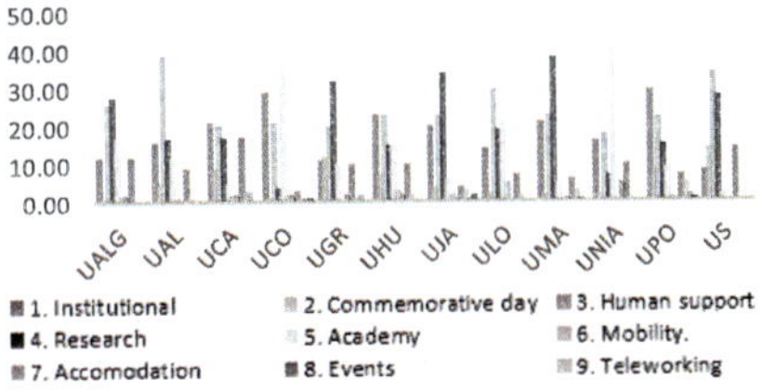

Fig. 4. Theme of the 2019/20 publications

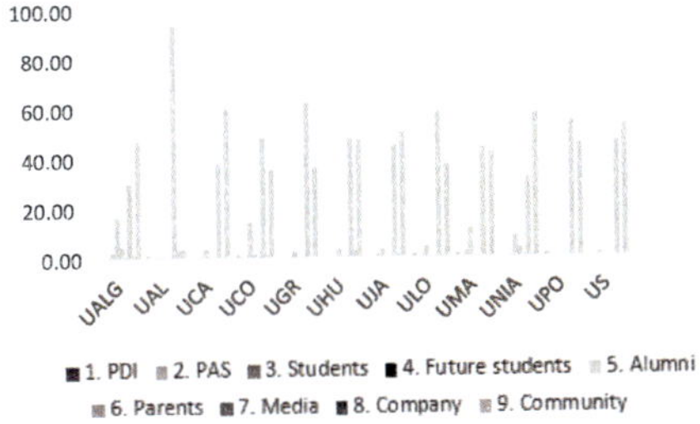

Fig. 5. Audience 2018/19

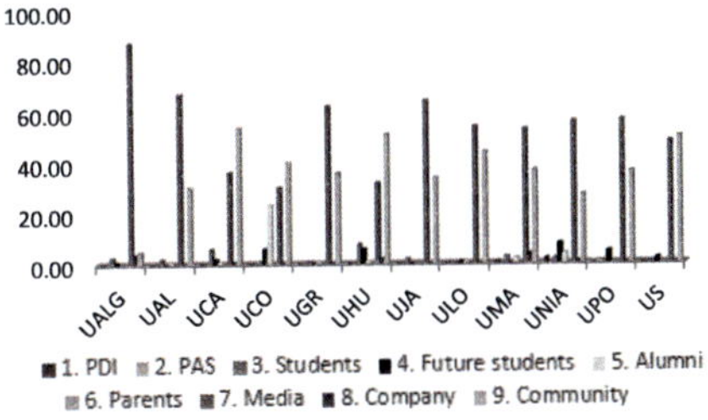

Fig. 6. Audience 2019/20

The following graphs (Fig. 5 and 6) show the results in percentages according to the type of audience to whom the publications are intended.

Publications destined for the PDI have decreased −0.17% on average in the 2019/20 academic year compared to the 2018/19 academic year. The results for each university are as follows: UALG, UCA, UGR, UHU, UJA and US have not had data in this category, UAL -1%, UCO -1%, ULO -1%, UMA 0% (remains at 1%), UNIA 2%, UPO -1%.

Publications for the PAS have slightly increased the average 0.08%. The UALG, UAL, UCA, UCO, UGR, UHU, UJA, ULO, UMA, UNIA, US universities have not obtained data in this category. Only the UPO university has increased its average with 1.01%.

The average number of publications aimed at current students has increased by 1.92%. The results for each of the universities are: UALG 1%, UAL 2%, UCA 6.06%, UCO 1%, UGR 1%, UHU 8%, UJA 1%, ULO 0% (no publications have been obtained for this category), UMA 1%, UNIA 2%, UPO 1.01%, US -1%.

On the contrary, the average number of publications aimed at future students has decreased −2.75%. The results for each of the universities are: UALG -15%, UAL 0% (no publications have been obtained for this category), UCA 1.01%, UCO -8%, UGR -2%, UHU 3%, UJA -3%, ULO -3%, UMA -11%, UNIA -1.08%, UPO 5.05%, US 2%.

Publications addressed to alumni audience (current students and potential students) has increased the average by 2.16%. The results for each of the universities are: UALG -4%, UAL 1%, UCA 1,01%, UCO 22%, UGR1%, UHU 1%, UJA, UPO and US, no publications have been found for this category, ULO 1%, UMA 2%, UNIA 0.97%.

No publications addressed to parents have been found at any university 0%.

The average number of publications directed to the media has increased 4.11%. The results for each of the universities are: UALG 57%, UAL -26%, UCA -1.01%, UCO -18%, UGR 0% (it remains constant at 62%), UHU -16%, UJA 19%, ULO -4%, UMA 9%, UNIA 24.69%, UPO 2.57%, US 2%.

The average number of publications for companies has also increased by 0.33%. The average has increased 0.33%. The results for each of the universities are: UALG 3%, UAL -3%, UCA 1.01%, UCO -1%, UGR has not had a%, UHU remains the same as the previous year with 2%, UJA - 1%, ULO, UPO and US have not had, UMA 4%, UNIA 1%. On the other hand, the average number of publications destined for the entire community has fallen -5.69%. The results for each of the universities are: UALG -42%, UAL 27%, UCA -6.06%, UCO 5%, UGR 0% (it remains the same as the previous year at 36%), UHU 4%, UJA -16%, ULO 7%, UMA -5%, UNIA -31.58%, UPO -8.64%, US -3%.

5 Conclusions

Visibility of the institutional image and content published by universities is important to attract and retain students [3]. The format, purpose, content of publications and the frequency with which it is published are increasingly being taken into account [24].

The type of content and the frequency of publication are factors that improve interaction [3, 24–29].

A good communication strategy that serves stakeholders helps to improve interaction, participation and increase the reach of your publications [25].

The trend in institutional social networks, according to reports from the best universities in the world, are publications whose objective is: to inform and promote [12]. Following this line and pressured by the social changes derived from the pandemic, the universities of the south of the peninsula have reflected the communication strategies of this trend in their social networks. Publications whose purpose is to inform, promote, inspire and motivate have been increased.

The recipients of the publications have varied from one course to the other. On the one hand, those publications aimed at future students and the entire community in general have decreased. However, there has been an increase in publications aimed at students enrolled in the current academic year (2019/20), and publications in the media, especially in the digital press.

Comparing the 2019/20 and 2018/19 courses, a trend is observed in the increase of publications whose themes are human support, institutional communication, teleworking and, to a lesser extent, fakes news. On the contrary, those that have decreased the most are academic subjects and, above all, events, the result of the reality that has been lived and as a consequence of the state of alarm due to the pandemic.

Research has played an important role that has transcended the media on many occasions, especially during the pandemic, and even publications on scientific advances have also served as support and inspiration for the entire community, such as the patent of the first artificial respirator developed by Andalusian universities and human and technical support to health workers.

It can also be concluded that in the period analyzed, universities have increased the visibility of their research related to the pandemic and the achievements of transfer to society and of public utility of their laboratories and researchers.

In summary, continuing to build effective, responsible and sustainable communication through social networks will imply continuing to forge new strategic alliances between all agents of the university communities where diversity and participatory inclusion are valued.

References

1. Rodríguez, A., Santamaría, P.: Análisis del uso de las redes sociales en internet: facebook y Twitter en las universidades españolas. Rev. ICONO14 Rev. Científica Comun. Tecnol. Emerg. **10**(2), 228 (2012)
2. Reina-Estévez, J., Fernández-Castillo, I., Noguer Jiménez, Á.: El uso de las Redes sociales en las Universidades andaluzas. El caso de Facebook y Twitter. Rev. Int. Relac. Públicas **4**(11), 123–144 (2012)
3. Peruta, A., Shields, A.B.: Social media in higher education: understanding how colleges and universities use Facebook. J. Mark. High. Educ. **27**(1), 131–143 (2017). https://doi.org/10.1080/08841241.2016.1212451
4. Simón-Onieva, J.E.: Uso de las redes sociales por las universidades públicas andaluzas. Análisis de contenido de la cuenta oficial de Twitter. Estud. Sobre Mensaje Periodístico **23**(1), 631–645 (2017)
5. Aldeanueva-Fernández, I., Arrabal-Sánchez, G.: La comunicación y medición de la responsabilidad Social Universitaria: Redes sociales y propuesta de indicadores. Rev. Digit. Invest. Docencia Univ. **2**(1), 121–136 (2018)
6. Garza-Salgado, E., Royo-Vela, M.: Brand Fan Pages experience and strength as antecedents to engagement and intensity of use to achieve HEIS' brand loyalty. J. Mark. High. Educ. **29**(1), 102–120 (2019)
7. Ashley, C., Tuten, T.: Creative strategies in social media marketing: an exploratory study of branded social content and consumer engagement: creative strategies in social media. Psychol. Mark. **32**(1), 15–27 (2015)
8. García-Gordillo, M.: Universidad y medios sociales. Gestión de la comunicación en la universidad española. Rev. Prisma Soc. **22**, 20–36 (2018)
9. Simancas-González, E., García-López, M.: Gestión de la comunicación en las universidades públicas españolas. El Prof. Inform. **26**(4), 735–744 (2017). https://doi.org/10.3145/epi.2017.jul.17

10. Salaverría, R., Buslón, N., López-Pan, F., León, B., López-Goñi, I., Erviti, M.-C.: Desinformación en tiempos de pandemia: tipología de los bulos sobre la Covid-19. El Prof. Inform. **29**(3) (2020). https://doi.org/10.3145/epi.2020.may.15
11. Valerio-Ureña, G., Herrera-Murillo, D., Madero-Gómez, S.: Analysis of the presence of most best-ranked universities on social networking sites. Informatics **7**(1), 9 (2020)
12. Segura-Mariño, A.G., Paniagua-Rojano, F.J., Sande, M.F.: Metodología para evaluar la comunicación universitaria en Facebook y Twitter. Prisma Soc.: Rev. Invest. Soc. (28), 127–144 (2020)
13. Manca, S., Bocconi, S., Gleason, B.: "Think globally, act locally": a glocal approach to the development of social media literacy. Comput. Educ. **160**, 104025 (2021)
14. Bolat, E., O'Sullivan, H.: Radicalising the marketing of higher education: learning from student-generated social media data. J. Mark. Manag. **33**(9–10), 742–763 (2017)
15. García-Domingo, M., Aranda, M., Fuentes, V.M.: Facebook use in university students: exposure and reinforcement search. Proc. Soc. Behav. Sci. **237**, 249–254 (2017)
16. Paniagua Rojano, F.J., Gómez Calderón, B., Fernández Sande, M.: La incorporación de los departamentos de comunicación de las universidades españolas al entorno digital. Un análisis cuantitativo. Estud. Sobre Mensaje Periodístico **18**(Nov 12), 691–701 (2012)
17. Igartua, J.J.: Métodos cuantitativos de investigación en comunicación. Bosch, Barcelona (2006)
18. Peruta, A., Shields, A.B.: Marketing your university on social media: a content analysis of Facebook post types and formats. J. Mark. High. Educ. **28**(2), 175–191 (2018)
19. Bellucci, M., Biagi, S., Manetti, G.: Dialogic accounting and stakeholder engagement through social media: the case of top-ranked universities. Rev. High. Educ. **42**(3), 1145–1184 (2019)
20. Brech, F.M., Messer, U., Vander Schee, B.A., Rauschnabel, P.A., Ivens, B.S.: Engaging fans and the community in social media: interaction with institutions of higher education on Facebook. J. Mark. High. Educ. **27**(1), 112–130 (2017)
21. Segura-Mariño, A.G.: Comunicación online de las universidades de Ecuador. Estudio de la estrategia en Facebook. Rev. Asoc. Española Invest. Comun. **5**(10), 81–89 (2018)
22. Gómez, B.J., Paniagua, F.J.: Las universidades españolas en Twitter. Hist. Comun. Soc. **19**(19), 681–694 (2014)
23. Lund, B.: Universities engaging social media users: an investigation of quantitative relationships between universities' Facebook followers/interactions and university attributes. J. Mark. High. Educ. 1–17 (2019).
24. Lund, B.D., Wang, T.: Information dissemination and interactions in higher education social media posts. J. Promot. Manag. **27**(4), 547–561 (2021)
25. del Rocío Bonilla Quijada, M., Muñoz, E.P., Corrons, A., Olmo-Arriaga, J.-L.: Engaging students through social media. Findings for the top five universities in the world. J. Mark. High. Educ. 1–18 (2021)
26. Assimakopoulos, C., Antoniadis, I., Kayas, O.G., Dvizac, D.: Effective social media marketing strategy: Facebook as an opportunity for universities. Int. J. Retail Distrib. Manage. (2017)
27. Akyildiz, M., Argan, M.: Using online social networking: students' purposes of Facebook usage at the university of Turkey. J. Technol. Res. **3**, 1–11 (2011)
28. Antoniadis, I., Koukoulis, I., Serdaris, P.: Social network sites' usage among Greek students in Western Macedonia. Int. J. Strategic Innov. Mark. **3**, 52–65 (2015). https://doi.org/10.15556/IJSIM.02.03.005
29. Eger, L., Egerová, D., Tomczyk, L., Krystoň, M., Czeglédi, C.: Facebook for Public Relations in the higher education field: a study from four countries Czechia, Slovakia, Poland and Hungary. J. Mark. High. Educ. 1–21 (2020)

The Perception of Cyberbullying by Adolescents in Rural and Urban Spain

Claudia Pardo Ramos[1], Angel Torres-Toukoumidis[2](✉), Mari Carmen Caldeiro Pedreira[1], and Tereza Havránková[3]

[1] Universidad de Santiago de Compostela, Praza do Obradoiro, 0, 15705 Santiago de Compostela, Spain
claudia.pardo@rai.usc.es, mcarmen.caldeiro@usc.es
[2] Universidad Politécnica Salesiana, Cuenca 010105, Ecuador
atorrest@ups.edu.ec
[3] University of West Bohemia, Univerzitní 2732/8, 301 00 Plzeň 3, Czechia

Abstract. Cases of bullying have become more serious from the use of information and communication technologies, especially with an immersion in social networks—creating the situation of cyberbullying. The objectives of our study are to analyze the relationship between cyber-victims and cyber-aggressors with respect to the use of Information and communication technology (ICT) and, finally, to identify the distribution by sex, type of center, and academic level of cases of cyber-bullying. The results we obtained show a significant relationship between cybervictims and the lack of parental supervision. Men are frequent aggressors within sexual cyberbullying, while women are equally aggressors in terms of identity usurpation, ignoring or marginalizing a partner especially in urban centers with no connection to academic level. In short, prevention policies must be incorporated into the classroom with the participation of students and teachers in order to mitigate this type of behavior in schools.

Keywords: Cyberbullying · Teenagers · Internet · Perception · Rural schools

1 Introduction

School bullying, also referred to as bullying or harassment among peers, is present in all schools today. Around 200 million children and young people worldwide are bullied by their peers [1]. The most widely used definition to refer to bullying was formulated by Olweus (1999). The author [2] defines bullying as "harassment of a person who is repeatedly exposed to adverse actions for a long time by one or more people who intentionally intend to cause him/her harm with an imbalance of power between the victim and aggressor".

The academic community distinguishes four types of harassment: physical, which corresponds to aggressive behavior against a person; verbal, which includes derogatory nicknames, insults or humiliating jokes; social, which consists of isolating and marginalizing the victim; and psychological, which includes behaviors that affect the individual's self-esteem, creating fear and insecurity [3].

© The Author(s), under exclusive license to Springer Nature Singapore Pte Ltd. 2022
Á. Rocha et al. (Eds.): ICOMTA 2021, SIST 259, pp. 573–582, 2022.
https://doi.org/10.1007/978-981-16-5792-4_56

According to the National Institute of Statistics (2017) [4], 84.60% of people between the age of 16 and 74 have accessed the Internet at some point. In addition, 80% of the people use the Internet at least once a week and thus can be considered as frequent users. According to the same study, the use of new information and communication technologies is closely linked to the age of users. The rate of ICT uses and internet access of young people between 16 and 24 is 98.00%. Also, 75.30% of adolescents accesses social networks frequently. The percentage increases to 90% when we add those who connect to social networks occasionally [5]. The same author affirms that social networks are accessed by 78.50% of adolescents and 71.80% by men. A different study [6] stresses the different use of social networks according to sexes. Girls spend most of the time online communicating through social networks, while boys mainly access online video game pages.

The extension of social life to the virtual sphere carries numerous advantages and risks [7]. One of these risks is bullying, also known as the phenomenon of cyberbullying [8] which is constantly evolving. The presence of cyberbullying has increased dramatically in recent years and has triggered concern in society.

In sum, Hinduja and Patchin (2014) [9] claim that cyberattacks occur when a child, a preadolescent or adolescent, is humiliated by person on the Internet, phone, or other digital tool. The authors add that cyberattacks take place among young people without any adult being involved. Also, cyberattacks intend to harm someone. In many cases, there can be a shift in roles where the victim becomes a stalker.

The repetition of cyberattacks and the widely available digital tools can prolong damage. This can happen with just with a single action or incident. An example could be videos or photos posted on the Internet [10]. In addition to the multiple definitions, it is vital to refer to the different forms of cyberbullying that are known today.

1.1 Prevalence of Cyberbullying

Cyberbullying has become a problematic phenomenon, shared by all developed countries. However, it is difficult to state exact figures of the number of victims and aggressors that reflect the prevalence among adolescents. Over the years, the data obtained from studies widely differs [11]. The studies differ in geographical areas of reference, age (10–18 years) of participants, degree of education, research methodology, evaluation instrument, the type of behaviors studied, and the time interval considered. Another critical point for the existence of these differences is whether or not repetition is considered a necessary characteristic for cyberbullying [12].

Some other studies link cyberbullying to the use of social networks. The studies state that adolescents who make greater use of ICT are more likely to be involved in cyberbullying as victims or aggressors [13]. There should be parental supervision when children and adolescents are connected to the Internet, restricting the time spent on the Internet. On the other hand, there are studies that relate to the use of social networks, in which adolescents who adhere to the use of ICT tend to be more likely to to become aggressors [14]. In relation to these tenders, parental supervision lasts at the time of connection to the Internet, which is currently centered on the time restriction [15].

In order to carry out more effective prevention of cyberbullying, it is critical to consider the variable of geography and rural and urban areas play a role in the discussion of cyberbulling. Few studies have taken this point into account. The one carried out by the Ombudsman-UNICEF (2007) [16] shows that no significant differences have been found between rural and urban areas, neither in traditional bullying nor in cyberbullying. It contradicts the studies on bullying reporting that violent behavior is more common in urban areas than in rural environments [17]. Basically, the same document also indicates that students from schools located in rural settings receive significantly fewer cyber-attacks than those located in urban settings.

In this sense, various reasons explain the difference and refer both to the environment and the characteristics of the areas. In the first place, there would be the impersonality that characterizes urban environments, which favors anonymity and lack of empathy, while rural environment favors prosocial attitudes [18]. In addition, the forms of leisure activities of adolescents can influence cyberbullying behaviors, such as the consumption of designer drugs [19], which are more linked to urban settings. On the other hand, rural areas are characterized by having fewer students than urban areas allowing teachers to pay more individual attention to both students and their families [20].

2 Methodology

The paper's main objective is to study the phenomenon of cyberbullying in students of third and fourth grade of Compulsory Secondary Education, making a comparison between rural and urban areas in the province of Lugo, Galicia, Spain. The specific objectives were established:

1. Analyze the relationship of cyber victims regarding ICT use.
2. Evaluate the relationship between cyberbullies regarding the use of ICT.
3. Identify the distribution by sex, area and academic level of cyberbullying cases.

The participants in this study are third and fourth-year students from two secondary schools in Lugo (Spain), one located in an urban area and the other in a rural area. The selection of the schools enables us to compare the results, despite the difference in the number of students since rural schools have a smaller number of students.

The total number of students surveyed was 238, of which 83 belonged to the rural school and the remaining 155 to the urban school. As previously specified, they belong to the third and fourth year of secondary and their ages are between 14 and 18, with a mean value of $\mu = 15.26$ years and a standard deviation of $\sigma = 0.81$. Regarding the distribution by sex, of the total number, 51.70% are women, and 48.30% are men, so the sample is very balanced.

When we differentiate the type of school, in the rural school, we have 39 students from the fourth grade and 44 from the third grade, whose ages are between 14 and 18 with the mean $\mu = 15.22$ years and the standard deviation $\sigma = 0.85$. Furthermore, 53.01% are women, and 46.99% are men. As for the courses, the fourth grade consists of 61.54% women and 38.46% men, and the ages are between 15 and 18 with the mean of $\mu =$ 15.84 years and the standard deviation of $\sigma = 0.72$. Regarding the third-year students, 44 students aged between 14 and 15 years, with the mean $\mu = 14$, 14.64 years, and the standard deviation $\sigma = 0.49$. Regarding the distribution by sex, 45.45% are women, and 54.55% are men.

In the urban school, 79 secondary students from the fourth year and 76 from the third year, whose ages are between 14 and 18, were surveyed, with a mean of $\mu = 15.29$ years and the standard deviation $\sigma = 0, 78$. In the fourth year, 53.16% are women, and 46.84% are men, whose ages are between 15 and 18 with a mean of $\mu = 15.81$ years, the standard deviation being $\sigma = 0.68$. Regarding the third year, we have 48.68% women and 51.32% men and the age range between 14 and 15 years with a mean of $\mu = 14.75$ years and the standard deviation $\sigma = 0.44$ (Table 1).

Table 1. Distribution of participants according to grade, gender and type of school.

	Gender	Rural	Urban	Total
4th grade	Women	24	42	66
	Men	15	37	52
3rd grade	Women	20	37	57
	Men	24	39	63
Total		83	155	238

An ad hoc self-report questionnaire was created to collect the data. According to Whitney and Smith (1993) [21], it is how the best results are obtained in this type of research. The Cyberbullying questionnaire: Peer harassment screening, developed by Garaigordobil (2013), and the DAPHNE Questionnaire questionnaire by Calmaestra (2011) were used as a starting point [10].

The questionnaire is configured in five parts, and with a total of 21 items, with a reliability index calculated using Cronbach's Alpha, in the SPSS statistical analysis software, of $\alpha = 0.844$.

The first part "Student data", which consists of two items was designed to classify students according to gender and age. In order to enhance anonymity, and as recommended by the experts, the type of the school and academic year was not collected by the interviewer and thus were not included in the questionnaire.

The second part, "Internet uses", has a total of nine items, which aimed to collect data on whether the adolescent has a mobile phone and/or computer with Internet access at home, whether he/she has Internet access outside the home and from home and how that connection is made. It also includes two questions about whether they are supervised by parents when accessing the Internet at home or school. This section also includes a frequency table with a 5-level Likert scale, in which the activities carried out by adolescents on the Internet are analyzed.

First, the schools were contacted to request their collaboration in the study. A meeting was held with the management team in which the objectives of the work were reported. Then the research and the ethical criteria were approved, and the questionnaires were passed to the students in the third quarter of the 2018/2019 academic year. The students were supervised by teachers while filling in the online questionnaire. The authors of the study opted for an online version of the questionnaire as it is economically and time convenient approach to data collection.

An analysis of the data collected was carried out using the statistical analysis software SPSS. As for the coding of the data coding, the authors of the study decided to follow Calmaestra (2011) [10] and defined the severity in such a way that it is considered occasional when cyber-attacks occur at most two or three times a month, and frequently after two or three times a month. For the codification of the data disclosed, we decided to delimit the severity of the effort that is considered appropriate when the episodes are produced as close as possible to each other, and the frequency of the part the three times the month.

3 Results

This portion describes the results of the research on cyberbullying. In the first place, the frequency with which the different cyberbullying situations occur for the three roles (observer, victim and aggressor) are addressed, taking into account the variables of gender and type the school (rural or urban). Subsequently, the prevalence of bullying is analyzed according to the role played by each of the participants in this research. Also, the authors analyze the relationship with the variables of gender, type of school, academic year, hours of Internet connection, involvement in cyberbullying and the presence of parental supervision.

3.1 Cyber Victims

This section aims to analyze the frequencies with which the participants have witnessed cyberbullying in the degrees established above, taking into account the variable of gender and type of school. According to the results obtained, the most frequent victims of cyberbullying receive messages with offences or insults via mobile phones or the Internet. The percentage is 11.3%, the rate of occasional victims is 29.0%. Regarding gender, the percentage of women who are frequent victims (12.2%) is higher than that of men (10.4%), while the opposite is the case for occasional cyber victims (38.3%). -20.3%). The differences between rural and urban schools are significant, with a percentage of frequent victimization higher in the rural school (12.0% -1.9%). In comparison, the percentage of occasional victimization is higher in the urban schools (32.9%). % -21.7%).

Cyberbullying through offensive or humiliating calls has a frequent victimization rate of 3.4% and an occasional of 18.9%. The differences by sex are quite wide, with the percentage of frequent victimization higher in women (4.9% -1.8%) and the percentage of occasional victimization higher in men (28.7% -9.8%). According to the type of school, the greatest difference appears in occasional cybervictimization in which the percentage of men is 28.7% and that of women is 9.8%. The onset of median offensive or humiliating substances is an indicator of a 3.4% and occasional victimization. 18.9%. The differences between sexes are often amplified, including the percentage of victimization in women (4.9% -1.8%) and the temporary victimization in men (28.7% -9.8%). According to the type of school, the most significant difference appears in occasional cyber victimization, in which the percentage of men is 28.7%, and that of women is 9.8%.

Threatening anonymous calls have a frequent victimization rate of 3.4%, while the occasional calls rise to 18.9%. In the differentiation by sex, the percentage of men is higher, both in the occasional variant (21.7% -4.9%) and in the frequent 4.3% -2.4%). Depending on the type of school, the differences are scarce, although the values obtained are slightly higher in the urban school.

Regarding blackmail via mobile or Internet, the frequent victimization rate is 3.8%, while the occasional one is 10.5%. In the differentiation by sex, we obtain slightly higher values of women as frequent victims (4.1% -3.5%), while in occasional victimization, the percentage of men is much higher than that of women (18.3% -3, 3%). Sexual harassment through ICT has a frequent victimization rate of 0.4% and an occasional 11.8%. In the differentiation by sex, women correspond to a higher percentage in the occasional variant (19.1% -4.9%) and the frequent variant (0.9% -0.0%). The rural center has slightly higher indices in the differentiation by the school than the urban one.

The percentages of victimization of defamation through lies or rumors is 2.1% in the frequent variant and 13.5% in the occasional variant. Women suffer more frequent victimization of this type (4.9% -0.9%), while the percentage of the occasional variant is higher in men (22.8% -4.9%). The differences between rural and urban schools are minor. The theft of the password of social networks, email or blog has a percentage of 8.0% of frequent victims and 11.0% of occasional victims. It presents higher percentages of male victims, both in the frequent variant (11.4% -4.8%) and in the occasional variant (17.5% -4.9%). The percentage of frequent victims of identity theft is 2.1% and the occasional 15.1%. In the differentiation by sex, the number of male victims in May, both in the frequent slope (2.6% -1.6%) and occasional (23.5% -7.3%). Depending on the type of school, the differences are minimal.

Being ignored or marginalized in a chat, social network, or instant message application represents a percentage of frequent victims of 7.6% and occasional victims of 18.1%. The frequent victimization is higher in women (13.9%) than in men (0.9%), while the opposite occurs with occasional victimization (24.3% -12.2%). In the differentiation according to the school, the center percentages of the urban school are slightly higher in both occasional and frequent victims.

3.2 Cyberbullies

The highest rate of cyberbullies occurs again in sending insulting or offensive messages via mobile phones or the Internet, with a frequent victimization rate of 3.4% and an occasional of 24.8%. The frequent variant is greater in men (7.0% -0.0%) and the occasional one in women (27.6% -21.7%). Regarding the differentiation by the school, frequent victims have a higher percentage in urban schools (3.8% -2.4%), the same as in occasional victims (27.7% -19.3%). In the category of offensive or insulting calls, the percentage of frequent aggressors is 0.4%, and occasional ones are 8.4%. The differentiation by gender indicates that men are more frequent cyberbullies (0.9% -0.0%) and occasional (13.9% -3.3%).

The urban school has a higher percentage of both frequent (0.6% -0.0%) and occasional (9.0% -7.2%) aggressors. Threatening anonymous calls have a frequent aggressor rate of 0.0% and occasional of 5.5%. According to gender, the percentage of occasional male aggressors is 11.3% and 0.0% of women. Depending on the type of school, occasional aggressors are 5.8% in the urban school and 4.8% in the rural school.

As for sexual harassment through mobile phones or the Internet, there are generally 0.0% frequent aggressors and 5.5% occasional. Men are the majority as occasional aggressors (10.4% -0.8%). The difference by type of school is minimal. The dissemination of photos or videos has a rate of frequent aggressors of 0.0% and an occasional 6.3%. Women are the majority as occasional aggressors (7.3% -5.2%), while the differences according to the type of school are minimal. Through lies or rumors through mobile phones or the Internet, defamation does not have aggressors in the frequent variant but the occasional variant (9.7%). The percentage of aggressors is higher in men (13.0% -6.5%) and the urban school (10.3 -8.4%).

Identity theft has only occasional aggressors in a percentage of 5.9%. All the aggressors are men with an index of 12.3%, and the differences according to the type of school are not very significant. Finally, ignoring or marginalizing a peer in a chat, social network, or instant message application has a rate of frequent aggressors of 1.3% and occasional aggressors of 16.0%. Women are the majority both in the frequent (2.4% -0.0%) and in the occasional (16.3% -15.7%) side. The percentage is also higher in the urban school for frequent (2.5% -0.0%) and occasional (17.4% -13.3%).

3.3 Cyberbullying by Gender, the School and Academic Year

The percentages of the different roles of cyberbullying presented by the participants in this research will be analyzed. In addition, the frequency of each role will be crossed with the variables of gender, type of school, academic year, hours on the Internet, presence of parental supervision and the roles played in cyberbullying by each participant in the study.

The analyzed sample presents a percentage of controls of 28.57%. Occasional victims are 22.27%, while the percentage of frequent victims rising to 24.37%. Regarding the aggressors, the occasional represent 0.84% of the sample and the frequent 0.42%. Also, the sample contains victimized aggressors, whose percentage in the occasional occurrence is 18.91% and in the frequent one, 4.62%.

The variable of the rural or urban school, a dependency relationship with involvement in cyberbullying has not been found either. The results show a very similar number of witnesses in the rural (28.9%) and the urban school (28.4%). There are more occasional and frequent victims in rural than in urban school, with percentages of 24.1% -21.3% for the occasional variant and 27.7% -22.6% for the frequent variant. Occasional aggressors are 2.4% in the rural school and non-existent in the urban school, while in the frequent variant they are 0.6% in the urban and 0.0% in the rural school. As for the victimized aggressors, they have a higher percentage in the urban school, both the occasional (21.3% -14.5%) and the frequent (5.8% -2.4%). A dependency relationship was not found with the academic year variable; again, there are differences between the third and fourth grade of secondary who participated in the survey. The number of witnesses is higher in the fourth grade, with a percentage of 30.5% compared to 26.7% in the third grade. The global number of victims is very similar in both courses/years, but in occasional and frequent victimization, the differences are appreciated. The occasional have a higher percentage in the fourth grade (22.9% -21.7%) and the frequent in third (25.0% -23.7%).

However, we have found a significant relationship between cyberbullying and time spent connected to the Internet [χ^2 (1) = 4,609, p < ,05]. According to the data obtained, the participants who spend less than an hour on the Internet are 100% occasional victims. Those included in the period of 1 to 2 h of connection, the percentage of witnesses is 36.3%, that of occasional victims is 37.5%, and that of frequent victims is 6.3%. There are no frequent aggressors, but 1.3% are occasional. Regarding the victimized aggressors, 13.8% are occasional and 5.0% frequent. With participants with a time range of 2 to 4 h of Internet connection, the percentage of witnesses is 24.7%, occasional victims 7.5% while frequent victims have a much higher rate than the two previous ranges, with 36.3%. We only found occasional aggressors with 1.1%.

Regarding the victimized aggressors, the percentage is also higher in both the occasional (23.7%) and the frequent (6.5%). For the most extended connection to the Internet is more than four hours, the percentage of witnesses is 28.3%. As for the victims, the occasional have a percentage of 14.0% and the frequent 33.3%. The percentage of occasional aggressors is zero, and that of frequent aggressors is 1.8%. Regarding the victimized aggressors, 21.1% are occasional and 1.8% frequent.

On the contrary, a significant link [χ^2 (6) = 12,832, p < ,05] between the involvement in cyberbullying and parental control. The results obtained in this study reflect that in those participants who do not have parental control, 28.3% are witnesses, 25% are occasional victims and 24.3% frequent, there are only frequent aggressors with 0.7%, and within the victimized aggressors, the percentage of occasional is 15.8%, and that of frequent is 5.9%. As for those who have parental supervision, 29.8% are witnesses, 17.9% occasional victims and 25% frequent. Occasional aggressors account for 2.4%, and frequent aggressors 8%. Among the victimized aggressors, there are only occasional ones that represent 25%.

4 Conclusions

Media and the inappropriate use of technological devices and tools increase the tendency towards harassment, especially among adolescents. In this sense, it is convenient to refer to the analysis of the prevalence of cyberbullying among students of the third and fourth year of compulsory secondary education. The authors of the paper conducted research analyzing the prevalence of cyberbullying in rural and urban schools.

The research objective was to analyze the relationship between cyber victims using mobile devices and/or a computer and the involvement in cyberbullying. The results show that 63.07% of all participants claim that they are not supervised when using a mobile device or a computer when accessing the Internet. 30.9% of the participants that do not have parental have direct involvement in cyberbullying at 25.00%. The authors observe a significant association between involvement in cyberbullying and parental control, as confirmed by Leung and Lee (2012), who consider parental control as an element of cyberbullying prevention.

The study's second objective followed Álvarez-García (2010), who notes that schools located in rural areas receive significantly fewer cyber-attacks than those located in urban areas. The percentage of participants from rural schools who experience cyberbullying is lower than in urban schools, taking into account cyber victims and victimized cyberbullies. Especially, men are frequent aggressors in sexual cyberbullying, while women are equally aggressors in terms of identity theft, or ignoring/marginalizing a partner, especially in urban schools.

The third objective of the research was to identify cyberbullying according to the distribution by gender, school, and degree of education. As for gender, the percentage of women is higher than that of men with a relatively wide difference. On the other hand, frequent victimization was highest in women, with 30.1% compared to 18.3% in men. These figures confirm research results of Estévez et al. (2011), Buelga et al. (2010), Garaigordobil and Aliri (2012), Capadoccia et al. (2013), Ortega et al. (2008) and Mateo et al., (2010). Frequent cyberbullies are common among men, with 0.9% compared to 0.0% of women, a result following other authors (Calvete et al., 2010; Finkelhor et al., 2010; Li, 2006; Estévez et al., 2011; Pelfrey and Weber, 2013; Ortega et al., 2008; Mateo et al., 2010). Victimized aggressors have a higher rate in men (7.0%) than in women (2.4%), contrasting Mishna et al. (2012). The latter confirms that the number of aggressive cyber victims is more significant in women than in men.

The limitation of the study is, in the first place, the size of the sample, which can be considered negligible, although, for an initial study, it has a relatively significant value. In this sense, the authors of the study propose extending the research to obtain broader results and conclusions that confirm or deny these initial findings.

Since the research analyzes information from adolescents, it would be interesting to contrast the data with both parents' and teachers' opinions and provide the study with a more significant adjustment to authenticity, since using a self-report questionnaire as a data collection instrument can lead to certain self-bias. Further research could aim at the causes of cyberbullying and the most effective prevention and detection measures. The authors also suggest implementing the questionnaire to different schools considering this study as the framework. Later the authors of the study could probe the opinion of the participating sample and contrast the results. In this sense, the study could be extended to other communities or geographic spaces with similar characteristics. A further study could help us establish synergies and contribute to the design of good practices that favour preventing cyberbullying behaviour or desirably the total eradication.

References

1. Salmivalli, C.: Bullying and the peer group: a review. Aggress. Violent Behav. **15**(2), 112–120 (2010)
2. Smith, K., Morita, Y., Junger-Tas, J., Olweus, D., Catalano, R., Slee, P.: The Nature of School Bullying: Across-national Perspective. Routledge, London (1999)
3. Garaigordobil, M.: Cyberbullying. Screening de acoso entre iguales. TEA, Madrid (2013)
4. Instituto Nacional de Estadística.: Población que usa Internet. INE, Madrid (2017)
5. Morduchowicz, R., Marcon, A., Sylvestre, V., Ballestrini, F.: Los adolescentes y las redes sociales. FCE, Buenos Aires (2012)
6. Holtz, P., Appel, M.: Internet use and video gaming predict problem behavior in early adolescence. J. Adolescence **34**, 49–58 (2011)
7. Pesántez, F., Torres-Toukoumidis, A., Álvarez Rodas, L.: COVIDA-20 Una coalición educativa para enfrentar la pandemia. Pearson, Lima (2021)

8. Garaigordobil, M., Aliri, J.: Ciberacoso en el País Vasco: Diferencias de sexo en víctimas, agresores y observadores. Psicol. Conductual **21**(3), 461–474 (2013)
9. Hinduja, S., Patchin, J.W.: Bullying Beyond the Schoolyard: Preventing and Responding to Cyberbullying. Corwin Press, EEUU (2014)
10. Calmaestra, J.: Cyberbullying: Prevalencia y características de un nuevo tipo de bullying indirecto. Servicio de publicaciones de la Universidad de Córdoba, Córdoba (2011)
11. Álvarez-García, D., Núnez, J.C., Álvarez, L., Dobarro, A., Rodríguez, C., González-Castro, P.: Violence through information and communication technologies in secondary students. Anales Psicol. **27**, 221–231 (2011)
12. Beran, T., Li, Q.: The relationship between cyberbullying and school bullying. J. Student Wellbeing **1**(2), 16–33 (2008)
13. Erdur-Baker, O.: Cyberbullying and its correlation to traditional bullying, gender and frequent and risky usage of internet-mediated communication tools. New Media Soc. **12**(1), 109–125 (2010)
14. Arnaiz, P., Cerezo, F., Giménez, A.M., Maquilón, J.J.: Conductas de ciberadicción y experiencias de cyberbullying entre adolescentes. Anales Psicol. **32**(3), 761–769 (2016)
15. De Morentin, J.I.M., Cortés, A., Medrano, C., Apodaca, P.: Internet use and parental mediation: a cross-cultural study. Comput. Educ. **70**, 212–221 (2014)
16. UNICEF. Violencia escolar: el maltrato entre iguales en la Educación Secundaria Obligatoria 1999–2006. Publicaciones de la Oficina del Defensor del Pueblo, Madrid (2007)
17. González, F.: Violencia y acoso en los/as escolares extremeños/as: Vías de solución. Campo Abierto **26**(2), 27–46 (2007)
18. Bierhoff, H.W.: Prosocial Behaviour. Psychology Press, Hove (2002)
19. Luukkonen, A.H., Riala, K., Hakko, H., Räsänen, P.: Bullying behaviour and substance abuse among underage psychiatric inpatient adolescents. Eur. Psychiatry **25**(7), 382–389 (2010)
20. Calvete, E., Orue, I., Estévez, A., Villardón, L., Padilla, P.: Cyberbullying in adolescents: modalities and aggressors' profile. Comput. Hum. Behav. **26**(5), 1128–1135 (2010)
21. Whitney, I., Smith, P.K.: A survey of the nature and extent of bullying in junior/middle and secondary schools. Educ. Res. **35**(1), 3–25 (1993)

Author Index

© The Editor(s) (if applicable) and The Author(s), under exclusive license
to Springer Nature Singapore Pte Ltd. 2022

Á. Rocha et al. (Eds.): ICOMTA 2021, SIST 259, pp. 583–585, 2022.
https://doi.org/10.1007/978-981-16-5792-4